DRUG DESIGN: STRUCTURE- AND LIGAND-BASED APPROACHES

Structure-based drug design (SBDD) and ligand-based drug design (LBDD) are active areas of research in both the academic and commercial realms. This book provides a current snapshot of the field of computer-aided drug design and associated experimental approaches. Topics covered include x-ray crystallography, nuclear magnetic resonance, fragment-based drug design, free-energy methods, docking and scoring, linear-scaling quantum calculations, quantitative structure/activity relationship, pharmacophore methods, computational absorption/distribution/metabolism/excretion-toxicity, and drug discovery case studies. Authors from academic and commercial institutions all over the world have contributed to this book, which is illustrated with more than 200 images. This book covers SBDD and LBDD, and it provides the most up-to-date information on a wide range of topics for the practicing computational chemist, medicinal chemist, or structural biologist.

Kenneth M. Merz, Jr., received his PhD in organic chemistry at the University of Texas at Austin and completed postdoctoral research at Cornell University and the University of California, San Francisco. He is a member of the Quantum Theory Project and Professor of Chemistry at the University of Florida, Gainesville.

Dagmar Ringe received her PhD in biochemistry at Boston University. She is Professor of Biochemistry and Chemistry in the Rosenstiel Basic Medical Sciences Research Center at Brandeis University, Waltham, Massachusetts.

Charles H. Reynolds received his PhD in theoretical organic chemistry at the University of Texas at Austin. He is a Research Fellow at Johnson & Johnson Pharmaceutical Research and Development, Spring House, Pennsylvania.

D1428898

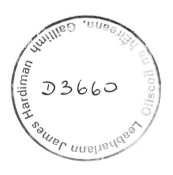

Drug Design

STRUCTURE- AND LIGAND-BASED APPROACHES

Edited by

Kenneth M. Merz, Jr.
University of Florida, Gainesville

Dagmar Ringe
Brandeis University, Waltham, Massachusetts

Charles H. Reynolds
Johnson & Johnson Pharmaceutical Research and Development,
Spring House, Pennsylvania

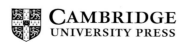
CAMBRIDGE
UNIVERSITY PRESS

CAMBRIDGE UNIVERSITY PRESS
Cambridge, New York, Melbourne, Madrid, Cape Town, Singapore,
São Paulo, Delhi, Dubai, Tokyo

Cambridge University Press
32 Avenue of the Americas, New York, NY 10013-2473, USA

www.cambridge.org
Information on this title: www.cambridge.org/9780521887236

First published 2010

Printed in China by Everbest

A catalog record for this publication is available from the British Library.

Library of Congress Cataloging in Publication data

Drug design : structure- and ligand-based approaches / edited by Kenneth M. Merz,
Dagmar Ringe, Charles H. Reynolds.
    p.   ;   cm.
Includes bibliographical references and index.
ISBN 978-0-521-88723-6 (hardback)
1. Drugs – Design.   2. Drugs – Structure-activity relationships.   I. Merz, Kenneth M., 1959–
II. Ringe, Dagmar.   III. Reynolds, Charles H., 1957–   IV. Title.
[DNLM: 1. Drug Design.   2. Ligands.   3. Structure-Activity Relationship.
QV 744 D79327 2010]
RS420.D793   2010
615′.19–dc22   2009051613

ISBN   978-0-521-88723-6 Hardback

Contents

PART III: APPLICATIONS TO DRUG DISCOVERY

Contributors

Frank U. Axe
Axe Consulting Services
Sutter Creek, California

Scott P. Brown
Department of Structural Biology
Abbott Laboratories
Abbott Park, Illinois

Stephen K. Burley
SGX Pharmaceuticals
San Diego, California

Peter J. Connolly
Vertex Pharmaceuticals Inc.
Cambridge, Massachusetts

Qiaolin Deng
Department of Molecular Systems
Merck Research Laboratories
Merck & Co. Inc.
Rahway, New Jersey

Fangyu Ding
Department of Chemistry
Center for Structural Biology
Stony Brook University
Stony Brook, New York

Steven L. Dixon
Schrodinger, Inc.
New York, New York

Arthur M. Doweyko
Research and Development
Computer-Assisted Drug Design
Bristol-Myers Squibb
Princeton, New Jersey

William J. Egan
Novartis Institutes for BioMedical Research
Cambridge, Massachusetts

Martha S. Head
Computational and Structural Chemistry
GlaxoSmithKline Pharmaceuticals
Collegeville, Pennsylvania

Gavin Hirst
SGX Pharmaceuticals
San Diego, California

M. Katharine Holloway
Molecular Systems
Merck Research Laboratories
West Point, Pennsylvania

William L. Jorgensen
Department of Chemistry
Yale University
New Haven, Connecticut

Christopher A. Lepre
Vertex Pharmaceuticals Inc.
Cambridge, Massachusetts

Nigel J. Liverton
Medicinal Chemistry
Merck Research Laboratories
West Point, Pennsylvania

Kenneth M. Merz, Jr.
Department of Chemistry and
Quantum Theory Project
University of Florida
Gainesville, Florida

David L. Mobley
Department of Chemistry
University of New Orleans
New Orleans, Louisiana

Jonathan M. Moore
Vertex Pharmaceuticals Inc.
Cambridge, Massachusetts

Andrew S. Murkin
Department of Biochemistry
Albert Einstein College of Medicine
Bronx, New York

Gregory A. Petsko
Department of Chemistry
Rosenstiel Basic Medical Sciences Research Center
Brandeis University
Waltham, Massachusetts

Siegfried Reich
SGX Pharmaceuticals
San Diego, California

Charles H. Reynolds
Johnson & Johnson Pharmaceutical Research and
    Development, LLC
Spring House, Pennsylvania

Dagmar Ringe
Department of Chemistry
Rosenstiel Basic Medical Sciences Research
    Center
Brandeis University
Waltham, Massachusetts

Vern L. Schramm
Department of Biochemistry
Albert Einstein College of Medicine
Bronx, New York

Michael R. Shirts
Department of Chemical Engineering
University of Virginia
Charlottesville, Virginia

Carlos Simmerling
Department of Chemistry
Center for Structural Biology
Stony Brook University
Stony Brook, New York

Paul Sprengeler
SGX Pharmaceuticals
San Diego, California

Alexander Tropsha
Laboratory for Molecular Modeling and
Carolina Center for Exploratory Cheminformatics Research
School of Pharmacy
University of North Carolina at Chapel Hill
Chapel Hill, North Carolina

Preface

Our goal in producing this book is to provide a broad overview of the most important approaches used in protein- and ligand-structure-based drug design. Beyond this we aim to illustrate how these approaches are currently being applied in drug discovery efforts. We hope this book will be a useful resource to practitioners in the field, as well as a good introduction for researchers or students who are new to the field. We believe it provides a snapshot of the most important trends and capabilities in the application of modeling and structural data in drug discovery.

Since the 1990s the role of structure and modeling in drug discovery has grown enormously. There have been remarkable scientific advances in both the experimental and computational fields that are the underpinnings of modern drug design. For example, x-ray capabilities have improved to the point that protein structures are now routinely available for a wide range of protein targets. One only need look at the exponential growth of the Protein Databank (RCSB) for evidence. Tremendous strides have been made in all aspects of protein structure determination, including crystallization, data acquisition, and structure refinement. Modeling has made similar gains. Recent years have brought more realistic force fields, new and more robust free-energy methods, computational models for absorption/distribution/metabolism/excretion (ADME)-toxicity, faster and better docking algorithms, automated 3D pharmacophore detection and searching, and very-large-scale quantum calculations. When coupled with the inexorable increase in computer power, new and improved computational methods allow us to incorporate modeling into the drug discovery process in ways that were not possible just a short time ago.

In addition to improvements in methods, academic and industrial groups have gained significant experience in the application of these approaches to drug discovery problems. Protein structures, docking, pharmacophore searches, and the like have all become a staple of drug discovery and are almost universally applied by large and small pharma companies. A recent example of a new approach that is gaining wider acceptance is fragment-based drug design. The goal of fragment-based design is to build up drug candidates from small low-affinity, but high-information-content, hit structures. As such, fragment-based design relies critically on structural, computational, and biophysical methods to identify, characterize, and elaborate small low-affinity ligands.

The book is divided into three broad categories: structural biology, computational chemistry, and drug discovery applications. Each section contains chapters authored by acknowledged experts in the field. Although no book of reasonable size can be completely comprehensive, we have attempted to address the most significant topics in each category, as well as some areas we see as emergent. We are fortunate to have an introductory chapter from Professor William Jorgensen that sets the tone for the book.

The structural biology section begins with a comprehensive review of the strengths and weaknesses of x-ray crystallography. This is the logical starting point for most protein-structure-based design programs, as crystallography is certainly the most common approach for obtaining the three-dimensional structures of therapeutically important proteins. This section also includes two chapters on fragment-based drug design, including one devoted to the important role nuclear magnetic resonance has played in this new approach.

The computational chemistry section covers a range of modeling techniques, including free-energy methods, dynamics, docking and scoring, pharmacophore modeling, quantitative structure/activity relationships, computational ADME, and quantum methods. Each topic was selected either because it is a commonly employed tool in drug discovery (e.g., docking and scoring) or because it is seen as an emerging technology that may have an increasing role in the future (e.g., linear-scaling quantum calculations). Taken together, these chapters provide a fairly comprehensive overview of the computational approaches being used in drug discovery today.

The final section on applications in drug discovery provides a few concrete examples of using the methods outlined in the first two sections for specific drug discovery programs. This is the ultimate validation of any experimental or computational approach, at least with regard to drug discovery. These examples from six diverse protein targets are useful to the expert as examples of best practices and to the novice as examples of what can be done. An overview of G-protein-coupled receptor (GPCR) modeling and structure is of keen current interest given that this class has historically been a rich source of drugs, and it has recently seen a major advance in access to experimental structures. This bodes well for the future application of structure-based design to GPCR targets.

Finally, we must thank all the authors who generously agreed to participate in this project for their efforts and patience. Without them, of course, there would be no book. We have been particularly fortunate to enlist such a talented group of authors.

DRUG DESIGN: STRUCTURE- AND LIGAND-BASED APPROACHES

Progress and issues for computationally guided lead discovery and optimization

William L. Jorgensen

INTRODUCTION

Since the late 1980s there have been striking advances, fueled by large increases in both industrial and NIH-funded academic research, that have revolutionized drug discovery. This period has seen the introduction of high-throughput screening (HTS), combinatorial chemistry, PC farms, Linux, SciFinder, structure-based design, virtual screening by docking, free-energy methods, absorption/distribution/metabolism/excretion (ADME) software, bioinformatics, routine biomolecular structure determination, structures for ion channels, G-protein-coupled receptors (GPCRs) and ribosomes, structure/activity relationships (SAR) obtained from nuclear magnetic resonance (SAR by NMR), fragment-based design, gene knockouts, proteomics, small interfering RNA (siRNA), and human genome sequences. The result is a much-accelerated progression from identification of biomolecular target to lead compound to clinical candidate. However, a serious concern is that the dramatic increase in drug discovery abilities and expenditures has not been paralleled by an increase in FDA approvals of new molecular entities.[1] High demands for drug safety, broader and longer clinical trials, too much HTS, too little natural products research, and effective generic drugs for many once-pressing afflictions have all been suggested as contributors.[2–4] Numerous corporate mergers and acquisitions may have also had adverse effects on productivity through distractions of reorganization and integration. Nevertheless, one should consider what the success would have been in the absence of the striking technical advances. Certainly, progress with some critical and challenging target classes such as kinases would have been greatly diminished, and the adverse impact on many cancer patients would have been profound. Indeed, further gains in the treatment and prevention of human diseases must require even more emphasis and commitment to fundamental research. As in other discovery enterprises, the answer is to drill deeper.

The topic of this volume focuses on one of the areas in drug discovery that has seen major transformation and progress: structure- and ligand-based design. The design typically features small molecules that bind to a biomolecular target and inhibit its function. The distinction stems from whether a three-dimensional structure of the target is available and used in the design process. Structure-based design can be carried out with nothing more than the target structure and graphics tools for building ligands in the proposed binding site. However, additional insights provided by evaluation of the molecular energetics for the binding process are central to most current structure-based design activities. Ligand-based design does not require a target structure but rather stems from analysis of structure/activity data for compounds that have been tested in an assay for the biological function of the target. One seeks patterns in the assay results to suggest potential modifications of the compounds to yield enhanced activity. The upside is that a target structure is not required; the downside is that substantial activity data are needed. My research group has focused on the development and application of improved computational methodology for structure-based design. Some of the experiences and issues that have been addressed are summarized in the following.

LEAD GENERATION

Both lead generation and lead optimization may be pursued through joint computational and experimental studies. As summarized in Figure 1.1, our approach has evolved to feature two pathways for lead generation, de novo design with the ligand-growing program BOMB (Biochemical and Organic Model Builder)[5] and virtual screening using the docking program GLIDE.[6] Fragment-based design, which involves the docking and linking together of multiple small molecules in a binding site, is another popular alternative.[7,8] Desirable compounds resulting from de novo design normally have to be synthesized, whereas compounds from virtual screening of commercial catalogs are typically purchased. In both cases, it is preferable to begin with a high-resolution crystal structure for a complex of the target protein with a ligand; though the ligand is removed, it is advisable to start from a complex rather than an apo structure, which may have side chains repositioned to fill partially the binding site. An extreme example occurs with HIV-1 reverse transcriptase (HIV-RT) for which the allosteric binding site for nonnucleoside inhibitors (NNR-TIs) is fully collapsed in apo structures.[9]

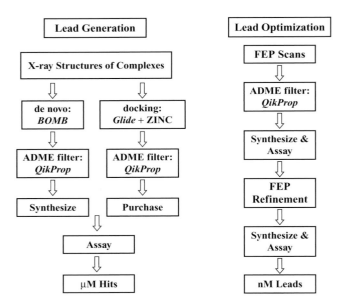

Figure 1.1. Schematic outline for structure-based drug lead discovery and optimization.

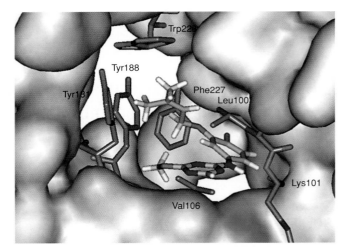

Figure 1.2. An inhibitor built using BOMB in the NNRTI binding site of HIV-RT.

De Novo design with BOMB

BOMB is used to construct complete analogs by adding 0–4 substituents to a core that has been placed in a binding site. A thorough conformational search is performed for each analog, and the position, orientation, and dihedral angles for the analog are optimized using the OPLS-AA force field for the protein and OPLS/CM1A for the analog.[10] The resultant conformer for each analog with the lowest energy is evaluated with a dockinglike scoring function to predict activity. The core may be as simple as, for example, ammonia or benzene, or it may represent a polycyclic framework of a lead series. For the example in Figure 1.2, ammonia was the original core, and it was positioned to form a hydrogen bond with the carbonyl group of Lys101. A library of molecules is then often built using a "template" that has been envisioned by the user to be complementary to the binding site and often to also be amenable to straightforward synthesis. For Figure 1.2, the template was Het-NH-34Ph-U, where Het represents a monocyclic heterocycle, 34Ph is a 3- or 4-substituted phenyl group, and U is an unsaturated hydrophobic group. The template specifies the components that constitute the desired molecules and the topology by which they are linked together.

BOMB includes a library of approximately 700 possible substituents, with code numbers from 1 to about 700, including most common monocyclic and bicyclic heterocycles and about 50 common U groups such as allyl, propargyl, phenyl, phenoxy, and benzyl derivatives. They are provided as groupings by the code numbers or the user can create a custom grouping with desired code numbers. The groupings correspond to template components such as Het, 5Het (just 5-membered ring heterocycles), 6Het, biHet, U, oPhX, mPhX, pPhX, mOPhX, pSPhX, OR, NR, SR, and C = OX. The program then builds all molecules that correspond to the template. In the example, if there were 50 Het and 20 U options, the program would build the 1,000 Het-NH-3-Ph-U and 1,000 Het-NH-4-Ph-U possibilities. This de novo design exercise with HIV-RT as the target resulted in identification of Het = 2-thiazolyl and U = dimethylallyloxy as a promising pair. Subsequent synthesis of the thiazole **1** in Figure 1.3 did provide a 10-μM lead in an MT-2 cell-based assay for anti-HIV activity. As described below, the lead was optimized to multiple highly potent NNRTIs, including the chlorotriazine in Figure 1.2 (31 nM), the corresponding chloropyrimidine (10 nM), and the cyanopyrimidine analog **2** (2 nM).[11–14]

Some additional details should be noted. The host, typically a protein, is rigid in the BOMB optimizations except for variation of terminal dihedral angles for side chains with

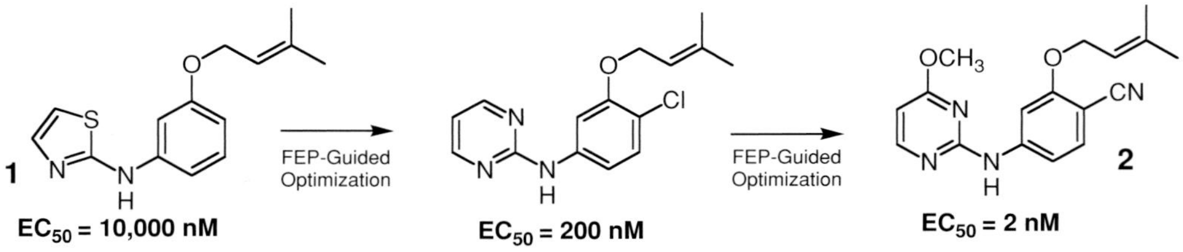

1 EC$_{50}$ = 10,000 nM → FEP-Guided Optimization → EC$_{50}$ = 200 nM → FEP-Guided Optimization → EC$_{50}$ = 2 nM **2**

Figure 1.3. Example of a 10-μM lead proposed by BOMB that was optimized to provide numerous potent anti-HIV agents.

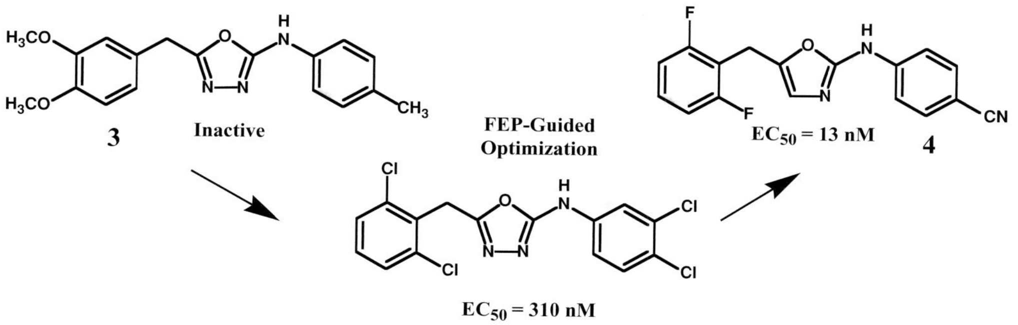

Figure 1.4. Progression of a false positive from docking to potent anti-HIV agents.

hydrogen-bonding groups, for example, the OH of tyrosine or serine and ammonium group of lysine. The current scoring function has been trained to reproduce experimental activity data for more than 300 complexes of HIV-RT, COX-2, FK506 binding protein, and p38 kinase.[5] It yields a correlation coefficient r^2 of 0.58 for the computed versus observed log(activities). The scoring function contains only five descriptors that were obtained by linear regression, including an estimate of the analog's octanol/water partition coefficient from QɪᴋPʀᴏᴘ (QPlog$P$),[15] the amount of hydrophobic surface area for the protein that is buried on complex formation, and an index recording mismatched protein/analog contacts, such as a hydroxyl group in contact with a methyl group. Interestingly, the most significant descriptor is QPlog$P$, which alone yields a fit with an r^2 of 0.47. Thus, the adage that increased hydrophobicity leads to increased binding is well supported, though it requires refinement for quality of fit using the host/ligand interaction energy or an index of mismatched contacts. Overdone, it also leads to ADME problems, especially poor aqueous solubility and high serum protein binding.

The results from a BOMB run include the structure for each protein/analog complex as a Protein Data Bank (PDB) file or BOSS/MCPRO Z-matrix (internal coordinate representation)[16] and a spreadsheet with one row for each analog summarizing computed quantities from the BOMB calculations, including host–analog energy components and surface area changes as well as predicted properties for the analog, including log $P_{o/w}$, aqueous solubility, and Caco-2 cell permeability from QɪᴋPʀᴏᴘ, which is called as a subroutine. The processing time for Het-NH-Ph-U using ammonia as the core is approximately 15 s per analog on a 3-GHz Pentium IV processor. The required time increases roughly linearly with the number of conformers that need to be constructed. For large libraries, multiple processors are used.

Virtual screening

The common alternative is to perform virtual screening on available compound collections using docking software. Many reviews and comparisons for alternative software and

scoring functions are available.[6,17–20] There is no question that there have been many successes with docking such that, given a target structure, it is expected to be competitive with and far more cost effective than HTS and is now an important component of lead discovery programs in the pharmaceutical industry. New success stories are reported regularly in the literature and at conferences. However, it is generally accepted that correct rank-ordering of compounds for activity is beyond the current capabilities. This is not surprising in view of the thermodynamic complexity of host/ligand binding, including potential structural changes for the host on binding, which have usually been ignored, and the need for careful consideration of changes in conformational free energetics between the bound and unbound states.[21]

In our experience, docking has been a valuable complement to de novo design (Figure 1.1). When large compound collections are docked, interesting structural motifs often emerge as potential cores that may have been overlooked otherwise. Our earliest docking effort started out well, was formally a failure, and then recovered to provide an interesting lead series that yielded potent anti-HIV agents.[5,22] Leads were sought by processing a collection of approximately 70,000 compounds from the Maybridge catalog, which was supplemented with twenty known NNRTIs. The screening protocol began with a similarity filter that retrieves 60% of the known actives in the top 5% of the screened library. The approximately 2,000 library compounds that were most similar to the known actives were then docked into the 1rt4 structure of wild-type HIV-RT, using Gʟɪᴅᴇ 3.5 with standard precision.[6] The top 500 compounds were then redocked and scored in Gʟɪᴅᴇ extraprecision (XP) mode.[23] The top 100 of these were postscored with a molecular mechanics/generalized Born/surface area (MM-GB/SA) method that was shown to provide high correlation between predicted and observed activities for NNRTIs.[22] Though known NNRTIs were retrieved well (ten were ranked in the top twenty), purchase and assaying of approximately twenty high-scoring compounds from the library failed to yield any active anti-HIV agents. Persisting, the highest-ranked library compound, the inactive oxadiazoles **3** in Figure 1.4, was pursued computationally to seek

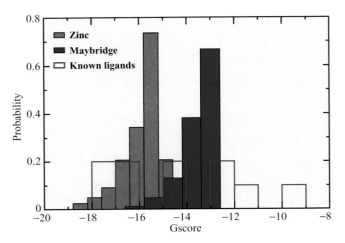

Figure 1.5. Distributions of the Glide XP scores for the top-ranked 1,000 ZINC compounds, the top-ranked 1,000 Maybridge compounds, and the 10 known tautomerase inhibitors.

constructive modifications. Specifically, the substituents were removed to yield the anilinylbenzyloxadiazole core. A set of small substituents was reintroduced in place of each hydrogen using BOMB; scoring with BOMB, followed by free-energy perturbation (FEP)-guided optimization, led to synthesis and assaying of several polychloro analogs with EC_{50} values as low as 310 nM in the MT-2 HIV-infected T-cell assay.[5] Further cycles of FEP-guided optimization led to novel, very potent NNRTIs, including the oxazole derivative **4**, as described more below.[24]

A more recent virtual screening exercise was strikingly successful.[25] New protocols had evolved, including use of the much larger ZINC database of approximately 2.1 million commercially available compounds.[26] The goal in this case was to disrupt the binding of macrophage migration inhibitory factor (MIF) to its receptor CD74, an integral membrane protein, and a major histocompatibility complex (MHC) class II chaperone. MIF is a pro-inflammatory cytokine that is released by T-cells and macrophages. It plays a key role in a wide range of inflammatory diseases and is involved in cell proliferation and differentiation and angiogenesis.[27,28] Curiously, MIF is also a keto-enol isomerase. There is evidence that the interaction of MIF with CD74 occurs in the vicinity of the tautomerase active site and that MIF inhibition is directly competitive with MIF/CD74 binding.[29] The docking was performed using GLIDE 4.0 and the 1ca7 crystal structure of the complex of MIF with p-hydroxyphenylpyruvate.[30] In addition to the ZINC collection, the Maybridge HitFinder library was screened, which provided an additional 24,000 compounds. After all structures were processed using SP GLIDE, the top-ranked 40,000 from ZINC and 1,000 from Maybridge were redocked and rescored using GLIDE in XP mode.[23] GLIDE XP scoring was also shown to provide good correlation with experimental data for 10 known inhibitors of MIF's tautomerase activity.

A key observation from the docking is illustrated in Figure 1.5, which shows the distributions of GLIDE XP scores for the top-ranked 1,000 compounds from ZINC, the top-ranked 1,000 Maybridge compounds, and the ten known MIF inhibitors. Clearly, the large ZINC collection yields many compounds with much more promising XP scores than the Maybridge HitFinder library. The average molecular weights for the two sets of 1,000 compounds are 322 for ZINC and 306 for Maybridge. The variation only amounts to one additional nonhydrogen atom for the ZINC set, so the improved performance with the ZINC collection presumably results from greater structural variety. In view of the sensitivity of activity to structure, as reflected in Figures 1.3 and 1.4, it is highly unlikely that active compounds can be found in small libraries like Maybridge HitFinder unless the assays can be run with the compounds at millimolar or higher concentrations, which is often precluded by solubility limits. Even with a viable core (Figure 1.4), the chance is low that a small library will contain a derivative with a substituent pattern that yields an active in a typical assay.

Finally, the GLIDE poses for approximately 1,200 of the top-ranked compounds were displayed and 34 compounds were selected by human evaluation of the poses with input from QIKPROP on predicted properties and structural liabilities. The filtering included rejection of poses where the conformation of the ligand was energetically unlikely or where there were overly short intramolecular contacts and compounds with generally undesirable features such as readily hydrolizable functional groups or substructures such as coumarins, which are promiscuous protein binders. Only 24 of the 34 selected compounds were, in fact, available for purchase, which represents a typical ratio. Ultimately 23 compounds were submitted to a protein-protein binding assay using immobilized CD74 and biotinylated human MIF with streptavidin-conjugated alkaline phosphatase processing p-nitrophenyl phosphate as substrate. Remarkably, eleven of the compounds were found to have inhibitory activity in the μM regime including four compounds with IC_{50} values below 5 μM. Inhibition of MIF tautomerase activity was also established for several of the compounds with IC_{50} values as low as 0.5 μM. Representative active compounds are shown in Figure 1.6; optimization of several of the lead series is being pursued. Notably, these are the most potent small-molecule inhibitors of MIF-CD74 binding that have been reported to date.

The first three compounds in Figure 1.6 were ranked in 285th, 696th, and 394th place by the XP scoring, so they were not "high in the deck." However, prior de novo structure building with BOMB had indicated that 6–5 fused bicyclic cores should be promising, so the selections were biased in this direction. The compound ranked first with XP GLIDE was also purchased and assayed; it turned out to be the 250-μM inhibitor in Figure 1.6. In addition, the compounds ranked 26th and 32nd were purchased and found to be inactive. Overall, it is expected that contributors to the success with the virtual screening in this case were

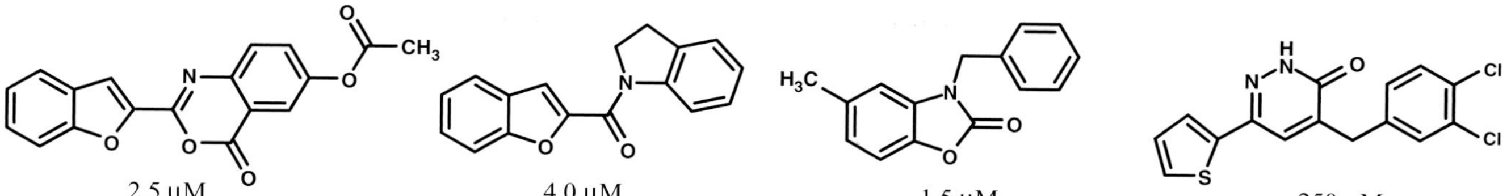

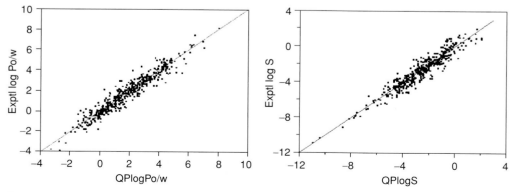

Figure 1.6. Structures and IC_{50} values for some inhibitors of MIF-CD74 binding discovered by virtual screening.

improvements with GLIDE 4.0 and the XP scoring, use of the large ZINC library, the relatively small binding site and consequently small number of rotatable bonds for potential inhibitors, and the human filtering.

ADME ANALYSES

As indicated in Figure 1.1, as one pursues leads it is important to be aware of potential pharmacological liabilities. The significance of this issue became increasingly apparent in the 1990s because of high failure rates for compounds in clinical trials that could be ascribed to ADME and toxicity problems.[31] This led to the introduction of Lipinski's rules and recognition that compounds developed in the post-HTS era frequently tended to be too large and hydrophobic, which is accompanied by solubility and bioavailability deficiencies.[32] In this atmosphere, more effort was placed on quantitative prediction of molecular properties beyond $\log P_{o/w}$ using statistical procedures such as regression analyses and neural networks, which were trained on experimental data.[33,34] The typical regression equation is a linear one, Equation (1.1), where the sum is over molecular descriptors i that have values c_i for the given structure and the coefficients a_i are determined to minimize the error with the experimental data:

$$property = \sum_i a_i c_i + a_0. \tag{1.1}$$

In Figure 1.1, the choice for ADME analyses is QIKPROP, which was among the earliest programs to predict a substantial array of pharmacologically relevant properties.

Version 1.0, which was released in March 2000, provided predictions for intrinsic aqueous solubility, Caco-2 cell permeability, and hexadecane/gas, octanol/gas, water/gas, and octanol/water partition coefficients. The required input for QIKPROP is a three-dimensional structure of an organic molecule, and it mostly uses linear regression equations with molecular descriptors such as surface areas and hydrogen-bond donor and acceptor counts. By version 3.0 from 2006, the output covered eighteen quantities, including log BB for brain/blood partitioning, log K_{hsa} for serum albumin binding, hERG K^+ channel blockage, primary metabolites, and overall percentage human oral absorption.[15] The prediction of primary metabolites is based on literature precedents and recognition of corresponding substructures; for example, methyl ethers and tolyl methyl groups are typically metabolized to the alcohols. Execution time with QIKPROP is negligible because the most time-consuming computation is for the molecule's surface area. Average root-mean-square (rms) errors for most quantities are about 0.6 log unit, as in Figure 1.7.

To gauge acceptable ranges of predicted properties, QIKPROP 3.0 was used to process approximately 1,700 known neutral oral drugs,[13] which were compiled by Proudfoot.[35] For submission to QIKPROP, the original two-dimensional structures were converted to three-dimensional structures and energy-minimized with BOSS using the OPLS/CM1A force field.[10,16] Some key results from the analyses are summarized as histograms in Figures 1.8 and 1.9. Consistent with the log $P_{o/w}$ limit of 5 in Lipinski's rules,[32] 91% of oral drugs are found to have

Figure 1.7. Experimental data and QikProp 3.0 results for 400–500 octanol/water partition coefficients (left) and aqueous solubilities (right). S is aqueous solubility in moles per liter. Correlation coefficients r^2 are 0.92 and 0.90 and the rms errors are 0.54 and 0.63 log unit, respectively.

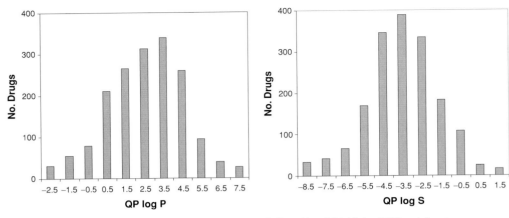

Figure 1.8. QikProp distributions for log $P_{o/w}$ (left) and log S (right) for 1712 oral drugs.

QPlog$P$ values below 5.0. However, values below zero are uncommon, presumably because of poor cell permeability, and the "sweet" range for log $P_{o/w}$ appears to be 1–5. For aqueous solubility, 90% of the QPlog$S$ values are above −5.7, that is, S is greater than 1 μM. QPlog$S$ values less than −6 or greater than −1 are undesirable. The QIKPROP results also state that 90% of oral drugs have cell permeabilities, P_{Caco}, above 22 nm/s and no more than six primary metabolites. These quantities and limits address important components of bioavailablility, namely, solubility, cell permeability, and metabolism.

For our design purposes (Figure 1.1), a compound is viewed as potentially ADME challenged if it does not satisfy all components of a "rule-of-three": predicted log $S > -6$, $P_{Caco} > 30$ nm/s, and maximum number of primary metabolites of 6. For central nervous system (CNS) activity requiring blood-brain barrier penetration, an addendum is that QPlogBB should be positive. Also, some caution is warranted for a compound with no metabolites because of possible clearance problems.[17] A further note is that QPlog$P$ and QPlog$S$ are correlated with an r^2 of 0.68, so there would be some redundancy in invoking limits on both. Among reasons for preferring solubility, there are quite a few examples of relatively small drugs that

have log $P_{o/w}$ values greater than 5 but have acceptable solubility, for example, meclizine, prozapine, clocinizine, bepridil, denaverine, bopindolol, phenoxybenzamine, and terbinafine. Of course, compounds with reactive functional groups, for example, those that are readily hydrolizable or strongly electrophilic, are flagged by QikProp and normally eliminated from inclusion in a lead structure. For example, in rofecoxib (Vioxx) concern could be expressed for possible nucleophilic attack and ring opening at the furanone carbonyl and for Michael addition to the α,β-double bond; metabolic oxidation at the allylic methylene group is also expected to yield the 5-hydroxy derivative (Scheme 1). For celecoxib (Celebrex), metabolic oxidation to the benzylic alcohol is noted by QIKPROP, and an "alert" is given that

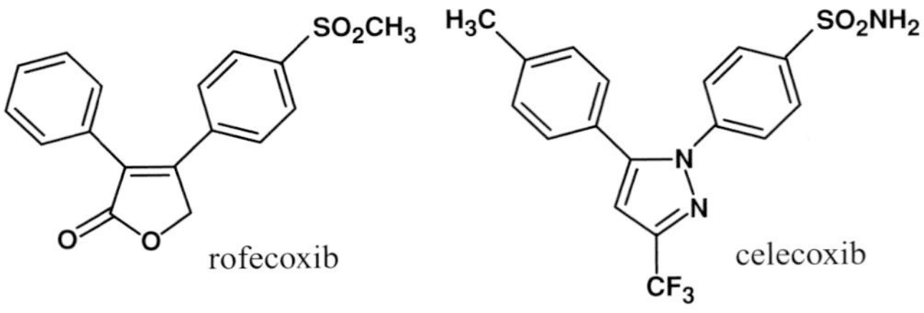

Scheme 1.

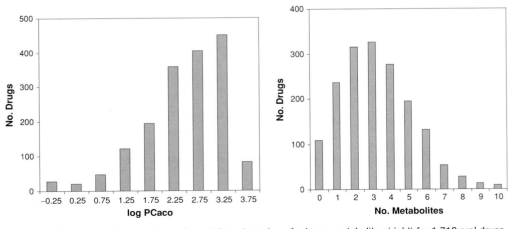

Figure 1.9. QikProp distributions for log P_{Caco} (left) and number of primary metabolites (right) for 1,712 oral drugs. P_{Caco} is the Caco-2 cell permeability in nm/s.

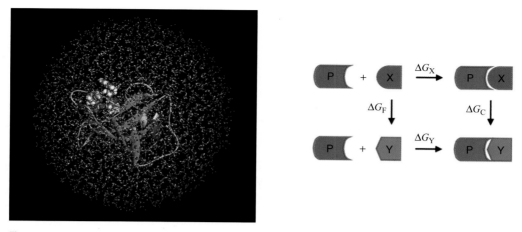

Figure 1.10. (Left) A protein/ligand complex surrounded by approximately 1,000 water molecules in a spherical shell or "cap." (Right) Thermodynamic cycle used to compute relative free energies of binding, $\Delta\Delta G_b$. P is a host and X and Y are two ligands.

the primary sulfonamide group can be associated with sulfa allergies and indiscriminant metal chelation.[36]

Overall, for the 1,712 oral drugs, 278 violate one or more of the four Lipinski rules (MW < 500, $\log P_{o/w} < 5$, H-bond donors ≤ 5, H-bond acceptors ≤ 10) with QPlog$P$ used for $\log P_{o/w}$. There are 178, 82, and 18 oral drugs with one, two, and three violations, respectively. The group with two violations includes macrolides such as erythromycin and azithromycin and some other well-known drugs like atorvastatin, amiodarone, chloramphenicol, ketoconazole, and telmisartan. These examples all fail one member of the rule-of-three, either the solubility limit or number of primary metabolites, for example, respectively, atorvastatin and the macrolides. The group with three rule-of-five violations includes the HIV-protease inhibitors ritonavir and saquinavir, which are known to have low bioavailability. There are exceptions to such rules because they are based on 90th-percentile limits. Nevertheless, in all stages of lead generation, it would be imprudent to ignore property distributions for known drugs such as those in Figures 1.8 and 1.9.

LEAD OPTIMIZATION

It is assumed that inhibitory potency increases with increasing biomolecule-inhibitor binding. So, on the computational side, the key for lead optimization is accurate prediction of biomolecule-ligand binding affinities. There are many approaches, but the potentially most accurate ones are the most rigorous.[17] At this time, the best that is done is to model the complexes in the presence of hundreds or thousands of explicit water molecules using Monte Carlo (MC) statistical mechanics or molecular dynamics methods (Figure 1.10).[17] Classical force fields[16] are used, and extensive sampling is performed for key external (translation and rotation) and internal degrees of freedom for the complexes, solvent, and any counterions. FEP and thermodynamic integration (TI) calculations then provide for-

mally rigorous means to compute free-energy changes.[37] For biomolecule/ligand affinities, perturbations are made to convert one ligand to another using the thermodynamic cycle in Figure 1.10. The conversions involve a coupling parameter, λ, that causes one molecule to be smoothly mutated to the other by changing the force field parameters and geometry.[38] The difference in free energies of binding for the ligands X and Y then comes from $\Delta\Delta G_b = \Delta G_X - \Delta G_Y = \Delta G_F - \Delta G_C$. Two series of mutations are performed to convert X to Y unbound in water and complexed to the biomolecule, which yield ΔG_F and ΔG_C.

Absolute free energies of binding are not obtained, but for lead optimization it is sufficient to assess the effects of making changes or additions to a core structure in the same spirit as synthetic modifications. Though the MC or MD plus FEP or TI calculations are rigorous, the accuracy of the results is affected by many issues, including the use and quality of force fields; missing energy terms, such as instantaneous polarization effects; and possible inadequate configurational sampling, which may be associated with, for example, infrequent conformational changes that are beyond the duration of the simulations. In the author's experience, more approximate methods are not accurate enough to provide satisfactory guidance in lead optimization.

The idea of using such calculations for molecular design goes back more than twenty years, at least to the report of the first FEP calculation for conversion of a molecule X to molecule Y in 1985[38] and to the earliest application of FEP calculations for protein-ligand binding by Wong and McCammon.[39] A final comment from McCammon's review on computer-aided molecular design in *Science* in 1987 was perspicacious: "The attentive reader will have noticed that no molecules were actually designed in the work described here."[40] The situation has remained basically unchanged since the late 1980s. As the convergence of FEP calculations was investigated, it was apparent that they were too computationally intensive for routine use in molecular

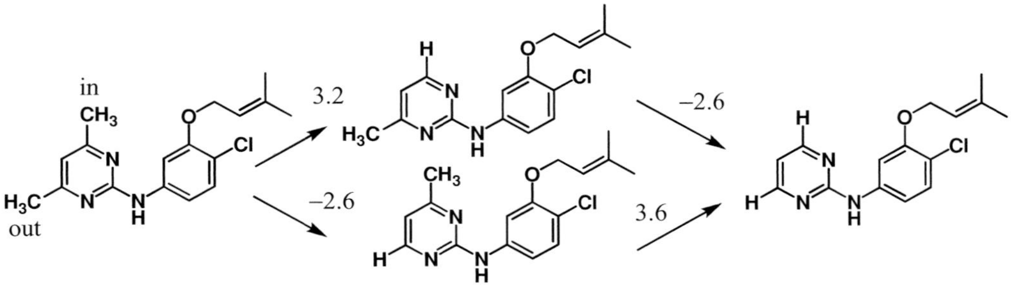

Figure 1.11. MC/FEP results for $\Delta \Delta G_b$ (kcal/mol) established a strong preference for a single methyl group oriented "in" toward Tyr188 in the NNRTI binding site. The precision of the calculations is reflected in the cycle's small hysteresis, 0.4 kcal/mol.

design given the computer resources available before ca. 2000. In 1985, the ethane-to-methanol FEP calculation in a periodic cube with 125 water molecules required two weeks on a Harris-80 minicomputer,[38] and the Wong/McCammon MD simulation for the trypsin-benzamidine complex covered only 29 ps but was performed on a Cyber 205 "supercomputer."[39]

Thus, until recently the application of FEP or TI calculations on protein-ligand systems predominantly featured retrospective calculations to reproduce known experimental inhibition data and generally addressed small numbers of compounds. Kollman was a strong advocate of the potential of free-energy calculations for molecular design, and he and Merz reported a rare, prospective FEP result on the binding of a phosphonamidate versus phosphinate inhibitor with thermolysin.[41,42] Pearlman also advanced the technology, though publications in 2001 and 2005 were still retrospective and confined to a simple congeneric series of 16 p38 kinase inhibitors.[43,44] In addition, Reddy and Erion have been steady contributors; they have used FEP calculations to evaluate contributions of heteroatoms and small groups to the binding of inhibitors to gain insights on directions for improvement.[45,46] Our own computations on protein/ligand binding began to appear in 1997 using MC/FEP methodology.[47,48] Many issues and systems were subsequently addressed, including substituent optimization for celecoxib analogs,[49] COX-2/COX-1 selectivity,[50] and heterocycle optimization for inhibitors of fatty acid amide hydrolase.[51] An additional series of publications used MC/FEP calculations to compute the effects of HIV-RT mutations on the activity of NNRTIs.[52–55] The latter work included predictions for the structures of the complexes of efavirenz and etravirine with HIV-RT, which were subsequently confirmed by x-ray crystallography.[52,54,56] Confidence in the predicted structures came from agreement between the FEP results and experimental activity data.

FEP-guided optimization of azines as NNRTIs

With this preparation, large increases in computer resources, the hiring of synthetic chemists, and collab-

oration with biologists, FEP-guided lead optimization projects were initiated in 2004. Early successes in the optimization of potent NNRTIs are reflected in Figures 1.2 and 1.3 for the Het-NH-3-Ph-U series.[11–13] MC/FEP calculations were used to optimize the heterocycle and the substituent in the 4-position of the phenyl ring. The calculations are run with MCPRO and all use the OPLS/CM1A force field for the ligands and OPLS-AA for the protein.[10,16] This quickly led to selection of 2-pyrimidinyl and 2-(1,3,5)-triazinyl for the heterocycle and chlorine or a cyano group at the 4-position. These combinations yielded NNRTIs with EC_{50} values near 200 nM.

Extensive FEP calculations then focused on optimization of substituents for the heterocycle.[13] For the 2-pyrimidines, the immediate question concerned whether 4,6-disubstitution would be favorable or if mono substitution at the 4- or 6-position is preferred. In complexes with HIV-RT, the 4- and 6-positions are not equivalent; for example, in Figure 1.2, the methoxy group could be directed toward the viewer ("out") or away ("in"), as shown. From display of structures of the complexes, the preferences for in or out were not obvious. This was clarified by MC/FEP results, which showed a strong preference for having a single small substituent on the pyrimidine ring and that the substituent would be oriented "in" (Figure 1.11). Synthesis of a variety of such mono-substituted pyrimidines and triazines yielded ten NNRTIS with EC_{50}s below 20 nM.[11–13] There was good correlation between the FEP results and the observed activities.[11,13] The methoxypyrimidine **2** in Figure 1.3 (2 nM) was the most potent, although it was also relatively cytotoxic ($CC_{50} = 230$ nM). The corresponding 1,3,5-triazine is also a potent anti-HIV agent (11 nM) and has a large safety margin ($CC_{50} = 42 \, \mu$M).

Heterocycle scans

FEP results also established the orientation of the methoxy methyl group in the pyrimidine and triazine derivatives shown in Figure 1.2, that is, pointing toward Phe227 rather than Tyr181. This suggested the possibility of cyclizing the methoxy group back into the azine ring to form 6–5 and 6–6 fused heterocycles in the manner indicated in Scheme 2.

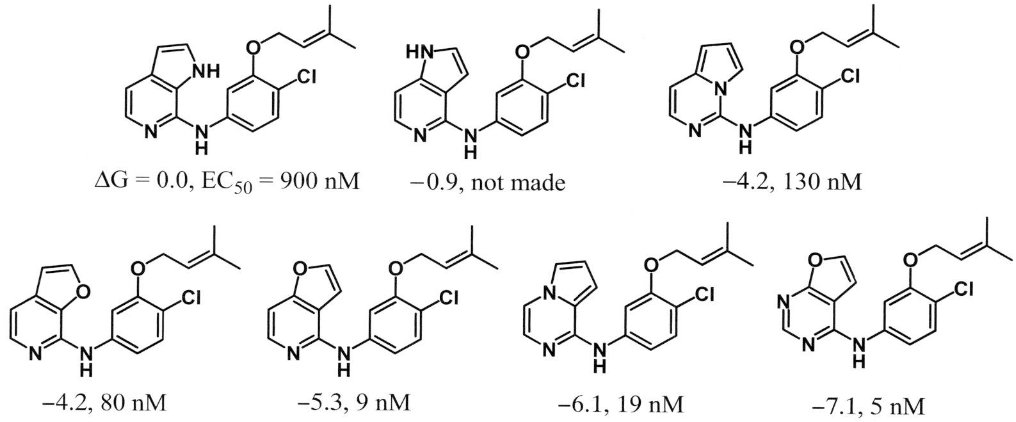

Figure 1.12. FEP results for relative ΔG_b (kcal/mol) and experimental anti-HIV activities (nM).

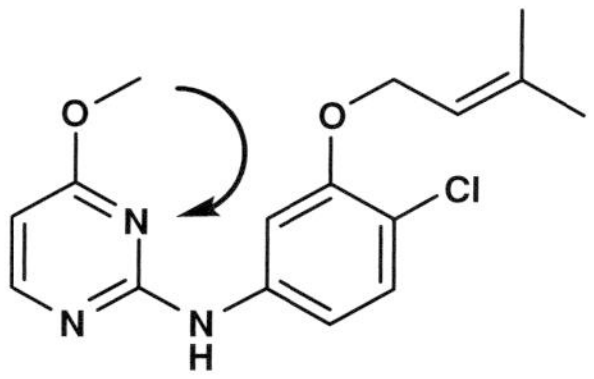

Scheme 2.

The decision on which analogs to pursue was driven by the prospective FEP results shown in Figure 1.12. Subsequent synthesis and assaying of the series of 6–5 compounds showed close parallel between the predicted and observed activities.[11] The illustrated furanopyrimidine derivative was predicted and observed to be the most potent; it is a highly novel and potent (5 nM) NNRTI. The results highlight the accuracy of the FEP predictions and again the sensitivity of activity to structure. The pyrrolopyrimidine (130 nM) and pyrrolopyrazine (19 nM) pair is particularly striking. After the fact, analyses showed a larger dipole moment for the bound pyrrolopyrazine and more negative charge on the pyrazinyl nitrogen leading to stronger hydrogen bonding with the backbone NH of Lys101.[14]

This procedure can be referred to as a heterocycle scan, which is clearly a powerful lead-optimization strategy.[51] It is also an area where computation is far easier than synthesis, so computational screening to focus the synthetic options is very beneficial. This is particularly true for polycyclic heterocycles, as in Figure 1.12, where there are many options and the synthetic challenges can be great. In this example, heteroaryl halides were needed for reaction with substituted anilines; several were not previously reported and required considerable synthetic effort.[14] Even with the notion of pursuing bicyclic heterocycles, in the absence of the FEP results, the synthetically less accessible ones might have been skipped.

Changing heterocycles in the center of a structure is also often challenging from a synthetic standpoint. For example, synthesis of the oxadiazoles and oxazole in Figure 1.4 requires fundamentally different procedures for the ring

construction.[24] This corresponds to a change in chemotype and there can be a significant delay as a viable synthetic route is found for the new target. In the case of this U-5Het-NH-*p*PhX series, FEP calculations were carried out for eleven alternative five-membered-ring heterocycles (5Het) by perturbation from the corresponding thiophene.[24] Remarkably, the only one that was predicted to be more active than the oxadiazole was the 2,5-substituted oxazole. The prediction was confirmed and provided a major step forward for the optimization of this series, as shown in Figure 1.13. It is noted that the approximately eight-fold activity improvement, which corresponds to a $\Delta \Delta G$ of about 1.2 kcal/mol, is less than the computed $\Delta \Delta G$ of 2.5 kcal/mol. This is a common pattern that likely results from the use of a cell-based assay, so the comparison is not with actual binding data (K_d). Moreover, it is also probable that the computed electrostatic interactions in the complexes are not properly damped because of the lack of explicit polarization effects.

In view of the synthetic challenges, only two alternatives were synthesized, the thiadiazole and thiazole analogs,

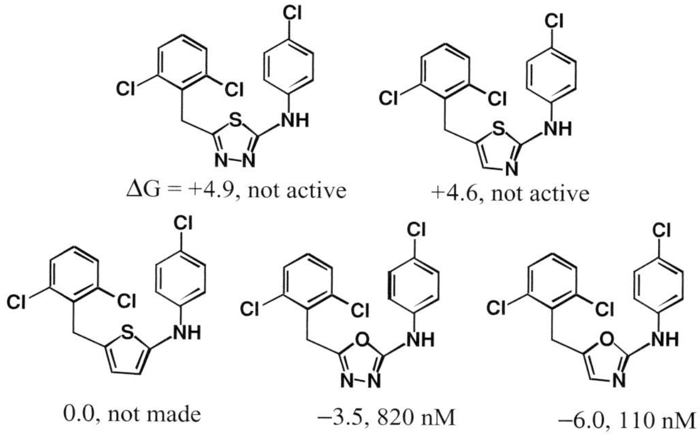

Figure 1.13. Heterocycle scan in the U-5Het-Ph X series; FEP results for ΔG_b (kcal/mol) relative to the thiophene analog and experimental anti-HIV activity (nM).

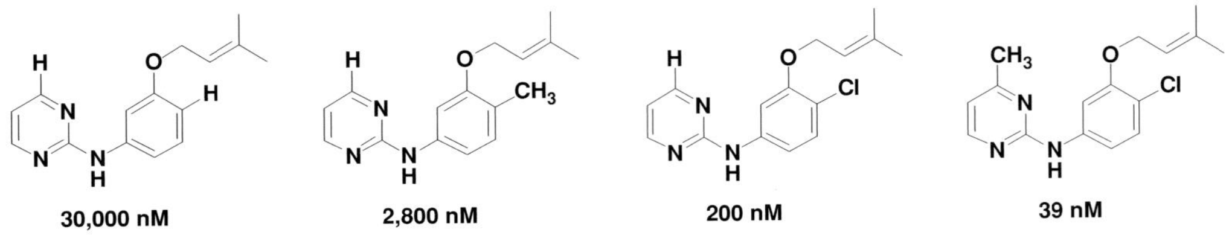

Figure 1.14. The power of chlorine and methyl scans; experimental EC_{50} values for anti-HIV activity in an MT-2 cell assay.

which were both predicted and found to be inactive (Figure 1.13). It is noted that the MT-2 assay is run to a maximum concentration of 100 μM; the thiadiazole showed no activity or cytotoxicity up to this concentration, whereas the thiazole has a CC_{50} of 24 μM and no anti-HIV activity to this point. Overall, this provides another example of the sensitivity of activity to structure and the desirability of rigorous computational guidance. Graphical display of modeled complexes is inadequate to gauge relative potency. In retrospect, the results indicate that the longer C-S bonds in the 2,5-disubstituted sulfur-containing heterocycles cause crowding of the dichlorobenzyl group and Tyr181, and the nitrogen in the 3-position has an electrostatically unfavorable interaction with Glu138.

An interesting aside is that in the original publication, it was thought that the 2,5-disubstituted thiazole in Figure 1.13 showed weak activity with an EC_{50} of 3.1 μM, which was out of line with the FEP results.[24] It was subsequently found that instead of the 2,5-isomer, the 2,4-isomer (S and N interchanged in the structure in Figure 1.13) was the actual compound that had been synthesized and assayed, as confirmed by a crystal structure. The two isomers are not unequivocally distinguishable by NMR. An alternative synthetic route was then pursued to yield the 2,5-isomer, which is indeed inactive, as predicted by the FEP calculations.

Small group scans

In addition to the heterocycle scans, small group scans are highly informative. These are performed routinely with BOMB to build the structures and provide initial scoring, followed by refinement with FEP calculations. A standard protocol with BOMB is to replace each hydrogen of a core, especially aryl hydrogens, with ten small groups that have been selected for difference in size, electronic char-

acter, and hydrogen-bonding patterns: Cl, CH_3, NH_2, OH, CH_2NH_2, CH_2OH, CHO, CN, $NHCH_3$, and OCH_3. This is generally adequate to define likely places for beneficial substitution of hydrogen by the least polar groups, Cl, CH_3, and OCH_3. The situation with the polar groups is less clear because of the competition for the ligand between hydrogen bonding in the complex versus unbound in water. As long as some hydrogens appear viable for substitution, a chlorine and/or methyl scan using FEP calculations is then desirable to obtain quantitatively reliable predictions. The potential value of using both a chlorine and methyl scan is well illustrated by the results in Figure 1.14; knowing the optimal position for a methyl group and a chlorine provides an activity boost from 30 μM to 39 nM in this case.[11-13]

A chlorine scan was also particularly helpful in evolving the inactive oxadiazole **3** in Figure 1.4 into potent anti-HIV agents. **3** had emerged in third place after the docking exercise and embedded among known, potent NNRTIs. The docking pose and the structure of the complex as built by BOMB also looked reasonable, although the score from BOMB was modest because of poor accommodation of the methoxy groups in the vicinity of Tyr181 and Tyr188. Assuming that the tricyclic core might be viable, the substituents were removed and a chlorine scan was performed using MC/FEP simulations.[5,24] The predicted changes in free energy of binding for replacing each hydrogen by chlorine are summarized in Figure 1.15; again formally equivalent positions become nonequivalent in the complexes. The scan indicated that the most favorable positions for introduction of chlorines were at C3 and C4 in the phenyl ring and at C2 and C6 in the benzyl ring. A series of polychloro analogs were then synthesized and the activities were found to closely parallel the predictions (Scheme 3). The core and, for example, the 4,4'-dichloro analog were inactive; however, the illustrated

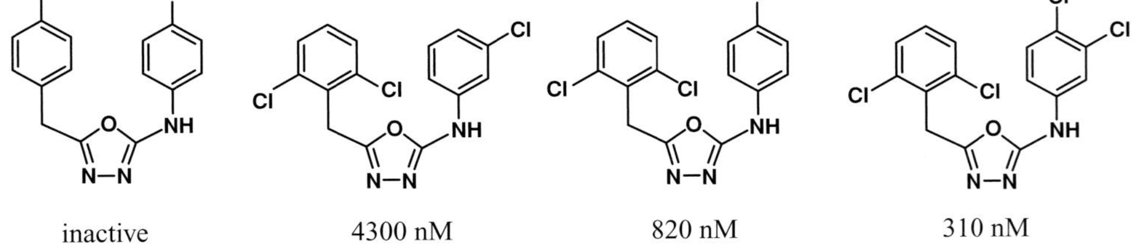

inactive   4300 nM   820 nM   310 nM

Scheme 3.

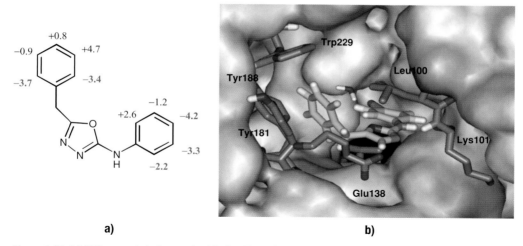

Figure 1.15. (a) FEP-computed changes in ΔG_b (kcal/mol) for replacement of the indicted hydrogens by chlorine. (b) Snapshot of the complex of the 13-nM NNRTI **4** bound to HIV-RT from the MC/FEP simulations.

trichloro and tetrachloro analogs followed the expectations from the FEP results and yielded sub-μM NNRTIs. Thus, with the aid of the FEP chlorine scan it was possible to evolve the false positive from the docking calculations into true positives.[5,24]

Small group and linker refinement

Given the positive outcome of chlorine and/or methyl scans, it is natural to consider further optimization at the replacement sites. This has been successfully guided by FEP results several times, for example, in the optimization of the substituent in the pyrimidine ring and at the 4-position in the phenyl ring for the Het-NH-3-Ph-U compounds in Figure 1.3.[11–13,24] More recent examples occurred with the azoles (Scheme 4). At C4 in the illustrated 2′,6′-dichlorobenzyloxadiazole, FEP calculations were performed and predicted relative ΔG_b values in kcal/mol for X = H (0.0), CH_2CH_3 (−0.3), CH_3 (−1.6), CH_2OCH_3 (−1.7), OCH_3 (−1.8), CF_3 (−2.2), F (−2.3), Cl (−4.0), and CN (−5.2). The X = CH_3, CH_2OCH_3, Cl, and CN analogs were synthesized and the assay results with EC_{50} values of 4, 4, 0.8, and 0.1 μM, respectively, conformed well to the expectations.[24]

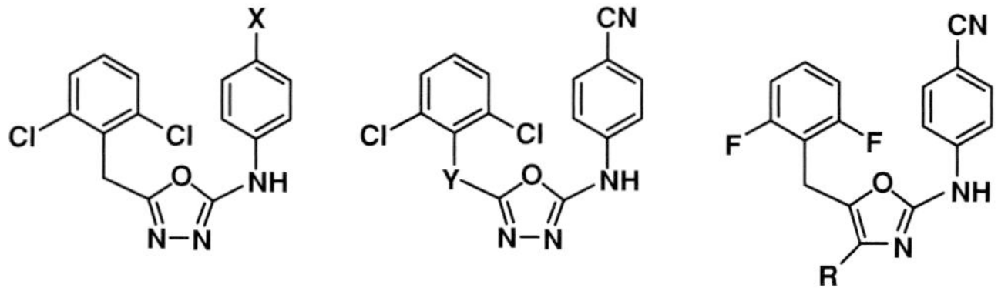

modification of the methylene group were all unfavorable except for minor improvement for the methylamino (−1.6) and thio (−1.4) alternatives. The Y = NH and racemic $CHCH_3$ analogs were synthesized and indeed found to be less active than the methylene compound; the methylamino compound turned out to have similar activity (0.2 μM) as the methylene analog (0.1 μM) with X = CN, and the oxo and thio options were not pursued. Overall, combination of the FEP-guided heterocycle, small substituent, and linker optimizations delivered the 13-nM difluorobenzyloxazole derivative **4**, which is shown in Figures 1.4 and 1.15(b).[24]

As a last thrust, FEP calculations were performed for possible replacement of the oxazole C4 hydrogen by R = F, Et, Me, CF_3, and CH_2OH. The five analogs were predicted to be less well bound than the unsubstituted compound by 0.8, 1.5, 1.8, 2.2, and 3.9 kcal/mol, respectively. Visual inspections of modeled structures were, once more, ambiguous. The qualitative FEP result was confirmed experimentally for the C4-methyl derivative, which was found to be seven-fold less potent than the unsubstituted compound. The other options were not pursued.

Overall approach and logistics

The experiences with FEP-guided lead optimization have led to the scheme in Figure 1.1. De novo design or virtual screening can be expected to provide one or more lead compounds with low-μM activity. The substituents in the lead are likely not optimal, especially from virtual screening. Consequently, removal of any small substituents from the core followed by chlorine and methyl FEP scans are then desirable. Synthesis and assaying of the most promising di- or trisubstituted compounds from the scans can provide significant activity improvements, as in Figures 1.13 and 1.14, often with modest synthetic effort. FEP-guided refinement of the small substituents, linkers, and heterocycles is

Scheme 4.

FEP-guided optimization of the linker Y between the oxadiazole and dichlorophenyl rings was also pursued. The options considered were Y = CH_2, (*R*)-$CHCH_3$, (*S*)-$CHCH_3$, NH, NCH_3, O, and S. Though display of the corresponding complexes appears reasonable, the FEP predictions for

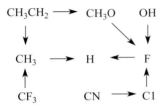

Figure 1.16. Possible series of FEP calculations to be run in parallel for optimization of a small substituent.

the logical next step; the order depends on the specific case. Optimization of peripheral rings and their substituents is likely to be easier synthetically than change of a central heterocycle. For the small groups, replacement of chlorine by fluorine (smaller, less lipophilic) and cyano (larger, more polar) can often be constructive, while replacements of methyl by OCH_3, CF_3, and CH_2OCH_3 can provide informative variety. It is straightforward to run a series of FEP modifications in parallel for optimization of a small substituent. A typical series is shown in Figure 1.16 for optimization of a substituent on an aromatic ring; the indicated conversions are intended to minimize steric and hydrogen-bonding changes. Avoidance of bromine, iodine, and nitro groups can be justified because of potential reactivity and metabolism drawbacks.

As a standard protocol, the necessary structure files are built using BOMB, and the nine indicated FEP calculations for the complexes are run simultaneously on nine processors; such calculations for an approximately 200-residue protein, 1,000 water molecules, and normal run lengths require six to seven days on a 3-GHz Pentium IV using MCPRO. A script is also used to extract the ligand from the complexes and to initiate the corresponding nine FEP calculations for the perturbations between the unbound ligands in water; these require one day each. So, with the commitment of eleven processors, the nine $\Delta\Delta G_b$ results are available in one week. For heterocycle optimization, it is convenient to use a reference that has the maximal number of hydrogens, for example, pyrrole, and perturb to other heterocycles with the same ring size and with the same or a smaller number of hydrogen atoms. Such isosteric FEP calculations converge well, and running about ten heterocycle perturbations in parallel is straightforward.[14,24] The default FEP procedure is to use eleven windows of overlap sampling (11-SOS), which is described in detail elsewhere.[57] If rapid turn-around is needed, it is easy to have a script distribute the eleven windows on eleven processors. An FEP calculation for a complex can then be completed in one day, and a twelfth processor can be used for the unbound leg of the cycle in Figure 1.10; that is, one $\Delta\Delta G_b$ result can be obtained in one day using twelve processors.

As noted in Figure 1.1, throughout the lead generation and optimization process it is also advisable to stay aware of the predicted ADME characteristics of the compounds to avoid potential bioavailability problems. It is often more difficult to change properties than potency

because potency is so locally sensitive. For example, the predicted solubilities, QPlog$S$, and octanol/water partition coefficients, QPlog$P$, for the four compounds in Figure 1.14 are within approximately 0.5 log unit, whereas the activity range is nearly 3 log units. Molecular design for some drug classes can be particularly challenging, for example, for CNS-active compounds in view of the simultaneous needs for good potency, solubility, cell permeability, and blood/brain barrier penetrability, and for Gram-negative antibacterial agents because of the outer membrane structure. In general, a common problem that needs to be avoided is being lured by the Siren of in vitro potency into the Charybdis of insolubility.

CONCLUSION

Great progress has been made in the development and application of methodology to facilitate both drug lead generation and lead optimization. Computational chemistry has contributed significantly through advances in de novo design, virtual screening, prediction of pharmacologically important properties, and the estimation of protein-ligand binding affinities. Docking of large commercial and in-house libraries has evolved into being an essential approach for structure-based lead generation. All pharmaceutical companies also routinely use software for predictive ADME profiling. Furthermore, as summarized here, the long-standing promise of the utility of free-energy calculations for molecular design including thorough lead optimization has been fulfilled. The methodology allows broad exploration of the effects of potential modifications to a compound without the need for synthesis and without conceptual constraints associated with ease of synthesis. Depending on the outcome of the computational explorations, synthetic and biological resources can be focused on the most promising directions. In view of the ever-pressing needs for efficiency, free-energy-guided molecular design can be expected to become a mainstream activity in many contexts.

ACKNOWLEDGMENTS

The work described here has been supported by grants from the National Institutes of Health (GM32136, AI44616) and the Alliance for Lupus Research. The contributions from the coworkers listed in the references were also essential.

REFERENCES

1. Hughes, B. 2007 FDA drug approvals: a year of flux. *Nat. Rev. Drug Discov.* **2008**, *7*, 107–109.
2. Lahana, R. How many leads from HTS? *Drug Discov. Today* **1999**, *4*, 447–448.
3. Posner, B. A. High-throughput screening-driven lead discovery: Meeting the challenges of finding new therapeutics. *Curr. Opin. Drug Disc. Dev.* **2005**, *8*, 487–494.

4. Ganesan, A. The impact of natural products upon modern drug discovery. *Curr. Opin. Chem. Biol.* **2008**, *12*, 306–317.

5. Barreiro, G.; Kim, J. T.; Guimarães, C. R. W.; Bailey, C. M.; Domaoal, R. A.; Wang, L.; Anderson, K. S.; Jorgensen, W. L. From docking false-positive to active anti-HIV Agent. *J. Med. Chem.* **2007**, *50*, 5324–5329.

6. Friesner, R. A.; Banks, J. L.; Murphy, R. B.; Halgren, T. A.; Klicic, J. J.; Mainz, D. T.; Repasky, M. P.; Knoll, E. H.; Shelley, M.; Perry, J. K.; Shaw, D. E.; Francis, P.; Shenkin, P. S. GLIDE: A new approach for rapid, accurate docking and scoring. 1. Method and assessment of docking accuracy. *J. Med. Chem.* **2004**, *47*, 1739–1749.

7. Leach, A. R.; Hann, M. M.; Burrows, J. N.; Griffen, E. J. Fragment screening: an introduction. *Mol. Biosyst.* **2006**, *2*, 429–446.

8. Congreve, M.; Chessari, G.; Tisi, D.; Woodhead, A. J. Recent developments in fragment-based drug discovery. *J. Med. Chem.* **2008**, *51*, 3661–3680.

9. Rodgers, D. W.; Gamblin, S. J.; Harris, B. A.; Ray, S.; Culp, J. S.; Hellmig, B.; Woolf, D. J. The structure of unliganded reverse transcriptase from the human immunodeficiency virus type 1. *Proc. Natl. Acad. Sci. U.S.A.* **1995**, *92*, 1222–1226.

10. Jorgensen, W. L.; Tirado-Rives, J. Potential energy functions for atomic-level simulations of water and organic and biomolecular systems. *Proc. Nat. Acad. Sci U.S.A.* **2005**, *102*, 6665–6670.

11. Jorgensen, W. L.; Ruiz-Caro, J.; Tirado-Rives, J.; Basavapathruni, A.; Anderson, K. S.; Hamilton, A. D. Computer-aided design of non-nucleoside inhibitors of HIV-1 reverse transcriptase. *Bioorg. Med. Chem. Lett.* **2006**, *16*, 663–667.

12. Ruiz-Caro, J.; Basavapathruni, A.; Kim, J. T.; Wang, L.; Bailey, C. M.; Anderson, K. S.; Hamilton, A. D.; Jorgensen, W. L. Optimization of diarylamines as non-nucleoside inhibitors of HIV-1 reverse transcriptase. *Bioorg. Med. Chem. Lett.* **2006**, *16*, 668–671.

13. Thakur, V. V.; Kim, J. T.; Hamilton, A. D.; Bailey, C. M.; Domaoal, R. A.; Wang, L.; Anderson, K. S.; Jorgensen, W. L. Optimization of pyrimidinyl- and triazinyl-amines as non-nucleoside inhibitors of HIV-1 reverse transcriptase. *Bioorg. Med. Chem. Lett.* **2006**, *16*, 5664–5667.

14. Kim, J. T.; Hamilton, A. D.; Bailey, C. M.; Domaoal, R. A.; Wang, L.; Anderson, K. S.; Jorgensen, W. L. FEP-guided selection of bicyclic heterocycles in lead optimization for non-nucleoside inhibitors of HIV-1 reverse transcriptase. *J. Am. Chem. Soc.* **2006**, *128*, 15372–15373.

15. Jorgensen, W. L. QIKPROP, v 3.0. New York: Schrödinger LLC; **2006**.

16. Jorgensen, W. L.; Tirado-Rives, J. Molecular modeling of organic and biomolecular systems using BOSS and MCPRO. *J. Comput. Chem.* **2005**, *26*, 1689–1700.

17. Jorgensen, W. L. The many roles of computation in drug discovery. *Science* **2004**, *303*, 1813–1818.

18. Kellenberger, E.; Rodrigo, J.; Muller, P.; Rognan, D. Comparative evaluation of eight docking tools for docking and virtual screening accuracy. *Proteins* **2004**, *57*, 225–242.

19. Leach, A. R.; Shoichet, B. K.; Peishoff, C. E. Prediction of protein-ligand interactions. Docking and scoring: successes and gaps. *J. Med. Chem.* **2006**, *49*, 5851–5855.

20. Zhou, Z.; Felts, A. K.; Friesner, R. A.; Levy, R. M. Comparative performance of several flexible docking programs and scoring functions: enrichment studies for a diverse set of pharmaceutically relevant targets. *J. Chem. Inf. Model.* **2007**, *47*, 1599–1608.

21. Tirado-Rives, J.; Jorgensen, W. L. Contribution of conformer focusing to the uncertainty in predicting free energies for protein-ligand binding. *J. Med. Chem.* **2006**, *49*, 5880–5884.

22. Barreiro, G.; Guimarães, C. R. W.; Tubert-Brohman, I.; Lyons, T. M.; Tirado-Rives, J.; Jorgensen, W. L. Search for non-nucleoside inhibitors of HIV-1 reverse transcriptase using chemical similarity, molecular docking, and MM-GB/SA scoring. *J. Chem. Info. Model.* **2007**, *47*, 2416–2428.

23. Friesner, R. A.; Murphy, R. B.; Repasky, M. P.; Frye, L. L.; Greenwood, J. R.; Halgren, T. A.; Sanschagrin, P. C.; Mainz, D. T. Extra precision GLIDE: Docking and scoring incorporating a model of hydrophobic enclosure for protein-ligand complexes. *J. Med. Chem.* **2006**, *49*, 6177–6196.

24. Zeevaart, J. G.; Wang, L.; Thakur, V. V.; Leung, C. S.; Tirado-Rives, J.; Bailey, C. M.; Domaoal, R. A.; Anderson, K. S.; Jorgensen, W. L. Optimization of azoles as anti-HIV agents guided by free-energy calculations. *J. Am. Chem. Soc.* **2008**, *130*, 9492–9499.

25. Cournia, Z.; Leng, L.; Gandavadi, S.; Du, X.; Bucala, R.; Jorgensen, W. L. Discovery of human macrophage migration inhibitory factor (MIF)-CD74 antagonists via virtual screening. *J. Med. Chem.* **2009**, *52*, 416–424.

26. Irwin, J. J.; Shoichet, B. K. ZINC: a free database of commercially available compounds for virtual screening. *J. Chem. Inf. Model.* **2005**, *45*, 177–182.

27. Morand, E. F.; Leech, M.; Bernhagen, J. MIF: a new cytokine link between rheumatoid arthritis and atherosclerosis. *Nat. Rev. Drug Discov.* **2006**, *5*, 399–411.

28. Hagemann, T.; Robinson, S. C.; Thompson, R. G.; Charles, K.; Kulbe, H.; Balkwill, F. R. Ovarian cancer cell-derived migration inhibitory factor enhances tumor growth, progression, and angiogenesis. *Mol. Cancer Ther.* **2007**, *6*, 1993–2002.

29. Senter, P. D.; Al-Abed, Y.; Metz, C. N.; Benigni, F.; Mitchell, R. A.; Chesney, J.; Han, J.; Gartner, C. G.; Nelson, S. D.; Todaro, G. J.; Bucala, R. Inhibition of macrophage migration inhibitory factor (MIF) tautomerase and biological activities by acetaminophen metabolites. *Proc. Natl. Acad. Sci. U.S.A.* **2002**, *99*, 144–149.

30. Sun, H. W.; Bernhagen, J.; Bucala, R.; Lolis, E. Crystal structure at 2.6-Å resolution of human macrophage migration inhibitory factor. *Proc. Natl. Acad. Sci. U.S.A.* **1996**, *93*, 5191–5196.

31. Egan, W. J.; Merz, K. M., Jr.; Baldwin, J. J. Prediction of drug absorption using multivariate statistics. *J. Med. Chem.* **2000**, *43*, 3867–3877.

32. Lipinski, C. A.; Lombardo, F.; Dominy, B. W.; Feeney, P. J. Experimental and computational approaches to estimate solubility and permeability in drug discovery and development settings. *Adv. Drug Deliv. Rev.* **2001**, *46*, 3–26.

33. Jorgensen, W. L.; Duffy, E. M. Prediction of solubility from structure. *Adv. Drug Deliv. Rev.*, *54*, 355–365.

34. Norinder, U.; Bergström, C. A. S. Prediction of ADMET properties. *ChemMedChem* **2006**, *1*, 920–937.

35. Proudfoot, J. R. The evolution of synthetic oral drug properties. *Bioorg. Med. Chem. Lett.* **2005**, *15*, 1087–1090.

36. Weber, A.; Casini, A.; Heine, A.; Kuhn, D.; Supuran, C. T.; Scozzafava, A.; Klebe, G. Unexpected nanomolar inhibition of carbonic anhydrase by COX-2-selective celecoxib: new pharmacological opportunities due to related binding site recognition. *J. Med. Chem.* **2004**, *47*, 550–557.

37. Chipot, C.; Pohorille, A. In *Springer Series in Chemical Physics: Free Energy Calculations: Theory and Applications in Chemistry and Biology*, Vol. 86, Chipot, C.; Pohorille, A.; Eds. Berlin: Springer-Verlag; **2007**, 33–75.

38. Jorgensen, W. L.; Ravimohan, C. Monte Carlo simulation of differences in free energies of hydration. *J. Chem. Phys.* **1985**, *83*, 3050–3054.

39. Wong, C. F.; McCammon, J. A. Dynamics and design of enzymes and inhibitors. *J. Am. Chem. Soc.* **1986**, *108*, 3830–3832.

40. McCammon, J. A. Computer-aided molecular design. *Science* **1987**, *238*, 486–491.

41. Kollman, P. A. Free energy calculations: applications to chemical and biochemical phenomena. *Chem. Rev.* **1993**, *93*, 2395–2417.

42. Merz, K. M.; Kollman, P. A. Free energy perturbation simulations of the inhibition of thermolysin: prediction of the free energy of binding of a new inhibitor. *J. Am. Chem. Soc.* **1989**, *111*, 5649–5658.

43. Pearlman, D. A.; Charifson, P. S. Are free energy calculations useful in practice? A comparison with rapid scoring functions for the p38 MAP kinase protein system. *J. Med. Chem.* **2001**, *44*, 3417–3423.

44. Pearlman, D. A. Evaluating the molecular mechanics Poisson-Boltzmann surface area free energy method using a congeneric series of ligands to p38 MAP kinase. *J. Med. Chem.* **2005**, *48*, 7796–7807.

45. Reddy, M. R.; Erion, M. D. Calculation of relative binding free energy differences for fructose 1,6-biphosphatase inhibitors using thermodynamic cycle perturbation approach. *J. Am. Chem. Soc.* **2001**, *123*, 6246–6252.

46. Erion, M. D.; Dang, Q.; Reddy, M. R.; Kasibhatla, S. R.; Huang, J.; Lipscomb, W. N.; van Poelje, P. D. Structure-guided design of amp mimics that inhibit fructose-1,6-bisphosphatase with high affinity and specificity. *J. Am. Chem. Soc.* **2007**, *129*, 15480–15490.

47. Pierce, A. C.; Jorgensen, W. L. Computational binding studies of orthogonal cyclosporin-cyclophilin pairs. *Angew. Chem. Int. Ed. Engl.* **1997**, *36*, 1466–1469.

48. Essex, J. W.; Severance, D. L.; Tirado-Rives, J.; Jorgensen, W. L. Monte Carlo simulations for proteins: binding affinities for trypsin-benzamidine complexes via free energy perturbations. *J. Phys. Chem.* **1997**, *101*, 9663–9669.

49. Plount-Price, M. L.; Jorgensen, W. L. Analysis of binding affinities for celecoxib analogs with COX-1 and COX-2 from docking and Monte Carlo simulations and insight into COX-2/COX-1 selectivity. *J. Am. Chem. Soc.* **2000**, *122*, 9455–9466.

50. Plount-Price, M. L.; Jorgensen, W. L. Rationale for the observed COX-2/COX-1 selectivity of celecoxib from Monte Carlo simulations. *Bioorg. Med. Chem. Lett.* **2001**, *11*, 1541–1544.

51. Guimarães, C. R. W; Boger, D. L.; Jorgensen, W. L. Elucidation of fatty acid amide hydrolase inhibition by potent α-ketoheterocycle derivatives from Monte Carlo simulations. *J. Am. Chem. Soc.* **2005**, *127*, 17377–17384.

52. Rizzo, R. C.; Wang, D.-P.; Tirado-Rives, J.; Jorgensen, W. L. Validation of a model for the complex of HIV-1 reverse transcriptase with Sustiva through computation of resistance profiles. *J. Am. Chem. Soc.* **2000**, *122*, 12898–12900.

53. Wang, D.-P.; Rizzo, R. C.; Tirado-Rives, J.; Jorgensen, W. L. Antiviral drug design: Computational analyses of the effects of the L100I mutation for HIV-RT on the binding of NNRTIs. *Bioorg. Med. Chem. Lett.* **2001**, *11*, 2799–2802.

54. Udier-Blagović, M.; Tirado-Rives, J.; Jorgensen, W. L. Validation of a model for the complex of HIV-1 reverse transcriptase with the novel non-nucleoside inhibitor TMC125 *J. Am. Chem. Soc.* **2003**, *125*, 6016–6017.

55. Blagović, M. U.; Tirado-Rives, J.; Jorgensen, W. L. Structural and energetic analyses for the effects of the K103N mutation of HIV-1 reverse transcriptase on efavirenz analogs. *J. Med. Chem.* **2004**, *46*, 2389–2392.

56. Das, K.; Clark, A. D., Jr.; Lewi, P. J.; Heeres, J.; de Jonge, M. R.; Koymans, L. M. H.; Vinkers, H. M.; Daeyaert, F.; Ludovici, D. W.; Kukla, M. J.; De Corte, B.; Kavash, R. W.; Ho, C. Y.; Ye, H.; Lichtenstein, M. A.; Andries, K.; Pauwels, R.; de Béthune, M.-P.; Boyer, P. L.; Clark, P.; Hughes, S. H.; Janssen, P. A. J.; Arnold, E. Roles of conformational and positional adaptability in structure-based design of TMC125-R165335 (Etravirine) and related non-nucleoside reverse transcriptase inhibitors that are highly potent and effective against wild-type and drug-resistant HIV-1 variants. *J. Med. Chem.* **2004**, *47*, 2550–2560.

57. Jorgensen, W. L.; Thomas, L. T. Perspective on free-energy perturbation calculations for chemical equilibria. *J. Chem. Theor. Comput.* **2008**, *4*, 869–876.

PART I

Structural biology

X-ray crystallography in the service of structure-based drug design

Gregory A. Petsko and Dagmar Ringe

Protein crystallography traditionally has been at the base of structure-based drug discovery (SBDD) by providing the structures of protein/ligand complexes that are often the starting point for the design and improvement of specific ligands. Consequently, an awareness of the strengths and weaknesses of this method is important for the success of ligand design. For instance, questions are often raised about the validity of a particular protein structure and whether that structure is relevant to the biological activity of the protein or about the conformation of a bound ligand and whether it represents a productive form. Some of these questions can be answered or at least addressed, whereas others cannot. There is an attempt to address those that can be addressed and to make some suggestions about those that cannot. Therefore, this chapter will focus more on the criteria that can be used to assess the quality of a structure determined by x-ray crystallography and less on the detailed methods used to achieve it.

BASIC CONCEPTS: CRYSTALLIZATION

The basic requirement for a crystal structure is a crystal. Although crystallization of proteins is still more of an art than a science, methods for routine searches of crystallization conditions are indeed available. Historically, the crystallization of proteins was a normal procedure used when working with an enzyme. Because of the known salting out effects of ammonium sulfate, this salt was used to induce selective crystallization, thereby purifying the protein. However, numerous other conditions exist that also promote or prevent crystallization, including pH, presence of counterions or organic compounds, additives with no known rationale, and temperature. A combination matrix of such conditions must be tested to find the best set of conditions that produce not only crystals but crystals of the size and quality required for x-ray diffraction.[1]

How much protein is needed for such a crystallization search? It could be anywhere from micrograms to buckets, depending on how readily conditions are found. What should these crystals look like for a crystallographic experiment? With today's x-ray sources, crystals as small as micrometers on a side are sufficient to obtain measurable diffraction. The most important criterion for successful crystals is the ability to diffract x-rays, and that criterion depends on well-ordered crystals. How to obtain such crystals in a predictable fashion is still not known precisely because each protein seems to have its own characteristics. However, in general, the purity and concentration of the protein, the stability of the protein, and the rate at which crystals form are the dominant features that lead to success (Figure 2.1).

It is a basic fact that if the protein does not crystallize the project cannot proceed. To obtain some structural information despite this roadblock, a number of avenues are available. The most obvious is to obtain a homologous protein from an organism that is different than the target organism and that behaves better with regard to the above criteria. Proteins from thermophiles are especially useful in this context, because they seem to be more thermally stable than their mesophilic counterparts. A number of other approaches are useful in individual cases, such as truncation of a protein to a core domain, selective mutations, and selective modifications. Finally, modification of the protein in a noncovalent fashion, specifically the binding of an inhibitor to an enzyme, often leads to successful crystallization when the apo enzyme is resistant.

For instance, to obtain a crystal structure for the human enzyme glucocerebrosidase, the protein could be purified from tissue directly, or, more commonly when possible, it can be cloned, expressed, and purified from another vector. In the case of glucocerebrocidase, both purified protein from tissue and, later, cloned material from COS cells has been used.[2,3] Mammalian proteins are often posttranslationally modified in their physiological environment, and these modifications, being heterogeneous as a rule, often interfere with crystallizations. Consequently, the proteins may have to be, for instance, deglycosylated to obtain crystals.[3] A protein obtained from a cloned source may lack these modifications or have different ones unique to the cloning cells, and such differences may spell success or failure for crystallization and a structure determination.

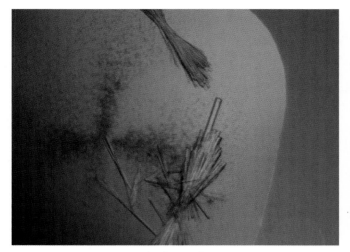

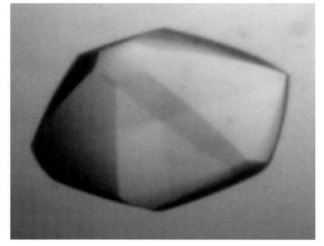

bad crystal   good crystal

Figure 2.1. Examples of crystallization trials. Proteins can aggregate in many ways but usually crystallize in only one form. The example on the left shows protein aggregation without forming a crystal (cloudy areas). Aggregation may be random protein association or denaturation of the protein under the conditions of the crystallization trial. Also shown is formation of crystals that do not diffract, possibly because they are too small in two dimensions or because they crystallized in a disordered fashion. The example on the right shows a beautifully formed protein crystal. On occasion, even such a lovely crystal may show poor or no diffraction because of internal systematic lattice disorder. In this case, the crystal diffracts to 0.9Å resolution.

DATA COLLECTION

Once crystals are obtained, they can be tested for their ability to diffract x-rays and data can be collected. There is a fundamental principle about diffraction that allows it to be transformed into structural information: the diffraction pattern of an object is the Fourier transform of the object (for details, see Stout & Jensen, 1989; Blow, 2002; Rhodes, 2006).[4-6] Conversely, the inverse Fourier transform of the diffraction pattern will give a model of the object.

In principle, a single object will diffract x-rays. Diffraction depends on the interaction of electromagnetic radiation with an object and the scattering of that radiation. Other scattering methods also exist, such as the scattering of neutrons from nuclei, but at present they constitute only a very tiny fraction of the diffraction experiments done today. For proteins or other organic molecules, x-rays are the electromagnetic radiation of choice because the typical wavelength of an x-ray is 0.15 nm, the approximate distance of bond lengths in such molecules. Consequently, it should be possible to detect such distances using x-ray diffraction.

Ideally, a single molecule should suffice for such an experiment. However, the use of a single molecule results in such a low intensity of the scattered beam that it is too weak to be measured by any detector available today. Consequently, scattering from many molecules is required to obtain a signal strong enough to measure. For a scattered beam to be measurable, somewhere in the vicinity of 10^{15} molecules are required. Not only are a large number of molecules required, but also they all have to be in the same or a limited number of orientations that repeat in a regular

pattern in three dimensions. That is the definition of a crystal in which the repeating unit that builds the crystal is the unit cell. When scattering comes from a crystal it is called diffraction. The fundamental principle of diffraction of a crystal of a protein states that the Fourier transform of the electron distribution of the protein in the crystal is the diffraction pattern and the inverse Fourier transform of the diffraction pattern is the electron density of the protein.

Just as the protein is three-dimensional, so is the diffraction pattern. In addition, the diffraction pattern mirrors the symmetry of the arrangements of the unit cells in the crystal and the protein in the unit cell. These arrangements are defined in terms of space groups and asymmetric units. The asymmetric unit is the smallest unit from which a unit cell can be constructed and represents the minimum number of independently determined structures in a crystal. Thus, an asymmetric unit may contain as few as one example of a protein or as many as twelve or more. Sometimes such arrangements make it possible to determine the oligomeric state of a protein, particularly if one subunit is not identical to another (Figure 2.2).

Because of the three-dimensional character of a diffraction pattern, a reflection, the effect of a diffracted beam on a detector, may lie closer to the center of the pattern or further away from it. The identity of a reflection is defined by its Miller indices, its position on a three-dimensional grid, starting with zero at the center and moving outward. The angles the diffracted beams make with the direction of the incident beam determines the level of information obtainable from them. The larger the angle, the more precise the information carried relative to the distances within the

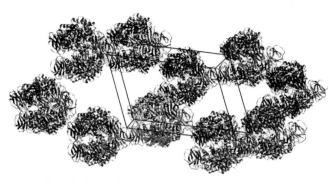

Protein Crystals Contain Solvent-Filled Channels

Figure 2.2. Because protein molecules are generally of irregular shapes, packing in the crystal leads to spaces and channels between molecules that are filled with solvent from the crystallization mother liquor. Consequently, small molecules, such as substrates and inhibitors, can diffuse into the crystal and reach the protein surface. Shown are several molecules of glucocerebrosidase, showing the arrangement of the packing, the unit cell, and the asymmetric unit. Data were taken from PDB code 1OSG.

crystal and the higher the resolution of the resulting electron density, thus, the higher the indices of the reflections that can be observed, the higher the resolution of the diffraction pattern, and the more precise the resulting electron density (Figure 2.3).

Ultimately, the quality of the diffraction pattern, in terms of the intensities of the reflections and the resolution of the data set, will determine the quality of the electron density map that can be obtained. A number of criteria are used to determine the quality of a data set: I(ntensity), R(adiation damage), O(verlap), Rm(erge), C(ompleteness) (Table 2.1) (a useful discussion of these parameters may be found in Wlodawer et al., 2008).[7]

(I) The intensities of the reflections will clearly influence the quality of the data. Intensity depends on a number of factors, mainly the size and quality of the crystal, the length of exposure to the x-ray beam, and the intensity of the x-ray beam. The quality of the intensity relative to background is given as the signal-to-noise ratio: $I/\sigma(I)$. Because proteins are subject to interactions with x-rays that lead to chemical changes, the latter two factors are counterproductive relative to the intensity of the reflection. Therefore, the $I/\sigma(I)$ criterion is sometimes used to define the resolution limits of the data, the diffraction limit defined where this value decreases to 2.0.

(R) Radiation damage is a significant factor for data quality and is usually dealt with by reducing the temperature of the crystal during data collection. The most common temperature is the "cryo" range, achieved by using liquid nitrogen to cool to approximately 100 K. Such a temperature requires special treatment of the crystal, because it contains water, which can freeze with disastrous results for the crystal. Flash freezing,

with and without additives to prevent crystallization of water, is used.

(O) Beyond intensity of a reflection, the ability to distinguish individual reflections from each other is also essential. The separation of reflections in a diffraction pattern depends primarily on the size of the unit cell: the larger the unit cell axes, the closer the reflections are to each other, and overlap of reflections leads to inaccurate intensity determination. Disorder in the crystal, either of packing or from mechanical damage (e.g., through freezing), can lead to a broadening of the reflections, and excessive broadening will produce overlap.

(R_m) Because the diffraction pattern contains elements of symmetry, and because of the method used to measure reflections, most reflections are measured more than once. Consequently, the reproducibility of these measurements is a measure of the precision to which the reflections can be determined. Statistically, the more often a reflection is measured, and the closer those measurements are to each other, the better the data set. The redundancies for the data are given in terms of an average, overall redundancy. The reproducibility of the reflection measurements is given in terms of a residual factor, R_{merge} (R_m, sometimes called R_{sym}), the difference between a measured intensity and the average intensity, divided by the average intensity, for all related reflections. This factor will change with resolution, so it should be given for all data and for data in the highest resolution shell for

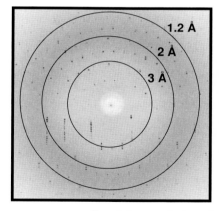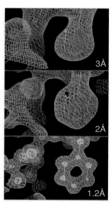

Resolution vs electron density

Figure 2.3. The resolution to which a structure can be determined depends on the reflections that can be measured. Shown at left is a diffraction pattern of a typical protein. The rings indicate levels of resolution. At right are electron densities for the same residue of a protein, calculated from the data within a resolution range. Thus, if only the data within the 3Å resolution circle are used, the electron density map lacks detail at the atomic level. On the other hand, if all of the data within the 1.2Å resolution circle are used, the electron density resolves the positions of individual atoms (shown are two levels of the electron density). Note that the reflections become weaker as the resolution gets higher (measured as $I/\sigma(I)$), and the total number of possible reflections measured becomes less (completeness).

Table 2.1. Data collection statistics for a typical protein structure determination. The numbers in parentheses refer to the highest resolution bin and are indicative of how well the higher resolution data are measured. (Data adapted from the structure determination of glucosidase at pH 4.5; PDB code 2NT0)[3]

Space group	P2$_1$
Cell dimensions	110.5,91.8,152.8Å
	90, 111.2, 90°
Resolution (Å)	34–2.2 (2.28–2.20)
R_{sym}	10.3 (47.3)
$I/\sigma(I)$	9.8 (2.2)
Completeness (%)	96.4 (91.2)
Redundancy	2.5 (1.8)

which data are included. A good data set is characterized by an overall R_{merge} value of about 5% or less. A value higher than ~10% suggests less than optimal data quality. At the highest resolution shell, R_{merge} can reach as high as 40% for low-symmetry crystals and 60% for high-symmetry crystals, the difference being a reflection of the level of redundancy, which is higher for high symmetry crystals.

(C) Finally, the completeness of the data is an important factor in determining data quality. Completeness is determined by comparison with the expected number of reflections for a particular space group and unit cell size, and given as a percentage. Because the ability to measure reflections decreases with resolution, completeness also decreases with resolution, so this parameter should be given for all data and for the highest resolution shell as defined for the R_{merge}.

In general, the data should have as high a resolution range as possible, with a high signal-to-noise ratio (>10), well-separated reflections, a low R_{merge} (<10), and high completeness (overall, it is acceptable to have relatively low completeness in the highest resolution shells). How well these factors interact with each other will determine the quality of the electron density map that is obtained. In practice, these measures may not be ideal, but in general, the higher the quality of the data, the greater the likelihood that they will lead to an interpretable electron density map.

However, the measures should never be used as a substitute for judgment in deciding whether to "believe" a structure or not. They are merely rough guidelines. There are many examples of acceptable structures from data of marginal quality, and, unfortunately, a few examples of wrong structures from excellent data. It is true, though, that the most important quantity is the resolution. The higher the resolution of the data the greater the likelihood that the electron density will have been interpreted correctly. Most serious mistakes in protein crystallography have resulted from overinterpretation of poor-quality electron density at relatively low resolution.

PHASING

Electromagnetic radiation can be defined in terms of waves that are defined in terms of an amplitude and a wavelength. The phase is the relative time of arrival of the crest of the wave at a reference point, compared with any other wave. Waves of identical phase will have their peaks and troughs in common and will sum accordingly. Waves with opposite phases will tend to cancel one another out, at least partially depending on their amplitudes. Both parameters are required to define a wave mathematically. To solve a crystal structure, in principle all one has to do is add up all of the diffracted waves; that is what a Fourier synthesis is. Before that can be done, however, the two parameters must be determined for every scattered wave (i.e., every reflection).

Experimentally, the amplitude manifests itself as the square root of the measured intensity of the reflection. That is easily determined with modern area detectors. However, when waves are added, they must be added with their correct phases. Consequently, to apply the Fourier transform to a reflection, both a measure of intensity and a correct phase are required. Unfortunately, in a diffraction experiment, although the intensities and positions of the diffracted waves are measurable, the phases of the reflections are not. X-rays travel at the speed of light, so as far as we are concerned, the relative time of arrival of all of the scattered waves from the crystal at the detector will appear to be the same. Consequently, the phases must be determined in some other way.

The most common method of phasing, particularly in drug design, is molecular replacement. The method relies on two factors: (1) that the structure of the protein of interest, or that of a very similar protein, has already been determined and (2) on the observation that the diffraction pattern of the object of interest is very similar to that of a related or similar object. In molecular replacement one measures the diffraction amplitudes from the crystal of the protein of interest but "replaces" their unknown phases with phases calculated from the previously determined structure of the related protein. The dominant issue that determines success with this method, and that makes it possible, is the level of similarity between the two objects. When determining the structure of a protein/ligand complex, for instance, the expectation that the binding of the ligand produces only minor changes in the structure of the protein is usually a good one, and in such cases the known structure of the apo protein or that of the protein with another ligand bound can be used as the model from which to obtain phases.

The importance of the phases in the determination of a structure cannot be overemphasized and can be demonstrated. An electron density map, calculated from the correct structure amplitudes but incorrect phases, is uninterpretable. Conversely, an electron density map determined from random structure amplitudes but correct phases is often interpretable, albeit very noisy. For the purposes of drug design, these two rules can be combined:

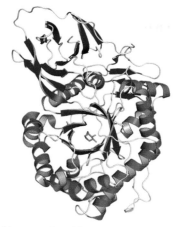

Glucocerebrocidase with IFG bound

Figure 2.4. Common representation of a protein molecule, in this case, acid β-glucosidase with the inhibitor isofagomine (IFG) bound.[3] The ribbon represents the polypeptide, whose path is shown in three dimensions. Secondary structural elements are shown by arrows (beta sheet), helices, and coils (no secondary structure). The position of the inhibitor indicates the location of the active site. Data were taken from PDB code 1OSG.

the structure amplitudes for a protein/ligand complex are combined with the phases for the protein alone, giving an electron density map of the protein with somewhat weaker electron density for the ligand but enough to interpret the structure of the added molecule (Figure 2.4).

How good does the model have to be for success in this process? The answer is not definitive but can be estimated from the figure. Clearly a protein/ligand complex falls into the acceptable range as long as the ligand is a small molecule. However, if the ligand produces major conformational changes to the protein, all bets are off. Our experience is that if the model structure has at least a 50% sequence identity to that of the new, unknown protein, molecular replacement often works (Figure 2.5). Below that rough dividing line, sometimes it works, but many times it does not.[8]

There are many other methods of phase determination that are available if molecular replacement fails or if no related structure exists, but these are outside the scope of this chapter. Suffice it to say that, in modern protein crystallography, phase determination is rarely the bottleneck. We personally have never failed to solve a structure once well-diffracting crystals have been obtained.

ELECTRON DENSITY INTERPRETATION

The electron density map is the end product of an experiment in x-ray diffraction followed by mathematical analysis of the data. It results from a Fourier synthesis with the measured diffraction amplitudes and experimentally determined or calculated phases of each reflection to the highest possible resolution. A number of smoothing operations can enhance the quality of the map but cannot make a silk purse out of a sow's ear. For instance, solvent flattening can sharpen the boundaries between solvent and molecule and

thereby improve the observed electron density. If more than one molecule is contained in the asymmetric unit, averaging of the electron densities of these molecules can increase the signal-to-noise ratio of the map. Once the best possible electron density map has been calculated, it must now be interpreted to extract a model of the molecule that produced it.

The electron density map is the objective result of a diffraction study. Now comes the subjective part, the part that is no longer experimental and requires some skill in shape fitting. Building a model into electron density requires interpretation on the part of the operator because more than one fit may be possible. The ability to interpret electron density therefore will depend on a number of the factors already mentioned. Probably the most important is the resolution. Resolution is a measure of the level of detail with which a protein is viewed, and different levels provide different kinds of information. For instance, at 5Å resolution, the limits of the protein (i.e., the protein/solvent boundary), the overall shape of the molecule, and elements of secondary structure are apparent; at 3Å resolution, the general course of the polypeptide chain and the shapes of side chains are interpretable; at 1Å resolution, individual atoms are recognizable not only as individual entities of electron density but also as identifiable atom types. The average structure determination does not achieve that level of resolution, but 1.5–2Å resolution is common, especially for ligand complexes. The electron density in such maps should be easily interpretable (Figure 2.6).

A number of factors contribute to the ease with which interpretation is possible. Because the electron density is an average of any position over all of the unit cells that make up the crystal, a sharp electron density depends on

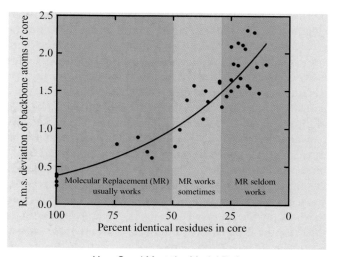

How Good Must the Model Be?
Irving, Whisstock and Lesk. Proteins **42**, 378-82 (2001).

Figure 2.5. The structural similarity between the model and the unknown determines the probability of success in a molecular replacement experiment. Some guidelines are available but are not absolute. Note that the comparison is made in terms of the identity of core residues, that is, those that are expected to be most similar in terms of sequence and structure between two related structures.[8]

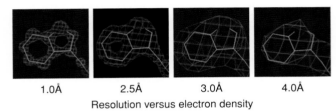

1.0Å   2.5Å   3.0Å   4.0Å

Resolution versus electron density

Figure 2.6. The ability to build a model into electron density depends on the quality of that electron density and the resolution at which it is calculated. Here the effect of resolution on the quality of the electron density is illustrated. At high resolution, such as 1.0Å resolution, individual atoms are visible to the extent that carbon and nitrogen atoms are distinguishable. At medium resolution, such as 2.5–3.0Å resolution, the shape of the residue side chain is clearly interpretable even though the individual atoms are not. At low resolution, such as 4Å resolution, the position of the side chain is clear, but the configuration is not and the fit of the model to the electron density is unclear.

perfect alignment of all the molecules, and all of the parts of molecules. If the electron density is unequivocal, there is only one molecule or residue, and the shape is unique, the model of the peptide or ligand may be "dropped" into the electron density without a problem. However, if the electron density is not so clear, if it is spread out or not quite connected everywhere, or there may be more than one molecule present in more than one orientation, interpretation becomes complicated.

For instance, a side chain or stretch of peptide may have more than one conformation. If the number is small (i.e., 2), both will usually be apparent if their occupancies are roughly equal. If the number becomes large (i.e., >3 or 4), the electron density may no longer be distinguishable from the noise of the map. A similar phenomenon applies if a ligand is bound to only some of the protein molecules in the crystal and not all. Such partial occupancy produces weak electron density for the ligand, and that may be hard to interpret. At low resolutions the spread of the electron density as a result of multiple conformations is accounted for by a term called the B factor or temperature factor: the greater the spread, the larger the B factor. Average B factors for protein atoms are in the range of 20–30A^2 depending on the resolution of the data. Occupancy is given in terms of a fraction between 0 and 1. These two are related to each other and at the resolutions generally observed for protein/ligand complexes they cannot be distinguished from each other. The B factor, which is given for each atom in the coordinate file, consequently takes both into account. It is not uncommon for the B factors for a ligand to be significantly higher than those for the protein, accounting at least in part for partial occupancy of the ligand (Figure 2.7).

Electron density maps can be displayed in a number of different ways: the most common for interpretation of protein/ligand complexes are those with coefficients Fo-Fc and 2Fo-Fc. The former displays the difference between the observed electron density and that calculated from a model. Such a difference map highlights missing parts of the model (positive difference electron density) and parts added by

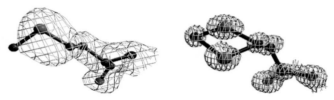

1.8 vs 0.9 Å resolution

Figure 2.7. Because the structure determined for a protein represents an average over all of the molecules in a unit cell, parts of the protein can have different conformations. The ability to deconvolute these different conformations depends partly on the resolution of the structure determination. Although the electron density at 1.8Å resolution clearly shows the direction in which the side chain points, it does not show the exact location of the end sulfur atom and methyl group. At 0.9Å resolution, this problem is resolved, showing that the sulfur atom can be in two possible conformations, in this case of approximately equal probability. It can also happen that a side chain may point in completely different directions or may have different conformations. Data were taken from PDB codes 1AMP (1.8Å resolution)[9] and 1RTQ (0.95Å resolution).[10]

the model that are not supported by the data (negative difference electron density). The latter displays the electron density emphasizing the difference between observed and calculated (Figure 2.8).

REFINEMENT

The key structures needed for the purposes of drug design are those of the protein, usually an enzyme, by itself and in the presence of a ligand; and those models should be as accurate as possible. The crystallographic experiment, however, does not provide an "accurate" model; it provides a precise model. The difference refers to the closeness with which the model can be fitted to the observed electron density and how well the two can be made to match, and the "real" structure. What the experimentalist can do is to align the model and the electron density as closely as possibly by a protocol of refinement in which the model is iteratively matched to the electron density, and the measure of fit is recalculated to determine success by the procedure. Iteration is continued until convergence occurs. Refinement is generally carried out with stereochemical restraints that

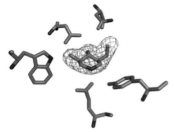

IFG/GCase with electron density

Figure 2.8. The electron density for the inhibitor isofagomine bound to glucocerebrosidase appears in an electron density map that has been calculated from the data for the enzyme-inhibitor complex and the phases from the protein alone. The electron density for the inhibitor has a shape that is consistent with only one orientation of the inhibitor in the active site. Data were taken from PDB code 2NSX.[3]

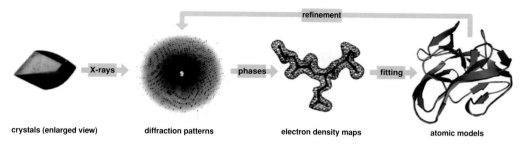

refinement

crystals (enlarged view)   diffraction patterns   electron density maps   atomic models

X-rays →   phases →   fitting →

Iterative process of refinement

Figure 2.9. The process of refinement is an iterative one, in which small changes are made to the atomic model, a new diffraction pattern is calculated from that model, and that pattern is compared to the measured diffraction pattern. The discrepancy between the two is expressed as the R factor. The lower the R factor, the better the agreement between the two. Taken from G. A. Petsko and D. Ringe, in *Protein Structure and Function*, New Science Press Ltd, London, 2004.

guide how far a molecule may deviate from ideality in attempting to fit an electron density feature. The limits are determined from what is known about the structures of small molecules that are representative of substructures of the protein (Figure 2.9).[11–14]

The measure of success for this fitting procedure is the R factor, a measure of the disagreement between model and experiment. Although the fitting of the model to the electron density, and the agreement between the two, is seen at the level of the electron density map, this measure of agreement can be calculated only at the level of the measurements made to obtain that map (i.e., the structure amplitudes). The calculation determines the difference between the calculated reflection amplitudes derived from the model and the measured ones derived from the x-ray experiment. Thus, R factors reflect not only the quality of the fit of the model but also the quality and resolution of the data. For protein macromolecules, R factors are usually within the range of 15% to the low 20% for data around 1.8–2.5Å resolution, which is a common resolution range for protein/ligand complexes. These numbers mean that roughly 80% of the measured scattering from the crystal has been accounted for by the model. In many cases, the unaccounted-for scattering will include not only errors of measurement but also the failure to model the disordered solvent in the channels within the crystal lattice (Figure 2.10).

Because of the overwhelming influence of the phases (calculated) over the reflection amplitudes (observed data) in determining the final electron density, the R factor can be manipulated. Consequently, it is now common practice to calculate an R factor from data that have not been used in the refinement process and therefore not been biased by calculated phases. This measure is called the R_{free} and usually uses 5–10% of the data, randomly chosen and excluded from all refinement steps, to calculate the measure of disagreement.[16] Because of the incompleteness of the data used, and the lack of phase bias, the R_{free} is always higher than the R factor by approximately 3–5% in the case of well-refined structures. In the early stages of refinement it may be 10% higher.

The molecules of protein in the crystal are packed in such a way that solvent channels are found between them. These are filled with the solution from which the protein was crystallized, and that solution may contain other ions and molecules that are associated with the protein. An estimate of the volume of the crystal that is attributable to solvent comes from the Matthews coefficient, calculated from the crystal data.[17] The most important component of the solvent is the bound water molecules that are found

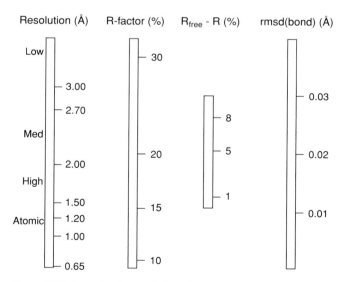

Figure 2.10. Approximate correlations between resolution of the data, the expected R factors for a refined structure, the expected differences between the R factor and R_{free} of the final refined structure, and the approximate precision of bond distances ascertainable from a structure.[7] These values can be used as criteria to assess the quality of a crystallographic model. For instance, a large difference between R and R_{free} could indicate possible overinterpretation of the data; if the difference is very low, it could mean that the test data set used to calculate R_{free} is not in fact "free." rmsd (root-mean-squared deviation) indicates the deviation of protein geometry from ideality. For instance, high rmsd(bonds) indicates model error. If it is too low, the refinement may have been dominated by strict adherence to geometry rather than refinement to experimental diffraction data. It should be noted that "ideal" bond lengths may have errors of approximately 0.02Å, so the expectation that a model is better than that is unreasonable. Redrawn from data in Wlodawer et al., 2008.[7]

in discreet locations, usually on the protein surface. Water molecules are placed according to a procedure that involves identifying electron density features that are not accounted for by protein. Are they necessarily all waters? Probably not: at very high resolution, some "waters" have been shown to be sodium or ammonium ions. But in the absence of other information, they are interpreted as water, usually based on criteria such as the height of the electron density peak and the position of the putative water molecule to protein atoms with which it can form hydrogen bonds. This does not rule out misidentification, but most ions that might be associated with a protein are sufficiently larger or have a shape or electronic properties that might rule out being a water molecule. Again, the number of water molecules that can be identified as associated with a given model will depend on the quality of the model, the quality of the data, and the resolution of the data. For instance, at 2Å resolution, the number of water molecules expected to be observable is very low and may include only those that are very tightly associated with the protein, often in the active or other functional site. Resolution of 1.8Å is usually required to place a significant number of water molecules on the surface with any precision. At this level of resolution, it is important to look for a certain ratio; namely there should be approximately as many water molecules as residues in the protein. Too many water molecules in a final model may mean that "extraneous" electron density is simply being fitted with water when in fact it may tell a different story. Because the R factor can be viewed as a measure of how much electron density is accounted for, such water molecules can drive an R factor down without adding accuracy to the model. The comparison between the R factor and R_{free} is therefore a good measure to assess the possibility of overfitting or misinterpretation (Figure 2.11, Table 2.2).

The second measure of misinterpretation relies on calculation of the biophysical data for the protein. If a model is well fitted to an electron density map, then it should reflect what we know about the properties of proteins. Those properties include the geometries of amino acids and secondary structures in terms of distances and angles. Atom-to-atom distances and angles for components of proteins are well known from small molecule structures and can be compared with those obtained for the model. The measure given is a root-mean-squared deviation (rmsd) for all such distances and angles. Such angles for the relationships of backbone atoms in specific secondary structures has been analyzed theoretically and is given in terms of allowed and disallowed values in a Ramachandran plot.[18] These can be calculated for the model and compared to the theoretical values (Figure 2.12).

A number of residues may fall outside of these criteria for different reasons. For instance, the values for glycine, because of the absence of a side chain, may fall outside the accepted ranges. Proline may fall outside these ranges because proline may exist in both *cis* and *trans* forms. Occasionally, particularly if the resolution is high enough

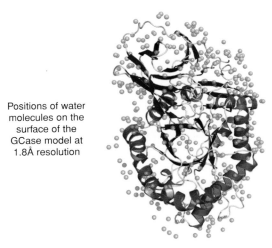

Positions of water molecules on the surface of the GCase model at 1.8Å resolution

Figure 2.11. Ribbon diagram of the glucocerebrosidase model with the positions of bound water molecules. The surface of a protein model has extraneous electron density that is modeled as water molecules. The gray balls show the positions of such water molecules that have been placed in spherical electron densities on the surface of the protein. An electron density has been interpreted as a water molecule only if the resulting water position (only the oxygen atom is interpretable) is within hydrogen bonding distance of a protein atom that can donate or accept a hydrogen bond. Some of these water molecules can be considered part of the protein structure because they are found in the same position in every structure determination of that protein. Data were taken from PDB code 1OGS.[2]

to allow for a precise interpretation, any residue may fall outside acceptable ranges. When that happens it is worth paying some attention to such a residue, because there is usually a functional reason for it to do so. The final coordinates from the model, together with the data from which it was obtained, can be made available by deposition into the Protein Data Base.[19,20]

These measures address the precision of the model. However, accuracy is the most important criterion for the quality of the model, and the only measure of accuracy is the agreement between the model of the protein and the biochemical data for its function. If the model does not explain those data, or at least agrees with them, the model is probably wrong, no matter how precise it may appear in terms of R factors, and so on. Does that mean that all correct models always explain all biochemical data? Certainly not, especially if the configuration of the model seen in the crystal represents only one possible form from a number of possible forms, only one of which is the functionally relevant one for the protein. But in general, the model should make biochemical sense in terms of what is already known about the protein. If it generally does, it is probably accurate (Figure 2.13).

STRENGTHS AND WEAKNESSES OF CRYSTALLOGRAPHY

From the above discussions it is clear that the crystallographic method has strengths and weaknesses. The greatest strength of the method is the ability to visually understand the binding of ligands and the conformational changes in both the protein and the ligand that are associated with such interactions. The interpretation of interactions in terms of geometry and distances between interacting parts is essential to the design of new interacting species that can take advantage of these and potentially new interactions, that is, the basis of structure-based drug design.

However, there are also obvious weaknesses in the method. Unless there is obvious disorder in the model of the protein, manifested as poor or absent electron density for parts of it, any one model is a rigid one that may not be an accurate representation of the plasticity of the protein. Thus, any one structure may represent only one form of the protein, of which there may be many. The conditions used for crystallization are rarely representative of the conditions under which the protein functions in the cell. Consequently, interpretation of function from the structure has to consider that the pH, ionic strength, and presence or absence of other molecular species in the model are most likely very different from the native conditions. This usually does not lead to misinterpretation but must be kept in mind nevertheless, because conformational changes may result from such conditions as well as from binding of ligands.

A number of strategies are available to attempt to address these problems. One is to find more than one set of crystallization conditions that vary the pH and constituents of the crystallization solution. Conditions that vary dramatically from high salt to low salt, or at extremes of pH, may provide some insight into the conformational changes that can be associated with such differences in solution conditions. Another is to determine the structure of the protein/ligand complex by two methods: one is to soak the ligand into an existing crystal, and the other is the form the protein/ligand complex in solution and then to crystallize it. If the binding site for the ligand happens to be at a protein/protein interaction site, binding may disrupt this interaction and the integrity of the crystal. Alternatively, the packing of the crystal may prevent the protein from undergoing conformational changes that would occur on ligand interactions in solution. Cocrystallization after binding in solution gets around both of these problems – if the complex crystallizes.

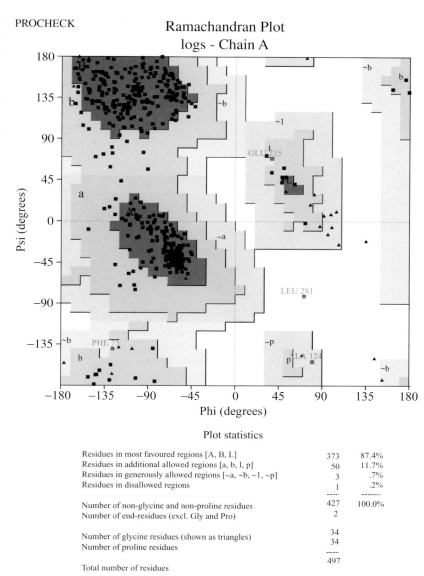

Plot statistics

Residues in most favoured regions [A, B, L]	373	87.4%
Residues in additional allowed regions [a, b, l, p]	50	11.7%
Residues in generously allowed regions [~a, ~b, ~l, ~p]	3	.7%
Residues in disallowed regions	1	.2%
	----	-------
Number of non-glycine and non-proline residues	427	100.0%
Number of end-residues (excl. Gly and Pro)	2	
Number of glycine residues (shown as triangles)	34	
Number of proline residues	34	

Total number of residues	497	

Based on an analysis of 118 structures of resolution of at least 2.0 Angstroms and R-factor no greater than 20%, a good quality model would be expected to have over 90% in the most favoured regions.

Figure 2.12. Ramachandran plot for glucosidase showing that four residues have angles that do not conform to the ones expected for amino residues in secondary structures. Three of these residues are close enough to be accepted as possible conformations. One of them, Leu281, is considered in an unusual conformation. Inspection of the structural model shows that this residue is in a hydrophobic pocket stabilizing several structural elements. Data were taken from PDB code 1OGS.[2]

FRAGMENT-BASED APPROACHES TO SURFACE MAPPING

Despite the limitations of the crystallographic method, it is clear that the association of small chemical entities can be visualized, just as large ones can, when bound to a protein. The most frequently assigned small molecule on the surface of a protein is water. Once all of the protein is assigned to electron density, and all of the side chains are accounted for, a significant amount of electron density scattered over the surface of the protein is left unaccounted for. Much of that

Table 2.2. Refinement statistics for a typical protein structure determination. (Data taken from the structure determination of glucosidase at pH 4.5; PDB code 2NT0)[3]

Resolution (Å)	20–2.2
Reflections	131814
R_{work}/R_{free}	22.0/27.6
No. of protein atoms	1988
Sulfate ions	28
Water	1181
B factors:	
Protein	24.6
rms deviations	
Bond lengths (Å)	0.016
Bond angles (°)	1.7

electron density has a spherical shape and is observed near the surface of the protein. When is such an electron density a water molecule and when is it something else? Unless the electron density feature has a nonspherical shape to indicate that it might be a compound or ion with more than one nonhydrogen atom, such as the commonly observed sulfate or phosphate ions, or glycerol used for cryo-protection, it is assigned to a water molecule. This assignment may not be correct because other individual ions can interact with the protein surface. The resolution range usually found for good protein structure determinations is from approximately 2 to 1.5Å. In this range, electron density for hydrogens is not

visible. In fact, resolution of better than 1Å is required to see electron density for hydrogens, and even that is not always sufficient. Consequently, identification of one ion from another is usually not possible, and, in the absence of hydrogen positions, distinguishing water from a cation or anion is usually not possible either.

This leaves an important question: When can the electron density feature be assigned to a water molecule or when is it part of the noise inherent in an electron density map? A number of criteria are applied to make this determination. The two most important ones are the height of the electron density peak (given in terms of the sigma level of the peak relative to the overall average electron density level of the map) and the interactions that a putative water molecule would make with nearby protein atoms if placed into that electron density. Different researchers apply different criteria. Because the height of an electron density peak depends on the occupancy and *B* factor (mobility) of an atom, assignment of a water molecule must take these two factors into account. In general, if an electron density is no longer visible at a σ level of 3, indicating poor occupancy, high mobility, or simply noise, it should not be assigned. Second, if the water molecule at any given position does not interact with the protein in terms of at least some putative hydrogen bonds, of which water is capable of a potential four, it is unlikely to be one. This still does not identify a water molecule unambiguously, but it is the best we can do (Figure 2.14).

It has been shown that small molecules, as small as two or more nonhydrogen atoms, can also interact with the surface of a protein.[21,22] Determining the orientation in which such a molecule binds depends on the shape of the electron

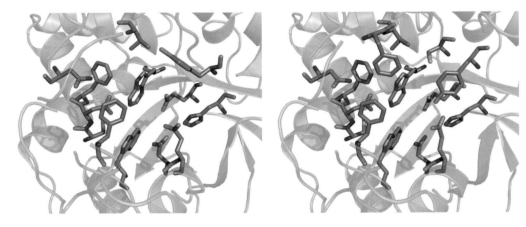

Comparison: structure of GCase at
pH 7.5 (er) vs pH 4.5 (lysosome)

Figure 2.13. The structure of a protein may not be relevant to its catalytic form. In this case, the structure of glucocerebrosidase is subject to changes in configuration as a response to environment, such as the binding of an inhibitor or pH. For instance, the active site of glucocerebrosidase has a different conformation at the pH at which it is synthesized in the endoplasmic reticulum from that at the pH of the lysozome. The conformational changes observed reflect the inactive and active forms of the enzyme in the different compartments of the cell. Data were taken from PDB codes 2NT1 (pH 7.5) and 2NT0 (pH 4.5).[3]

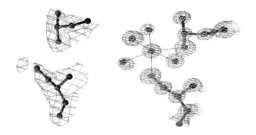

Interpretation of electron density at different resolutions:
2.0Å resolution vs 0.95Å resolution

Figure 2.14. Water molecules are placed in electron density features based on a number of criteria. In the lower resolution structure, the water molecule is assigned based on the height of the electron density feature of a magnitude realistic for an oxygen atom and the location of that feature near hydrogen bonding partners (a carbonyl oxygen atom in this case) if it were a water molecule. At ultrahigh resolution, where the feature is more clearly defined, that "water" molecule turns out to be a cation, probably a sodium ion, identified on the basis of the dominant ion in the mother liquor from which the crystal was obtained. Data were taken from PDB codes 1AMP (1.8Å resolution)[9] and 1RTQ (0.95Å resolution).[10]

density feature, and, if the shape is not definitive, the chemical interactions that atoms of the molecule can make with atoms of the protein. The obvious interaction is a hydrogen bonding one, but hydrophobic or polar interactions are equally useful to define orientation.

The sites at which small molecules bind can be random. However, some spots on the protein are more prone to interaction with such compounds than others,[23–25] for instance, the active site of an enzyme or an allosteric site on a protein. These are sites that are designed to interact with molecules – substrates or inhibitors or activators – in such a way as to confer specificity to the interaction. Often more than one part of such a site interacts with the recognized molecule. Any one part may therefore be prone to a different type of interaction, such as electrostatic or hydrophobic, depending on the characteristics of the overall compound recognized. Small molecules may make such interactions individually and therefore be attracted to a particular subsite within a larger interaction site.

Any organic ligand can be decomposed into substructures (fragments) that are reminiscent of smaller molecules. Such a small molecule may therefore occupy the same site on a protein as the substructure that it represents. The position of such a small molecule may therefore be used to characterize a particular site on the protein that has a specific affinity for the chemical group represented by the small molecule. If a set of such fragments is found bound to an overall site on the protein, they should map out the binding surface of a region of the protein. The basic assumption is that a specific chemical group will interact with a specific site on a protein in the absence of the rest of a larger ligand molecule. If that is true, the small molecules can be linked together to make a large molecule that fits all of the

regions defined by such a mapping procedure. This method was first proposed by Fitzpatrick et al.[21]:

> Thus, acetonitrile may act as a probe to map the amphiphilic regions of the enzyme surface, which would suggest an experimental approach to mapping the complete binding surface of any crystalline protein. By the methods described here, crystals would be transferred to a series of organic solvents, each designed to mimic a particular functional group (e.g., benzene can be used to map binding sites for aromatic groups). Such experiments are directly analogous to computational methods that map the interaction energies of small probe molecules to protein surfaces, thus providing a direct experimental test of such theoretical methods. Once the interaction surface has been mapped by a series of solvent experiments, the various functional groups can be connected to provide specific lead compounds for drug design. Unlike conventional substrate analogues, which interact only with the active center, compounds designed by solvent mapping can exploit additional regions of the protein surface to provide greater specificity and affinity.

Once a set of small molecules are found that associate with a region on the surface of the protein, in principle they can be linked to make a larger compound that contains the combined affinities of the smaller parts as well as the synergistic affinity of the combination (Figure 2.15). Alternatively, the method can be used to build onto an existing framework to optimize the affinity of a starting compound that already binds to the protein. One of the earliest uses of this strategy at the experimental level is the structure/activity relationship by nuclear magnetic resonance (SAR by NMR)

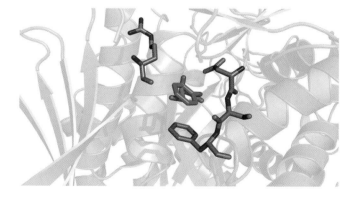

Binding of solvent molecules to the surface of GCase

Figure 2.15. Results of solvent mapping of glucocerebrosidase. A molecule of glycerol (blue) and one of phenol (green) bind to a site on the surface of the protein. Solvent molecules are placed into electron density the same way as inhibitor or water molecules are placed, based on the shape and size of the electron density feature. If several solvent molecules bind in or near the same site on the protein, such a cluster can be used to identify hot spots such as active sites, allosteric sites, or simply binding sites. Data were taken from unpublished structure determinations by Raquel Lieberman.

method,[26] in which the binding positions of molecules, representing fragments, are determined by NMR. Fragments that interact closely are then linked to make a larger ligand.

But the real power of the method comes from more recent computational application of the method. In this approach, the binding of fragments is determined computationally, and the compounds derived from the mapping of such fragments are then synthesized and tested.[27-29] The accuracy of these computations is matched against the experimental results.

An extension of these methods is to use either the experimental or the computational method to identify binding sites that can then be probed by molecular docking procedures[30,31] to find compounds that will bind at a particular site. In all cases, the success of the methods is determined by the effect of the final compound on the biological system being studied. Examples of such procedures are found in other chapters in this book.

ACKNOWLEDGMENTS

Figure 2.1 was taken by Walter Novak; Figures 2.8 and 2.12 were made by Cheryl Kreinbring; Figures 2.11 and 2.13 were made by Melissa Landon; Figure 2.15 was made by Melissa Landon from unpublished data from Raquel Lieberman.

REFERENCES

1. Jancarik, J.; Kim, S.-H. Sparse matrix sampling: a screening method for crystallization of proteins. *J. Appl. Crystallogr.* **1991**, *24*, 409–411.

2. Dvir, H.; Harel, M.; McCarthy, A. A.; Toker, L.; Silman, I.; Futerman, A. H.; Sussman, J. X-ray structure of human acid-beta-glucosidase, the defective enzyme in Gaucher disease. L. EMBO Rep. **2003**, *4*, 704–709.

3. Lieberman, R. L.; Wustman, B. A.; Huertas, P.; Powe, A. C., Jr.; Pine, W. P.; Khanna, R.; Schlossmacher, G.; Ringe, D.; Petsko, G. A. Structure of acid beta-glucosidase with pharmacological chaperone provides insight into Gaucher disease. *Nat. Chem. Biol.* **2007**, *3*, 101–107.

4. Stout, G. H.; Jensen, L. H. *X-Ray Structure Determination: A Practical Guide*, 2nd ed. New York, NY: Wiley & Sons, **1989**.

5. Blow, D. *Outline of Crystallography for Biologists*. New York, NY: Oxford University Press; **2002**.

6. Rhodes, G. *Crystallography Made Crystal Clear*. Burlington, VT: Academic Press; **2006**.

7. Wlodawer, A.; Minor, W.; Dauter, Z.; Jaskolski, M. Protein crystallography for non-crystallographers, or how to get the best (but not more) from published macromolecular structure. *FEBS J.* **2008**, *275*, 1–21.

8. Irving, J. A.; Whisstock, J. C.; Lesk, A. M. Protein structural alignments and functional genomics. *Proteins* **2001**, *42*, 378–382.

9. Chevrier, B.; Schalk, C.; D'Orchymont, H.; Rondeau, J. M.; Moras, D.; Tarnus, C. Crystal structure of *Aeromonas proteolytica* aminopeptidase: a prototypical member of the co-catalytic zinc enzyme family. *Structure* **1994**, *2*, 283–291.

10. Desmarais, W.; Bienvenue, D. L.; Bzymek, K. P.; Petsko, G. A.; Ringe, D.; Holz, R. C. J. The high-resolution structures of the neutral and the low pH crystals of aminopeptidase from *Aeromonas proteolytica*. *Biol. Inorg. Chem.* **2006**, *11*, 398–408.

11. Hendrickson, W. A. Stereochemically restrained refinement of macromolecular structures. *Methods Enzymol.* **1985**, *115*, 252–270.

12. Kleywegt, G. J.; Jones, A. T. Where freedom is given, liberties are taken. *Structure* **1995**, *3*, 535–540.

13. Engh, R. A.; Huber, R. Accurate bond and angle parameters for X-ray protein structure refinement. *Acta Crystallogr. D. Biol. Crystallogr.* **1991**, *47*, 392–400; and Engh, R. A.; Huber, R. Bond lengths and angles of peptide backbone fragments. In: *Structure Quality and Target Parameters*, International Tables of Crystallography, Vol. F, Rossman, M. G.; Arnold, E.; Eds. Dordrecht: Kluwer, **2001**, 382–392.

14. Allen, F. H. An experimental approach to mapping the binding surfaces of crystalline proteins. *Acta Crystallogr. D Biol. Crystallogr.* **2002**, *58*, 380–388.

15. Petsko, G. A.; Ringe, D. *Protein Structure and Function*. London: New Science Press; **2004**.

16. Brunger, A. T. Free R value: a novel statistical quantity for assessing the accuracy of crystal structures. *Nature* **1992**, *355*, 472–474.

17. Matthews, B. W. *J. Mol. Biol.* **1968**, *33*, 491–497.

18. Ramakrishnan, C.; Ramachandran, G. N. Stereochemical criteria for polypeptide and protein chain configuration – part II. Allowed conformations for a pair of peptide units. *Biophys. J.* **1965**, *5*, 909–933.

19. Bernstein, F. C.; Koetzle, T. F.; Williams, G. J. B.; Meyer, E. F., Jr.; Brice, M. D.; Rogers, J. R.; Kennard, O.; Shimanouchi, T.; Tasumi, M. The Protein Data Bank. A computer-based archival file for macromolecular structures. *J. Mol. Biol.* **1977**, *112*, 535–547.

20. Berman, H. M.; Wetbrook, J.; Feng, Z.; Gilliland, G.; Bhat, T. N.; Weissig, H.; Shindyalov, I. N.; Bourne, P. E. The Protein Data Bank. *Nucleic Acids Res.* **2000**, *28*, 235–242.

21. Fitzpatrick, P. A.; Steinmetz, A. C. U.; Ringe, D.; Klibanov, A. M. Enzyme crystal structure in a neat organic solvent. *Proc. Natl. Acad. Sci. U.S.A.* **1993**, *90*, 8653–8657.

22. Mattos, C.; Ringe, D. Locating and characterizing binding sites on proteins. *Nat. Biotechnol.* **1996**, *14*, 595–599.

23. Allen, K. N.; Bellamacina, C.; Ding, C.; Jeffrey, C.; Mattos, C.; Petsko, G. A.; Ringe, D. The Cambridge Structural Database: a quarter of a million crystal structures and rising. *J. Phys. Chem.* **1996**, *100*, 2605–2611.

24. Mattos, C.; Bellamacina, C. R.; Peisach, E.; Vitkup, D.; Petsko, G. A.; Ringe, D. Multiple solvent crystal structures: probing binding sites, plasticity and hydration. *J. Mol. Biol.* **2006**, *357*, 1471–1482.

25. Ringe, X.; Mattos, X. Location of binding sites on proteins by the multiple solvent crystal structure method. In: *Fragment-Based Approaches in Drug Discovery*, Jahnke, W.; Erlanson, D. A.; Eds. Weinheim: Wiley-VCH; **2006**.

26. Shuker, S. B.; Hajduk, P. J.; Meadows, R. P.; Fesik, S. W. Discovering high-affinity ligands for proteins: SAR by NMR. *Science* **1996**, *274*, 1531–1534.

27. Guarnieri, F. Computational protein probing to identify binding sites. U.S. Patent 6735530, **2004**.

28. Clark, M.; Guarnieri, F.; Shkurko, I.; Wiseman, J. Grand canonical Monte Carlo simulation of ligand-protein binding. *J. Med. Inf. Model.* **2006**, *46*, 231–242.

29. Landon, M. R.; Lancia, D. R., Jr.; Yu, J.; Thiel, S. C.; Vajda, S. Identification of hot spots within druggable binding regions by computational solvent mapping of proteins. *J. Med. Chem.* **2007**, *50*, 1231–1240.

30. Graves, A. P.; Shivakumar, D. M.; Boyce, S. E.; Jacobson, M. P.; Case, D. A.; Shoichet, B. K. Rescoring docking hit lists for model cavity sites: predictions and experimental. *J. Mol. Biol.* **2008**, *377*, 914–934.

31. Repasky, M. P.; Shelley, M.; Friesner, R. A. Flexible ligand docking with Glide. *Curr. Protoc. Bioinformatics* **2007**, June; Chapter 8: Unit 8.12.

3

Fragment-based structure-guided drug discovery: strategy, process, and lessons from human protein kinases

Stephen K. Burley, Gavin Hirst, Paul Sprengeler, and Siegfried Reich

INTRODUCTION

The experimental roots of fragment-based drug discovery can be found in the work of Petsko, Ringe, and coworkers, who were the first to report flooding of protein crystals with small organic solutes (e.g., compounds such as benzene with ten or fewer nonhydrogen atoms) to identify bound functional groups that might ultimately be transformed into targeted ligands.[1] The concept of linking fragments together to increase binding affinity was described as early as 1992 by Verlinde et al.[2] Computational screening of fragments, using tools such as DOCK[3,4] or MCSS,[5] was also described in the early 1990s. Pharmaceutical industry application of fragment screening began at Abbott Laboratories, where Fesik and coworkers pioneered "SAR by NMR" (structure/activity relationship by nuclear magnetic resonance).[6] In this spectroscopic approach, bound fragments are detected by NMR screening and subsequently linked together to increase affinity, as envisaged by Verlinde and coworkers.[2] Application of x-ray crystallography to detect and identify fragment hits was also pursued at Abbott.[7]

Fragment-based drug discovery has now been under way for more than a decade. Although Fesik and coworkers popularized the notion of linking fragments (as in their highly successful BCL-2 program), tactical emphasis appears to have largely shifted from fragment condensation to fragment engineering (or growing the fragment) to increase binding affinity and selectivity. Various biotechnology companies, including SGX Pharmaceuticals, Astex, and Plexxikon, have recently demonstrated that fragment-based approaches can indeed produce development candidates suitable for Phase I studies of safety and tolerability in patients (www.clinicaltrials.gov). Within many larger pharmaceutical companies, detection and optimization of fragments as a path to discovering new chemical entities appears to be gaining acceptance.

Before describing the SGX fragment-based drug discovery strategy, process, and lessons from human protein kinases, we review our current understanding of the nexus between chemical diversity of screening libraries and the challenges of compound screening that explain both the utility of starting the search for clinical development candidates with small fragments and the pharmaceutical industry's failure to realize the much-vaunted potential of combinatorial chemistry/high-throughput screening. Traditional drug discovery usually begins with a search for small molecule "hits" that demonstrate modest inhibition ($IC_{50} \sim 10$ μM) of the molecular target in an in vitro biochemical assay. Promising hits are subsequently optimized into development candidates using iterative, trial-and-error methods and/or structure-guided design. The most commonly used approaches for finding hits have involved either high-throughput screening (HTS) of large compound libraries [typically 100,000–2,000,000 compounds with molecular weights (MW) of about 350–550] or opportunistic modification of substrate analogs and/or published active compounds. Although these methods have yielded a number of successfully marketed drugs, annual rates of new drug approval over the past decade have remained essentially unchanged despite dramatically increased research budgets at large pharmaceutical companies.

The fundamental shortcoming of any conventional HTS campaign derives from the reality that even the largest screening library exhibits only limited chemical diversity. For reference, the number of potential druglike molecules is predicted to be $\sim 10^{60},$[8] which is comparable to accepted estimates for the total number of atoms comprising the universe. Such limitations effectively bias sampling of potential starting points for drug discovery and, therefore, may not yield the best lead series. Proprietary screening libraries are often biased toward certain structural classes, because these collections are composed of molecules synthesized for targets of historical importance rather than molecules chosen to sample leadlike chemical space.

Typical HTS libraries also consist of molecules (MW $\sim$350–550) larger than fragments (MW < $\sim$250), deliberately chosen because they yield more potent starting points for synthetic chemistry than do fragments (i.e., $IC_{50} < \sim 10$ μM versus $IC_{50} < \sim 10$ mM). Regrettably, subsequent optimization of these larger molecules is often complicated by the need to identify and remove functional groups to minimize molecular weight and hydrophobicity, while other functional groups must be added or modified to increase binding affinity. Thus, optimization of larger HTS hits into development candidates may require retrospective disassembly into smaller pieces. Another significant weakness of the traditional drug discovery approach is the poor compliance of most screening hits with what we now recognize as being highly advantageous leadlike properties.[9–12] Such poor compliance frequently complicates and prolongs the lead optimization process and contributes, at least in part, to the relative paucity of new chemical entities plaguing the pharmaceutical industry. Finally, HTS hit rates tend to be very low (i.e., < 0.01%), which we now appreciate to be a direct consequence of screening libraries of compounds with MW ~350–550.[5]

Screening of small fragments (i.e., simple one- or two-ring heterocycles with MW < ~250) instead of larger HTS library compounds overcomes all three of the shortcomings enumerated above. First, well-designed fragment libraries embody significantly more potential for chemical diversity than even the largest HTS libraries. For example, a 1,000-compound fragment library (each compound bearing two or more sites of chemical modification) can be readily elaborated into more than 10^8 accessible analogs (MW < ~500). This extremely conservative estimate dwarfs even the largest HTS screening collections assembled within the pharmaceutical industry. Second, fragment libraries can be assembled with leadlike compounds exclusively, thereby maximizing the likelihood of successful optimization. Finally, small fragments exhibit an increased probability of binding to a given target (hit rates for many targets ~ 1–5%) versus larger, more complex molecules.[9] For a 1,000-compound fragment library such hit rates yield ten to fifty starting points for medicinal chemistry elaboration.

Such bounty does come at the expense of initial potency. Small fragment hits identified using various screening methods typically exhibit binding affinities of ~10 μM to 10 mM or even greater and are in some cases not measurable. The relatively weak character of fragment hits is deemed so unpalatable in some circles that adoption of fragment-based drug discovery approaches has been effectively inhibited within some organizations. Many medicinal chemists believe it more reasonable to attempt optimization from ~10 μM than an apparently 1,000-fold weaker starting point. Experience at both SGX and other fragment-based drug discovery companies has shown that 10 mM screening hits can in fact be rapidly optimized to better than 10 nM (see below).

The relationship between molecular weight and binding affinity has been explored intensively in various quarters. Astex has popularized the concept of ligand efficiency (LE),[13] which represents an indirect measure of the number of constituent atoms that participate in interactions with the target protein:

$$LE = -\Delta G/(\text{no. of nonhydrogen atoms})$$
$$\sim -RT\ln(IC_{50})/(\text{no. of nonhydrogen atoms}).$$

In general, even weakly bound fragment hits are ligand efficient (LE > 0.3), whereas most HTS hits are not (LE < 0.3). During optimization of a fragment hit to generate nanomolar potency lead compounds, ligand efficiency can be monitored with the goal of maintaining/improving the balance between binding affinity and molecular weight (i.e., adding only atoms that contribute substantially to improved binding affinity).

As heralded by the MIT group's successful studies of protein crystals flooded with small organic solutes,[1] x-ray crystallographic screening has proven ideally suited to fragment-based drug discovery. The three-dimensional structure of the hit interacting with the target protein is the product of its detection. (Unlike NMR spectroscopy, x-ray crystallography provides a "direct look" at the protein/ligand complex.) A promising hit can be immediately qualified for further effort by establishing that it binds to the protein target in a well-defined orientation that is compatible with synthetic optimization. Such hits have been optimized by various structure-guided medicinal chemistry approaches.[13–16] Without three-dimensional structure validation and subsequent structural guidance, optimization of weakly bound fragments is extremely challenging because of the high propensity for nonspecific binding and false positives detected by biochemical assays. Application of x-ray crystallographic screening and/or cocrystallization with fragment hits has made fragment-based approaches to drug discovery both practical and successful.

SGX *FAST* FRAGMENT-BASED STRUCTURE-GUIDED DRUG DISCOVERY STRATEGY

Design of the SGX core fragment library

Recent studies of hit-to-lead optimization proposed a general definition of "leadlike" properties that increase the probability of successful optimization of hits to clinical candidates and successful prosecution of clinical development. These concepts have their origin in Lipinski's "rules,"[17] which describe properties of approved orally administered drugs: MW < 500, calculated log P or Clog P < 5, hydrogen-bond donors < 5, and nitrogens+oxygens < 10. Powerful though they are, Lipinski's rules are not appropriate for either HTS hits or evolving leads.[11,12] Hits usually increase in molecular weight, Clog P, and in number of rings and freely rotatable bonds during initial lead optimization and during subsequent development candidate optimization. Screening hits and leads should, therefore, be smaller than the molecular weight range embodied within Lipinski's rules. Teague et al.[12] initially proposed that leads should satisfy the following criteria: MW < 350 and Clog P < 3.0. Hann and Oprea[10] more recently proposed that leadlike molecules should have the following properties: MW ≤ 460, Clog P ≤ 4.2, freely rotatable bonds ≤ 10, ≤ 4 rings, hydrogen-bond donors ≤ 5, and hydrogen-bond acceptors ≤ 9.

"Leadlike" properties were originally proposed for molecules with binding affinities in the low micromolar range derived from HTS or combinatorial chemistry approaches. Fragment hits have binding affinities in the low micromolar to low millimolar range, thereby requiring

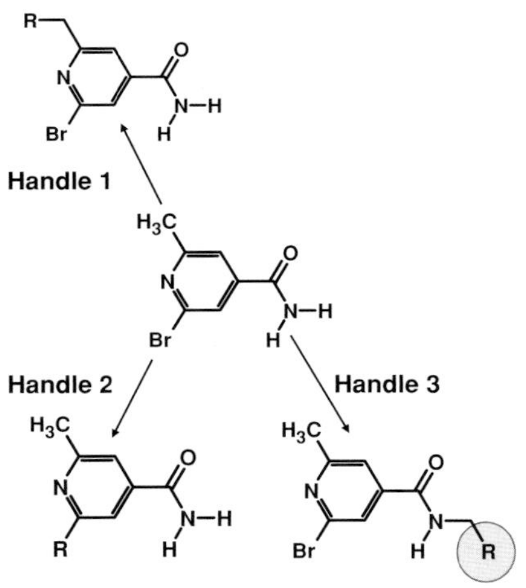

Figure 3.1. A typical member of the SGX core fragment library showing three chemical handles that support rapid R group elaboration.

screening library selection criteria that focus on yet smaller, simpler molecules. Hann and Oprea[10] proposed a "reduced complexity" screening set, with the following properties: MW $\leq$ 350, Clog $P \leq 2.2$, freely rotatable bonds ≤ 6, heavy atoms ≤ 22, hydrogen-bond donors ≤ 3, and hydrogen-bond acceptors ≤ 3. Congreve et al.[18] proposed a similar "rule-of-three": MW < 300, Clog $P < 3$, hydrogen-bond donors < 3, and freely rotatable bonds < 3. General conclusions from these studies provided guidance for the initial design and ongoing refinement of the SGX core fragment library, which follows a "rule-of-two" (Figure 3.1).

We have exploited two other important considerations in the design and ongoing refinement of the SGX core fragment library. First, hits from HTS and literature sources are not infrequently incompatible with efficient follow-on syntheses and may require substantial custom, labor-intensive chemistry for optimization. In practice, the probability of optimizing a hit increases with the synthetic amenability of the hit to follow-up elaboration. We, therefore, enriched the SGX core fragment screening library with compounds that support rapid, forty-eight- or ninety-six-at-a-time, automated parallel synthesis using liquid handling robotics and well-established synthetic routes. Second, aromatic bromine is a particularly useful substituent for an x-ray crystallographic approach to fragment discovery and optimization. The anomalous dispersion signal from one or more bromine atoms enhances the utility of fragment x-ray screening if the x-ray energy can be tuned to the bromine absorption edge. In addition, a bromide can act as a leaving group during carbon-carbon bond formation via Suzuki coupling and related reactions.

Enabling the target, fragment screening, initial SAR optimization, and the end game

Our FAST (Fragments of Active STructures) fragment-based structure-guided drug discovery process encompasses the following steps: (1) target enablement; (2) screening of

the core fragment library and selected fragments derived from other sources; (3) structural guided selection of fragments for SAR exploration; (4) SAR exploration design/prioritization; (5) initial chemical elaboration of selected fragments; (6) analysis of the results of initial fragment elaboration with x-ray crystallography and in vitro biochemical assays of potency; (7) subsequent rounds of fragment elaboration/evaluation, now including cellular potency assays, selectivity profiling, in vitro and in vivo pharmacokinetic studies, and in vivo efficacy studies; and (8) further focused optimization of development candidates versus the target product profile, now including rat toxicology studies.

Properties of the deliverable

Recently published studies[19,20] have documented that the likelihood of success in clinical trials depends critically on compound molecular weight. Specifically, clinical candidates with MW ≤ 400 have a 50% greater probability of obtaining approval as compared to those with MW >400. Paolini et al. extended these analyses to a second dimension by analyzing both MW and Clog P for approved orally administered compounds.[21] Their work identified a "sweet spot" for oral drugs, falling within the following MW and Clog P ranges: $300 < $ MW $ < 400$ and $2.5 < $ Clog $P < 4.5$. Insights from these studies provided general guidance for the prosecution of the SGX fragment-based structure-guided drug discovery process against all of our targets.

SGX FAST FRAGMENT-BASED STRUCTURE-GUIDED DRUG DISCOVERY PROCESS

Properties of the SGX core fragment library

A diverse screening library of ~1,500 leadlike compound fragments has been assembled over the past five years in various stages. Most library members possess two to three built-in synthetic handles to aid rapid elaboration of structurally validated fragment hits (Figure 3.1). Approximately one-third of library members contain one or more bromine atoms to facilitate detection and routine synthetic elaboration of crystallographic screening hits. The bulk of the library was assembled with no bias toward particular targets or target classes. During the most recent stage of library expansion, however, ~100 unrewarding fragments were removed and ~500 fragments biased toward protein kinases were added. Figure 3.2 illustrates five histograms summarizing various properties of the SGX core fragment library. (See Blaney et al. for a detailed account of library inclusion criteria.[22])

The current size of our core library reflects the balance struck among potential chemical diversity, the time required to screen the library using x-ray crystallography, and target screening hit rates. At present, screening can be completed in two to three days of x-ray beam time by dividing the ~1,500-compound core fragment library

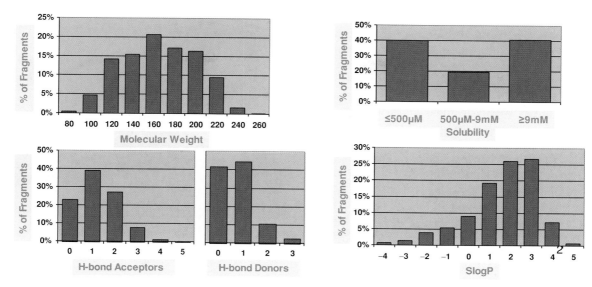

Figure 3.2. Properties of the SGX core fragment library.

into 150 shape-diverse mixtures of 10 compounds each. As discussed earlier, the estimated number of possible druglike molecules that could be included in an HTS library is $\sim 10^{60}$.[8] In contrast, the estimated number of all possible leadlike molecules with MW $<$ 160 is only about 14,000,000.[23] A fragment library containing a modest number of compounds (i.e., $\sim$1,500) can, therefore, be used to sample leadlike compound space much more efficiently than an HTS library samples the space of druglike molecules. A fragment library of 1,000–10,000 small compounds (MW $<$ 160) represents $\sim$0.001–0.01% of all possible leadlike compound spaces. In stark contrast, a typical HTS library, containing 10^5–10^6 compounds, encompasses $\sim 10^{-55}$ of the total estimated druglike space. Empirically, we have observed that hit rates for x-ray screening of our core fragment library fall in the range of 1–5%, thereby providing fifteen to seventy-five possible hits for subsequent fragment optimization. Taken together, these arguments/ observations document that our $\sim$1,500-compound core fragment library represents an efficient means of generating a reasonable number of starting points for fragment elaboration from a not insubstantial fraction of the total leadlike chemical space.

The potential chemical diversity of the SGX core fragment library is estimated to fall in the range of 10^8–10^{17} compounds. Intrinsic to most of the $\sim$1,500 fragments are two to three sites for R-group addition or chemical handles. For each chemical handle, the number of commercial reagents available for chemical modification ranges from a minimum of $\sim$400 to a maximum of $\sim$40,000. In the most pessimistic scenario (i.e., use of only two chemical handles with only 400 possible independent modifications at each handle), $\sim$1,500 fragments can be elaborated into $\sim$2.4$\times 10^8$ distinct compounds. In the most optimistic scenario (i.e., use of all three chemical handles with 40,000 possible independent modifications at each handle), $\sim$1,500 frag-

ments can be elaborated into $\sim 10^{17}$ distinct compounds, which is comparable to accepted estimates for the age of the universe in minutes.

Enabling the target, fragment x-ray screening, complementary biophysical screening, SAR optimization, and the end game

Enabling the target

At SGX, de novo protein crystal structures are determined using a gene-to-structure platform that supports prosecution of multiple protein samples in parallel. Our platform consists of modular robotics and a comprehensive laboratory information management system (SGX LIMS) that facilitates data entry and electronic data capture at all stages of the process. The SGX LIMS system also permits comprehensive data mining for troubleshooting and project management. The SGX target-to-structure platform has facilitated high-resolution (typically better than $\sim$2Å resolution) structure determinations for a large number of drug discovery targets, including more than sixty unique human protein kinases, more than twenty unique human and pathogen protein phosphatases, a large number of nuclear hormone receptor ligand binding domains, and many bacterial and viral proteins. Successes have included many targets not represented in the public domain Protein Data Bank (PDB; www.pdb.org), some of which have been regarded as being extremely difficult if not "impossible" to express, purify, and crystallize (e.g., the IκB kinases). Modular SGX platform robotics encompasses gene cloning, protein expression and purification, crystallization, and structure determination. Most of this work is conducted using ninety-six-well-format liquid-handling robotics to process multiple expression constructs for many protein targets in parallel. Multiple constructs for a given target typically express various truncations of the N- and C-terminus and/or internal loop deletions. Precise truncations are defined with the results of bioinformatics analyses of target protein sequences and/or by experimental domain mapping via limited proteolysis combined with mass spectrometry.[24] For a typical target of unknown structure, a minimum of twenty to thirty constructs are prepared in multiple expression vectors (encoding N- and C-terminal hexahistidine tags and a removable N-terminal hexahistidine/Smt3 tag). Well-expressed, soluble versions of the target protein are purified in parallel and then tested for crystallizability, using a predetermined set of ~1,000 crystallization conditions at two temperatures (4° and 20°C). Rapid, fine sampling during the early stages of the process allows us to express the right truncated form(s) of a difficult target that are amenable to crystallization, thereby enabling structure determination.

Once an initial crystal structure is obtained, additional experiments are conducted to enable the target for fragment screening. This process encompasses the transition from small-scale crystal growth and data collection, required to determine a de novo crystal structure, to a robust large-scale process for x-ray screening. Typical requirements for crystallographic screening include the ability to routinely produce and soak crystals on a large scale (~300 diffraction quality crystals/screen) and to obtain reproducible diffraction data to better than 2.5Å resolution. In most cases, the crystal form used for de novo structure determination suffices for crystallographic screening of our core fragment library. In extreme cases, the process may require using information from the initial structure to engineer a new crystal form. Such protein reengineering may be necessary to improve crystal stability [particularly in the presence of dimethyl sulfoxide (DMSO)] and/or the packing of target molecules within the crystal lattice (to permit fragments to diffuse through solvent channels within the crystal and reach the enzyme active site).

After obtaining a suitable crystal form, the system is validated by soaking "control" compounds known to bind and/or inhibit the target of interest. In the absence of reference inhibitors, substrate analogs, cofactors, or other known ligands (i.e., ATP analogs and staurosporine for protein kinases) serve as controls. If the reference compound(s) is readily visible in difference electron density maps, the soaking system is considered validated. After validation of the crystal form, the ability to soak mixtures into the system is tested. In some cases, crystallization and/or soaking conditions must be further optimized to permit efficient soaking of mixtures.

Fragment x-ray screening

Once a target is enabled for crystallographic screening, crystals are prepared for data collection at our dedicated x-ray beamline at the Advanced Photon Source (APS; SGX-CAT). Duplicate crystals are soaked with mixtures of ten

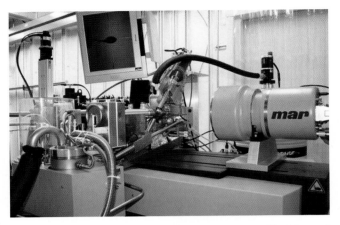

Figure 3.3. SGX-CAT beamline data collection apparatus at the Advanced Photon Source (APS). Shown are the x-ray beam carriage tubes, the cryogenic gaseous nitrogen stream, the sample stage, the Mar sample stage/automated sample changer, and the Mar CCD x-ray area detector.

structurally dissimilar fragments (typically with each fragment present at ~5–10 mM, DMSO concentration ~5%), flash-frozen, and stored in liquid nitrogen. All experiments are tracked within the SGX LIMS system, which is accessible from SGX-CAT. Direct T3 line connectivity permits rapid data transfer between the two SGX facilities. Once the frozen crystals are transported to SGX-CAT by courier, pertinent sample information is accessed from the SGX LIMS system and the samples are manually loaded into data collection carousels. Multiple data collection carousels are then stored in liquid nitrogen and queued for automated data collection. When a carousel is ready for analysis, it is automatically transferred from the storage dewar to the crystal mounting robot. Figure 3.3 shows the SGX-CAT x-ray diffraction facility on the 31-ID beamline at the APS, which includes x-ray optical elements (for focusing and wavelength selection), beam carriage tubes, a crystal mounting robot, cryogenic nitrogen gas stream for crystal cooling, and a MarCCD detector. To facilitate unattended data collection, crystal centering software was developed by SGX in conjunction with Mar Research.

Data collection/processing parameters are retrieved from the SGX LIMS system to control both the progress of the diffraction experiment and data processing in real time. Reduced diffraction data are automatically transferred back to SGX headquarters in San Diego via the T3 line and experimental parameters are captured by the SGX LIMS database. This system permits routine, unattended data collection from approximately fifty crystalline samples per day, enabling data acquisition for the entire SGX fragment library in about three days (recording diffraction data from the better of each pair of duplicate soaked crystals). Fragment screening results are analyzed automatically using a multi-CPU linux cluster located at SGX San Diego. Automated processing of diffraction data is performed using a system that combines proprietary SGX software and the CCP4[25] program package. For each screening attempt with a ten-compound, shape-diverse mixture, the structure of the target protein is automatically redetermined by molecular replacement using a reference target structure predefined in the SGX LIMS. Once this step is complete, the structure is partially refined and a difference Fourier synthesis is calculated to reveal any superficial electron density features that cannot be explained by either the structure of the protein target or surrounding water molecules. For each unexplained electron density feature, an attempt is made to automatically identify the fragment within the mixture that best corresponds to the shape of the electron density feature.

Once the automated processing/fragment identification is complete, "snapshots" of each difference electron density feature, with accompanying ligand atomic stick-figure interpretation, can be accessed via the SGX LIMS. Visual inspection of these images represents the first point at which manual intervention by a protein crystallographer is required. Expert inspection of the electron density images facilitates prioritization of the three-dimensional map viewing process and assessment of the results of automated fragment fitting. This combination of proprietary and public domain software tools provides an efficient process for analyzing the results of SGX core fragment library x-ray screening.

In addition to providing the all important "direct look" at the fragment binding to the target, x-ray screening has proven remarkably sensitive. Fragments with measurable IC_{50} values up to 50 mM have been detected, and in some cases we have not even been able to measure the binding affinity of a fragment hit. The sensitivity of the x-ray screening approach obtains from the very high local protein concentration within a typical crystal ($\sim$0.1 M). The other advantage of x-ray screening comes, paradoxically, from the limitation of the crystallographic method itself. Visualization of fragment hits via difference Fourier syntheses depends critically on the fraction of individual protein molecules comprising the crystal to which ligand is bound (i.e., fractional occupancy) and on how well the fragment is anchored to its binding site on the surface of the protein. Average occupancy levels must exceed $\sim$30% for a ligand to be detectable by x-ray screening. The ligand must also bind to the target with a single, well-defined set of intermolecular interactions. If a fragment binds to multiple subsites within an enzyme active site, the resulting electron density feature(s) will be weak and blurry and will, therefore, be scored as an uninterpretable negative. Thus, fragment hits detected by x-ray screening exhibit both high fractional occupancy and well-defined anchoring to the surface of the target protein.

Complementary biophysical screening

As a complement to crystallographic screening, SGX frequently conducts both biochemical and surface plasmon resonance (SPR) screening of the $\sim$1,500-compound core fragment library. Biochemical screening is performed using a Beckman BioMek FX liquid-handling system equipped with a Sagian rail. Our core fragment library can be screened one compound at a time via the appropriate biochemical assay in less than a day to complement results from crystallographic screening. It is often challenging to use biochemical assays to characterize weakly binding ligands, because of the problem of spectral interference. We screen the SGX core fragment library at 500 μM ligand concentration, using biochemical assays formatted to minimize spectral interference, while maximizing throughput. IC_{50} values are determined for all biochemical hits (defined as >$\sim$50% inhibition). Spectral interference is not a shortcoming of SPR screening, which is performed with a Biacore T-100 instrument using either 96- or 384-well compound array formats. Our core fragment library can be screened one compound at a time in a week to complement results from both crystallographic screening and biochemical assays. Data from biochemical/SPR screening are automatically imported into the SGX LIMS for comparison with the results of x-ray screening.

Comparison of x-ray, biochemical, and SPR screening

Combining x-ray screening with biochemical assays and SRP studies typically reveals compound hits common to all three approaches plus hits limited to two of three methods and hits peculiar to a single method. Follow-up x-ray crystallographic studies of individual fragment soaks or cocrystallization are used as the final arbiter of the utility of hits coming independently from biochemical assays and/or SPR screens. X-ray validated biochemical/SPR hits are retained for further evaluation. Biochemical/SPR hits that cannot be confirmed by crystallography are abandoned. Although rare, because the hit rate is $\sim$1–5%, x-ray screening sometimes fails to detect a fragment hit because of masking by the presence of a more potent compound in the same shape-diverse fragment screening mixture. Biochemical assays and/or SPR screening of single fragments can overcome this shortcoming. The following section discusses criteria used to select fragment hits for structure-guided optimization.

Structure/activity relationship optimization

As discussed above, a typical crystallographic screen yields approximately fifteen to seventy-five hits per target with binding affinities (IC_{50}) ranging from low micromolar to low millimolar levels. A fragment hit is useful only if it can be elaborated through efficient synthesis in directions that rapidly lead to dramatic improvements in activity. Computational prediction of which fragments represent the best candidates for optimization is not feasible because of the huge number of possible analogs that can be generated from each fragment and the computational time required for predicting binding free energies. Instead, we select four to five of the most promising fragments to optimize in parallel. Our experience has shown that careful selection and prioritization of fragment hits typically provides two to three orders of magnitude enhancement in activity during the first round of fragment elaboration.

The primary determinant for choosing a fragment for chemical elaboration is a high-quality, unambiguous crystal structure of the target-fragment complex at better than 2.5Å resolution, which clearly reveals the orientation of the bound ligand and the conformation of the polypeptide chain segments forming the ligand binding site. As discussed earlier, the ligand efficiency of the fragment hit represents an important parameter with which to prioritize among potential starting points for medicinal chemistry elaboration. Biochemical measurements of IC_{50} and/or SPR measurements of binding kinetics (k_{on} and k_{off}) permit estimation of ligand efficiency. In aggregate, fragment hits are prioritized for synthetic elaboration based on the following criteria: location of the fragment binding site, fragment binding mode, structural accessibility of chemical handles for synthesis, a preliminary evaluation of synthetically accessibility, potential novelty in terms of patentability, the conformation of the protein, and ligand efficiency.

Ideally fragment hits will bind to either the active site or a known allosteric site. Fragments that bind at previously unknown sites remote from a lattice packing interface represent opportunities for discovery of novel/selective lead compounds, but such sites require validation through fragment elaboration into more potent compounds with which to perform definitive biochemical or cellular assays. The mode of fragment binding must orient synthetic handles toward pockets or subsites on the surface of the target protein. If the intrinsic synthetic handles of the fragment hit are oriented only toward solvent or are sterically blocked, alternative handles may be found by searching for available fragment analogs or introduced via synthesis of a fragment analog. Synthetic feasibility is assessed by considering the diversity of available reagents that are compatible with the fragment hit and related synthons. Ligand efficiency is assessed by examining the ratio of biochemical activity to the size of the fragment (see above). Novelty is evaluated in terms of both the fragment hit and its binding mode. A familiar fragment can be observed to bind in an unusual way, which can provide novel elaboration opportunities. Observing a common binding mode for similar fragments sometimes provides an initial SAR and gives support, albeit indirectly, for fragment hit selection. Previous experience with the same or a related target and the same or a similar scaffold represented by the fragment hit can also help support the choice of a fragment hit. Fragment biochemical activity is usually less important than the criteria described above, because poorly oriented or ligand-inefficient fragments can be difficult if not impossible to optimize.

A detailed account of how we use computational chemistry tools to plan fragment elaboration chemistry has been published by Blaney et al.[22] Our current methods of predicting binding free energies of partially elaborated fragment hits are used to compare different elaboration routes for the selected fragment hits, to select the best of these routes, and to prioritize analogs for synthesis. This approach is currently too expensive from the computational standpoint to apply to all of the possible virtual libraries for all fragment hits.

Our goals for the first stage of fragment optimization are to improve binding affinity by at least 100-fold for each chemical handle (i.e., $IC_{50} \sim 1-10\,mM \rightarrow \sim 10-100\,\mu M$), to validate the selected fragment by establishing an initial SAR at each available synthetic handle, and to correlate this SAR with observed cocrystal structures and computational predictions of potency. As discussed previously, optimization of fragment hits into nanomolar leads typically requires an increase in binding energy of $\sim$4–9 kcal/mol (three to six orders of magnitude). Without appeal to structural information, this task would be daunting.

With timely access to the right cocrystal structures, weakly binding fragments have been successfully optimized into potent lead compounds. At SGX, access to our proprietary x-ray beamline at the APS provides very rapid turnaround between compound synthesis and cocrystal structure determination. The median time required for x-ray data collection and structure determination is forty-eight hours, with 90% of requested cocrystal structures being delivered to the project team within ninety-six hours. With such rapid turnaround our multidisciplinary design teams (consisting of medicinal chemists, computational chemists, and protein crystallographers) can make decisions regarding the next round of compound synthesis with a full three-dimensional view of the SAR for the evolving lead series.

SGX has had considerable success with the fragment engineering method, wherein optimization involves "growing" each fragment with small focused analog libraries at each synthetic handle, followed by synthesis of multiply elaborated fragments using the better substituents identified for each chemical handle. This approach is stepwise, systematic, and lends itself to maintaining and even improving ligand efficiency. Once fragments have been selected for synthesis, available reagents are assembled to generate various small focused analog libraries. Compounds are prioritized for synthesis using predicted binding free energies for each fragment analog and on the basis of medicinal chemistry SAR considerations. In silico docking of fragments is not part of the SGX fragment-based drug discovery strategy. Experience has shown that much more reliable results can be obtained using experimentally determined structures of protein-fragment complexes as starting points for planning synthetic chemistry.

The resource needs of such an exercise depend on the particulars of the target. SGX metrics for this initial SAR exploration are as follows: duration = 2–8 months (average 4 months), number of fragment analogs synthesized = 10–150 (average 60 analogs), potency gain = 500–10,000 fold (average 3,500 fold). Following experimental validation of the optimization potential of a given fragment hit, further chemistry is executed to improve the druglike properties of the evolving lead series, including selectivity, cell permeability, cellular activity, and liver microsome and hepatocyte clearance. Again, the time required to complete this stage of the process is a function of the particular target.

End game

The final stages of any drug discovery process are focused on identifying one or more compounds suitable for development candidate nomination, thereby committing significant resources to preparation of an investigational new drug (IND) application. At SGX, there is no "bright line" between SAR optimization and development candidate seeking. Structure-guided optimization of lead series continues with added feedback from the results of in vivo intravenous and oral pharmacokinetic studies in both mouse and rat, demonstrations of in vivo efficacy using various mouse xenograft tumor models, and preliminary fourteen-day toxicology studies in rat. The duration of the end game, simply put, is as long as it takes to achieve the desired balance among in vitro cellular potency, selectivity, oral bioavailability, half-life, in vivo efficacy, and absorption/distribution/metabolism/excretion (ADME)/safety properties [cytochrome P450 inhibition and induction, receptor inhibition profile, genotoxicity, and human ether-à-go-go related gene (hERG) channel binding].

Postscript

In closing this section, it is remarkable that the SGX fragment-based structure-guided drug process is entirely pragmatic in terms of when and where fragment information is exploited. Insights from cocrystal structures of fragments bound to the target of interest (and for some protein kinases, critical off targets) influence not only fragment elaboration but also lead series SAR optimization. Cocrystal structures coming from the initial x-ray screen of our core fragment library and fragments from other sources provide valuable information regarding possible interactions between small-molecule ligands and many of the functional groups comprising the enzyme active or allosteric site. In some cases, fragment hits that were not subject to elaboration later serve as the inspiration for choice of R groups during fragment/lead optimization. We have also developed proprietary computational chemistry software to overlay and merge experimentally identified fragments to create entirely new fragments (also commonly referred to as scaffolds) using a tool designated SMERGE (Scaffold MErging via Recursive Graph Exploration). The products of SMERGE have provided new starting points for structure-guided optimization that build rapidly on a wealth of information regarding the SAR implications of adding a particular R group to a particular site of a previously elaborated scaffold. For certain lead series, such merged fragments have helped us overcome unattractive druglike properties or navigate intellectual property constraints.

Lessons from FAST

Key experiences coming from application of the SGX fragment-based structure-guided drug discovery process to twenty-four protein targets, twenty of which are protein kinases, are presented below. Three "lessons" central to fragment-based approaches are reviewed, including (1) the importance of fragment library design, (2) the selectivity of fragment hits identified in x-ray screens of protein kinases, and (3) that the optimization potential of a fragment hit is not correlated with initial binding affinity.

Lesson 1: Fragment library design

Figure 3.4 illustrates three histograms that compare various properties of the SGX core fragment library and the hits obtained from twenty-four targets drawn from four protein families. It is remarkable that the properties of the fragment hits closely mirror those of the entire fragment library. This finding reflects the target agnostic nature of the composition of our core fragment library. We consciously sought to create a fragment screening library with maximum potential for chemical diversity that was not biased toward any one particular target class. As we continue to add fragments to our screening library, we will seek to further increase the potential for chemical diversity with ongoing attention to tractability in terms of synthetic elaboration.

Lesson 2: Fragment selectivity revealed by x-ray screens of protein kinases

Figure 3.5 summarizes our x-ray screening experience across twenty protein kinase targets. When we embarked on this odyssey, we naively assumed that fragment hits would be intrinsically nonselective and that selectivity would come only during the course of elaboration of such hits. Our experience with the protein kinases argues otherwise. Nearly 75% of the fragment hits detected by x-ray screening of protein kinases bound to only one of the twenty targets. Under the conditions of this very stringent screening process, we appear to be identifying "privileged" ligands (or scaffolds). This unanticipated benefit of our strong reliance on x-ray screening may well explain our success in elaborating fragment hits under structural guidance to produce highly selective kinase inhibitors. During the iterative design/chemical elaboration/biochemical assay/cocrystal structure determination process of optimizing attractive fragment hits, we strive to preserve the original anchoring interactions between the growing fragment and its target. With timely access to structural information we can monitor the impact of synthetic changes to the growing fragment to ensure that we do so. In rare cases (~5%), we have detected alterations in the mode of fragment binding, some of which have been exploited as opportunities with which to pursue alternative SAR regimes.

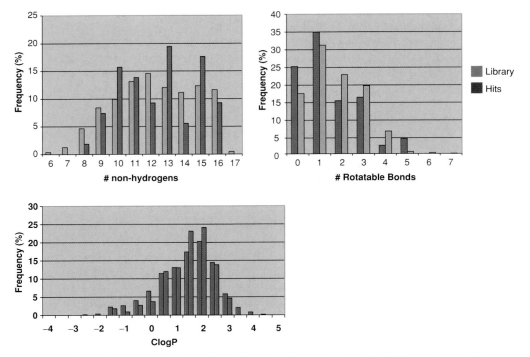

Figure 3.4. Comparison of selected properties of fragment hits versus those of the SGX core fragment library.

Lesson 3: Fragment optimization potential is not correlated with binding affinity

Figure 3.6 summarizes our experience with initial synthetic optimization of various fragments for some protein kinase targets. For each fragment we have plotted the relationship between the initially measured binding affinity of the fragment itself and the results of elaboration at one chemical handle. These data conclusively demonstrate that there is no correlation between the strength of initial binding and the optimization potential of a fragment. There is, therefore, no rational basis for preferentially devoting synthetic chemistry resources to fragment hits with higher affinities versus those that bind the target more weakly. Ligand efficiency is the issue, not affinity.

Future prospects

Notwithstanding the flurry of activity in fragment-based approaches since 2004, practitioners of this new strategy for drug discovery would appear to have only scratched the surface. There are many more target classes that should be pursued with fragment screening. Of particular interest

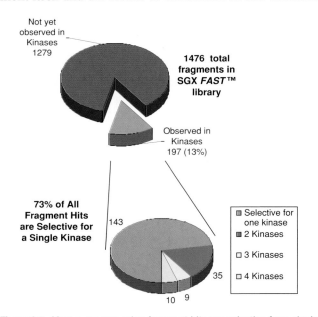

Figure 3.5. Most x-ray screening fragment hits are selective for a single protein kinase.

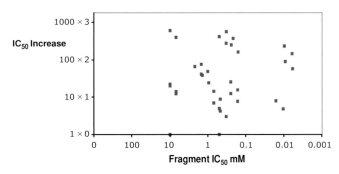

Figure 3.6. Relationship between initial binding affinity (IC$_{50}$) and increase in potency following elaboration at individual chemical handles for fragment hits obtained with five targets.

to biotechnology and pharmaceutical companies are ion channels and G-protein-coupled receptors, both of which have lately proven more amenable to x-ray crystallographic study. There is still much work to be done in terms of the design of fragment libraries. At present, we do not know with any certainty the optimum library size or the best way to maximize the potential of a library to generate chemical diversity during synthetic elaboration of fragment hits. Moreover, we do not yet know how best to screen fragment libraries. Various organizations have their respective biases, which reflect institutional memory, resource constraints, experience base, and the availability of particular skills, and so on. There is always the sobering possibility that fragment approaches will go the way of HTS, which appears to have fallen well short of expectations. We think it unlikely that fragment approaches will disappoint and we remain committed to exploring the potential of the method and continuously evolving our own process to maximize the likelihood of discovering development candidates suitable for entry into oncology clinical trials of targeted therapeutic agents.

ACKNOWLEDGMENTS

We thank all members of the SGX organization, past and present, who contributed to the manifold aspects of our FAST fragment-based structure-guided drug discovery process both as innovators and practitioners. We also acknowledge contributions to the field by competitors, who are too numerous to identify individually. Use of the Advanced Photon Source was supported by the U.S. Department of Energy, Office of Science, Office of Basic Energy Sciences, under Contract No. DE-AC02–06CH11357. SGX Pharmaceuticals, Inc., constructed and operates the SGX Collaborative Access Team (SGX-CAT) beam line at Sector 31 of the Advanced Photon Source.

REFERENCES

1. Allen, K. N.; Bellamacina, C. R.; Ding, X.; Jeffery, C. J.; Mattos, C.;Petsko, G. A.; Ringe D. An experimental approach to mapping the binding surfaces of crystalline protein. *J. Phys. Chem.* **1996**, *100*, 2605–2611.

2. Verlinde, C. I. M. J.; Rudenko, G.; Hoi, W. G. J. In search of new lead compounds for trypanosomiasis drug design: a protein structure-based linked-fragment approach. *J. Comput. Aided Mol. Des.* **1992**, *6*, 131–147.

3. Kuntz, I. D. Structure-based strategies for drug design and discovery. *Science* **1992**, *257*, 1078–1082.

4. Kuntz, I. D.; Meng; E. C.; Shoichet, B. K. Structure-based molecular design. *Acc. Chem. Res.* **1994**, *27*, 117–123.

5. Caflisch, A.; Miranker, A.; Karplus, M. Multiple copy simultaneous search and construction of ligands in binding sites: application to inhibitors of HIV-I aspartic proteinase. *J. Med. Chem.* **1993**, *36*, 2142–2167.

6. Shuker, S. B.; Hajduk, P. J.; Meadows, R. P.; Fesik, S. W. Discovering high affinity ligands for proteins: SAR by NMR. *Science* **1996**, *274*, 1531–1534.

7. Nienaber, V. I.; Richardson, P. I.; Klighofer, V.; Bouska, J. J.; Giranda, V. I.; Greer J. Discovering novel ligands for macromolecules using x-ray crystallographic screening. *Nat. Biotechnol.* **2000**, *18*, 1105–1108.

8. Bohacek, R. S.; McMartin, C.; Guida, W. C. The art and practice of structure-based drug design: a molecular modelling perspective. *Med. Res. Rev.* **1996**, *16*, 3–50.

9. Hann, M. M.; Leach, A. R.; G. Harper, G. Molecular complexity and its impact on the probability of finding leads for drug discovery. *J. Chem. Inf. Comput. Sci.* **2001**, *41*, 856–864.

10. Hann, M. M.; Oprea, T. I. Pursuing the lead likeness concept in pharmaceutical research. *Curr. Opin. Chem. Biol.* **2004**, *8*, 255–263.

11. Oprea, T. I.; Davis, A. M.; Teague, S. J.; Leeson, P. D. Is there a difference between leads and drugs? A historical perspective. *J. Chem. Inf. Comput. Sci.* **2001**, *41*, 1308–1315.

12. Teague, S. J.; Davis, A. M.; Leeson, P. D.; Oprea T. The design of leadlike combinatorial libraries. *Angew. Chem. Int. Ed.* **1999**, *38*, 3743–3748.

13. Congreve, M.; Chessari, G.; Tisi, D.; Woodhead A. J. Recent developments in fragment based drug discovery. *J. Med. Chem.* **2008**, *51*, in press.

14. Gill, A. I.; Frederickson, M.; Cleasby, A.; Woodhead, S. J.; Carr, M. G.; Woodhead, A J.; Walker, M. T.; Congreve, M. S.; et al. Identification of novel p38ct MAP kinase inhibitors using fragment-based lead generation. *J. Med. Chem.* **2005**, *48*, 414–426.

15. Lesuisse, D.; Lange, G.; Deprez, P.; Benard, D.; Schoot, B.; Delettre, G.; Marquette, J.-P; Broto, P.; et al. SAR and X-ray: a new approach combining fragment-based screening and rational drug design: application to the discovery of nanomolar inhibitors of Src SH2. *J. Med. Chem.* **2002**, *45*, 2379–2387.

16. Card, G. I.; Blasdel, I.; England, B. P.; Zhang, C.; Suzuki, Y.; Gillette, S.; Fong, D.; Ibrahim, P. N.; et al. A family of phosphodiesterase inhibitors discovered by cocrystallography and scaffold-based drug design. *Nat. Biotechnol.* **2005**, *23*, 201–207.

17. Lipinski, C. A.; Lombardo, F.; Dominy, B. W.; Feeney, P. J. Experimental and computational approaches to estimate solubility and permeability in drug discovery and development settings. *Drug Deliv. Res.* **1997**, *23*, 3–25.

18. Congreve, M.; Carr, R.; Murray, C.; Jhoti, H. A "rule of three" for fragment-based lead discovery? *Drug Discov. Today* **2003**, *8*, 876–877.

19. Wenlock, M. C.; Austin, R. P.; Barton, P.; Davis, A M.; Leeson P. D. A comparison of physiochemical property profiles of development and marketed oral drugs. *J. Med. Chem.* **2003**, *46*, 1250–1256.

20. Vieth, M.; Siegel, M. G.; Higgs, R. E.; Watson, I. A.; Robertson, D. H.; Savin, K. A.; Durst, G. I.; Hipskind P. A. Characteristic physical properties and structural fragments of marketed oral drugs. *J. Med. Chem.* **2004**, *47*, 224–232.

21. Paolini, G. V.; Shapland, R. H. B.; van Hoorn, W. P.; Mason, J. S.; Hopkins A. L. Global mapping of pharmacological space. *Nat. Biotechnol.* **2006**, *24*, 805–815.

22. Blaney, J.; Nienaber, V.; Burley, S. K. In: *Fragment-Based Approaches in Drug Discovery*, Jahnke, W.; and Erlanson, D. A.; Eds. Weinheim: Wiley VCH; **2006**, 215–248.

23. Fink, T.; Bruggesser, H.; Reymond, J.-L. Virtual exploration of the small molecule chemical universe below 160 daltons. *Angew. Chem. Int. Ed.* **2005**, *44*, 1504–1508.

24. Xie, X.; Kokubo, T.; Cohen, S. I.; Mirza, U. A.; Hoffman, A.; Chait, B. T.; Roeder, R. G.; Nakatani, Y.; et al. Structural similarity between TAFs and the heterotetrameric core of the histone octamer. *Nature* **1996**, *380*, 287–288.

25. Collaborative Computational Project. The CCP4 suite: programs for protein crystallography. *Acta Cryst.* **1994** *D50*, 760–763.

4

NMR in fragment-based drug discovery

Christopher A. Lepre, Peter J. Connolly, and Jonathan M. Moore

AN INTRODUCTION TO FRAGMENT-BASED LEAD DISCOVERY

For decades, molecular starting points for drug discovery have been found by screening large numbers of natural and synthetic compounds for biological activity in phenotypic and biochemical assays. Then, beginning in the mid to late 1990s, several pharmaceutical groups developed new approaches [such as structure/activity relationship by nuclear magnetic resonance (SAR by NMR),[1] the SHAPES strategy,[2] and needle screening[3]] in which simple, low-molecular-weight compounds were screened for binding to the target of interest, and these relatively weak binding molecules were then used to systematically construct larger, more potent, drug leads. Such small screening molecules are now commonly called fragments and the related processes collectively called fragment-based lead discovery (FBLD).

NMR was the first experimental method used to screen fragments, and although a variety of other techniques (including x-ray crystallography, surface plasmon resonance, high concentration bioassays, and mass spectroscopy) have also been applied, NMR is still the most widely used. This chapter reviews the use of NMR for FBLD, beginning with an explanation of the principles behind fragment screening. NMR screening methods are then described, followed by a series of examples that illustrate the process through which fragment screening hits are converted into leads.

Defining fragments

To explain the principles of FBLD, it is first necessary to define what molecules are considered to be fragments. Molecules are often classified using their physicochemical properties, such as molecular weight (MW), number of hydrogen bond donors and acceptors (HBD and HBA), calculated $\log P$ (Clog$P$), and number of rotatable bonds. A popular rule of thumb for classifying molecules as "drug-like" is the "rule-of-five" first described in a well-known article from Pfizer.[4] This study reported that a compound is more likely to exhibit poor oral absorption and cell permeability when its properties exceed limits (Table 4.1) defined by four simple rules (dubbed the "rule-of-five" because the values are multiples of five). Approximately 90% of the approximately 2,000 Phase II clinical candidates analyzed satisfied at least three of the four rules.

Because lead optimization by medicinal chemists typically results in molecules that are larger and more lipophilic than the starting lead, it has been proposed[5,6] that the compounds screened should be "leadlike" rather than "drug-like," with properties well within the rule-of-five limits to allow room for subsequent improvements in potency, selectivity, and absorption/distribution/metabolism/excretion (ADME) properties (Table 4.1).

Fragment-based screening evolved in parallel with the practice of classifying compounds as drug- or leadlike according to their physicochemical properties, so the much smaller molecules used for FBLD were defined using the same parameters. The term *fragment* originates from the practice of computationally dividing known biologically active molecules into their basic building blocks[7,8] and then using those components for screening. Although there is a general consensus among practitioners of FBLD regarding which properties should be used to define fragments, there is some disagreement about the preferred values. The group at Astex Therapeutics has reported that the hits obtained from crystallographic screening of their MW = 100- to 250-Da fragment library seem to conform to a "rule-of-three" (Table 4.1).[9] The rule-of-three has been adopted by many groups and commercial vendors for designing fragment libraries, particularly those used for crystallography-based screening. Some groups, particularly those using NMR-based screening methods, find that rule-of-three compliant libraries are too limited and produce hits that are so small and simple that they are difficult to optimize synthetically, because of very weak (e.g., multimillimolar) affinities, a lack of synthetically accessible functional groups, and the need for structural information to guide synthesis. To address this, they employ higher limits for molecular weight, HBA, and rotatable bonds to create libraries of "reduced complexity" leads or scaffolds (Table 4.1).[10–12] A minimum MW cutoff of ~150 Da is also often used to avoid the possibility of binding in multiple orientations, a problem that occurs more frequently for the smallest and simplest fragments.[13–15] In addition to the properties listed in

Table 4.1. Property ranges used to define druglike compounds, leadlike compounds, fragments, and scaffolds

	Druglike (rule-of-five) properties[4]	Leadlike properties[6]	Fragment-like (rule-of-three) properties[9]	Scaffold-like properties[10]
Molecular weight	$\leq$500	$\leq$450	<300	$\leq$350
ClogP	$\leq$5	−3.5 to 4.5	$\leq$3	$\leq$2.2
Hydrogen bond donors (e.g., NH, OH)	$\leq$5	$\leq$5	$\leq$3	$\leq$3
Hydrogen bond acceptors (e.g., N, O)	$\leq$10	$\leq$8	$\leq$3	$\leq$8
Rotatable bonds	(Not defined)	$\leq$9	$\leq$3	$\leq$6

Table 4.1, many other factors are considered when selecting fragments for screening, including solubility (a critical factor due to the high concentrations necessary to detect weak binding), chemical stability, low reactivity, commercial availability of compounds and analogs, synthetic accessibility, and the presence of preferred binding motifs.

The three principles of FBLD: Efficiency, efficiency, and efficiency

Conventional methods for lead discovery using phenotypic or biochemically based assays have produced many success stories. So why use fragment-based methods? Along with the successes of conventional methods, there have been many cases where leads could not be found or could not be developed into drugs because of inadequate potency; rapid metabolism or excretion; toxicity or off-target effects; difficulties with synthesis or formulation; and poor solubility, oral availability, or cell permeability.

Fragment-based lead discovery produces more choices, and potentially better choices, for lead optimization than conventional methods alone. FBLD is a complementary approach that generates independent sets of leads from which medicinal chemists may choose, and the pursuit of multiple chemically distinct lead classes for any given program increases the likelihood that at least one will succeed. Furthermore, by starting from leads that have lower molecular weights and bind more efficiently than typical high-throughput screening (HTS) hits, it is more likely that the final, optimized compounds will have desirable physicochemical (and hence ADME) properties. It has been argued that fragment-derived drug candidates, in addition to having lower molecular weights, tend to be more polar and water soluble. For example, the mean ClogP value for fragment-derived molecules patented by Astex in 2006 was 2.4, compared to a range of 3.5 to 4.2 for conventionally derived compounds from four major pharmaceutical companies.[16,17]

The key advantage of FBLD lies in its efficiency, as embodied by three principles, each of which will be discussed in detail in the following sections:

Chemical efficiency: Fragments sample chemical space more effectively than large molecules.

Searching efficiency: Fragments probe protein binding sites more efficiently and produce higher hit rates than large molecules.

Binding efficiency: By starting from fragments that bind very efficiently, it is possible to construct highly efficient lead molecules and thus better drug candidates.

The chemical efficiency of fragments

The number of possible druglike compounds containing up to thirty C, N, O, and S atoms is enormous and has been estimated to comprise around 10^{63} molecules.[18] It is impossible to effectively sample such a vast and diverse "chemistry space" with a screening library (to begin with, there is not enough matter on Earth to make that many molecules). Furthermore, maximizing chemistry diversity alone is an inherently inefficient strategy for library design. If biologically active molecules were uniformly distributed throughout chemistry space, then it has been estimated that at least 10^{14} compounds would have to be screened to find a single hit.[19] The fact that libraries of 10^5 to 10^6 molecules routinely produce multiple hits simply reflects the well-known empirical observation that biologically active molecules are actually clustered within small regions of chemistry space.

The number of possible fragments is, however, many orders of magnitude smaller than the number of possible druglike compounds. For example, a virtual library of all 26.4 million possible molecules containing up to eleven C, N, O, and F atoms has been computationally enumerated, and approximately half of the molecules conform to the rule-of-three.[20] It is therefore possible to sample more of the available chemistry space with much smaller libraries of compounds by screening fragments instead of larger molecules. Furthermore, fragments can be combined to make larger compounds, vastly expanding the represented chemical space. For example, if a receptor contains two binding sites that are close together, then rather than screen large molecules containing two components intended to bind to both sites simultaneously, fragments capable of binding to one or the other site individually can be screened and any hits subsequently linked together. Assuming that the binding modes of the individual fragments mimic that of a linked molecule, a 1,000-fragment library with several possible synthetic linkers could represent the chemistry space of a multimillion-member combinatorial library.

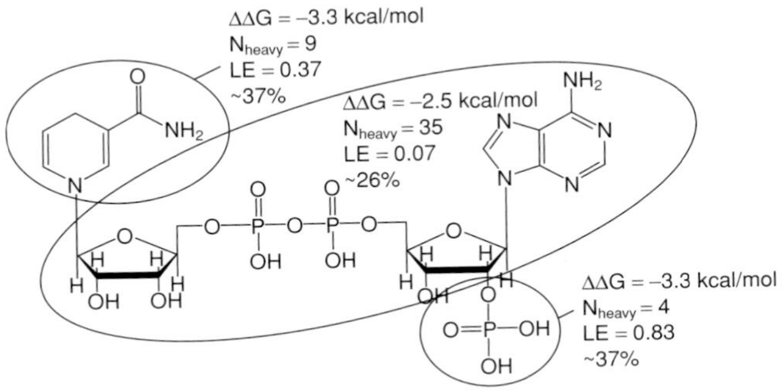

$\Delta\Delta G = -3.3$ kcal/mol
$N_{heavy} = 9$
LE = 0.37
~37%

$\Delta\Delta G = -2.5$ kcal/mol
$N_{heavy} = 35$
LE = 0.07
~26%

$\Delta\Delta G = -3.3$ kcal/mol
$N_{heavy} = 4$
LE = 0.83
~37%

Figure 4.1. Contributions by individual functional groups to the binding of NADPH to KPR (adapted from Cuilli et al.[34]). $\Delta\Delta G$: estimated contribution to the binding energy by the group calculated from the difference in the Gibbs free energy of binding[34] for fragments that differ only by that group (e.g., the contribution by 2'-phosphate was calculated from ΔG (NADPH) − ΔG (NADH). N_{heavy}: number of heavy atoms in the group. LE: ligand efficiency for the group (in kcal/mol-atom) calculated from $\Delta\Delta G/N_{heavy}$. Percentage of the total binding energy contributed by the group was calculated by dividing the $\Delta\Delta G$ by the total binding energy of NADPH (−9 kcal/mol).

To exploit the clustering tendency of bioactive molecules, a popular library design strategy has been to select diverse sets of fragments from within biologically active regions of chemistry space. For example, some groups have selected compounds for their fragment screening libraries based on the fragments commonly found in known drugs. Computational chemists at Vertex have found that just thirty-two simple graph frameworks are represented in approximately half of known drugs.[7] This result suggests that a relatively small collection of scaffolds could be used as a universal screening library for a wide variety of therapeutic targets.[2] A detailed discussion of fragment library design lies outside the scope of this review, but accounts have been published of the various methods used at Vertex,[21,22] Novartis,[12,23] Vernalis,[24,25] Astex,[26] SGX,[27] Astra-Zeneca,[28] and ZoBio/Pyxis.[15]

The searching efficiency of fragments

A high proportion of the binding energy driving the formation of protein/ligand and protein/protein complexes comes from relatively small regions of the protein surface, often termed *hot spots*.[29-32] Binding is thought to begin when a "molecular anchor" motif on the ligand recognizes a hot spot on the receptor. The binding of peripheral groups on the ligand to nearby regions of the protein serves to further increase affinity and confer specificity.[33] In principle, fragments are more capable than large molecules of probing binding hot spots and they can serve as molecular anchors from which more potent and selective ligands may be constructed.[13] In practice, fragments bind almost exclusively to hot spots and can be used to identify them and evaluate the "druggability" of new targets.[34,35]

The hot spot concept is clearly illustrated by the binding of NADPH ($K_d = 0.26$ μM, $\Delta G = -9$ kcal/mol) and its fragments to ketopantoate reductase (KPR).[34] Calorimetry

experiments reveal that most of the binding energy comes from two hot spots on the enzyme. From the results reported, we estimate that the 2'-phosphate and nicotinamide groups (comprising only thirteen heavy atoms) together contribute approximately three-quarters of the ligand binding energy of NADPH (Figure 4.1). As Ciulli et al. conclude, the phosphoribose portion of the ligand contributes little binding energy and serves mainly to connect and orient the two hot spot groups, which bind 13–14Å apart.[36]

The very fact that measurable binding can be observed for a small fragment suggests that it makes highly favorable contacts with the receptor. On binding, ligands lose a significant amount of rigid body rotational and translational entropy that must be outweighed by favorable binding interactions.[37,38] Because this entropic penalty is only weakly dependent on molecular weight, it is much more significant for small fragments. Low-molecular-weight fragments with millimolar affinities can thus possess very high intrinsic affinities for the receptor[37] and may bind in highly optimal orientations. Such fragments represent better starting points for chemistry than larger, more potent molecules whose affinities reflect the sum of multiple low-affinity, suboptimal interactions spread out across the molecule.

Because they are less complex, small molecules are less likely to be sterically blocked from binding to a receptor and will therefore produce higher hit rates. Using a computational model, Hann and coworkers at GlaxoSmithKline[13] predicted that the total probability of ligand binding (dashed line in Figure 4.2) is highest for the simplest molecules and decreases with increasing complexity. This total binding probability includes the possibility of a ligand binding to the receptor in multiple positions.

For drug discovery, it is preferable to find fragments that bind in one distinct position. The probability of such "unique binding" (Figure 4.2) peaks at some intermediate level of complexity and then drops off in concert with the total binding probability. The likelihood of observing "measurable inhibition" starts to rise at the detection threshold of the measurement method and increases with ligand complexity before leveling off. For binding to be useful, it must be both unique and measurable, and the "useful binding" curve is thus the product of the latter two probabilities.

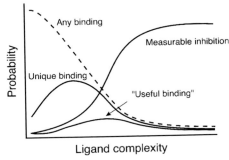

Figure 4.2. Ligand binding probability as a function of molecular complexity (adapted from Hann et al.[13]).

The higher probability of binding by fragments predicted by the Hann model is borne out experimentally. At Novartis, the hit rates for NMR screens of fragments (MW = 100 to 300 Da) were 3 to 30%, compared to 0.001 to 0.151% for HTS screens of full-sized compounds (200 to 600 Da).[12] Similarly, plotting hit rate versus complexity for the combined results of five fragment screens run at ZoBio[15] produced a profile resembling the "useful binding" curve of Figure 4.2. Because fragments bind more weakly than full-sized HTS compounds, the higher fragment hit rates are thought to be real and not just an artifact of the higher concentrations used in fragment screens.[39] The group at Abbott has claimed that fragment screening may thus "deliver more hits against larger numbers of protein targets" than conventional HTS screening.[39] For a set of forty-five Abbott targets screened using both fragment screening and HTS, the fragment screens identified interesting, chemically tractable hits for 76% of the targets, compared to 53% for HTS.

Binding efficiency of fragments

Because fragment hits have relatively weak affinities, they can easily be overlooked when compared to more complex and more potent molecules, even though the latter may be too large to serve as good starting points for lead optimization. For this reason, it is useful to compare hits according to their ligand efficiency (LE), defined as the free energy of binding per heavy atom in the molecule[40]:

$$\text{Ligand efficiency (LE)} = \Delta G / N_{\text{heavy}}$$

where $\Delta G = -RT \ln(K_d)$, where K_d is the dissociation constant and N_{heavy} is the number of nonhydrogen atoms in the molecule. Alternatively, the binding efficiency index (BEI) is a unitless metric that is simpler to calculate[41]:

$$\text{BEI} = -(\text{pKi, pKd, or pIC50}) / \text{MW (in kilodaltons)}.$$

These two metrics will be used interchangeably in this chapter.

Using ligand or binding efficiency, it is possible to rank hits that have dramatically different potencies and molecular weights. For example, even though it is 100-fold less potent, a 200-Da fragment hit (15 heavy atoms) with $K_d = 100 \, \mu M$ is a much more efficient binder (LE = 0.37 kcal/mol-atom, BEI = 20) than a 400-Da HTS hit (30 heavy atoms) with $K_d = 1 \, \mu M$ (LE = 0.27 kcal/mol-atom, BEI = 15).

Because molecular weight invariably increases during the process of synthetically optimizing leads to improve potency, and large molecules typically have poorer oral bioavailability, it naturally follows that, all other considerations being equal, the best leads are those with the highest ligand efficiencies. In a study of eighteen highly optimized drug leads at Abbott,[42] pK_d was found to increase linearly with molecular weight, with an average increase of 1 pK_d unit for every 64 Da added, as the fragment leads (average MW = 224) progressed to final compounds (average MW = 463). The binding efficiency, however, usually remained constant or decreased, even as the potencies

increased by over three orders of magnitude. Other groups have also reported that ligand efficiency usually does not increase during lead optimization.[16]

A linear relationship between potency and molecular weight makes it possible to predict the molecular weight of a final drug candidate based on the MW and potency of the lead.[42] For example, the 400-Da, $K_d = 1 \, \mu M$ HTS hit from the previous example might initially seem to be an attractive starting point, but optimization to a potency of 10 nM (maintaining the starting BEI of 15) would result in a final compound of MW = 666 Da, well above the rule-of-five limit. The 200-Da, $pK_d = 100 \, \mu M$ fragment (BEI = 20), however, would be expected to produce a 10 nM final compound with MW = 500. This example underscores the importance of starting optimization from the most efficient fragment lead.

Another argument in favor of screening fragments is the observation that ligand efficiency varies with size and is higher, on average, for small ligands. Reynolds and coworkers[43] analyzed published pK_d and pIC_{50} data for 8,653 ligands and found that ligand efficiency dropped dramatically as the number of heavy atoms increased from 10 to 20 and then leveled off for ligands with more than twenty-five heavy atoms. A heavy atom count of twenty-five corresponds to a molecular weight around 333, a value that is close to the average molecular weight (~340) for marketed oral drugs.[44,45] It is tempting to speculate that twenty-five heavy atoms may mark the point of diminishing returns for lead optimization, after which adding more molecular weight results in smaller potency improvements at the expense of potential decreases in oral bioavailability.

Reynolds et al.[43] attribute the intrinsically higher ligand efficiency of fragments to two primary causes. First, small fragments are able to freely adopt orientations that make ideal interactions with the receptor (e.g., optimal hydrogen bond and salt bridge geometries), while larger, more complex molecules are sterically constrained, forcing them into suboptimal, energetically strained orientations. Second, small ligands present more accessible surface area for interaction per heavy atom than large ligands, resulting in a higher average binding energy per atom.

Building from fragments

Once fragment hits have been identified, they must be validated, preferably using multiple methods. When NMR is used for the primary screen, initial validation of the hits is often obtained at the time of the screen from NMR experiments that provide information about the binding site: competition studies using known ligands or binding site maps obtained using heteronuclear chemical shift perturbation experiments. Other popular methods for confirming binding and measuring affinity include biochemical (activity) assays, SPR, and isothermal titration calorimetry (ITC). A crystal structure of the receptor with a ligand bound in the active site is, of course, also proof of binding, but provides no affinity information.

Once the fragment hits have been validated, the hit-to-lead process begins. It is essential for the success of this process to have an assay that can reliably measure the affinities of very weak binders, is robust enough to tolerate high concentrations of compounds and solvent [i.e., dimethyl sulfoxide (DMSO)], and has sufficient throughput to test tens to hundreds of compounds. Hits are typically ranked on the basis of ligand efficiency and other factors (e.g., synthetic attractiveness, availability of structural information), and analogs are screened to expand the scaffold classes, find more potent compounds, and identify structure/activity relationships. In choosing hits for follow-up, an LE > 0.3 kcal/mol-atom cutoff is sometimes imposed because this is the minimum LE value predicted to produce a 10 nM final inhibitor that conforms to the MW = 500 (rule-of-five) limit.

The most desirable result from the hit-to-lead process is to find multiple scaffolds that bind to the same hot spot on the receptor using a similar pattern of interactions and that offer chemically tractable sites for adding functional groups that can access nearby subsites. Using the bound structures of overlapping hits it is sometimes possible to design hybrid molecules that combine the features of multiple molecules. As fragments are optimized into potent inhibitors, they usually maintain the original binding mode of the fragment hit. Caution is indicated if the hits are found to bind at multiple locations in the active site and/or in a variety of different orientations, without making a consistent set of interactions with the receptor, or if the binding mode changes dramatically during optimization. These observations indicate that the fragments can bind in many different modes that have approximately the same energy, rather than a single mode that is much lower in energy than the rest, and the binding energy landscape of the receptor may not offer a suitable hot spot for placing a molecular anchor.[33] We suspect that proteins exhibiting a high degree of conformational flexibility may be particularly susceptible to this problem, because they are more likely to possess multiple conformational states that have similar energies.

For cases where two or more fragments are found to bind in close proximity, the additivity of binding energies[37,46,47] favors linking them together (e.g., linking two millimolar fragments to make a micromolar binder). Because the linked molecule suffers an entropic penalty on binding of just one rather than two molecules, it is expected to be much more potent than the sum of the fragments. Although the linking approach is conceptually elegant, it is seldom used because of the practical difficulty of connecting two fragments using the limited set of synthetically accessible bond lengths and angles provided by nature, without straining or perturbing the favorable interactions of either fragment or introducing unfavorable entropic or enthalpic effects from the linker. In practice, the actual potency gained by linking fragments is usually significantly less than theory (in one study the gains were, on average, fivefold lower than expected).[48] Also, in many cases the binding site contains only one hot spot consistently targeted by fragments, so a set of independent second site binders is not available. For these reasons, it is far more common for fragments to be optimized by elaborating or building out from scaffolds bound to a single site.

EXPERIMENTAL METHODS: DETECTION OF FRAGMENT BINDING BY NMR

In the early development of NMR fragment-based screening techniques, literature descriptions of new experiments focused on methods of detection rather than the lead generation strategies. As the number of studies grew, and real drug discovery problems were addressed, it became apparent that experimental approaches and fragment follow-up strategies could be combined in many different ways to uniquely address each target and drug design program. For this reason, it is best to consider the physical methods used to detect binding in NMR-based screening separately from the strategies used to elaborate fragment hits into medicinal chemistry leads. In the following sections, the most commonly used experimental techniques are reviewed.

NMR has long been established as a sensitive method for detecting binding of small molecules to macromolecular targets. Methods for detecting ligand binding by NMR can be either target directed or ligand directed. Target-directed methods rely on observing a change in an observable NMR parameter of the target biomolecule that results from its interaction with a ligand. Alternatively, ligand-directed techniques rely on the observation of a change in an NMR parameter of the ligand, which arises as a consequence of its interaction with the target receptor. Each method has advantages and disadvantages, and choosing the optimal approach will depend on a number of factors such as the molecular weight of the macromolecule, solubility and expression yield of the target protein, and, most importantly, the overall requirements of the drug discovery project.

Target-directed methods

Target-directed detection of ligand binding is most often accomplished by observing differences between the chemical shift of one or more resonances of the receptor spectrum in the presence of a mixture of ligands relative to those of a reference spectrum of the receptor in the unliganded state. When differences are observed, additional spectra are then acquired using the individual components of the ligand mixture to deconvolute the mixture spectrum and determine the identity of the binding ligand. In principle, any NMR spectrum can be acquired for this purpose, but the high sensitivity and resolution of two-dimensional ^{15}N-^{1}H correlation spectroscopy using uniformly ^{15}N labeled protein makes it the most frequently chosen method. If sequence-specific resonance assignments are available for the target protein, the amino acid residues at the interaction site of the ligand can be readily identified by comparison with resonances observed to undergo chemical shift perturbations.

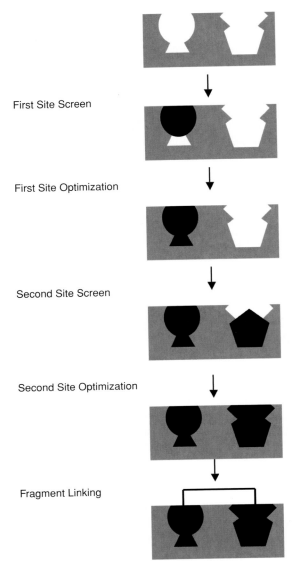

First Site Screen

First Site Optimization

Second Site Screen

Second Site Optimization

Fragment Linking

Figure 4.3. Outline of the SAR by NMR method. The SAR by NMR method consists of several steps. First, a molecule is identified that binds to one subsite. This scaffold is then optimized for affinity to the first subsite. A second compound is then identified that binds to an adjacent subsite. The second ligand is then optimized for maximum affinity. Finally, based on structural input, a linker is designed to optimally connect the two scaffolds (adapted from Shuker et al.[1]).

Direct detection of ligand binding can be a powerful technique in providing information for the drug discovery process. Because the sequence-specific assignments of the spectrum are usually determined before screening takes place, localization of ligand binding is revealed by the observed chemical shift perturbations. In addition, this information allows the discrimination of nonspecific and nonrelevant ligand binding from binding that affects the activity of the target protein and can be used as input to processes to develop more potent binding ligands, such as SAR by NMR.[1] This approach (illustrated in Figure 4.3)

relies on the identification of two distinct fragment binding sites on the target protein that are close in proximity. Optimal linking of the two fragments may result in a high-affinity ligand. SAR by NMR has become the principal motivation for target-directed detection of fragment binding using uniformly labeled proteins. Numerous applications of SAR by NMR and similar target-directed strategies have been reviewed in the literature.[11,49–56]

The use of chemical shift perturbation in uniformly labeled proteins to detect binding is limited by several factors. Because many ^{15}N-^{1}H correlation spectra are required to both screen the library and deconvolute the binding mixtures, a relatively large quantity of ^{15}N labeled protein must be available before studies can be undertaken. Furthermore, the target of interest must be sufficiently soluble and present in high concentrations so that data can be acquired without the need for excessive signal averaging. The actual quantity of protein required will depend on the library size and composition as well as the sensitivity of the available NMR instrumentation. For example, if reasonable data can be acquired at a target protein concentration of 100 μM on a 25-kDa protein, then screening 200 NMR samples of a 500-μl volume would require 250 mg of labeled protein. This would be sufficient to screen a library of 1,000–2,000 compounds (neglecting deconvolution) if each mixture contained five to ten fragments. Additional labeled protein would be required to obtain spectra of individual compounds from the "hit" mixtures to identify the binding ligand. For these reasons, some groups have developed strategies to minimize protein consumption and labeling costs, such as using NMR flow systems.[57]

To take full advantage of the information provided by target-directed screening methods, it is advantageous to have the sequence-specific resonance assignments of the target protein available. This requirement imposes further limitations on the method. For well-behaved, highly soluble proteins with molecular masses below approximately 25 kDa, three-dimensional triple resonance spectra of doubly labeled proteins can often be used efficiently to provide these assignments. At higher molecular masses, the requirement to perdeuterate the target protein to acquire triple resonance spectra[58] creates additional difficulties in protein expression. The lengthy data acquisition process, combined with complexity of obtaining resonance assignments of these large proteins, may make the process so time-consuming as to reduce the impact of information generated by NMR detected fragment screening approaches.

One technique to circumvent many of the limitations associated with uniformly labeled target protein has been described previously.[59] Provided that the binding site of interest is known independently (for example, by mutagenesis or structural studies) and it contains a sequentially unique pair of amino acids, an amino acid–specific labeling strategy may be employed to detect relevant binding without the need for determining complete sequence-specific resonance assignments. In this method, the *i*th residue is labeled with ^{13}C while the ith+1 amino acid is labeled with ^{15}N. Acquisition of a two-dimensional HNCO spectrum (which correlates the H and N resonances of the ith residue with the CO resonance of the ith-1 residue)[60,61] will consist of a single peak, which acts as a "spy" on the state of the binding site of interest. Because only one peak is observed, the demands on the sensitivity and resolution of the data can be relaxed, increasing both the molecular mass and solubility range of the method relative to that of the uniformly labeled approach. Another approach, described later in this chapter, that bypasses the need for full resonance assignments of the target is to use a well-characterized test ligand, for example, a known inhibitor, to induce perturbations in the ^{15}N-^{1}H correlation spectrum and then screen for new ligands that perturb the same resonances. This approach was used successfully for screening and fragment-based design of potent inhibitors for prostaglandin D synthase.[62]

Ligand-directed methods

Because of the limitations of target-directed methods described in the previous section, ligand-directed methods have become the most widely applied detection scheme for fragment screening by NMR. Although they contain less information about the ligand binding site than target-directed methods, they are more generally applicable and more rapidly implemented, making them highly valuable in the early drug discovery process. Ligand-directed methods enjoy a significant advantage, in that there are no limitations on the molecular mass of the target (and in fact are usually better suited to large targets). In addition, the protein required for ligand-directed methods need not be isotopically labeled, which provides more flexibility in the choice of expression systems that can be used to generate the sample. Finally, because it is the ligand that is observed, and the experimental mixtures contain a large excess of ligand relative to the protein, experiments can be performed with much less protein than in target-directed experiments, thus reducing the amount of protein that must be expressed and purified and also extending the solubility range of the targets that can be screened.

Despite these advantages, ligand-directed methods have two disadvantages relative to target-directed methods that should be considered before studies are undertaken. The first is that these methods require the ligand to be in rapid exchange between the bound and free state and are consequently limited to weakly binding fragments ($K_d > \sim 10^{-7}$ M). This is usually not a serious limitation as low MW fragments are expected to bind weakly and have been prescreened for good solubility. The second disadvantage is that these methods do not provide information about the nature of the binding site on the target receptor and as a result cannot distinguish nonspecific and/or biologically irrelevant association from binding at the desired site of the target.

Saturation transfer difference methods

Ligand-directed methods may be divided into to two distinct classes of experiments. One type of experiment relies on detecting a difference in an NMR observable parameter that is dependent on a change in the rotational correlation time (τ_c) of the small molecule ligand, resulting from interaction with the target receptor. Another class of experiments is based on transfer of magnetization between the target receptor and ligand that occurs during the time that the two molecules are bound to one another. In either method, the off rate of the ligand/protein complex must be fast on the NMR time scale ($K_{off} > \sim 100$ s^{-1}), such that the signal observed represents the population weighted average of the free and bound states of the ligand.

An example of the latter type of experiment is saturation transfer difference (STD) spectroscopy,[63] which is one of the most robust, and frequently employed, methods for detecting fragment binding by NMR. In this method, a train of frequency selective ^{1}H radio frequency (RF) pulses is applied for a number of seconds at a frequency that excites some resonances of the protein target but none of the ligand resonances of the fragment (or mixture of fragments) (Figure 4.4). During this saturation time, magnetization is transferred by spin diffusion from the selectively irradiated nuclei to all protons of the protein. In addition, this magnetization is transferred from the target protein to any small molecules that bind to the target. Provided that the ligand is in fast exchange on the NMR time scale, many target/ligand binding events will take place during the saturation time, resulting in a partial saturation of the fragments that have bound. A 90° pulse is then applied and a proton spectrum is recorded. A second data set is then acquired, this time applying the same selective ^{1}H RF saturation, except at a frequency that does not disturb the magnetization state of the nuclei of either the target protein or ligands. Ligands that do not interact with the protein do not have their proton magnetization perturbed in either spectrum, and subtraction of the data sets results in a null difference spectrum. For ligands that do interact with the target protein, a difference spectrum is observed and is used to determine the identity of the binding compound in the mixture of compounds (Figure 4.5). STD experiments (and virtually all other NMR-detected fragment screening methods) are most often applied to systems containing a soluble, purified protein but can be extended to more challenging and heterogeneous systems. For example, Claasen et al.[64] have reported using a double difference STD experiment to observe peptide binding to the membrane protein integrin expressed on the surface of intact platelets. Ligand binding can also be observed to integrin reconstituted into liposomes.[65]

WaterLOGSY

An alternative method to transfer magnetization from the target protein to the binding ligand has been described by Dalvit and coworkers.[66,67] In the WaterLOGSY (Water/Ligand Observed via Gradient SpectroscopY) experiment,

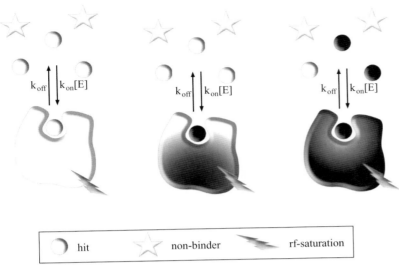

the bulk solvent is employed to create nonequilibrium magnetization on the target receptor, which is then transferred to a weakly binding ligand. At the beginning of the experiment, the magnetization of the bulk solvent (and protons of the target receptor whose resonance frequency is near that of bulk water) is either saturated or inverted by a selective 180° RF pulse. During the mixing time of the experiment, magnetization is transferred to the target protein by chemical exchange of the labile HN and OH protons of the target protein, as well as via cross-relaxation between the bulk solvent and protein protons. Magnetization is also transferred to ligands by either direct cross-relaxation with bulk solvent or relayed cross-relaxation via the target receptor. The magnetization transfer pathways are depicted in Figure 4.6. The resulting spectrum contains resonances from all the ligands in the fragment mixture. The binding ligands can be distinguished from the nonbinding ligands from the difference in the sign of the resonance peak as shown in Figure 4.7. Although a somewhat more technically challenging approach than STD methods, the WaterLOGSY experiment provides an excellent alternative when spin diffusion in the target receptor is inefficient. This situation typically arises where the target has a low proton density (i.e., nucleic acids).[68,69]

Relaxation and diffusion-based methods

There are also a number of ligand-directed methods that do not rely on intermolecular magnetization transfer between the fragment and target receptor but instead take advantage of a change in the translational and/or rotational mobility of the small molecule resulting from target binding. For example, the apparent diffusion coefficient of a small molecule is altered as a consequence of its interaction with a large molecule, while that of a noninteracting molecule is unaffected. Pulsed-field-gradient stimulated-echo experiments may be used to measure the difference in diffusion rates for ligands in the presence and absence of target protein receptor and thus detect binding ligands in a mixture of compounds.[70,71]

Interaction of a ligand with a large target molecule also alters the average rotational correlation time of the small molecule, and as a result, its relaxation properties. Shortened transverse relaxation times (due to longer average rotational correlation times and chemical exchange processes) are manifested in line broadening of the spectrum, which is often easily observable in a one-dimensional proton spectrum. Alternatively, the same phenomena can be observed by employing a CPMG (Carr-Purcell-Meiboom-Gill) pulse train (or, in the case of measuring $T_{1\rho}$, a spin lock) and determining the difference in peak intensity of ligand resonances in the presence and absence of the target of interest.[72] This effect can be enhanced by incorporation of one or more paramagnetic spin labels on the target protein by covalent modification of side chains such as lysine, tyrosine, cysteine, histidine, and methionine. This method (known as SLAPSTIC or Spin Labels Attached to Protein Side chains as a Tool to identify Interacting Compounds)[73,74] has a distinct advantage in sensitivity over detecting exchange line broadening in native proteins. Because the magnitude of the proton/electron dipole-dipole interaction is much larger than the proton-proton interaction, the effect extends over a much larger distance and allows lower bound ligand fractions, resulting in a lower protein concentration requirement. To apply this method, it must first be demonstrated that attachment of the spin label does not affect the binding properties or activity of the target receptor, which in turn requires detailed knowledge of the target's three-dimensional structure.

Longitudinal relaxation rates (R_1) can also be affected by binding to the target receptor and can be used to identify fragment binding in mixtures. As described by Peng et al.,[52] only selective R_1 measurements are useful in detecting ligand binding. However, it is impractical to have a different selective inversion RF pulse for every compound in a fragment library. An alternative method is to collect two-dimensional nuclear overhauser effect (NOE) spectra to identify those ligands that exhibit transferred

NOEs.[2] Interproton NOEs of small molecules are positive and have cross-peaks with signs that are opposite to those of the diagonal peaks. When a small molecule binds to a high-molecular-weight receptor, a transferred NOE can be observed, which is negative and has the same sign as the diagonal peak. Thus, binding ligands are easily recognized by a change in the sign of ligand NOEs. This method is less sensitive than other methods, such as STD spectroscopy; however, it is capable of providing information regarding the structure of the bound ligand. Moreover, intermolecular NOEs can be detected if two fragments bind in close proximity. Generally speaking, it is impractical to collect a large number of 2D spectra for screening purposes, and this method is not widely employed.

Competition binding methods

Competitive binding studies can be used to address some of the shortcomings of ligand-directed methods in a number of ways. As previously mentioned, the problem of nonspecific binding must be addressed when applying ligand-directed methods. Because of the large ligand-to-protein ratio, nonspecific binding of fragments to hydrophobic patches on the protein surface is common and can generate false positive results. To properly interpret the results of a ligand-directed fragment screen, low-affinity specific binding to the target site of interest must be distinguished from binding to other, nonfunctional sites. Although this could be accomplished by dilution/titration studies,[75] employing a competitive binding strategy is the most straightforward method for identifying specific binding. In this case, the aim is to displace the weakly binding ligand with a high-affinity ligand that is known to bind to the desired site on the target. If the fragment is displaced, the original NMR signal that indicated binding is eliminated, and it can be concluded with some confidence (assuming the absence of an allosteric effect) that the fragment was bound specifically and with low affinity to the active site of the target. Conversely, if the NMR signal is unchanged on addition of a high-affinity ligand, it is likely that nonspecific binding is being observed. It should be noted that the competing ligand itself is usually not detected as a binder directly, because a high-affinity ligand is not expected be in fast exchange between the bound and unbound states.

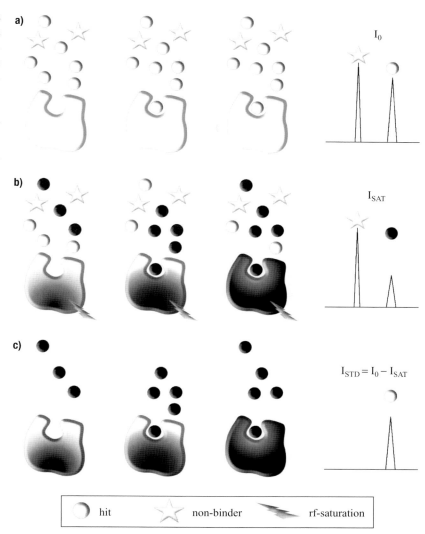

Figure 4.5. Schematic diagram depicting difference spectroscopy in the STD experiment. Circles and stars indicate binding and nonbinding compounds, respectively. STD involves two experiments: an off-resonance and an on-resonance experiment. (a) Off-resonance (reference) applies RF irradiation off-resonance from both receptor and compound protons. Detection produces spectra with intensity I_0. (b) In the on-resonance experiment, the RF irradiation (lightning bolt) selectively saturates receptor and any binding compounds (indicated by dark shading). This manifests as the decreased signal intensity I_{SAT}. (c) The STD response is the spectral difference $I_{STD} = I_0 - I_{SAT}$, which yields only resonances of the receptor and binding compounds. Receptor resonances are usually invisible due to either low concentration or relaxation filtering. The STD sensitivity depends on the number of ligands receiving saturation from the receptor and can be described in terms of the average number of saturated ligands produced per receptor molecule. Reprinted with permission from *Chemical Reviews* (2004), 104 (8) 3641–3675. © 2004 American Chemical Society.

Competitive binding may also be used to extend the affinity range that can be detected via ligand-directed methods. A weakly binding ligand that is known to interact with the target specifically, and in the desired binding site, is selected as a "spy" on the binding state of the receptor. A series of ligands is then screened against the target/weak ligand mixture. If a reduction or elimination of the binding signal from the reference ligand is observed, then it

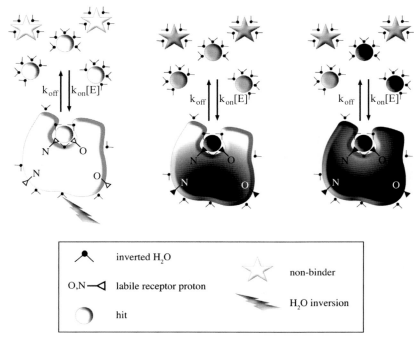

inverted H$_2$O

O,N —◁ labile receptor proton

◐ hit

non-binder

H$_2$O inversion

Figure 4.6. Magnetization transfer mechanisms underlying WaterLOGSY.[66,67] Magnetization transfer from bulk water to ligand occurs via labile receptor protons within and remote from the ligand binding site as well as from long-lived water molecules within the binding pocket. Dark gray and light gray shading indicate magnetization transfer from inverted water to ligand protons in the slow tumbling (i.e., receptor/ligand complex) and fast tumbling (i.e., free ligand) limits, respectively. Only the hits experience both types of magnetization transfer. The pool of free ligands having experienced inversion-transfer from bulk water builds up as ligand continues to exchange on and off the receptor. Reprinted with permission from *Chemical Reviews* (2004), 104 (8) 3641–3675. © 2004 American Chemical Society.

can be concluded that a compound in the sample has displaced the spy ligand. This method is capable of discriminating between specific and nonspecific binding as well as being sensitive to high-affinity ligands, and there are a number of examples in the literature applying this strategy using both relaxation[76] and magnetization transfer[77] experimental approaches. It is also possible to determine a rank order of binding of ligands and, if the affinity of the reporter ligand is independently known, to make good estimates of the K_d of competing ligands in a single measurement.

APPLICATIONS OF NMR FRAGMENT-BASED SCREENING: ILLUSTRATIVE EXAMPLES

Although the early literature focused primarily on proof-of-concept studies with model systems[1,2] and development of the experimental techniques required to detect ligand binding by NMR,[52] much of the published work from the past few years describes applications of fragment-based screening in bona fide discovery programs. Some of these studies are "NMR-centric," whereas others use NMR (or other methods) to detect binding and x-ray crystallography to guide hits-to-leads chemistry. Regardless of the strategy chosen, however, the ultimate goal is to turn low-molecular-weight fragments that bind receptor "hot spots" into potent,

elaborated leads with the potential to be further optimized into drug molecules. From a literature survey alone, it is difficult to assess the probability of success for fragment-based screening efforts, because many published studies describe low-potency leads from failed discovery programs. Many interesting drug leads, even those with high potencies, will eventually fail at a later stage for reasons that cannot be addressed at the hits-to-leads stage, for example, inadequate selectivity against other isoforms of the target (or closely related proteins) or, more commonly, unacceptable ADME properties or animal toxicity. However, it is valuable to understand and recognize situations in which a fragment-based strategy has a lower chance of success and, if possible, employ alternative approaches in parallel as a hedge. For example, consider the case where a target is screened by HTS and no hits are identified. Although the possibility exists that not enough compounds were screened, or the diversity of the library was not optimal for the target, in cases where large corporate compound collections were screened, these explanations are less likely. Alternatively, the target may not possess the hot spots required to accommodate a potent drug molecule (i.e., the target is simply not druggable).[35] Another caveat when considering targets for fragment-based design concerns the validity of the structural models used for elaboration of weak fragment hits. For example, if one is using x-ray crystallographic

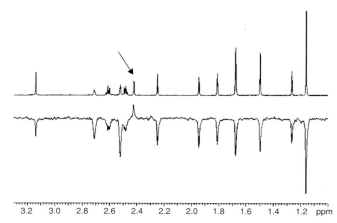

Figure 4.7. Example of the WaterLOGSY experiment. One-dimensional reference (upper) and WaterLOGSY (lower) spectra recorded for a ten-compound mixture in the presence of 10 μM cdk2. Positive and negative signals in the lower spectrum identify ckd2 binding and nonbinding compounds, respectively. The arrow indicates the methyl group resonances of the cdk2 ligand ethyl α-(ethoxycarbonyl)-3-indoleacrylate. Figure and legend are reprinted with permission from *J. Biomol. NMR* **18**: 65–68 (2000). The figure was kindly provided by Dr. Claudio Dalvit.

structures to suggest ways to grow or link bound fragments, it is usually assumed that the protein structure in the presence of the bound fragment is the same as with a more fully elaborated molecule. This might not be the case at all for compounds soaked into crystals of an apo protein. For example, are ligand-induced conformational changes necessary to access additional subsites via linked or elaborated substituents? Conformational heterogeneity, either intrinsic or related to mechanism, should be recognized and taken into account when choosing an appropriate structural model. In such cases, having NMR structural and dynamic data to complement the crystallographic data can be useful.[78] Alternatively, having x-ray structures from multiple crystal forms might provide insight.[78]

Having discussed both the advantages and the potential pitfalls of fragment-based design, we now turn to describing the different strategies that may be used to develop fragment hits into more potent leads. The transformation of validated hits into viable drug leads has been addressed using several approaches, generally described as combining, elaborating, or varying the molecular fragments.[22,69] Initially, the different methods for detecting ligand binding were primarily associated with a particular strategy (e.g., SAR by NMR[1] was associated with fragment combination and SHAPES[2] with fragment elaboration), but these distinctions have faded as new methods and studies have evolved. We therefore find that classifying applications by the hit development strategy is more generally useful than classifying by detection method. This classification, however, is also imperfect because more than one strategy is often applied in a given application. This reflects the flexibility and ease with which these methods may be tailored to address the problem at hand. The following sections present examples of applications of each of the three strategies.

Applications of fragment linking: The combination strategy

Combining multiple, weakly binding molecular fragments into larger, more complex molecules may potentially increase binding affinity by orders of magnitude, because binding energies are expected to be approximately additive.[1,48] To achieve this in practice, structural information that can describe the relative orientations of and distances between the bound fragments is required and is commonly derived from NOE measurements,[2,79–81] chemical shift perturbation mapping experiments,[56,82–85] or from x-ray crystallographic structures.[3,69,78,86–91] Structural information can also be inferred when fragments bind at overlapping subsites, such that the relative positions of their functional groups are apparent from the molecular topology, a procedure called *fragment fusion*.[2,69,87]

The earliest work in NMR-based fragment linking used the SAR by NMR method, in which protein-detected heteronuclear single-quantum correlation (HSQC) based methods were employed to characterize binding, and either x-ray crystallography or NOE-derived NMR structures were used to determine the bound fragment orientations. Early SAR by NMR examples were mostly proof-of-concept cases and have been extensively reviewed.[11,39,49] More recent SAR by NMR work, such as the design of Bcl-x_L[92,93] and Hsp90 inhibitors,[78] are significantly more relevant from a pharmaceutical perspective and illustrate the real potential of these methods in the ideal research environment.

Perhaps the best success story to date using the fragment linking strategy involves the design of Bcl-x_L inhibitors by the Abbott group. Although many interesting case studies have been reported by this group,[39] this is the first in which potent inhibitors of a protein/protein interaction were designed. In an initial study,[93] NMR chemical shift perturbation screening identified a biaryl acid with $K_d = 300$ μM (LE = 0.30 kcal/mol-atom) for the BH3 peptide binding groove (Figure 4.8). Using the SAR by NMR linking strategy, a second fragment was identified that bound near the first-site ligand, and a linked compound was synthesized possessing $K_i = 1.4$ μM. The NMR structure and a parallel synthesis approach were used to further optimize the linked Bcl-x_L lead to produce a compound with $K_i = 36$ nM and LE ∼ 0.27 kcal/mol-atom. In a second study,[92] the affinity of this compound was shown to be attenuated by a factor of >280 in the presence of 1% human serum. To suggest ways to reduce serum albumin binding, the x-ray structure of the compound bound to HSA was solved, leading to the addition of a basic 2-dimethylaminoethyl group to the thioethylamino linker, and replacement of a fluorophenyl group with a substituted piperazine. To further improve binding to Bcl-2, an additional lipophilic group was added to the piperazine to occupy an additional binding pocket unique to Bcl-2 inhibitor complexes.[94] The final compound, ABT-737, bound to Bcl-x_L, Bcl-2, and Bcl-w with $K_i < 1$ nM and retained nanomolar potency against Bcl-X_L (IC$_{50}$ = 35 nM) in the presence of 10% human serum. ABT-737 was active in killing cells from lymphoma, small-cell lung carcinoma, and patient-derived cell lines and also showed efficacy in improving survival and tumor regression and effecting cures in mouse cancer models.[92]

Another study from the Abbott group used a dual strategy of fragment linking and fragment elaboration to design inhibitors of Hsp90.[78] Initial NMR-based screening yielded two related chemotypes, an aminotriazine and an aminopyrimidine (Figure 4.9). Both fragments were shown to bind with affinities <20 μM and high ligand efficiencies (BEI = 21 and 27, respectively). Using a fragment elaboration strategy guided by x-ray crystallographic structures and high-throughput organic synthesis, the authors discovered a 60 nM inhibitor (Compound 5, BEI = 26), which bound to the open state of the Hsp90 protein. An alternative approach, using SAR-by-NMR-style fragment linking, resulted in two additional leads with K_i in the low micromolar range [Compound 6, $K_i = 1.9$ μM (BEI = 15); Compound 7, $K_i = 4$ μM (BEI = 17)] (Figure 4.9). The lack of binding synergy and lower affinities of Compounds 6 and 7 compared to Compound 5 are attributed to less than optimal

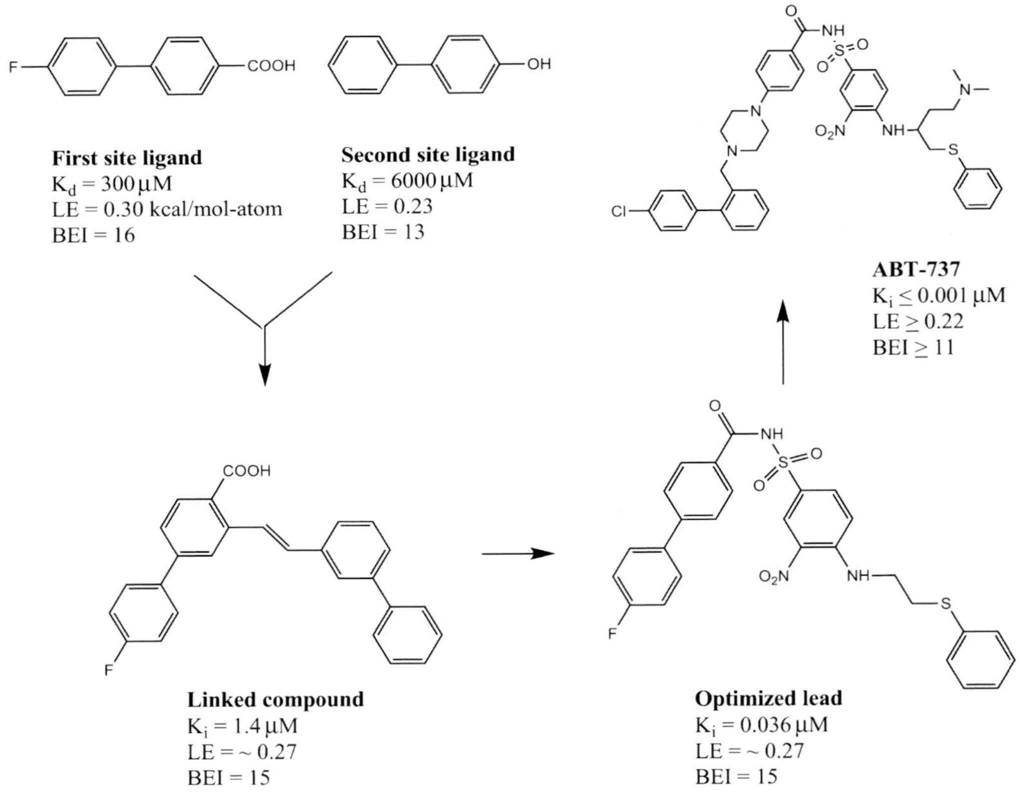

Figure 4.8. Compound flow chart showing fragment linking and optimization of Bcl-X$_L$ inhibitors.

chemical exploration of potential linkers for these fragments. What is unique about this study is that two unique binding modes were observed for several of the fragments when bound simultaneously to Hsp90 (Figure 4.10). Each of these modes led to the different linked leads targeting the closed (Compound 6) or open (Compound 7) state of the protein. The authors also reveal that Hsp90 is a particularly dynamic target, with many conformations sampled by the protein as shown by both NMR measurements and

crystallographic observations. This intrinsic flexibility, and ability of Hsp90 to access multiple conformational states as determined by NMR (line broadening for residues 105–121) and x-ray crystallography (multiple observed conformations from multiple crystal forms), led to different binding modes of fragments observed by crystallography versus NMR. Based on these findings, the authors caution against "rigid interpretation of any single piece of structural data."[78]

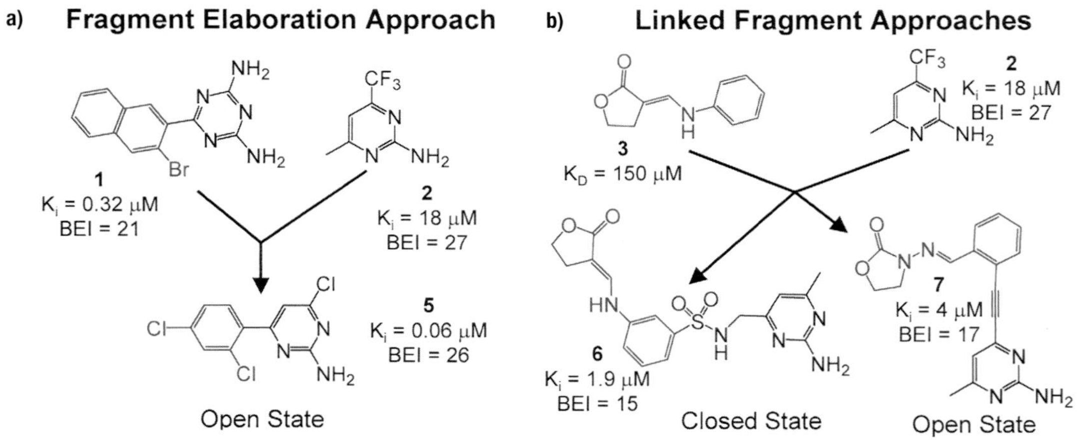

Figure 4.9. Compound flow chart for design of Hsp90 inhibitors. Reprinted from Huth et al.[78] with permission. The figure was kindly provided by Dr. Phil Hajduk.

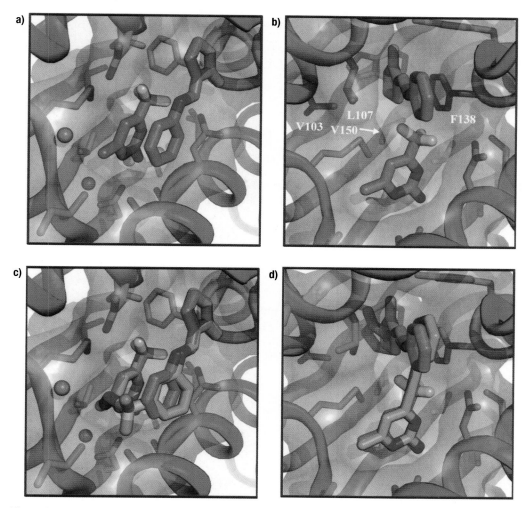

Figure 4.10. Binding of fragment hits compared to binding of linked compounds to Hsp90. Atom coloring for the fragment hits: carbons in magenta, nitrogens in blue, oxygen in red, and fluorines in light blue. Atom coloring for the linked compounds is the same except that carbons are in orange. (a) X-ray crystallographic structure of a ternary complex with Compounds **2** and **3** (compound chemical structures shown in Figure 4.9). (b) NOE-based model of the same ternary complex with Compounds **2** and **3** showing an alternate binding mode in solution. The side chains of L107, L103, F138, and V150 are colored in red to indicate key NOEs from HSP90 to **3** that were used to construct the model. (c) X-ray crystallographic structure of a binary complex with Compound **6** overlaid with the ternary complex shown in (a). Note the near perfect alignment of the linked and unlinked fragments. (d) X-ray crystallographic structure of a binary complex with Compound **7** overlaid with the model of the ternary complex shown in (b). Note that the oxazolidinone accesses the back of the pocket in an "open" conformation of HSP90 as suggested by the NOE-based model (shown in B). Figure and legend reprinted with permission from Huth et al.[78] The figure was kindly provided by Dr. Phil Hajduk.

Elaboration and variation of fragment hits

In the elaboration strategy, relatively simple primary hits are elaborated by adding chemical functionality, producing more complex molecules. The more elaborate molecules can make additional ligand/protein interactions, leading to higher potency. In the variation strategy, selected portions of a primary screening hit are systematically modified. The goal of this strategy is to identify and screen compounds that are of similar complexity to the primary hits but possess more optimal interactions with the target.

Both strategies may be pursued by purchasing analogs, screening similar scaffolds from corporate compound collections, or synthesis of second generation compounds. The elaboration strategy is particularly amenable to parallel synthesis strategies.[21,95–98] In both cases, structural information is not required but can be highly valuable for optimizing ligand/protein contacts and for selecting the type and location of functionalities to be added.

One of the first reported methods using fragment elaboration was the SHAPES strategy, an adaptable approach that follows ligand-detected NMR screening of druglike

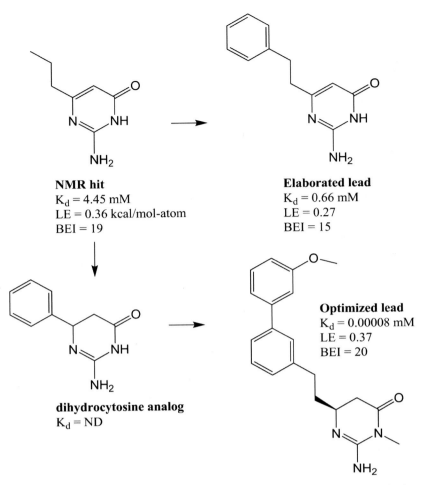

NMR hit
$K_d = 4.45$ mM
LE = 0.36 kcal/mol-atom
BEI = 19

Elaborated lead
$K_d = 0.66$ mM
LE = 0.27
BEI = 15

dihydrocytosine analog
K_d = ND

Optimized lead
$K_d = 0.00008$ mM
LE = 0.37
BEI = 20

Figure 4.11. Compound flow chart showing fragment variation, elaboration, and optimization of β-secretase inhibitors. Adapted from Edwards et al.[100]

molecules with successive rounds of activity assays and structure-based optimization.[2,69,87] A classical example of the elaboration strategy is the SHAPES screen of fatty acid binding protein (FABP-4).[11,69] Based on the crystal structures of two primary screening hits with low micromolar potencies, a follow-up library of 134 elaborated analogs was screened calorimetrically, which in turn produced nine leads with low micromolar to nanomolar affinities. The crystal structures of five more bound ligands were subsequently solved, mapping out the essential ligand/protein interactions and defining the binding pharmacophore. Other early examples of fragment elaboration include the design of urokinase inhibitors[88,99] and the discovery of new zinc-binding motifs for metalloprotease inhibitors.[85]

More recent publications report lead generation efforts targeting β-secretase (BACE-1)[100,101] and prostaglandin D synthase.[62] In the β-secretase example, an isocytosine fragment, a weak but efficient hit ($K_d = 4.45$ mM, LE = 0.36 kcal/mol-atom, BE = 19) from an NMR-based screen (Figure 4.11), was elaborated with larger substituents at the C6 position, yielding an approximately sevenfold improvement in potency, although at the expense of lower efficiency

($K_d = 0.66$ mM; LE = 0.27 kcal/mol-atom).[101] These scaffolds, despite their low affinity, represent reasonable starting points for further optimization based on their better ligand efficiency compared to known BACE-1 inhibitors (for example, substrate analog OM99–2 has $K_i = 1.6$ nM and LE ~0.19 kcal/mol-atom, BEI = 10). Also, like a previous scaffold class of interest, the aminopyrimidines,[102,103] the isocytosines possess a cyclic amidine capable of recognizing catalytic aspartate residues, as well as a hydrophobic substituent to access the S1 subsite of BACE-1. Additional testing of analogs, using a variation strategy,[100] identified the dihydroisocytosines as a more potent class of BACE-1 inhibitors, with some smaller dihydroisocytosines showing 1,000-fold improvement over similar isocytosines. The most potent optimized lead possessed an $IC_{50} = 80$ nM and is highly efficient (LE ~ 0.37 kcal/mol-atom, BEI = 20), representing an excellent lead for further optimization.

Another recent study from researchers at AstraZeneca with the target prostaglandin D_2 synthase (PGDS)[62] provides an excellent example of fragment-based design using both variation and elaboration strategies. An initial NMR fragment screen was carried out using two libraries, a general 2,000-compound NMR screening library, and a targeted library of 450 compounds selected based on the x-ray crystallographic structure of PGDS. NMR screening of these libraries yielded twenty-four primary hits (six from the targeted library), with affinities in the range K_d ~50–500 μM (Figure 4.12). The screening procedure was unusual, in that a target-directed screen was carried out on ^{15}N-labeled protein but without chemical shift assignments. However, it was clear based on perturbations from reference compounds titrated against ^{15}N-labeled PGDS that the screening compounds were binding at the same site as the reference compounds, because the same resonances were being perturbed. X-ray structures with a known inhibitor and a primary NMR screening hit identified key pharmacophore interactions and helped guide selection of follow-up compounds for further screening. In this first iteration, compounds were selected from the corporate library based on the initial NMR hits, as well as one hit from virtual screening ($IC_{50} = 0.99$ μM). Hits from this first iteration showed an increase of up to 200-fold over the primary hits, with affinities (IC_{50}) ranging from ~0.14 to 50 μM. In a second iteration, x-ray structures suggested that the pyrazole group of an NMR screening hit could be combined with the thiazole of an elaborated lead (Figure 4.12). Several compounds in this series were submicromolar, with one combined

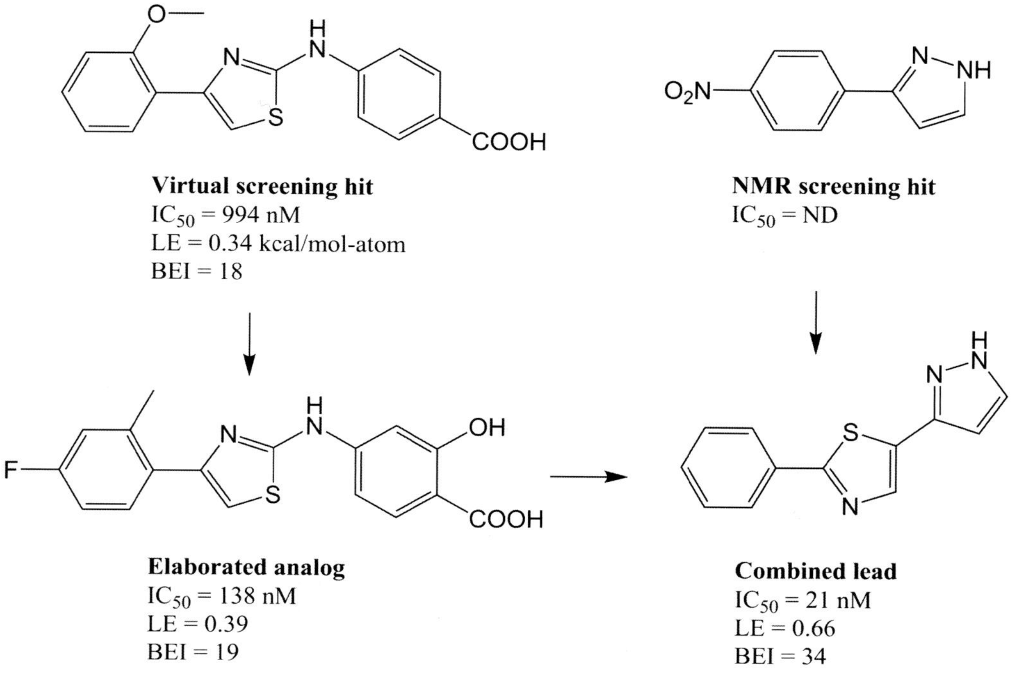

Figure 4.12. Compound flow chart showing fragment variation, elaboration, and optimization of prostaglandin D synthase inhibitors. Adapted from Hohwy et al.[62]

compound possessing an IC_{50} of 21 nM and a binding efficiency of 0.66 kcal/mol-atom, representing an optimal starting point for lead optimization of more druglike PGDS inhibitors.

CONCLUSIONS

It has been more than a decade since NMR fragment-based screening was introduced, and in that time the discipline has grown from a collection of experimental methods and drug design concepts into a mature discipline, one that provides a viable, and often preferred, alternative to HTS methods in early drug discovery. For each drug target and design challenge, detection of binding by NMR provides a starting point, but using that binding information to identify lead compounds with desirable, druglike properties requires a more complete strategy integrating computational, biochemical, biophysical, and synthetic tools and technologies. For this reason, we have forgone an exhaustive examination of NMR methods and their application in drug discovery and instead attempted to provide a synopsis of the more widely adopted NMR approaches. Beyond the physical and technical descriptions of the NMR experiments, we have also provided examples of how fragments have been linked, varied, elaborated, and optimized creatively in successful lead generation programs. Hopefully, the examples provided and references to the significant body of literature now available will enable researchers to implement these methods in their own laboratories and

develop drug design strategies uniquely matched to their own drug targets and program goals.

REFERENCES

1. Shuker, S. B.; Hajduk, P. J.; Meadows, R. P.; Fesik, S. W. Discovering high-affinity ligands for proteins: SAR by NMR. *Science* **1996**, *274*, 1531–1534.
2. Fejzo, J.; et al. The SHAPES strategy: an NMR-based approach for lead generation in drug discovery. *Chem. Biol.* **1999**, *6*, 755–769.
3. Boehm, H. J.; et al. Novel inhibitors of DNA gyrase: 3D structure based biased needle screening, hit validation by biophysical methods, and 3D guided optimization. A promising alternative to random screening. *J. Med. Chem.* **2000**, *43*, 2664–2674.
4. Lipinski, C. A.; Lombardo, F.; Dominy, B. W.; Feeny, P. J. Experimental and computational approaches to estimate solubility and permeability in drug discovery and development settings. *Adv. Drug Deliv. Rev.* **1997**, *23*, 3–25.
5. Teague, S. J.; Davis, A. M.; Leeson, P. D.; Oprea, T. The design of leadlike combinatorial libraries. *Angew. Chem. Int. Ed.* **1999**, *38*, 3743–3747.
6. Oprea, T. I.; Davis, A. M.; Teague, S. J.; Leeson, P. D. Is there a difference between leads and drugs? A historical perspective. *J. Chem. Inf. Comput. Sci.* **2001**, *41*, 1308–1315.
7. Bemis, G. W.; Murcko, M. A. The properties of known drugs. 1. Molecular frameworks. *J. Med. Chem.* **1996**, *39*, 2887–2893.
8. Lewell, X. Q.; Judd, D. B.; Watson, S. P.; Hann, M. M. RECAP – retrosynthetic combinatorial analysis procedure: a powerful new technique for identifying privileged molecular fragments

with useful applications in combinatorial chemistry. *J. Chem. Inf. Comput. Sci.* **1998**, *38*, 511–522.

9. Congreve, M.; Carr, R.; Murray, C.; Jhoti, H. A 'rule of three' for fragment-based lead discovery? *Drug Discov. Today* **2003**, *8*, 876–877.

10. Hann, M. M.; Oprea, T. I. Pursuing the leadlikeness concept in pharmaceutical research. *Curr. Opin. Chem. Biol.* **2004**, *8*, 255–263.

11. Lepre, C. A.; Moore, J. M.; Peng, J. W. Theory and applications of NMR-based screening in pharmaceutical research. *Chem. Rev.* **2004**, *104*, 3641–3676.

12. Schuffenhauer, A.; et al. Library design for fragment based screening. *Curr. Top. Med. Chem.* **2005**, *5*, 751–762.

13. Hann, M. M.; Leach, A. R.; Harper, G. Molecular complexity and its impact on the probability of finding leads for drug discovery. *J. Chem. Inf. Comput. Sci.* **2001**, *41*, 856–864.

14. Shoichet, B. K. Interpreting steep dose-response curves in early inhibitor discovery. *J. Med. Chem.* **2006**, *49*, 7274–7277.

15. Siegal, G.; Ab, E.; Schultz, J. Integration of fragment screening and library design. *Drug Discov. Today* **2007**, *12*, 1032–1039.

16. Congreve, M.; Chessari, G.; Tisi, D.; Woodhead, A. J. Recent developments in fragment-based drug discovery. *J. Med. Chem.* **2008**, *51*, 3661–3680.

17. Leeson, P. D.; Springthorpe, B. The influence of drug-like concepts on decision-making in medicinal chemistry. *Nat. Rev. Drug Discov.* **2007**, *6*, 881–890.

18. Bohacek, R. S.; McMartin, C.; Guida, W. C. The art and practice of structure-based drug design: a molecular modeling perspective. *Med. Res. Rev.* **1996**, *16*, 3–50.

19. Lipinski, C. A. Drug-like properties and the causes of poor solubility and poor permeability. *J. Pharmacol. Toxicol. Methods* **2000**, *44*, 235–249.

20. Fink, T.; Reymond, J. L. Virtual exploration of the chemical universe up to 11 atoms of C, N, O, F: assembly of 26.4 million structures (110.9 million stereoisomers) and analysis for new ring systems, stereochemistry, physicochemical properties, compound classes, and drug discovery. *J. Chem. Inf. Model* **2007**, *47*, 342–353.

21. Lepre, C. A. Library design for NMR-based screening. *Drug. Discov. Today* **2001**, *6*, 133–140.

22. Lepre, C. A. Strategies for NMR screening and library design. In: *BioNMR Techniques in Drug Research*, Zerbe, O.; Ed. Weinheim: Wiley-VCH; **2002**, 1349–1364.

23. Jacoby, E.; Davies, J.; Blommers, M. J. Design of small molecule libraries for NMR screening and other applications in drug discovery. *Curr. Top. Med. Chem.* **2003**, *3*, 11–23.

24. Baurin, N., et al. Design and characterization of libraries of molecular fragments for use in NMR screening against protein targets. *J. Chem. Inf. Comput. Sci.* **2004**, *44*, 2157–2166.

25. Hubbard, R. E.; Davis, B.; Chen, I.; Drysdale, M. J. The SeeDs approach: integrating fragments into drug discovery. *Curr. Top. Med. Chem.* **2007**, *7*, 1568–1581.

26. Hartshorn, M. J.; et al. Fragment-based lead discovery using X-ray crystallography. *J. Med. Chem.* **2005**, *48*, 403–413.

27. Blaney, J.; Nienaber, V.; Burley, S. Fragment-based lead discovery and optimisation using X-ray crystallography, computational chemistry, and high-throughput organic synthesis. In: *Fragment-Based Approaches in Drug Discovery: Methods and Principles in Medicinal Chemistry*, Vol. 34, Jahnke, W.; Erlanson, D.; Eds. Wennheim: Wiley–VCH; **2006**, 215–248.

28. Albert, J. S.; et al. An integrated approach to fragment-based lead generation: philosophy, strategy and case studies from AstraZeneca's drug discovery programmes. *Curr. Top. Med. Chem.* **2007**, *7*, 1600–1629.

29. Bogan, A. A.; Thorn, K. S. Anatomy of hot spots in protein interfaces. *J. Mol. Biol.* **1998**, *280*, 1–9.

30. Clackson, T.; Wells, J. A. A hot spot of binding energy in a hormone-receptor interface. *Science* **1995**, *267*, 383–386.

31. Moreira, I. S.; Fernandes, P. A.; Ramos, M. J. Hot spots–a review of the protein-protein interface determinant amino-acid residues. *Proteins* **2007**, *68*, 803–812.

32. Reichmann, D.; et al. Binding hot spots in the TEM1-BLIP interface in light of its modular architecture. *J. Mol. Biol.* **2007**, *365*, 663–679.

33. Rejto, P. A.; Verkhivker, G. M. Unraveling principles of lead discovery: from unfrustrated energy landscapes to novel molecular anchors. *Proc. Natl. Acad. Sci. U.S.A.* **1996**, *93*, 8945–8950.

34. Ciulli, A.; Williams, G.; Smith, A. G.; Blundell, T. L.; Abell, C. Probing hot spots at protein-ligand binding sites: a fragment-based approach using biophysical methods. *J. Med. Chem.* **2006**, *49*, 4992–5000.

35. Hajduk, P. J.; Huth, J. R.; Fesik, S. W. Druggability indices for protein targets derived from NMR-based screening data. *J. Med. Chem.* **2005**, *48*, 2518–2525.

36. Lobley, C. M.; et al. The crystal structure of *Escherichia coli* ketopantoate reductase with NADP+ bound. *Biochemistry* **2005**, *44*, 8930–8939.

37. Murray, C. W.; Verdonk, M. L. The consequences of translational and rotational entropy lost by small molecules on binding to proteins. *J. Comput. Aided Mol. Des.* **2002**, *16*, 741–753.

38. Page, M. I.; Jencks, W. P. Entropic contributions to rate accelerations in enzymic and intramolecular reactions and the chelate effect. *Proc. Natl. Acad. Sci. U.S.A.* **1971**, *68*, 1678–1683.

39. Hajduk, P. J.; Greer, J. A decade of fragment-based drug design: strategic advances and lessons learned. *Nat. Rev. Drug Discov.* **2007**, *6*, 211–219.

40. Hopkins, A. L.; Groom, C. R.; Alex, A. Ligand efficiency: a useful metric for lead selection. *Drug Discov. Today* **2004**, *9*, 430–431.

41. Abad-Zapatero, C.; Metz, J. T. Ligand efficiency indices as guideposts for drug discovery. *Drug Discov. Today* **2005**, *10*, 464–469.

42. Hajduk, P. J. Fragment-based drug design: how big is too big? *J. Med. Chem.* **2006**, *49*, 6972–6976.

43. Reynolds, C. H.; Tounge, B. A.; Bembenek, S. D. Ligand binding efficiency: trends, physical basis, and implications. *J. Med. Chem.* **2008**, *51*, 2432–243.

44. Vieth, M.; et al. Characteristic physical properties and structural fragments of marketed oral drugs. *J. Med. Chem.* **2004**, *47*, 224–232.

45. Wenlock, M. C.; Austin, R. P.; Barton, P.; Davis, A. M.; Leeson, P. D. A comparison of physiochemical property profiles of development and marketed oral drugs. *J. Med. Chem.* **2003**, *46*, 1250–1256.

46. Dill, K. A. Additivity principles in biochemistry. *J. Biol. Chem.* **1997**, *272*, 701–704.

47. Jencks, W. P. On the attribution and additivity of binding energies. *Proc. Natl. Acad. Sci. U.S.A.* **1981**, *78*, 4046–4050.

48. Hajduk, P. J.; Huth, J. R.; Sun, C. SAR by NMR: an analysis of potency gains realized through fragment-linking and fragment elaboration strategies for lead generation. In: *Fragment-Based Approaches in Drug Discovery*, Jahnke, W.; Erlanson, D. A.; Eds. Wennheim: Wiley-VCH; **2006**, 181–192.

49. Hajduk, P. J.; Meadows, R. P.; Fesik, S. J. NMR-based screening in drug discovery. *Q. Rev. Biophys.* **1999**, *32*, 211–240.

50. Moore, J. M. NMR screening in drug discovery. *Curr. Opin. Biotechnol.* **1999**, *10*, 54–58.

51. Pellecchia, M.; Sem, D. S.; Wuthrich, K. NMR in drug discovery. *Nat. Rev. Drug Discov.* **2002**, *1*, 211–219.

52. Peng, J. W.; Moore, J. M.; Abdul-Manan, N. NMR experiments for lead generation in drug discovery. *Prog. Nucl. Mag. Reson. Spectrosc.* **2004**, *44*, 225–256.

53. Roberts, G. C. Applications of NMR in drug discovery. *Drug Discov. Today* **2000**, *5*, 230–240.

54. Stockman, B.; Dalvit, C. NMR screening techniques in drug discovery and drug design. *Prog. Nucl. Mag. Reson. Spectrosc.* **2002**, *41*, 187–231.

55. van Dongen, M.; Weigelt, J.; Uppenberg, J.; Schultz, J.; Wikstrom, M. Structure-based screening and design in drug discovery. *Drug Discov. Today* **2002**, *7*, 471–478.

56. Wyss, D. F.; McCoy, M. A.; Senior, M. M. NMR-based approaches for lead discovery. *Curr. Opin. Drug Discov. Devel.* *5*, 630–647.

57. Ross, A.; Schlotterbeck, G.; Klaus, W.; Senn, H. Automation of NMR measurements and data evaluation for systematically screening interactions of small molecules with target proteins. *J. Biomol. NMR* **2000**, *16*, 139–146.

58. Salzmann, M.; Pervushin, K.; Wider, G.; Senn, H.; Wuthrich, K. TROSY in triple-resonance experiments: new perspectives for sequential NMR assignment of large proteins. *Proc. Natl. Acad. Sci. U.S.A.* **1998**, *95*, 13585–13590.

59. Weigelt, J.; van Dongen, M.; Uppenberg, J.; Schultz, J.; Wikström, M. Site-selective screening by NMR spectroscopy with labeled amino acid pairs. *J. Am. Chem. Soc.* **2002**, *124*, 2446–2447.

60. Grzesiek, S.; Bax, A. Improved 3D triple-resonance NMR techniques applied to a 31 kDa protein. *J. Magn. Reson.* **1992**, *96*, 432–440.

61. Ikura, M.; Kay, L.E.; Bax, A. A novel approach for sequential assignment of 1H, 13C, and 15N spectra of proteins: heteronuclear triple-resonance three-dimensional NMR spectroscopy. Application to calmodulin. *Biochemistry* **1990**, *29*, 4659–4667.

62. Hohwy, M.; et al. Novel prostaglandin D synthase inhibitors generated by fragment-based drug design. *J. Med. Chem.* **2008**, *51*, 2178–2186.

63. Mayer, M.; Meyer, B. Characterization of ligand binding by saturation transfer difference NMR spectroscopy. *Angew. Chem. Int. Ed.* **1999**, *38*, 1784–1788.

64. Claasen, B.; Axmann, M.; Meinecke, R.; Meyer, B. Direct observation of ligand binding to membrane proteins in living cells by a saturation transfer double difference (STDD) NMR spectroscopy method shows a significantly higher affinity of integrin alpha(IIb)beta3 in native platelets than in liposomes. *J. Am. Chem. Soc.* **2005**, *127*, 916–919.

65. Meinecke, R.; Meyer, B. Determination of the binding specificity of an integral membrane protein by saturation transfer difference NMR: RGD peptide ligands binding to integrin $\alpha_{IIb}\beta$. *J. Am. Chem. Soc.* **2001**, *44*, 3059–3065.

66. Dalvit, C.; Fogliatto, G.; Stewart, A.; Veronesi, M.; Stockman, B. WaterLOGSY as a method for primary NMR screening: practical aspects and range of applicability. *J. Biomol. NMR* **2001**, *21*, 349–359.

67. Dalvit, C.; et al. Identification of compounds with binding affinity to proteins via magnetization transfer from bulk water. *J. Biomol. NMR* **2000**, *18*, 65–68.

68. Johnson, E. C.; Feher, V. A.; Peng, J. W.; Moore, J. M.; Williamson, J. R. Application of NMR SHAPES screening to an RNA target. *J. Am. Chem. Soc.* **2003**, *125*, 15724–15725.

69. Lepre, C. A.; et al. Applications of SHAPES screening in drug discovery. *Comb. Chem. High Throughput Screen.* **2002**, *5*, 583–590.

70. Lin, M. L.; Shapiro, M. J.; Wareing, J. R. Diffusion-edited NMR: affinity NMR for direct observation of molecular interactions. *J. Am. Chem. Soc.* **1997**, *119*, 5349–5250.

71. Bleicher, K.; Lin, M.; Shapiro, M.; Wareing, J. Diffusion edited NMR: screening compound mixtures by affinity NMR to detect binding ligands to vancomycin. *J. Org. Chem.* **1998**, *63*, 8486–8490.

72. Hajduk, P. J.; Olejniczak, E. T.; Fesik, S. W. One-dimensional relaxation- and diffusion-edited NMR methods for screening compounds that bind to macromolecules. *J. Am. Chem. Soc.* **1997**, *119*, 12257–12261.

73. Jahnke, W.; et al. Second-site NMR screening with a spin-labeled first ligand. *J. Am. Chem. Soc.* **2000**, *122*, 7394–7395.

74. Jahnke, W.; Rudisser, S.; Zurini, M. Spin label enhanced NMR screening. *J. Am. Chem. Soc.* **2001**, *123*, 3149–3150.

75. Murali, N.; Jarori, G. K.; Landy, S. B.; Rao, B. D. Two-dimensional transferred nuclear Overhauser effect spectroscopy (TRNOESY) studies of nucleotide conformations in creatine kinase complexes: effects due to weak nonspecific binding. *Biochemistry* **1993**, *32*, 12941–12948.

76. Dalvit, C.; et al. High-throughput NMR-based screening with competition binding experiments. *J. Am. Chem. Soc.* **2002**, *124*, 7702–7709.

77. Wang, Y.-S.; Liu, D.; Wyss, D. F. Competition STD NMR for the detection of high-affinity ligands and NMR-based screening. *Magn. Reson. Chem.* **2004**, *42*, 485–489.

78. Huth, J. R.; et al. Discovery and design of novel HSP90 inhibitors using multiple fragment-based design strategies. *Chem. Biol. Drug Des.* **2007**, *70*, 1–12.

79. Li, D.; DeRose, E. F.; London, R. E. The inter-ligand Overhauser effect: a powerful new NMR approach for mapping structural relationships of macromolecular ligands. *J. Biomol. NMR* **1999**, *15*, 71–76.

80. Lugovskoy, A. A.; et al. A novel approach for characterizing protein ligand complexes: molecular basis for specificity of small-molecule Bcl-2 inhibitors. *J. Am. Chem. Soc.* **2002**, *124*, 1234–1240.

81. Pellecchia, M.; et al. NMR-based structural characterization of large protein-ligand interactions. *J. Biomol. NMR* **2002**, *22*, 165–173.

82. Medek, A.; Hajduk, P. J.; Mack, J.; Fesik, S. W. The use of differential chemical shifts for determining the binding site location and orientation of protein-bound ligands. *J. Am. Chem. Soc.* **2000**, *122*, 1241–124.

83. McCoy, M. A.; Wyss, D. F. Alignment of weakly interacting molecules to protein surfaces using simulations of chemical shift perturbations. *J. Biomol. NMR* **2000**, *18*, 189–198.

84. McCoy, M. A.; Wyss, D. F. Spatial localization of ligand binding sites from electron current density surfaces calculated from NMR chemical shift perturbations. *J. Am. Chem. Soc.* **2002**, *124*, 11758–11763.

85. Klaus, W.; Senn, H. Strategies for hit finding using NMR. In: *BioNMR in Drug Research*, Zerbe, O.; Ed. Weinheim: Wiley-VCH; **2003**, 417–437.

86. Liepinsh, E.; Otting, G. Organic solvents identify specific ligand binding sites on protein surfaces. *Nat. Biotechnol.* **1997**, *15*, 264–268.

87. Fejzo, J.; Lepre, C.; Xie, X. Applications of NMR screening in drug discovery. *Curr. Top. Med. Chem.* **2002**, *2*, 1349–1364.

88. Hajduk, P. J.; et al. Identification of novel inhibitors of urokinase via NMR-based screening. *J. Med. Chem.* **2000**, *43*, 3862–3866.

89. Nienaber, V. L.; et al. Discovering novel ligands for macromolecules using x-ray crystallographic screening. *Nat. Biotechnol.* **2000**, *18*, 1105–1108.

90. Carr, R.; Jhoti, H. Structure-based screening of low-affinity compounds. *Drug Discov. Today* **2002**, *7*, 522–527.

91. Lesuisse, D.; et al. SAR and X-ray. A new approach combining fragment-based screening and rational drug design: application to the discovery of nanomolar inhibitors of Src SH2. *J. Med. Chem.* **2002**, *45*, 2379–2387.

92. Oltersdorf, T.; et al. An inhibitor of Bcl-2 family proteins induces regression of solid tumours. *Nature* **2005**, *435*, 677–681.

93. Petros, A. M.; et al. Discovery of a potent inhibitor of the anti-apoptotic protein Bcl-xL from NMR and parallel synthesis. *J. Med. Chem.* **2006**, *49*, 656–663.

94. Bruncko, M.; et al. Studies leading to potent, dual inhibitors of Bcl-2 and Bcl-xL. *J. Med. Chem.* **2007**, *50*, 641–662.

95. Hajduk, P. J.; et al. Novel inhibitors of Erm methyltransferases from NMR and parallel synthesis. *J. Med. Chem.* **1999**, *42*, 3852–3859.

96. Park, C. M.; et al. Non-peptidic small molecule inhibitors of XIAP. *Bioorg. Med. Chem. Lett.* **2005**, *15*, 771–775.

97. Hochgurtel, M.; Lehn, J.-M. Dynamic combinatorial diversity in drug discovery. In: *Fragment-Based Approaches in Drug Discovery*, Vol. 34, Jahnke, W.; Ed. Wennheim: Wiley-VCH; **2006**, 341–364.

98. Roper, S.; Kolb, H. Click chemistry for drug discovery. In: *Fragment-Based Approaches in Drug Discovery*, Vol. 34, Jahnke, W.; Ed. Wennheim: Wiley-VCH; **2006**, 313–339.

99. Huth, J. R.; Sun, C. Utility of NMR in lead optimization: fragment-based approaches. *Comb. Chem. High Throughput Screen.* **2002**, *5*, 631–643.

100. Edwards, P. D.; et al. Application of fragment-based lead generation to the discovery of novel, cyclic amidine beta-secretase inhibitors with nanomolar potency, cellular activity, and high ligand efficiency. *J. Med. Chem.* **2007**, *50*, 5912–5925.

101. Geschwindner, S.; et al. Discovery of a novel warhead against beta-secretase through fragment-based lead generation. *J. Med. Chem.* **2007**, *50*, 5903–5911.

102. Congreve, M.; et al. Application of fragment screening by x-ray crystallography to the discovery of aminopyridines as inhibitors of beta-secretase. *J. Med. Chem.* **2007**, *50*, 1124–1132.

103. Murray, C. W.; et al. Application of fragment screening by x-ray crystallography to beta-secretase. *J. Med. Chem.* **2007**, *50*, 1116–1123.

PART II

Computational Chemistry Methodology

5

Free-energy calculations in structure-based drug design

Michael R. Shirts, David L. Mobley, and Scott P. Brown

INTRODUCTION

The ultimate goal of structure-based drug design is a simple, robust process that starts with a high-resolution crystal structure of a validated biological macromolecular target and reliably generates an easily synthesized, high-affinity small molecule with desirable pharmacological properties. Although pharmaceutical science has made significant gains in understanding how to generate, test, and validate small molecules for specific biochemical activity, such a complete process does not now exist. In any drug design project, enormous amounts of luck, intuition, and trial and error are still necessary.

For any small molecule to be considered a likely drug candidate, it must satisfy a number of different absorption/distribution/metabolism/excretion (ADME) properties and have a good toxicological profile. However, a small molecule must above all be active, which in most cases means that it must bind tightly and selectively to a specific location in the protein target before any of the other important characteristics are relevant. To design a drug, large regions of chemical space must be explored to find candidate molecules with the desired biological activity. High-throughput experimental screening methods have become the workhorse for finding such hits.[1,2] However, their results are limited by the quality and diversity of the preexisting chemical libraries, which may contain only molecules representative of a limited portion of the relevant chemical space for a given target. Combinatorial libraries can be produced to supplement these efforts, but their use requires careful design strategies and they are subject to a number of pitfalls.[3] More focused direct in vivo or in vitro measurements provide important information about the effect of prospective drugs in the complete biological system but provide relatively little information that can be directly used to further engineer new molecules. Given a small number of molecules, highly accurate assays of binding, such as surface plasmon resonance (SPR) or isothermal calorimetry (ITC), are relatively accessible though rather costly.

Ideally, small molecules with high potential biological activity could be accurately and reliably screened by computer before ever being synthesized. The degree of accuracy that is required of any computational method will depend greatly its speed. A number of rapid structure-based virtual screening methods, generally categorized as "docking," can help screen large molecular libraries for potential binders and locate a putative binding site (see Chapter 7 for more information on docking). However, recent studies have illustrated that although docking methods can be useful for identifying putative binding sites and identifying ligand poses, scoring methods are not reliable for predicting compound binding affinities and do not currently possess the accuracy necessary for lead optimization.[4–6]

Atomistic, physics-based computational methods are appealing because of their potential for high transferability and therefore greater reliability than methods based on informatics or extensive parameterization. Given a sufficiently accurate physical model of a protein/ligand complex and thorough sampling of the conformational states of this system, one can obtain accurate predictions of binding affinities that could then be robustly incorporated into research decisions. By using a fundamental physical description, such methods are likely to be valid for any given biological system under study, as long as sufficient physical detail is included. Yet another advantage of physics-based models is that the failures can be more easily recognized and understood in the context of the physical chemistry of the system, which cannot be easily done in informatics-based methods.

Despite this potential for reliable predictive power, few articles exist in the literature that report successful, prospective use of physics-based tools within industrial or academic pharmaceutical research. Some of the likely reasons for such failures are the very high computational costs of such methods, insufficiently accurate atomistic models, and software implementations that make it difficult for even experts to easily set up with each new project. Until these problems are resolved, there remain significant obstacles to the realization of more rigorous approaches in industrial drug research.

There have been a number of important technical advances in the computation of free energies since the late 1990s that, coupled with the rapid increase in computational power, have brought these calculations closer to the goal of obtaining reliable and pharmaceutically useful binding energies. In this chapter, we briefly review these latest advances, with a focus on specific applications of these methods in the recent literature. Under "How Accurate Must Calculations of Affinity Be to Add Value" we first discuss the level of reliability and accuracy that binding calculations must have to add some degree of value to the pharmaceutical process. Under "Free Energy Methodologies" we give an overview of the methods currently used to calculate free energies, including recent advances that may eventually lead to sufficiently high throughput for effective pharmaceutical utility. Under "MM-PBSA Calculations" and "Alchemical Calculations" we review recent ligand binding calculations in the literature, beginning with relatively computationally efficient methods that are generally more approximate but still attempt to calculate a true affinity without system-dependent parameters and then address pharmaceutically relevant examples of most physically rigorous methods. We conclude with a discussion of the implications of recent progress in calculating ligand binding affinities on structure-based drug design.

HOW ACCURATE MUST CALCULATIONS OF AFFINITY BE TO ADD VALUE?

Physics-based binding calculations can be very computationally demanding. Given these time requirements, it is important to understand quantitatively what levels of precision, throughput, and turnaround time are required for any computational method to systematically effect the lead-optimization efforts of industrial medicinal chemists in a typical work flow. To be useful, a method does not necessarily need to deliver perfect results, as long as it can produce reliable results with some predictive capacity on time scales relevant to research decision-making processes. These issues are frequently addressed anecdotally, but rarely in a quantitative manner, and we will try to sketch out at least one illustration of what the requirements of a computational method might be.

A recent analysis of more than 50,000 small-molecule chemical transformations spanning over 30 protein targets at Abbott Laboratories found that approximately 80% of the resulting modified molecules had potencies lying within 1.4 kcal/mol (i.e., 1 pK_i log unit) of the starting compound.[7] Potency gains greater than 1.4 kcal/mol from the parent were found to occur approximately 8.5% of the time, whereas gains in potency greater than 2.8 kcal/mol were found with only 1% occurrence. Losses in binding affinity on modification were approximately equal in magnitude and probability to the gains for most types of modifications; presumably wholly random chemical changes would result in a distribution with losses in binding that are much more common than gains. We treat this distribution as typical of lead-optimization affinity gains obtained by skilled medicinal chemists and use this distribution to examine the

ability of accurate and reliable computational methods to influence drug research productivity.

Suppose our chemist sits down each week and envisions a large number of modifications of a lead compound he or she would like to make and test. Instead of simply selecting only his or her best guess from that list, which would lead to a distribution in affinity gains similar to the one described above, this chemist selects N compounds to submit to an idealized computer screening program. The chemist then synthesizes the top-rated compound from the computer predictions. What is the expected distribution of affinities arising from this process for different levels of computational error?

To model this process, we assume the medicinal chemist's proposals are similar to the Abbott data and we approximate this distribution of binding affinity changes as a Gaussian distribution with mean zero and standard deviation of 1.02 kcal/mol, resulting in 8.5% of changes having a pK_i increase of 1.0. We assume the computational predictions of binding affinity have Gaussian noise with standard deviation ϵ. In our thought experiment, we generate N "true" binding affinity changes from the distribution. The computational screen adds Gaussian error with width ϵ to each measurement. We then rank the "noisy" computational estimates and look at distribution of "true" affinities that emerge from selecting the best of the corresponding "noisy" estimates. Repeating this process a number of times (for Figure 5.1, one million), we can generate a distribution of affinities from the screened process.

Shown in Figure 5.1 is the modeled distribution of experimental affinity changes from the chemist's predictions (blue) versus the distribution of the experimental affinity changes after computationally screening $N = 10$ compounds with noise $\epsilon = 0.5$ (pink), $\epsilon = 1.0$ (red), and $\epsilon = 2.0$ (purple). In other words, the blue distribution of affinities is what the medicinal chemist would obtain alone; the redder curves what the chemist would obtain synthesizing the computer's choice of his N proposed modification. The shaded area represents the total probability of a modification with affinity gain greater than 1.4 kcal/mol.

With 0.5 kcal/mol computational noise, screening just ten molecules results in an almost 50% chance of achieving 1 pK_i binding increase in a single round of synthesis, versus an 8.5% chance without screening. With 1 kcal/mol error, we still have 36% chance of achieving this binding goal with the first molecule synthesized. Surprisingly, even with 2 kcal/mol, computational noise almost triples the chance of obtaining a 1 pK_i binding increase. Similar computations can be done with large numbers of computer evaluations; unsurprisingly, the more computational evaluations can be done, the more computational noise can be tolerated and still yield useful time savings. For example, even with 2 kcal/mol error, screening 100 molecules results in the same chance of producing a 1 pK_i binding increase that is the same as if ten molecules are screened with 0.5 kcal/mol error.

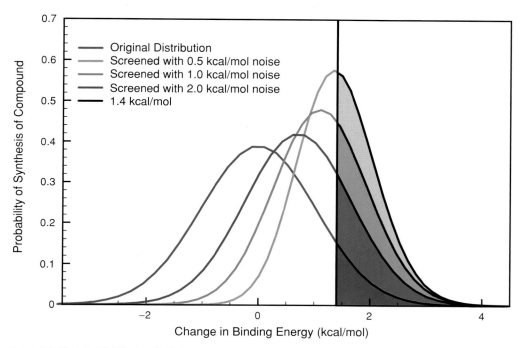

Figure 5.1. Modeled distribution of affinity changes of the proposed modifications (blue) compared to the distribution of affinity changes after computational screening with Gaussian error $\epsilon = 0.5$ (pink), $\epsilon = 1.0$ (red), and $\epsilon = 2.0$ (purple). The shaded area represents the total probability of a proposed modification with affinity gain greater than 1.4 kcal/mol. Hence, in many situations, even with moderate error, a reliable method of filtering compounds could significantly improve the efficiency of synthesis in lead optimization.

So even relatively small numbers of moderately accurate computer predictions may be able to give significant advantage in the pharmaceutical work flow. When we translate the chance of obtaining binding improvement into the number of rounds of synthesis required to obtain that improvement, then screening 100 molecules with 2 kcal/mol noise or 10 screened molecules with 0.5 kcal/mol noise in this model reduces the number of molecules to be synthesized by almost an order of magnitude. Clearly, these calculations assume the simulations are not biased against active compounds, and errors that are highly dependent on the binding system would result in less reliable advantages. The type of computation matters as well – computing relative binding affinities would require only one calculation to compare affinity changes, whereas absolute binding affinities would require two, increasing the effective error. But physically based prediction methods should in principle be more reliable than parameterized methods, as the basic physics and the atomistic details are transferable between drug targets.

This analysis is in agreement with informal discussions with pharmaceutical chemists, who mentioned reliability as being more important than pure speed or the highest accuracy. Many thought they could fit methods that took as much as a month into a work flow, as long as they truly converged reliably with 1 kcal/mol variance error. Even a slight decrease in reliability, for example, being off by several kcal/mol more than 20% of the time, greatly decreased the amount of time that scientists would be willing to wait, perhaps down to a day or two.

FREE-ENERGY METHODOLOGIES

A very large number of methods for computing binding free energies with atomistic molecular models have been developed. Most of them are still under active study, and each has different trade-offs between accuracy and computational efficiency. Because of the scale, complexity, and speed of methodological developments, choosing and applying methods can be confusing even to experienced practitioners. Here, we focus on an overview of some of the key methods available for computing binding affinities, emphasizing references to primary literature. A number of useful recent reviews have focused specifically on free energy methods.[8–14] Of particular note is a recent, fairly comprehensive book on free-energy methods, specifically Chapters 1–7.[15] Several molecular simulation and modeling textbooks have useful introductions to free-energy calculations as well.[16–18]

In this discussion of methods, we will assume standard classical molecular mechanics models, with harmonic bond and angle terms, periodic dihedral terms, and nonbonded terms consisting of point charges and Lennard–Jones repulsion/dispersion terms. In the vast majority of ligand-binding free-energy methods, calculations have been performed with these types of models. Adding classical polarizability terms has seldom been done, though we will briefly mention attempts to include these. Computing free energies using mixed QM/MM simulations can be done but its use has been even more restricted and so will not be discussed here.[19]

Basic equations

The binding affinity K_d of a small molecule ligand L to a protein P can be expressed simply by

$$K_d = \frac{[L][P]}{[PL]}, \qquad (5.1)$$

where the brackets denote an equilibrium concentration, L is the ligand, P is the protein, and PL is the protein/ligand complex. This definition makes the assumption that the difference between bound and unbound states can be well defined, an assumption that is essentially always valid for tight, specific binders but becomes more complicated for very weak and nonspecific binders.

This binding affinity can then be related to the free energy of binding by

$$\Delta G_{\text{Bind}} = -kT \ln \frac{K_d}{C^\circ}, \qquad (5.2)$$

where C° indicates the standard state concentration (by convention, 1 M for solutions). We use the Gibbs free energy G in our equations, because situations of pharmaceutical interest are usually under constant pressure.

The free energy of binding can also be expressed as

$$\Delta G_{\text{Bind}} = -kT \ln \frac{Z_P Z_L}{C^\circ Z_{PL}}, \qquad (5.3)$$

where Z represents the partition function of the system. It is this quantity that we wish to calculate via simulation.

MM-PBSA

As a compromise between speed and accuracy for physics-based estimates of protein/ligand binding affinities, we first discuss the end-point free-energy method molecular mechanics with Poisson–Boltzmann and surface area (MM-PBSA).[20] As an end-point method, MM-PBSA requires direct simulation of only the bound and unbound states. This simplification comes with the expectation of significantly larger intrinsic errors with MM-PBSA than with other more rigorous methods we will address later in the chapter.

The free energy of binding can be written as a difference in the solvation free energies of each of the components:

$$\Delta G_{\text{Bind}} \Delta G_{\text{PL-solv}} - \Delta G_{\text{L-solv}} + \Delta G_{\text{P-solv}}. \qquad (5.4)$$

Each of these solvation energies can be written as

$$\Delta G_{\text{solv}} = \Delta H_{\text{solv}} - T \Delta S_{\text{solv}}. \qquad (5.5)$$

If we average out the coordinates of the solvent over all the configurations, then we can approximate each of these free energies as

$$\Delta G_{\text{X-solv}} = \langle E_{\text{X-MM}} \rangle + \Delta G_{\text{X-solvent}} - T \Delta S_{\text{X-MM}}, \qquad (5.6)$$

where $\langle E_X \rangle$ is the average molecular mechanics energy of X alone (without water), ΔS_X is the internal entropy of

X (without water), and $\Delta G_{\text{X-solvent}}$ is the energy and entropy due to the solvation of X waters. These solvation energies for P, L, and PL can then be combined to compute a full binding energy.

In practice, a variety of implementations of the MM-PBSA protocol have been reported, and particular care needs to paid to a number of details in setting up the calculations. In general, protocols can be separated into three steps. First, coordinate sampling [such as molecular dynamics (MD)] is performed on the protein/ligand complex to sample configurations for energy analysis. In the next step, calculation of gas-phase potential energies and solvation free energies is performed on each structure collected from the previous step to produce ensemble averages. Finally, some measure of estimated change in solute entropy is computed for the set of structures. The final binding free energy is then obtained by combining these various components.

To generate the structures in the first step, one can perform separate MD simulations for the isolated ligand, apo protein, and bound protein/ligand complex. Alternatively, one can use a single trajectory of the bound complex as the source of conformations for the unbound (and bound) states.[21] This second case is equivalent to assuming that the conformations explored in the protein/ligand complex in solution are sufficiently similar to those conformations explored by the apo protein and isolated ligand. This assumption is not necessarily reasonable and in fact is guaranteed to be grossly incorrect in some contexts; however, the amount of noise added when taking differences between averages produced from independent bound and unbound trajectories substantially increases the sampling required for convergence, so by simulating one structure, lower variance is traded for some bias.[22,23] In theory, one could then perform a single MD run of the apo protein, and all additional runs would involve only isolated ligands. In any case, determining arrival at a stable average can be challenging.[24] A possible alternative formulation for the case of running the three separate trajectories is to disregard all energies but the interaction energies in an attempt to dampen the contributions to noise due to noncanceling internal-energy differences.

The potential energy $E_{\text{X-MM}}$ is that of only the protein and ligand and consists of

$$E_{\text{X-MM}} = E^{\text{elec}} + E^{\text{vdW}} + E^{\text{int}}, \qquad (5.7)$$

where E^{elec} is the electrostatic energy, E^{vdW} is the van der Waals dispersion and repulsion, and E^{int} is composed of internal-energy terms for the ligand and protein, such as bond, angle, and torsion terms.

The solvation energy term $\Delta G_{\text{X-solvent}}$ is subdivided into a sum of two components, one due to electrostatic interaction and the other due to nonpolar interactions:

$$\Delta G_{\text{X-solvent}} = \Delta G_{\text{PBSA}} = \Delta G_{\text{PB}} + \Delta G_{\text{SA}}, \qquad (5.8)$$

where ΔG_{PB} represents the polar contribution and ΔG_{SA} represents the nonpolar contribution to the solvation free energy.

The polar term in Equation (5.8) represents the energy stored in the continuum dielectric in response to the presence of the solute's charge distribution and is typically obtained by solution of the Poisson–Boltzmann (PB) equation. The PB equation provides a rigorous framework for representing discrete solute molecules embedded in a uniform dielectric continuum and has been shown to be capable of producing relatively robust predictions of electrostatic contributions to solvation free energies of small molecules as well as biological macromolecules.[25,26] The PB solutions are obtained in separate calculations for the ligand, protein, and bound protein/ligand complex, and the final solvation free-energy values are assembled using the thermodynamic cycle for association in solution.[27,28]

For any PB calculation, one must choose a particular representation of the dielectric boundary between solute and solvent, which can involve a number of subtleties.[29,30] In addition to the boundary representation, dielectric functions for the solute and solvent must also be chosen. For typical protein/ligand systems, constant values of 1.0 for solutes and 80.0 for solvent are most commonly used,[31] though there are also other arguments that using 2.0, 4.0, or a residue-based dielectric for the solute may give superior performance.[32,33] It should be noted that most force fields have been parameterized using an internal dielectric of 1.0.

Finally, the last term in Equation (5.8) is the nonpolar component of solvation free energy, which is usually treated as being proportional to the solvent exposed surface area[34] of the solute,

$$G^{SA} = \gamma \Delta SA, \tag{5.9}$$

where ΔSA is the change in accessible molecular surface area on binding, and γ is a microscopic surface free energy for formation of a cavity in water.[35] The form of this equation derives from empirical data on transfer free energies for linear, cyclic, and branched hydrocarbons.[36,37] The precise value of γ depends on the particular method used to probe the solvent-accessible surface of the solute.[25] The equation implicitly assumes that the nonpolar component has negligible contributions from dispersion interactions between solute and solvent relative to the energy required in displacing solvent molecules to create the cavity. A number of objections to this expression point out its oversimplification,[38–40] and a number of models have been proposed to attempt to address these shortcomings with more sophisticated frameworks.[39–41]

The last term on the right-hand side of Equation (5.6) is the entropic cost of confining the free ligand, which represents a significant fraction of the total change in solute entropy ΔS_{solute} for formation of the bound complex. Additional estimates of solute entropy can be performed, which typically use some form of normal-mode analysis and that are very computationally expensive to perform.[42,43] Alternatively, one could use empirical estimates of average entropic costs, such as the entropy required to constrain rotation around any given torsional degree of freedom.[44] However, neither of these approaches produce quality estimates of solute entropy; instead, they tend to add a significant random scatter to results.[21]

Because of the complications in dealing with entropy, it is often neglected for computational convenience. This approximation may be reasonable in cases where we are only interested in rank-ordering, and the amount of entropy/enthalpy compensation remains roughly constant across ligands. It will certainly be unreasonable for any case where absolute comparisons of free energy are desired across protein targets and in situations for which non-negligible perturbations in binding modes and pocket geometries occur across a ligand set. Recent developments for treating the entropy more properly show significant promise.[45]

In systems where there are relatively few populated states, it may be sufficient to perform PB calculations alone to generate robust affinity estimates. In a number of situations, PB solutions have been successfully used to estimate affinities,[28,46–48] although some implementations begin to resemble empirical scoring methods.[49] A major criticism of these approaches is their potential inaccuracy in situations where conformational flexibility plays a significant role.[50]

In generating the dynamics trajectories for the MM-PBSA analysis explicit representation of water molecules are typically used. Although explicit water molecules give the most detailed glimpse into structural dynamics, it has been shown that there can be pathologies in certain situations when using implicit-solvent theory to "score" explicit water configurations,[21,51] because the ensemble average energies should be computed with the same energy function used to generate the ensemble structures. An alternative to this is to sample in implicit solvent directly.[52]

As PB solutions are in general computationally demanding calculations, a number of groups have put significant efforts into developing faster approximations, such as the suite of generalized Born (GB) approaches.[53–56] However, there are numerous examples of pathologies using GB methods.[57–59]

Other implicit solvent methods

Another approach requiring only simulations of the bound and unbound states is to compute the partition function directly. The partition function of a molecular system can be computed as the sum of the integral of Boltzmann factors over neighborhoods of only the low-energy states, which are a relatively small fraction of the total configurations of the molecules.[60]

With the full partition function for the protein, ligand, and the complex in the case of absolute free energies, or for two ligands and two complexes in the case of relative free energies, the binding free energy or changes in binding free energy can be computed directly from these end states. At least two methods for computing the configuration integrals in the neighborhood of minima have been developed that have been applied to ligand binding systems: mode integration (MINTA),[61] and the Mining Minima approaches of Gilson and coworkers. Both start out with a method for enumerating minima. In MINTA importance sampling Monte Carlo integration is used to calculate the configuration integrals. It has been used to screen for the free-energy difference between ligand enantiomers, where its accuracy was comparable to alchemical methods, but was more efficient,[62,63] though there are important caveats in the original implementation.[64] Gilson and coworkers have emphasized calculating the integrals in bond/angle/torsion coordinates to minimize errors.[68] They have applied such methods successfully to a number of simplified binding systems.[65–68]

The methods' two shared main problems are the need to find all minima contributing to the partition function and the correct computation of entropies of neighborhoods near minima. Minima searches of proteins the size of typical drug targets are notoriously difficult, and hence the studies noted above focus mostly on problems where many of the errors may cancel out or on smaller model systems. The problems of estimating entropy in these methods has much in common with the same problem in MM-PBSA calculations, though because these methods are perhaps more sensitive to the correct entropy calculation, the problems have been investigated to a significant degree.[45,61,69,70] However, significantly fewer people are investigating these alternative end-point methods than MM-PBSA, and they are generally more computationally expensive, so the short-term prospects are not necessarily particularly encouraging despite the strong theoretical underpinnings.

Alchemical methods

The methods described above are designed primarily for implicit solvent systems and represent relatively computationally cheap approximations to the binding free energy. However, implicit water models are unsuitable for a fully molecular description of phenomena such as the formation of correlated hydrogen bonding networks in binding active sites and there are many protein/ligand systems where the atomic detail of the water in the binding site plays an important role in the binding process.[71] For free-energy calculations to include these phenomena, more expensive explicit water simulations must be used. Using explicit water, the free-energy terms in MM-PBSA become dominated by statistical noise from the water. The standard approach for solvation free energies in explicit solvent simulations is instead to compute the free energy of a particular change of state directly, while holding the rest of the system fixed, which does not depend directly on the energies of the rest of the system. We note that although these methods

are the techniques of choice for explicit water simulations, they can be performed equally easily for continuum water simulations.

"Free-energy perturbation" is a very common term for these methods that directly compute the free-energy difference as a function of changing molecular structure. "Perturbation" usually refers to an approximate theory that can be written as a series of more easily calculated terms. Free-energy perturbation (frequently abbreviated FEP), however, is exact. The term *perturbation* here instead refers to the changes in the chemical identity, as simulations frequently involve changes in chemical identity, such as an amine to an alcohol or a methyl group to a chlorine. Additionally, FEP is sometimes used to refer specifically to application of the Zwanzig relationship (discussed below). To avoid confusion, we will use the term *alchemical* to refer to this class of methods, as the chemical identity of the atomic models will change, appear, or disappear during the process, and use EXP to refer to the Zwanzig relationship.

Zwanzig relationship

The most well-known method historically for calculating free energies, and still a very common one, is the Zwanzig relationship.[72] The free energy between two Hamiltonians $H_0(x)$ and $H_1(x)$ over a coordinate and momentum space (x) can be calculated as

$$\Delta G = \beta^{-1} \ln \left\langle e^{-\beta[H_1(x) - H_0(x)]} \right\rangle_0 = \beta^{-1} \ln \left\langle e^{-\beta \Delta H(x)} \right\rangle_0, \quad (5.10)$$

where $\beta = (kT)^{-1}$. We will denote this method EXP, for exponential averaging. Although the equation is exact, many studies have demonstrated that except in the case of rather small changes, EXP convergence as a function of the amount of data collected is far from ideal, and an average that appears to have converged may only indicate very poor overlap between the two states studied.[73,74]

Overlap in configuration space in the direction of decreasing entropy is usually greater, and thus EXP in this direction will generally be more efficient.[75,76] For example, inserting a molecule into a dense fluid is a more effective way to compute the chemical potential than deleting molecules from the same fluid, because the important conformations for both ensembles are actually easiest to sample in simulations without the molecule present.

Multiple intermediates

In some cases, such as computing the chemical potential of bulk fluids, the symmetry of the problem can be used to greatly improve computational efficiency of FEP.[77] However, in most instances where the states of interest are very far from having any phase-space overlap, the transformation can be broken into a series of free-energy calculations with nonphysical intermediates – for example, turning off the atomic charges or turning a carbon into an oxygen. The total free energy can simply be written as a sum of the individual free energies between intermediate states, which can be completely nonphysical. We will first assume the existence of these intermediates, and the ability to perform simulations at these intermediates and then discuss the best choice of intermediate states.

If phase-space overlap between consecutive intermediates is very high, then EXP can work well. For example, if an ether is changed to a thioether, there is relatively little change in phase-space, and EXP will be effective with a small number of intermediates. However, if an entire heavy atom is disappearing or appearing or if the charge of an atom is changing significantly, phase-space overlap will not be significant, and EXP is almost guaranteed to do poorly without a large number of intermediates. Because of the large number of intermediates required, computations with EXP can be very inefficient, requiring the simulation of many states for computing the free energy of a single alchemical transformation.

Double-wide sampling is a commonly used technique that consists of simulating only at every other intermediate state and computing EXP in both directions from these intermediates.[78] The biases of free energy computed from EXP in different directions have opposite signs, so alternating directions will tend to cancel bias somewhat. This method nominally reduces the number of simulations necessary by half, but because the variance in the direction of increasing entropy is usually lower, this twofold gain in efficiency is rarely obtained. Fortunately, there are a number of alternatives that are more efficient than EXP in most cases.

Thermodynamic integration

By taking the derivative of the free energy with respect to some continuous parameter λ describing a series of intermediate alchemical states, we can see that

$$dG/d\lambda = \frac{d}{d\lambda} \int e^{-\beta H(\lambda, \boldsymbol{x})} d\boldsymbol{x} = \left\langle \frac{dH(\lambda, \boldsymbol{x})}{d\lambda} \right\rangle_{\lambda}$$

$$\Delta G = \int_0^1 \left\langle \frac{dH(\lambda, \boldsymbol{x})}{d\lambda} \right\rangle_{\lambda}, \tag{5.11}$$

where the pathway of intermediates between the states of interest is parameterized between $\lambda = 0$ and $\lambda = 1$. This formula can also be obtained by expanding the Zwanzig relationship in a Taylor series. Computing free energies using this formula is typically called thermodynamic integration (TI). In the rest of the discussion, we will denote $H(\lambda, \boldsymbol{x})$ by simply $H(\lambda)$. Note that when the end states have different masses, the momenta will have λ dependence as well, which must also be included in the derivative, but we omit this detail for clarity in the discussion.

Thermodynamic integration essentially trades variance for bias. Averaging over $\langle \frac{dH}{d\lambda} \rangle$ will require fewer uncorrelated samples to reach a given level of relative error than averaging $e^{-\beta \Delta H(x)}$, as as long as $\langle \frac{dH}{d\lambda} \rangle$ is well behaved, an important condition we will address later in the section "Choice of

Alchemical Pathways." However, to compute the total free energy from a series of individual simulations, we must use some type of numerical integration of the integral, which by definition introduces bias. A number of different numerical techniques have been applied.[79,80] A simple trapezoidal rule is usually used or, occasionally, Simpson's rule. Higher order integration methods converge more quickly in the distance between integration points, but this error term is proportional to the derivatives of the function, which can become large in some situations, such as when repulsive atomic centers are removed from the system entirely. Other techniques such as Gaussian integration have been used[79] but require knowledge about the variance to determine the Gaussian weighting and so become cumbersome to use.

For alchemical changes that result in smooth, monotonic curves for $\langle dH/d\lambda \rangle$, TI can be quite accurate using a relatively small number of points. However, if the curvature becomes large, as can frequently be the case in alchemical simulations where Lennard–Jones potentials are turned on or off, then the bias introduced by discretization of the integral can become large.[73,81,82] Even in the case of small curvature (i.e., charging of SPC water in water) reasonably large errors can be introduced (i.e., 5–10% of the total free energy with 5 λ values).[83]

Many early free-energy calculations approximated the integral by varying λ throughout the simulation, called "slow growth." The total free energy is then estimated as

$$\Delta G \approx \int_{t=t_0}^{t_1} \left\langle \frac{dH}{d\lambda} \right\rangle_{\lambda(t)} \frac{d\lambda}{dt} dt. \tag{5.12}$$

This, however, proved to be a very bad approximation in most molecular simulations, introducing large speed-dependent biases even for relatively long simulations. Forward and reverse simulations show significant hysteresis.[84,85] This method should always be avoided, except when used in the context of Jarzynski's relationship, which we will now discuss.

Jarzynski's relationship

If we have a physical or alchemical process that takes place in finite time, the amount of work performed will not be reversible and hence will not be equal to the free energy. Equation (5.12) can then be identified as the nonequilibrium work W for this transformation, not the equilibrium free energy ΔG. Jarzynski noticed that the free energy of the transformation can be written as the average of the nonequilibrium trajectories that start from an equilibrium ensemble:

$$\Delta G = \beta^{-1} \ln \left\langle e^{-\beta W} \right\rangle_0. \tag{5.13}$$

If the switching is instantaneous, then Equation (5.13) becomes identical to EXP because the instantaneous work is simply the change in potential energy. A number of studies have compared nonequilibrium pathways to single-step perturbations. However, in both theory and practice it appears that under most circumstances, equilibrium simulations are about the same or slightly more efficient than free energies calculated from ensembles of nonequilibrium simulations.[73,86,87] It is thus not clear that free energy calculations using Jarzynski's relationship will have much role in ligand-binding calculations in the future. There has been extensive research in this topic recently, partly because this formalism has proven useful in treating nonequilibrium experiments as well as simulations.

Bennett acceptance ratio

The free energy computed using EXP in either direction between two intermediate states converges to the same result with sufficient samples. The biases from opposite directions will cancel, which suggests that simple ways to improve EXP are to simply perform the calculation in both directions and average the results or to perform double-wide sampling. However, because of a direct relationship between the distributions of potential energy in the forward and reverse directions,[88] there is a significantly more robust and in fact provably statistically optimal way to use information in both directions. Bennett's original formulation started with a simple relationship for the free energies:

$$\Delta G_{0 \to 1} = \ln kT \frac{Z_0}{Z_1} = kT \ln \frac{\langle A(\boldsymbol{x}) \exp[-\beta(H_0 - H_1)] \rangle_1}{\langle A(\boldsymbol{x}) \exp[-\beta(H_1 - H_0)] \rangle_0},$$

(5.14)

which is true for any function $A(\boldsymbol{x})$. Bennett then used variational calculus to find the choice of $A(\boldsymbol{x})$ that minimizes the variance of the free energy,[89] resulting in an implicit function of ΔG that is easily solvable numerically. A separate approach demonstrates that the same formula provides the maximum likelihood estimate of the free energy given the observations of the potential energy differences between the two states.[90] Either derivation additionally gives a robust estimate for the variance of free energy. Studies have demonstrated both the theoretical and practical superiority of BAR over EXP in molecular simulations.[73,74] Significantly less overlap between the configurational space of each state is required to converge results than in the case of EXP, although some overlap must still exist.

It is difficult to directly compare TI and BAR on a theoretical basis. However, it appears that TI can be as efficient as BAR under conditions where the integrand is very smooth,[12,73] such as charging or small changes in molecular size, but BAR appears to be significantly more efficient than TI or EXP for free energies of larger molecular changes, sometimes by almost an order of magnitude.[73,74,91] If the intermediate states can be written as functions of the final states, as discussed previously, then the calculations of the potential energy in these alternate states can be very efficient, as only two computations of pairwise interactions are needed. Otherwise, the energies of changing parts of the system must be calculated for each state, which unfortunately is not necessarily implemented in most simulation codes currently.

WHAM

In most cases, alchemical free-energy computations require simulation at a number of different intermediates, and we would prefer to obtain as much thermodynamic information as possible from all of these simulations simultaneously. If one intermediate is relatively similar to a number of other intermediates, and not just the nearest neighbors, then all of this information can be used to calculate the free energy more precisely. Histogram weighting techniques were first introduced by Ferrenberg and Swendsen[92] to capture all of this information to compute free energies. A version called the weighted histogram analysis method (WHAM) was introduced in 1992 by Kumar and collaborators for alchemical simulations.[93] WHAM is provably the lowest uncertainty method to calculate the free energy for samples collected from discrete states. However, it introduces biases in continuous states (such as those obtained with atomistic simulations) because it requires discretization into bins. Other variations of WHAM based on maximum likelihood[94] and Bayesian methods[95] have also been developed. A version of WHAM-based free-energy calculation is available within the CHARMM molecular mechanics package.[96,97]

MBAR

It was noted[93,96] that one can reduce the histogrammed equations of WHAM to a simpler form by reducing the width of the histogram to zero, yielding a set of iterative equations to estimate the K free energies:

$$G_i = -\beta^{-1} \ln \sum_{k=1}^{K} \sum_{n=1}^{N_k} \frac{\exp[-\beta H_i(\boldsymbol{x}_{kn})]}{\sum_{k'=1}^{K} N_{k'} \exp[\beta G_{k'} - \beta H_{k'}(\boldsymbol{x}_{kn})]},$$

(5.15)

where i runs from 1 to K, the G_i are the free energies, and the H_i are the Hamiltonians of these K states. This approximation is somewhat suspect, as the derivation of WHAM involves finding the weighting factors that minimize the variance in the occupancy of the bins, which are undefined as the width goes to zero.

A recent mutitstate extension of the BAR has been derived that solves this problem. In this derivation, a series of $N \times N$ weighting functions $A_{ij}(\boldsymbol{x})$ are adjusted to minimize the free energies of all N states considered simultaneously. The lowest variance estimator can be seen to exactly be the WHAM equation in the limit of zero-width histograms [Equation (5.15)]. WHAM can therefore be seen as a histogram-based approximation to this multistate Bennett's acceptance ratio (or MBAR).[91] This MBAR derivation additionally gives the uncertainty of the calculated free energies, which is not available in WHAM.

Choice of alchemical pathways

A key point in these methods is that for almost all alchemical transformations between the initial and final

Hamiltonian, there must be a series of intermediates with mutual phase-space overlap leading connecting the two physical end states. The simplest choice for most transformations between two Hamiltonians H_0 and H_1 is the linear pathway:

$$H(\lambda, \boldsymbol{x}) = (1 - \lambda) H_0(\boldsymbol{x}) + \lambda H_1(\boldsymbol{x}). \qquad (5.16)$$

A significant problem with this formulation is that equal spacing in λ does not actually lead to equal spacing in phase-space overlap. If a Lennard–Jones function is used to represent the atomic exclusion and dispersion interaction, as is typically the case in biomolecular force fields, then when $\lambda = 0.1$, nearly at the disappearing end state, the excluded volume (i.e., the volume with energy above 2–3 kT) will still occupy 60–70% of the original volume, depending on the original Lennard–Jones well depth.

Additionally, this choice of parameterization with an r^{-12} potential leads to a singularity in $\langle dH/d\lambda \rangle$ at $r = 0$, which can be integrated formally but not numerically. By using a power of $\lambda \geq 4$ instead of a strictly linear parameterization [such as $H(\lambda) = (1 - \lambda)^4 H_0 + \lambda^4 H_1$], $\langle dH/d\lambda \rangle$ can be numerically integrated correctly. However, it will still converge slowly.[80,99] For any nonzero λ, whatever the power, there will be small "fenceposts," particles with a small impenetrable core.[99] One possible way to avoid issues with these fenceposts has been to shrink the entire molecular structure. However, this can create problems with nonbonded interactions as the molecular framework shrinks, causing instabilities in integration in molecular dynamics,[99–101] and is generally not practical for large numbers of bonds. A correction term must also be added for these bond length changes, which can be complicated if the bonds lengths are constrained.[102]

There are better ways to handle this transformation. The concept of a "soft core" was introduced around 1994,[82,103] with the infinity at $r = 0$ in the r^{-12} interaction being "smoothed out" in a λ-dependent way. The most common parameterizations for turning off the Lennard–Jones function are of the form

$$H(\lambda, r) = 4\epsilon\lambda^n \left\{ \left[\alpha(1 - \lambda)^m + \left(\frac{r}{\sigma}\right)^6 \right]^{-2} + \left[\alpha(1 - \lambda)^m + \left(\frac{r}{\sigma}\right)^6 \right]^{-1} \right\}$$
$$(5.17)$$

where ϵ and σ are the standard Lennard–Jones parameters, α is a constant (usually 0.5), with the original choice of $n = 4$ and $m = 2$.[82] Further research has shown that using $n = 1$ and $m = 1$ noticeably improves the variance.[80,99,104] The more flexible the molecule, the more using a soft atomic core improves the efficiency of the free-energy calculation. Approaches using a soft core for the Coulombic term[82,105] or making all the interactions disappear into an imaginary fourth dimension have also been tried,[106] but it can be difficult to choose parameters for these approaches that are transferable between systems.

Recent studies have demonstrated that one highly reliable, relatively high efficiency pathway for an alchemical

change where an atomic site disappears is to turn off the charges linearly and then turn off the Lennard–Jones terms of the uncharged particles using a soft-core approach. The same pathway can be followed in reverse for atomic sites that are introduced.[97,99] It is the treatment of the singularities at the center of particles that is the real challenge; atomic sites that merely change atom type can be handled with linear interpolation of the potential energy, as the phase-space overlap changes are relatively small with respect to phase-space changes with introduction of particles. The variance due to changes in the bonding terms is not generally a problem; although the energy changes for these terms can be quite large, the time scale of the motions means that they converge quite quickly.

It is likely that further optimizations of pathways may lead to additional efficiency gains. But they will probably not increase efficiency by much more than a factor of 2 as there are limits to the lowest possible variance path.[105] Studies of optimal pathways have focused on minimizing the variance in TI,[82,105] but it appears that highly optimal pathways for TI work well for all other methods.

Pulling methods

Another choice of pathway for determining the free energy of protein/ligand association is to physically pull the molecule away from the protein. If the final state is sufficiently far from the original protein, the free energy of this process will be the free energy of binding. This can be done either by nonequilibrium simulations, using the Jarzynski relationship, or by computing a PMF using umbrella sampling with different overlapping harmonic oscillators at specified distances from the binding site.[107–110]

There are a number of complications with pulling methods. Pulling a ligand out of a buried site can pose problems, and it can be difficult to pull the ligand sufficiently far away from the protein with a simulation box of computationally tractable size. In the latter case, some analytical or mean-field approximation must be applied for the free energy of pulling the ligand to infinity. However, it has been argued that pulling may be significantly more efficient for highly charged ligands.[108]

Promising methods not yet routine

Researchers are experimenting with a number of intriguing methods that have significant potential to make ligand-binding calculations much more efficient but that are not yet routine. It is likely that many or all of these will become much more commonplace in the near future. We will give only brief a introduction along with references for further investigation.

Using umbrella sampling for convergence

A general problem for any free-energy simulation method is sampling important configurations. One standard method for improving sampling in atomistic simulations is umbrella sampling,[111] where bias terms are added to constrain the simulation in some way and their effect is then removed. This procedure can be used to either lower potential energy barriers or to restrain simulations to slow-interconverting configurations that are relevant to the binding affinity (for example, different torsional states), allowing each of the component energies to be properly computed and then combined.[97,112,113] Another application is computing the free energy of constraining the free ligand into the bound conformation directly before computing the free energy of binding and then releasing these restraints, usually decreasing the correlation times for sampling of the intermediate states and thus increasing the efficiency of the simulation.[97,108]

Expanded ensemble, Hamiltonian exchange, and λ dynamics

Alchemical simulations usually include a number of intermediate states. It is possible to bring these intermediates together in a single simulation system, either as series of coupled simulations of the intermediate states, usually called Hamilton exchange, or as a single simulation that visits all of the intermediate states, called expanded ensemble simulation. A number of studies have shown that Hamiltonian exchange and expanded ensembles can speed up simulations by allowing the system to go around barriers by going through alchemical states where those barriers are not as pronounced, significantly speeding up free-energy simulations.[114–120] Alternatively, the alchemical variable λ can be treated as a dynamic variable, which adds complications by introducing a fictitious mass corresponding to the λ degree of freedom but is essentially equivalent to Monte Carlo techniques.[118,121–123] There are a number of variations of sampling in λ that may show promise in the future, but such methods are still in the preliminary stages of development.[124–128]

Multiple ligands simulations

If binding calculations of multiple ligands with a single protein target can be performed in the same simulation, this can significantly speed up the efficiency of calculations. This has been most successfully done by running a single simulation of a nonphysical reference state and then computing the free energy via EXP to a large number of potential ligands.[97,129,130] However, this frequently fails to work when the ligands are too dissimilar.[131] More sophisticated multiligand approaches will most likely be necessary.

RECENT HISTORY IN LIGAND BINDING CALCULATIONS FOR PHARMACEUTICALLY RELEVANT SYSTEMS

MM-PBSA calculations

MM-PBSA has been used in a range of applications for exploring the free energetics of biologically relevant molecules, and reports in the literature appear for a variety of nontrivial, structure-related problems. Although early applications focused on rationalizing relative conformational stabilities in DNA[132] and RNA,[133] it was not long before attempts to analyze protein/ligand interactions began to appear. For instance, MM-PBSA was used to verify a hypothesis that electrostatic interactions were the primary driver for hapten association with Fab fragments of antibody 48G7.[134] It was also used to elucidate situations in which hydrogen bonding was postulated to be an important contributor to protein/ligand association,[135] to gain insights into the role of hydrophobic interactions in cAMP-dependent protein kinase,[47] and to investigate carbohydrate recognition in concanavalin.[37] Other uses of MM-PBSA include rationalizing the role of pK_a shifts in protein/ligand binding,[137] and demonstrating the importance of the choice of proper protonation states in the active site.[138] Structure-based ligand design methods have also been built on top of MM-PBSA. One technique, called computational alanine scanning,[139] probes potential interaction sites in receptor binding pockets, and an analogous method was developed for small molecules called fluorine scanning.[140]

The wide range of applications of MM-PBSA reported in the literature reflect its increasing penetration into the scientific community. Based on results from a search of a life sciences citation database maintained by *Entrez*, the number of publications reporting some use of MM-PBSA to perform binding analysis has steadily increased from fourteen total in the two years from 2001 to 2002 to fifty total in the years 2006–2007. The consistent increase in the use of MM-PBSA is likely due to several factors. MM-PBSA has relatively low computational cost compared to other (more rigorous) binding free-energy methods, which broadens the number of systems to which it can be reasonably applied. Several initial reports on MM-PBSA appearing in the literature showed significant potential for the method. In particular, one of the earliest results demonstrated impressive affinity predictions for the protein target avidin binding a set of biotin analogs.[141] Subsequent reports showed equally promising results for affinity predictions for other systems.[142–146]

Because of the early reports a large number of groups have applied MM-PBSA to a wide variety of systems. We can investigate one aspect of the evolution of the use of MM-PBSA by inspecting the literature reports that have appeared over the years from 2001 to 2007. Shown in Figure 5.2 are values (estimated where possible from the publications found in the aforementioned citation search) for the mean-square error (MSE) in reported affinity predictions, as a function of the publication year.

From 2000 to 2003, MM-PBSA reports contained significantly smaller average MSE values in the literature, compared to averages from the span of 2004 to 2007. There are a number of possible explanations for this trend. Early applications may have been restricted to more well-behaved systems appropriate for initial verification and later studies were more representative of the average over many systems.

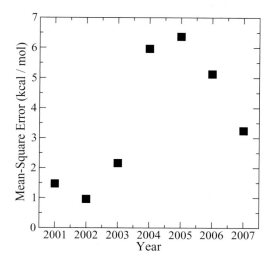

Figure 5.2. Errors obtained from literature data showing the progression of estimated mean-square errors for MM-PBSA affinity predictions.

It could also be that MM-PBSA has arrived in the hands of less experienced practitioners, who are less familiar with the subtleties involved. It also may be the case that people are currently more willing to publish less successful applications than has been the case in the past. Whatever the root cause, it seems safe to conclude that (at least for the published reports) there is a different expectation for the potential magnitudes of errors produced by MM-PBSA today than was initially apparent.

To explore the general question of reliability of MM-PBSA, its performance must be examined in a variety of systems. Shown in Figure 5.3 is the change in experimental binding affinity (relative to a known reference compound) plotted versus the percentage change in MM-PBSA "score" (relative to the same reference compound) from an internal Abbott study. The specific procedure used for these calculations has been detailed elsewhere.[146] Briefly, conformational sampling is performed in implicit solvent during which a set of structures are saved and subsequently analyzed for energetics as described under "MM-PBSA." All solute entropic changes on binding are ignored in these calculations. The MM-PBSA energies are referred to as "scores" to reflect the fact that they are not true free energies. To generate the data in Figure 5.3 MM-PBSA calculations were performed on 480 structures (based on 292 structures obtained from Abbott x-ray crystallography) that spanned eight protein targets, including representatives from a number of families, such as kinases, proteases, peptide signaling proteins, and phosphatases. For the compounds that did not have explicit x-ray crystal structures of the bound small molecule, the binding modes were prepared by selecting a (similar) existing crystal structure and performing a three-dimensional overlay of the small molecule onto the crystallographic binding mode.

The data in Figure 5.3 are partitioned into false positives (FP), false negatives (FN), true positives (TP), and

true negatives (TN). The relatively small number of FN produced in the calculations is worth noting, as FN are highly undesirable in a drug discovery setting, due to the fact that they represent missed opportunities. The presence of FP is less problematic as the threshold for desired MM-PBSA score can be altered to accommodate a desired FP rate. To illustrate this we describe several thresholds for percentage change in MM-PBSA score, yielding differing numbers of FP and TP, as shown in Figure 5.3. It can be seen that to reduce the rate of FP to below 10%, one must accept only those compounds exhibiting positive changes in MM-PBSA score greater than 40%. Given the results obtained with MM-PBSA in this study, it appears that it could be used for virtual library triage to produce enriched lists of ranked compounds. An inspection of the spread of $\Delta\Delta G_{Bind}$ values at various thresholds reveals that a probable value for an anticipated relative error might be in the 2–3 kcal/mol range, which is comparable to recent errors reported in the literature (see MSE for 2007 in Figure 5.2). Based on analysis presented in the introduction to this chapter, incorporating this level of calculation into the work flow of medicinal chemists might begin to add value to synthetic efforts by reducing the average number of compounds that need to be made.

There have been several recent studies investigating the use of MM-PBSA as a potential routine tool in drug discovery. Kuhn et al. found that small-molecule potency predictions with MM-PBSA are generally unreliable at predicting differences smaller than around 3–4 kcal/mol of relative potency,[147] which is in rough agreement with the conclusions presented above. The authors did find MM-PBSA to be useful as a postdocking filter. In a different study, Pearlman found that MM-PBSA performed extremely poorly, and

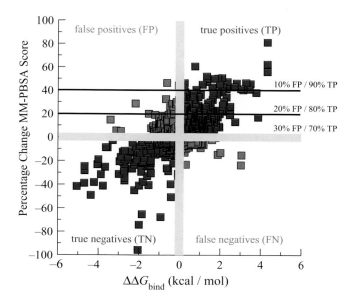

Figure 5.3. Data showing change in compound potency (relative to a reference compound) versus percentage change in MM-PBSA score (relative to same reference compound) for 480 compounds across eight targets, which span 292 x-ray crystallographic complexes.

in fact somewhat nonintuitively.[148] This study is somewhat difficult to interpret, as mixed small-molecule force fields were used in addition to normal-mode entropy estimates for all the of data points. In a later publication it was noted that both of the above studies selected molecules with insufficiently wide potency ranges[149]; however, the ranges of potencies in the reports of Pearlman and Kuhn et al. are around 3 kcal/mol, consistent with our findings that MM-PBSA, in general, cannot be expected to reliably resolve compounds within 2–3 kcal/mol. For a sufficiently wide range of potencies careful application of MM-PBSA may provide help and bias discovery effort toward the more potent compounds.[150]

The literature reports other issues with MM-PBSA, for example, in systems including in the presence of a metal ion in the binding site.[151] Inadequacies of MM-PBSA to accurately represent first-solvation-shell effects were shown to introduce significant error into direct potency prediction.[170] However, despite the first-solvation-layer error, MM-PBSA was still able to successfully rank-order the ligands.

There appears to be an emerging consensus that MM-PBSA likely has some applicability and utility in drug discovery. However, results have ranged too widely, from promising to poor to difficult, to interpret unambiguously. There is as of yet insufficient data to conclusively demonstrate the scope, the limitations of MM-PBSA, and the fundamental reliability in industrial drug discovery research, though the studies described here demonstrate enough promise to focus more effort on these methods in the future.

Alchemical calculations

Alchemical free energies are substantially more rigorous than MM-PBSA calculations but also significantly more computationally demanding. They were first applied to protein/ligand systems in the early to mid-1980s. Tembe and McCammon[152] laid out some of the basic theory for applying these calculations to protein/ligand interactions and used them to examine the "binding" of two Lennard–Jones spheres in a small bath of Lennard–Jones spheres in 1984. This was probably the first "alchemical" free-energy calculation, although the term itself originated somewhat later. The first applications to true protein/ligand complexes followed shortly, with Wong and McCammon computing relative binding free energies of three trypsin inhibitors[153] with some success, and Hermans and Subramaniam computing the binding free energy of xenon to myoglobin.[154] This and related work from others ushered in a wave of alchemical applications in the late 1980s and early 1990s.

However, in a recent review, David Pearlman noted that some of the early success with alchemical methods may have been simply luck. He argues, "[W]e are now at a point that is, in reality, where we thought we were 20 years ago!"[155] At the very least, performing accurate alchemical free-energy calculations has turned out to be a great deal more difficult and computationally demanding than originally

thought,[8,156] so enthusiasm waned after the initial success before undergoing a resurgence since the early 2000s. This recent change has been described as a "coming of age."[165] Alchemical methods have yet to see widespread use in pharmaceutical applications, however.

Part of the recent increase in enthusiasm for free-energy calculations has been due to some of the methodological innovations addressed above, including the movement away from EXP, and another large part has been due to steadily increasing computer power bringing new problems into range. Together, these factors mean that much of the work on alchemical methods before the early 2000s is woefully out of date, so in this discussion we focus mostly on work since 2000. As noted above, alchemical free energies can be calculated by TI, EXP (exponential averaging), or BAR, among other methods, but the basic ideas remain the same. Here we highlight some key applications areas of alchemical methods without focusing on methodological issues highlighted above.

Relative free energies

Relative binding free energies were one of the earliest applications of alchemical methods, and they have remained a traditional application of alchemical free-energy methods. Relative free-energy calculations involve alchemically transforming one ligand into another, allowing direct calculation of the relative binding free energies from an appropriate thermodynamic cycle. This may be substantially more efficient than computing two absolute binding free energies and subtracting in cases where the ligands are relatively similar, as it eliminates statistical noise due to transformation of the rest of the ligands. If the limiting factor in the precision of the calculations is a long time-scale conformational fluctuation of the protein, however, the relative efficiency of relative free-energy calculations may be lessened considerably.

There have been a number of practical success stories with these calculations. One particularly interesting and comprehensive set of studies has been work from the Jorgensen lab on binding of HIV-1 nonnucleoside reverse transcriptase inhibitors (NNRTIs).[157–163] One study used docking and molecular dynamics equilibration to generate a model structure of sustiva bound to HIV-1 reverse transcriptase and then alchemical free-energy methods with Monte Carlo conformational sampling to compute the change in binding affinity of sustiva due to several known drug resistance mutants. Because the computed drug resistance profile matched well with experiment (with relative binding free energies accurate to 1–2 kcal/mol), this suggested that the model binding mode was indeed correct, a fact that was subsequently confirmed crystallographically.[157] Two other studies examined effects of known drug resistance mutations on several inhibitors and derivatives[158,159]; both were accurate to within 1 kcal/mol in relative binding free energies. One issue with these calculations concerns the approximations made, including the fact that the protein backbone was fixed and only side chain atoms within 15Å of the ligand were allowed to move, which is worrisome given the fact that HIV-1 NNRTIs allosterically disrupt enzymatic activity at a site that neighbors the binding pocket. Three other studies describe the application of free-energy calculations to lead optimization and the resulting compounds' activity in a cell-based assay; no affinity measurements were made, so no quantitative assessment of accuracy is possible.[160,161,163]

In several other cases, relative free-energy calculations have been used to validate models and suggest mechanisms. As noted above, relative free-energy calculations were used to validate the modeled binding mode of sustiva in HIV-1 reverse transcriptase. Relative free-energy calculations were also used to validate a homology model of a G-protein-coupled receptor by computing relative binding affinities of several known inhibitors[164] with errors of less than 1 kcal/mol. This approach was suggested to be a general one for validating homology models.[156–164] On the mechanism side, Yang et al. used relative free-energy calculations to help identify the tight binding site for ATP in F1-ATPase,[165] and Banerjee et al. used relative free-energy calculations to elucidate the recognition mechanism of oxo-guanine by a DNA repair enzyme.[166]

There has also been a significant amount of work with relative free-energy calculations on the estrogen receptor, mostly using artificial intermediate states designed to allow rapid estimation of free energies of multiple different inhibitors from just one or two simulations.[87,129,167] The downside is that phase-space overlap issues due to the limited number of simulations can present convergence problems, so the quality of the results has been very mixed depending on the choice of reference state, with errors ranging from nearly 0 kcal/mol up to more than 20 kcal/mol.[87]

Another system of interest is fructose 1,6-bisphosphatase, where alchemical free-energy calculations have been used over many years to help guide lead optimization with some degree of success. A recent discussion is provided by Reddy and Erion.[168] Though extremely short simulations were used, with some other methodological limitations, alchemical calculations appear to have helped the lead optimization process.

Alchemical calculations have also been applied successfully to inhibitors of neutrophil elastase. A multistep procedure involving docking, then MM-PBSA scoring to identify binding modes, followed by thermodynamic integration to calculate relative binding free energies, gave results for relative binding free energies within 1 kcal/mol.[169] In a follow-up study, alchemical calculations were used to predict a modification to an inhibitor to increase the affinity. When synthesized, the new inhibitor had an IC$_{50}$ value that was a factor of 3 better.[213]

Alchemical calculations have given good correlations with experimental relative free energies for relative binding free energies of theophylline and analogs to an RNA aptamer.[170,171] One recent study also examined two trypsin inhibitors with a polarizable force field,[172] and another study with a polarizable force field examined a series of inhibitors of trypsin, thrombin, and urokinase and observed an excellent correlation with experimental relative binding affinities.[173] A series of relative free-energy studies have also examined binding of peptide and nonpeptide inhibitors of Src SH2 domains with mixed results.[174–177]

Several other studies have focused on the practical utility of free-energy calculations. Pearlman and Charifson compared alchemical free-energy calculations with more approximate methods on a challenging system and suggested that they have reached the point where they can be useful, and more predictive than other methods, in drug discovery applications; the test examined p38 MAP kinase.[178] A follow-up study showed that alchemical methods compared favorably with MM-PBSA in terms of accuracy and computational efficiency.[148] Another study by Chipot argues that the accuracy of alchemical methods is now sufficient to be useful in drug discovery, and the main remaining hurdle for their widespread application is how difficult they are to set up.[156] A further study by Chipot and coauthors shows that these calculations can be in some cases done quite rapidly and still yield accurate rank-ordering,[176] further highlighting the potential utility of alchemical methods. Another particularly interesting application was the computation of implicit solvent alchemical free energies of several different protein/ligand systems, where free-energy methods compare very favorably with docking, with much greater speed than with explicit solvent methods.[229]

Absolute free energies

Alchemical binding free-energy calculations have mostly been restricted to computing relative binding free energies. Computing the absolute binding free energy of a single ligand to a particular protein introduces two additional complexities not ordinarily encountered in relative free-energy calculations. An early (1986) article on protein/ligand binding highlighted both of these issues.[154] First, absolute binding free energies are reported relative to a standard state or reference concentration of ligand, so a reference concentration must somehow be introduced into the relevant thermodynamic cycle. Second, if a ligand does not interact with the rest of the system (as in an alchemical absolute binding free-energy calculation) it will need to sample the whole simulation box for convergence, presenting potential sampling problems that are discussed in more detail elsewhere.[153] The authors' solution to these problems was to introduce biasing restraints that both kept the ligand in the binding site when noninteracting and simultaneously introduced the standard state when the effect of the restraints is analytically accounted for. The clearest and most detailed discussion of these issues is provided by the excellent review of Gilson,[180] which laid the foundation for recent applications of binding free-energy calculations. A recent review of absolute free-energy calculations is provided by Deng and Roux.[181]

Despite the fact that these issues were raised in the 1986 work, a variety of "absolute" binding free-energy calculations since then have neglected one or both of these issues. Nevertheless, beginning in the mid-1990s, there have been a number of successful applications of absolute binding free-energy calculations. These cluster in three general categories that each merit individual discussion: (1) binding of water within buried sites or binding sites of proteins, (2) binding of nonpolar ligands in a designed binding cavity within T4 lysozyme, and (3) binding of ligands to FKBP.

Water binding. The area of water binding is particularly interesting (and challenging) because it is extremely difficult to access the thermodynamics of water binding experimentally, meaning that computation uniquely provides access to important and interesting information. It represents an important application of free-energy calculations that does not simply serve to predict a binding affinity but also adds physical insights about the binding process that can also be used in the further design. One important computational challenge is to ensure that the water molecule being removed is not replaced by any other water molecules while being removed, or else the net result of the calculation will simply be to remove a water molecule from bulk. This methodological issue is not always addressed in work on water binding and in some cases may be a concern.

Work in the area of water binding was begun with the absolute binding free-energy calculations of Helms and Wade in 1995. They found that a crystallographic water bound in a cavity in cytochrome P450cam with a particular inhibitor had a binding free energy around -2.8 ± 1.6 kcal/mol while transferring a water into the cavity with the natural substrate (camphor) would cost 3.8 ± 1.2 kcal/mol. A follow-up study found the preferred number of water molecules in the cavity in the absence of ligand,[182] finding that six waters is thermodynamically preferable over five and seven or eight by 1–2 kcal/mol. A third study then computed the absolute binding free energy of camphor by replacing it with six waters in the binding site.[183] More recently, Deng and Roux applied alchemical free-energy calculations in combination with a grand canonical Monte Carlo scheme to replace camphor with water molecules while removing camphor from the cavity.[184] Their computed binding free energy for camphor agreed fairly well with that of Helms and Wade, but they differed slightly on the number of water molecules in the cavity.

Another water binding free-energy study examined the binding of crystallographic waters in the subtilisin Carlsberg complex with eglin-C and found that only some of the waters appeared to bind favorably.[185] Another study (on bovine pancreatic trypsin inhibitor and a barnase mutant) reached similar conclusions about crystallographic waters,[186] and a more recent study has also observed unfavorable binding energies for crystallographic waters.[187]

The reasons for this apparent discrepancy are so far unclear, but one suggestion has been limitations in the force field,[186,187] partly because the crystallographic waters are often conserved across several different structures of the same complex or binding site, suggesting that crystal structure uncertainties may not be the problem.

Several studies have examined binding of a specific water (water 301) in the complex of HIV-1 protease with inhibitor KNI-272. Two studies agreed on the binding free energy of this water (around -3.3 kcal/mol for one protonation state of the protease),[188,189] while a third study disagreed by about 7 kcal/mol,[187] possibly due to methodological differences relating to the treatment of protein flexibility. The active site protonation state appears to substantially modulate the binding free energy of this water molecule.[189]

There have been a variety of other examinations of water energetics as well. Roux et al. looked at binding of several waters within bacteriorhodopsin and found that transfer of waters from bulk to the proton channel was thermodynamically favorable (in some cases by up to 6 kcal/mol), suggesting implications for proton transfer.[190] De Simone et al. looked at water binding within the prion protein.[191] An extensive study looked at binding free energies of fifty-four water molecules in binding sites of six proteins, with and without ligands present. As validation, some results were compared with previously published work before moving to new binding sites. Overall, water binding free energies varied substantially, with a mean binding free energy of -6.7 kcal/mol, substantially more favorable than the mean binding free energy of water molecules that are displaced by ligands (-3.7 kcal/mol). The range of binding free energies runs from slightly positive to around -10 kcal/mol.[187] One major conclusion from this and the other studies in this area is that water molecules make a highly variable contribution to the thermodynamics of ligand binding, and factoring water molecules into ligand design is likely not to be an intuitive process, thus increasing the need for computational methods that can account for variable contributions of bound waters.

A final study worthy of note for its novelty and potential practicality for drug discovery is the work of Pan et al., which used a grand canonical Monte Carlo technique to qualitatively predict locations around binding sites where waters can easily be displaced, suggesting routes for lead optimization.[192] Although this is not an application of absolute alchemical free-energy methods, it is nevertheless an extremely interesting application of free-energy methods to water binding.

T4 lysozyme ligand binding. Another important set of systems for studying binding free-energy calculations are the two model binding sites in T4 lysozyme created by point mutations. The first of these, the L99A mutant, introduces a simple nonpolar cavity, while the second (L99A/M102Q) adds a polar group at the margin of the cavity and introduces the possibility of more hydrogen bonding. Both have been extensively characterized experimentally.[113,193–199] Because these binding sites are relatively simple and rigid, and structural data are so easy to obtain, they have been attractive sites for the development and testing of absolute free-energy methods. Most of the work has been on the apolar version of this cavity.

One early absolute free-energy study, in 1997, examined the binding of benzene in the apolar cavity.[200] Depending on the computational details, calculated values range from −4.0 to −5.1 kcal/mol, and the experimental absolute binding free energy is −5.2 kcal/mol. A follow-up study examined binding of noble gases in the cavity, especially xenon, which binds under pressure, in agreement with computed binding free energies.[201]

The lysozyme cavity was also used as a test system for the methodological work of Boresch et al. in 2003, which fell short of actually computing a binding free energy, but laid out a clear and straightforward thermodynamic cycle for computing binding free energies; the cycle involves the use of both orientational restraints and distance restraints.[202] Work on the polar cavity extended some of the arguments in favor of using orientational restraints and found that large kinetic barriers can separate ligand orientations, so considering multiple candidate bound orientations can help when computing absolute binding free energies.[179]

More recent work done by Deng and Roux[203] looked at a series of known binders to the lysozyme cavity, with somewhat mixed success; some binding free energies were too negative by a few kcal/mol. Another study used grand canonical Monte Carlo techniques on the same system, but while neglecting protein flexibility,[204] again with mixed success. A third looked at binding of a single ligand in the lysozyme cavity and quantified the contributions of a slow side-chain motion to ligand binding. It found that a single side-chain rearrangement could affect binding free energies by a few kcal/mol and that including the free energies associated with this conformational change was key for obtaining accurate binding free energies.[205]

The most extensive study to date has been the joint theory-experiment work of Mobley, Graves, and others,[113] which studied a variety of previously measured ligands and reached a root-mean-square error of roughly 1.9 kcal/mol after dealing with problems relating slow sampling of ligand orientational changes, protein conformational changes, and ligand electrostatics parameters. A unique feature of this study was that bound crystal structures were not used as starting points for the calculations, except for comparison purposes. Absolute free-energy methods were then applied successfully to predict binding affinities, with errors less than 0.7 kcal/mol, and orientations of five previously untested small molecules. The contribution of protein flexibility was also assessed and turned out to be key for the accuracy of the results.

Overall, a message from the lysozyme work has been that even simple binding sites can present significant sampling problems for molecular simulations, especially concerning ligand orientations and side-chain degrees of freedom and

that a proper accounting of the thermodynamics here is key for obtaining predictive results.

FKBP binding calculations. The FK506 binding protein (FKBP) has been another popular test system for absolute free-energy methods, in part because of the relative rigidity of its backbone. FKBP-12 was important in the development of the immunosuppresive drug cyclosporin and has remained popular because of its role in the development of the field of chemical biology. A series of ligands studied experimentally by Holt et al. have been studied particularly closely by a number of researchers.[206]

Absolute alchemical free-energy methods were first applied to the system by Shirts,[207] who obtained root-mean-square error of 2.0 kcal/mol and a correlation coefficient (R^2) of 0.75. A follow-up study by Fujitani and collaborators[208] achieved a root-mean-square difference from a linear fit of only 0.4 kcal/mol, but with a large offset of −3.2 kcal/mol relative to experiment. As previously noted,[10] care must be taken when comparing this study directly with other absolute free-energy studies, because it neglects any treatment of the standard state, which could be part of the reason for the offset.[179]

A further study by Wang, Deng, and Roux using the same parameters as Shirts obtained a root-mean-square error around 2.0–2.5 kcal/mol,[97] but despite the fact that the results used the same parameters, they were significantly different from those of Shirts,[207] suggesting methodological or convergence differences. Another study by Jayachandran and coworkers obtained a root-mean-square error of 1.6 kcal/mol using a novel parallelized free-energy scheme that allows for contributions of multiple kinetically distinct ligand orientations.[209]

Two other smaller studies also applied absolute free-energy methods to the same system, although not alchemical free-energy methods. The work of Lee and Olson used PMF techniques to compute binding free energies of two inhibitors[106] with accuracies of 1–2 kcal/mol depending on the solvent model, and Ytreberg used nonequilibrium pulling techniques for two inhibitors with accuracies around 1 kcal/mol.[109]

In many cases, computed values have varied substantially, even when using the same parameters. Likely, full convergence has not yet been truly reached. This provides a warning for computations on the many systems that have significantly more conformational flexibility and an indication that higher accuracy with systems that have not been studied as systematically might result from some degree of coincidence.

Other interesting binding calculations. Absolute free-energy methods have also been applied in several other interesting cases where there is less of a body of work. Recently, Jiao et al. calculated the absolute binding free energy of benzamidine binding to trypsin using AMOEBA, a polarizable force field, and then computed the relative binding free energy of a benzamidine derivative[172] with accuracies to within than 0.5 kcal/mol. Due to the small size of the study, it is difficult to be sure whether the high accuracy here is fortuitous or because of the use of a polarizable force field itself.

Dixit and Chipot also applied absolute free-energy calculations to compute the binding free energy of biotin to streptavidin; they obtained -16.6 ± 1.9 kcal/mol compared to an experimental value of -18.3 kcal/mol.[210]

Solvation free energies

Alchemical free-energy methods have often been tested by or applied to computing hydration free energies of small molecules like amino acid side-chain analogs or other small neutral compounds,[81,205,211] occasionally in a predictive context.[212] These tests can provide insight into the fundamental level of accuracy that can be expected of current force fields and also provide guidance for improvements to force fields. Also, several studies have highlighted the fact that solvation of small molecules can play an important role in determining binding free energies. One recent study found that the affinity of two trypsin inhibitors for water was very different, but these differences nearly canceled with differences in the binding site.[172] Another study suggested that solvation free energies played a substantial role in determining the change in binding affinity when optimizing fructose 1,6-bisphosphatase inhibitors.[168]

Predictive tests

Predictive tests of alchemical free-energy methods have been relatively rare, but at the same time are especially valuable for two reasons. First, to apply these methods in the context of drug discovery, they need to be predictive, and so testing them in a predictive context is a more realistic. Second, when doing retrospective studies, it is easy to be unintentionally influenced by the existing experimental results. For example, one might perform several sets of binding free-energy calculations with altered parameters and conclude that the "correct" set is the set that agrees best with experiment. Was any variation with parameters due to (a) the parameters themselves or (b) random errors due to poor convergence? And how would one proceed in a predictive setting?

However, alchemical free-energy methods have been applied predictively (together with or in advance of experiment) in a few studies. Here we focus especially on cases where experimental results are known and pass over those where we are not aware of any experiment that tests the computational results.

A number of studies have applied alchemical methods in the context of lead optimization. Some of the work from the Jorgensen lab on HIV-1 NNRTI has been predictive,[157,160,161] where free-energy calculations were used to help identify a binding mode and guide lead optimization. Similarly, the work on fructose 1,6-bisphosphatase has been predictive and applied in drug discovery.[168] Alchemical methods have been used to

successfully predict an optimization of a neutrophil elastase inhibitor that was subsequently synthesized and tested.[213] Another application in lead optimization used grand canonical Monte Carlo techniques to guide lead optimization.[192]

Alchemical free-energy calculations were also used predictively, or at least in a joint theory-experiment study, in examining binding of benzamidium derivatives and their binding to trypsin.[214] The computational results correctly captured experimental trends, though falling short of quantitative accuracy. A joint theory-experiment study that examined relative binding free energies of inhibitors to a GPCR was used to help validate a homology model; the computational results proved accurate to less than 1 kcal/mol.[164] Alchemical free-energy calculations were also used to predict the tight binding site of ATP in F1-ATPase,[165] a prediction subsequently confirmed experimentally.[215]

The only predictive absolute binding free-energy calculation we are aware of to date is the work on the T4 lysozyme system by Mobley, Graves, and collaborators, where absolute free energies were used to predict binding affinities and binding modes of several new ligands.[113]

Pitfalls and negative results

Negative results and failures can in some cases be extremely informative, especially when it is possible to identify failures with specific issues, because in such cases the failures highlight the importance of certain factors. Unfortunately, negative results and failures are not always published, so it can be difficult to gather information in this area, and it is often even more difficult to trace failures back to specific issues. Nevertheless, there are several articles that highlight issues in this area – either by tracing failure to a specific cause or by identifying and avoiding a potential pitfall.

One major, common pitfall is a dependence of computed free energies on starting structure. Because a binding free energy is a ratio of partition functions, it involves integrals over all of the relevant configurations of several systems and thus must be independent of the starting configurations of the system. Unfortunately, computed results often depend on the starting configuration of the system – for example, different starting ligand orientations or different starting protein structures may give different results, as noted in a number of studies. This kinetic trapping is inevitable whenever energy barriers are sufficiently large.[217] Mobley et al. found that results could depend significantly (by more than 1 kcal/mol, in some cases) on starting ligand orientation.[179] In FKBP, Shirts[206] and Wang et al.[97] found that computed binding free energies could differ by more than 1 kcal/mol depending on the choice of starting protein/ligand configuration, and Fujitani et al. also observed a dependence on starting structure.[208] An even larger dependence on the starting protein conformation was observed in lysozyme, where computed values could differ by 3–5 kcal/mol depending on the starting configuration of a valine side chain.[112,113,203] In another study of HIV-1 NNRTIs, computed relative binding free energies had the wrong sign (an error of roughly 4 kcal/mol) when beginning from a crystal structure with an alternate rotamer conformation near the active site.[63] As noted previously, these are not simply issues of having a wrong protein structure: when protein conformational changes occur on binding, multiple metastable configurations are relevant.[112] Thus, some authors have suggested starting simulations from different regions of phase space as a test for these sorts of issues[111,155] or have in some cases performed this test.[112,155]

Another potential pitfall is the possibility of multiple potentially relevant bound ligand orientations that can be separated by kinetic barriers.[179] This has been observed not only in absolute free-energy calculations on the lysozyme binding site, where interpretation and analysis is simplest,[113,179] but also in relative free-energy calculations for ligands binding to neutrophil elastase[169] and the estrogen receptor.[129] Ligand symmetries can also play a complicating role.[167,179]

In many cases, failures are more difficult to interpret. In a recent study on squalene-hopene cyclase inhibitors, relative free energies computed with a single-step perturbation method had large errors and in some cases had the wrong sign;[131] this was also the case in a study by some of the same authors on phosphodiesterase inhibitors.[216] Another study with single-step methods found results of varied quality depending on the (in principle arbitrary) choice of reference state, indicating poor convergence,[87] and in some cases resulting in very large errors. These errors may mostly be due to poor phase-space overlap with the single-step approach.

Using multiple routes around the same thermodynamic cycle can be a helpful way to check for errors when doing relative free-energy calculations. This approach was used by de Graaf et al.[218] and found very different results depending on the choice of pathway (indicating convergence problems along at least some pathways); cycle closure errors were up to 4.9 kcal/mol and for some paths and mutations, the sign of the relative free energies was even incorrect. Cycle closure errors were also large in the work of van den Bosch et al.[219] Of course, cycle closures only provide a lower bound on the error, and in some cases true errors are much larger than the cycle closure error, as is the case with the large cycle closure error and even larger true error in the work of Dolenc et al.[220]

In many cases, studies may have simply been somewhat too ambitious. Donnini and Juffer attempted to use absolute free-energy calculations to examine binding free energies between peptides and proteins and concluded that "it generally proved rather difficult to predict the absolute free energies correctly, for some protein families the experimental rank order was reproduced. . . ."[221]

Other types of binding free-energy studies

There are several other types of rigorous binding free-energy calculations that have occasionally been applied to interesting biomolecular problems. Grand canonical Monte Carlo (GCMC) techniques have been used in several applications to compute insertion free energies; in one study these techniques were used to compute favorable sites for displacing waters around a ligand in a binding site,[192] and in another case GCMC techniques were used to estimate binding free energies of ligands to the lysozyme model binding site, though in the absence of protein flexibility.[204] More recently, grand canonical techniques were used to insert water molecules into a protein/ligand binding site while the ligand was being alchemically removed, thereby speeding convergence.[184] Potential of mean force (PMF) methods have also been applied to several protein/ligand systems, including the binding affinities of FKBP inhibitors[107] and the binding affinity of a phosphotyrosine peptide to the SH2 domain of Lck.[108] Nonequilibrium free-energy methods have also been applied to FKBP inhibitors and peptides binding to the SH3 domain.[109,110]

As mentioned previously, the mining minima approach of Gilson and collaborators is also particularly interesting and has given promising results in calculations of binding free energies for host/guest systems[66] and ligands to artificial receptors.[164] However, because of computational limitations, it is difficult to apply it to the protein/ligand systems that are of interest in drug discovery. One recent study used this approach, however, to assess changes in HIV protease inhibitor configurational entropy on binding.[68]

DIRECTIONS FOR LIKELY IMPROVEMENT

There are a number of different aspects in which free-energy calculations will need to improve to become more accurate and reliable. One of the most important is in the realistic treatment of the environment of the protein/ligand systems. Typical ligand binding simulations include only the protein, the ligand, water, and perhaps a few ions to neutralize the simulated system. But many ligand binding affinities have significant dependence on pH, salt concentration, and metal-ion concentration. None of these additional aspects are typically modeled in ligand binding free-energy calculations and will need to be treated better in the future.

It is also likely that there will need to be further advances in atomistic force field parameters. A number of tests of solvation free energies have demonstrated that the current generation of force fields have fundamental problems that may restrict the ability of these force fields to obtain binding free energies that are accurate to within 1 kcal/mol.[81,104,205,222] Most common force field protein parameters are more than ten to fifteen years old, and only the torsions have generally been improved.[223,224] The criteria used for validity of protein parameters is usually proper structural conformational preferences, which may not be sufficiently accurate for their use in protein/ligand binding calculations. A recent version of the GROMOS force field, 53A6 has parameters that were fit to free-energy calculations of the free energies of transfer between water and cyclohexane, a first for an atomistic force field.[232] It seems likely that parameterizing to phase transfer properties should result in higher accuracy for binding affinity calculations, which are essentially transfers to a heterogeneous liquid phase, though direct comparisons between force fields optimized to pure liquid properties and transfer free energies have yet to be made.

Even more problematic are sufficiently accurate ligand parameters, as the number of functional groups is significantly higher than for protein systems and the amount of time that has been invested for parameterization significantly lower. Typical ligand parameters might be taken from the generalized Amber force field (GAFF),[225] usually using the ANTECHAMBER program in the AMBER distribution for atomtyping, although it is also sometimes done by hand, and the AM1-BCC method[226,227] (implemented in a variety of software codes) to determine the charges. Schrödinger also has automatic tools to assign atom types of novel compounds within the OPLS-AA parameterization system. Relatively few force fields have associated tools or even algorithms for determining compatible (let alone validated) ligand parameters.[228]

A number of research groups are actively developing polarizable potential functions,[228] which have the potential to greatly improve macromolecular force fields' abilities to predict binding affinities by adding an extra level of physical detail. However, at this point, it is not clear that any of them yet are quantitatively better than fixed charge force fields, as few of them have been validated to the extent that fixed charge models have. Polarizable molecular models are significantly slower than fixed charge models, and therefore both the iterative improvement of such force fields and the development of tools useful for production runs for free-energy calculations will be substantially behind that of fixed change force fields.

CONCLUSIONS

As we have seen in this chapter, free-energy calculations are not at the present time generally reliable methods to predict binding affinity and are not currently truly a part of standard structure-based drug design methods. And they certainly are not, and will not anytime in the near future, "black-box" methods that will "automagically" allow determination of free energies without significant investment in the physical chemistry and biology of the system. Although many papers are being published computing binding free energies in retrospective case studies, there is still a lack of comparative studies presenting results over large numbers of systems, with even fewer purely predictive studies. Partly

for these reasons, quantitative free-energy calculations are not a vital part of the discovery work flow of most major pharmaceutical company as far as we aware.

However, such calculations are certainly much closer to usability than they have been in the past. In particular, several recent studies mentioned in this chapter have highlighted the advantages of alchemical relative free-energy calculations compared to approximate methods like MM-GBSA and docking.[130,178,229] Alchemical methods have also been successfully applied in a lead-optimization context[161,230] (and see references therein). It appears that in this area free-energy calculations are already becoming useful but with large remaining hurdles to their more widespread adoption. Such hurdles include not only the computer time needed but also the human time and biochemical knowledge required to set up these simulations.[156,176,218,229]

As we have presented in this chapter, the methods used for free-energy calculations are changing rapidly. Major molecular simulation codes, such as AMBER, CHARMM, NAMD, GROMACS, and GROMOS, are undergoing major improvements and changes in the features used to compute binding free energies. Although these changes will likely greatly improve the ability to perform free-energy calculations, ongoing changes make it difficult to put together stable work flows for preparing ligands and simulation structures and determining ideal free-energy protocols without significant human effort, and it is difficult to recommend particular codes for the easiest use at the present time. MCPRO, developed in the Jorgensen lab, which has recently begun to be distributed by Schrödinger as MCPRO+, although not including much of the most recent methodology (such as Bennett Acceptance Ratio methods or soft-core alchemical pathways), is likely the easiest to use and set up and was used successfully for the HIV-1 NNRTI work in the Jorgensen lab described in this chapter.

One ongoing problem has been the lack of extensive experimental high-accuracy ligand binding affinities. As we have discussed, a desirable goal for free-energy calculations is to reach an accuracy threshold of 1 kcal/mol. However, the majority of experimental measurements, unless using highly accurate methods like ITC or SPR or extremely well-tuned competitive binding affinity assays, many not be more accurate than this, making large-scale validation of computational methodologies difficult. A number of academic databases of protein/ligand structures and interactions have been created, such as http://www.bindingmoad.org/ and http://lpdb.chem.lsa.umich.edu/ at the University of Michigan, http://www.bindingdb.org at Johns Hopkins, http://www.agklebe.de/affinity at Phillips-Universität Marburg,[230] and http://www.pdbcal.org at Indiana, but the degree of validation and utility of these databases are not well established.

In the United States, a recently announced NIH NIGMS RFA to establish a national Drug Docking and Screening Data Resource represents an attempt to increase the public availability of high-quality experimental data sets required for developing, validating, and benchmarking computational screening, docking, and binding affinity prediction, including both curating crystal structures and experimental binding affinities (see NIH NIGMS RFA-GM-08-008). NIST has recently become interested in developing and curating such data as well. Most importantly, there is a much larger wealth of data in proprietary pharmaceutical databases that no longer has significant intellectual property value, and a system for releasing such data to the broader community would be immensely valuable for development of improved drug design methods.

Another problem in the development of free-energy techniques is that most large-scale validations and comparisons of methodologies have been retrospective. There are relatively few opportunities to participate in large-scale prospective trials, as confidence of experimentalists in quantitative predictions made by computer is usually not high enough to motivate the high-quality experiments that can validate the computational results.

The quality of techniques for protein structure prediction has increased since the introduction of CASP (Critical Assessment of Structure Prediction) in 1994. Despite some criticisms about some aspects of the program,[232] it is considered to have played an important role in developing computational structure prediction. Other successful ongoing prospective computational challenges have been CAPRI (Critical Assessment of PRedicted Interactions) for protein/protein complexes,[233] the Industrial Fluid Properties Simulation Collective (IFPSC) (at http://www. fluidproperties.org), the Cambridge Crystallographic Data Centre's blind tests of small-molecule crystal structure prediction,[234] and the McMasters high-throughput screening competition.[235] It is clear that providing an opportunity for truly blind predictions of chemical and biological properties structure has been beneficial for the computational methodology community. There has therefore naturally been an interest in developing a similar true prospective trial for prediction of ligand binding affinities.

One such attempt called CATFEE (Critical Assessment of Techniques for Free Energy Evaluation) was attempted in 2000 but failed because the experimental data never became available.[236] A more recent attempt, called SAMPL (Statistical Assessment of the Modeling of Proteins and Ligands), run by OpenEye Software, was conducted in late 2007 to early 2008, with two protein targets (urokinase, with data contributed by Abbott, and JNK3 kinase, with data contributed by Vertex) and sixty-three ligand binding points determined by IC_{50}s, but with the same assay for each target. The competition consisted of virtual screening against decoys, pose prediction of known actives, and prediction of binding affinity from crystal structures. Although the summary of the results is still in preparation, by almost all measures they were somewhat discouraging, with correlations to predictions using various physically based methods significantly worse than 1 kcal/mol

root-mean-square error. Interestingly, the best method was a less computationally demanding approximation to MM-PBSA that essentially ignored the entropy contribution[237] but even this method was very unreliable. The initial SAMPL generated significant participation and interest and is very likely to continue.

In the foreseeable future, fully atomistic free-energy calculations may be most important not solely for reliable predictions of binding affinity, but for a wealth of additional atomistic information such as probabilities of occupation of binding pose and water structure in the binding site that are impossible to gather from either experiment or more approximate methods. Free-energy calculations may also be of use in the future for the computation of octanol/water partition coefficients of molecules that are difficult to predict by standard rule-based algorithms like CLOGP or for even more direct membrane permeability simulations. Calculating the free energy, and thus stability, of different tautomers represents another important application of fully physical simulations. Questions of ligand-binding specificity can frequently be seen as a multivariate optimization problem, with binding to the intended target maximized, while binding to the alternative targets is minimized.

For further information, readers are encouraged to read a number of reviews on the subject of free-energy calculations published more recently,[8–11,13,238–240] useful textbooks,[15–17,231] as well as older reviews and books that may provide more historical perspective.[32,241,242]

A number of the reviews on the subject of free-energy calculations in ligand binding since the late 1980s conclude that free-energy calculations of ligand binding have finally overcome the problems and false starts of the past and that the time for free energies in pharmaceutical industry is nearly here or has already arrived. We will not make nearly as strong a claim here. An extensive survey of the latest results is somewhat mixed, and it is not clear that these methods will necessarily be an important part of the pharmaceutical work flow anytime in the near future. In some cases, computational simulations may be approaching the level of accuracy that they can provide some additional utility in some aspects of lead optimization, but the accuracy and speed of the methods presented in this chapter must both be improved drastically. Many computational chemists working in industry that were questioned by the authors thought that rigorous free-energy methods may eventually become a routine part of drug discovery methods but perhaps not for another twenty years.

It does, however, appear that improvements in computational power and methodologies have made it possible to compute increasingly reliable relative and absolute binding affinities, albeit with significant computational and human effort. Continuing improvements in techniques will make physics-based simulations more and more attractive, leading to improved simulation tools and eventually to a vital place in the pharmaceutical work flow.

REFERENCES

1. Houston, J. G.; Banks, M. N.; Binnie, A.; Brenner, S.; O'Connell, J.; Petrillo, E. W. Case study: impact of technology investment on lead discovery at Bristol Myers Squibb, 1998–2006. *Drug Discov. Today* **2008**, *13*, 44–51.

2. Keseru, G. M.; Makara, G. M. Hit discovery and hit-to-lead approaches. *Drug Discov. Today* **2006**, *11*, 741–748.

3. Koppitz, M.; Eis, K. Automated medicinal chemistry. *Drug Discov. Today* **2006**, *11*, 561–568.

4. Perola, E.; Walters, W.; Charifson, P. S. A detailed comparison of current docking and scoring methods on systems of pharmaceutical relevance. *Proteins* **2004**, *56*, 235–249.

5. Warren, G. L.; Andrews, C. W.; Capelli, A.-M.; Clarke, B.; LaLonde, J.; Lambert, M. H.; Lindvall, M.; Nevins, N.; Semus, S. F.; Senger, S.; Tedesco, G.; Wall, I. D.; Woolven, J. M.; Peishoff, C. E.; Head, M. S. A critial assessment of docking programs and scoring functions. *J. Med. Chem.* **2006**, *49*(20), 5912–5931.

6. Enyedy, I.; Egan, W. Can we use docking and scoring for hit-to-lead optimization? *J. Comput. Aided Mol. Des.* **2008**.

7. Hajduk, P. J.; Sauer, D. R. Statistical analysis of the effects of common chemical substituents on ligand potency. *J. Med. Chem.* **2008**, *51*, 553–564.

8. Shirts, M. R.; Mobley, D. L.; Chodera, J. D. Alchemical free energy calculations: ready for prime time? *Annu. Rep. Comput. Chem.* **2007**, *3*, 41–59.

9. Huang, N.; Jacobson, M. P. Physics-based methods for studying protein-ligand interactions. *Curr. Opin. Drug Di. De.* **2007**, *10*, 325–331.

10. Gilson, M. K.; Zhou, H.-X. Calculation of protein-ligand binding affinities. *Annu. Rev. Biophys. Biomed.* **2007**, *36*, 21–42.

11. Meirovitch, H. Recent developments in methodologies for calculating the entropy and free energy of biological systems by computer simulation. *Curr. Opin. Struc. Biol.* **2007**, *17*, 181–186.

12. Ytreberg, F. M.; Swendsen, R. H.; Zuckerman, D. M. Comparison of free energy methods for molecular systems. *J. Chem. Phys.* **2006**, *125*, 184114.

13. Rodinger, T.; Pomès, R. Enhancing the accuracy, the efficiency and the scope of free energy simulations. *Curr. Opin. Struc. Biol.* **2005**, *15*, 164–170.

14. Brandsdal, B. O.; Österberg, F.; Almlöf, M.; Feierberg, I.; Luzhkov, V. B.; Åqvist, J. Free energy calculations and ligand binding. *Adv. Prot. Chem.* **2003**, *66*, 123–158.

15. Chipot, C.; Pohorille, A.; Eds. *Free Energy Calculations: Theory and Applications in Chemistry and Biology*, Vol. 86. New York: Springer, **2007**.

16. Frenkel, D.; Smit, B. *Understanding Molecular Simulation: from Algorithms to Applications*. San Diego, CA: Academic Press; **2002**.

17. Leach, A. R. *Molecular Modelling: Principles and Applications*. Harlow, Essex, England: Addison Wesley Longman Limited; **1996**.

18. Allen, M. P.; Tildesley, D. J. *Computer Simulation of Liquids*. New York: Oxford University Press; **1987**.

19. Woods, C. J.; Manby, F. R.; Mulholland, A. J. An efficient method for the calculation of quantum mechanics/molecular mechanics free energies. *J. Chem. Phys.* **2008**, *128*(1), 014109.

20. Kollman, P. A.; Massova, I.; Reyes, C.; Kuhn, B.; Huo, S.; Chong, L.; Lee, M.; Lee, T.; Duan, Y.; Wang, W.; Donini, O.; Cieplak, P.; Srinivasan, J.; Case, D. A.; Cheatham, T. E. Calculating structures and free energies of complex molecules: combining molecular mechanics and continuum models. *Acc. Chem. Res.* **2000**, *33*, 889–897.

21. Lee, M. S.; Olson, M. A. Calculation of absolute protein-ligand binding affinity using path and endpoint approaches. *Biophys J.* **2006**, *90*, 864–877.

22. Gohlke, H.; Case, D. A. Converging free energy estimates: Mm-pb(gb)sa studies on the protein-protein complex ras-raf. *J. Comput. Chem.* **2004**, *25*, 238–250.

23. Swanson, J. M. J.; Henchman, R. H.; McCammon, J. A. Revisiting free energy calculations: a theoretical connection to MM/PBSA and direct calculation of the association free energy. *Biophys J.* **2004**, *86*, 67–74.

24. Daggett, V. Long timescale simulations. *Curr. Opin. Struc. Biol.* **2000**, *10*, 160–164.

25. Sitkoff, D.; Sharp, K.; Honig, B. H. Accurate calculation of hydration free energies using macroscopic solvent models. *J. Phys. Chem.* **1994**, *98*, 1978–1988.

26. Honig, B. H.; Nicholls, A. Classical electrostatics in biology and chemistry. *Science* **1995**, *268*, 1144–1149.

27. Gilson, M. K.; Sharp, K.; Honig, B. H. Calculating the electrostatic potential of molecules in solution: method and error assessment. *J. Comput. Chem.* **1987**, *9*, 327–335.

28. Gilson, M. K.; Honig, B. H. Calculation of the total electrostatic energy of a macromolecular system: solvation energies, binding energies, and conformational analysis. *Proteins* **1988**, *4*, 7–18.

29. Rubinstein, A.; Sherman, S. Influence of the solvent structure on the electrostatic interactions in proteins. *Biophys J.* **2004**, *87*, 1544–1557.

30. Swanson, J. M. J.; Mongan, J.; McCammon, J. A. Limitations of atom-centered dielectric functions in implicit solvent models. *J. Phys. Chem. B* **2005**, *109*, 14769–14772.

31. Schutz, C. N.; Warshel, A. What are the dielectric "constants" of proteins and how to validate electrostatic models? *Proteins* **2001**, *44*, 400–417.

32. Archontis, G.; Simonson, T.; Karplus, M. Binding free energies and free energy components from molecular dynamics and Poisson-Boltzmann calculations: Application to amino acid recognition by aspartyl-tRNA. *J. Mol. Biol.* **2001**, *306*, 307–327.

33. Sharp, K.; Honig, B. H. Electrostatic interactions in macromolecules: theory and applications. *Annu. Rev. Biophys. Biol.* **1990**, *19*, 301–332.

34. Richards, F. M. Areas, volumes, packing and protein structure. *Annu. Rev. Biophys. Biol.* **1977**, *6*, 151–176.

35. Sharp, K.; Nicholls, A.; Fine, R. F.; Honig, B. H. Reconciling the magnitude of the microscopic and macroscopic hydrophobic effects. *Science* **1991**, *252*, 106–109.

36. Hermann, R. B. Theory of hydrophobic bonding. II. The correlation of hydrocarbon solubility in water with solvent cavity surface area. *J. Phys. Chem.* **1972**, *76*, 2754–2759.

37. Reynolds, J. A.; Gilbert, D. B.; Tanford, C. Empirical correlation between hydrophobic free energy and aqueous cavity surface area. *Proc. Natl. Acad. Sci. U.S.A.* **1974**, *71*, 2925–2927.

38. Gallicchio, E.; Kubo, M. M.; Levy, R. M. Enthalpy-entropy and cavity decomposition of alkane hydration free energies: Numerical results and implications for theories of hydrophobic solvation. *J. Phys. Chem. B* **2000**, *104*, 6271–6285.

39. Wagoner, J. A.; Baker, N. A. Assessing implicit models for nonpolar mean solvation forces: the importance of dispersion and volume terms. *P. Natl. Acad. Sci. U.S.A.* **2006**, *103*, 8331–8336.

40. Tan, C.; Tan, Y.-H.; Luo, R. Implicit nonpolar solvent models. *J. Phys. Chem. B* **2007**, *111*, 12263–12274.

41. Levy, R. M.; Zhang, L. Y.; Gallicchio, E.; Felts, T. On the nonpolar hydration free energy of proteins: surface area and

continuum solvent models for the solute-solvent interaction energy. *J. Am. Chem. Soc.* **2003**, *125*, 9523–9530.

42. Luo, H.; Sharp, K. On the calculation of absolute macromolecular binding free energies. *Proc. Natl. Acad. Sci. U.S.A.* **2002**, *99*, 10399–10404.

43. Brooks, B. R.; Janezic, D.; Karplus, M. Harmonic analysis of large systems. I. Methodology. *J. Comput. Chem.* **2004**, *16*, 1522–1542.

44. Bohm, H. J. The development of a simple empirical scoring function to estimate the binding constant for a protein-ligand complex of known three-dimensional structure. *J. Comput. Aid. Mol. Des.* **1994**, *8*, 243–256.

45. Hnizdo, V.; Tan, J.; Killian, B. J.; Gilson, M. K. Efficient calculation of configurational entropy from molecular simulations by combining the mutual-information expansion and nearest-neighbor methods. *J. Comput. Chem.* **2008**, *29*(10), 1605–1614.

46. Froloff, N.; Windemuth, A.; Honig, B. H. On the calculation of binding free energies using continuum methods: application to MHC class I protein-peptide interactions. *Protein Sci.* **1997**, *6*, 1293–301.

47. Hünenberger, P. H.; Helms, V.; Narayana, N.; Taylor, S. S.; McCammon, J. A. Determinants of ligand binding to camp-dependent protein kinase. *Biochemistry* **1999**, *38*, 2358–2366.

48. Jian Shen, J. W. Electrostatic binding energy calculation using the finite difference solution to the linearized Poisson-Boltzmann equation: assessment of its accuracy. *J. Comput. Chem.* **1996**, *17*, 350–357.

49. Schapira, M.; Torrv, M. Prediction of the binding energy for small molecules, peptides and proteins. *J. Mol. Recognit.* **1999**, *12*, 177–190.

50. Mobley, D. L.; Dill, K. A.; Chodera, J. D. Treating entropy and conformational changes in implicit solvent simulations of small molecules. *J. Phys. Chem. B* **2008**, *112*, 938–946.

51. Olson, M. A. Modeling loop reorganization free energies of acetylcholinesterase: a comparison of explicit and implicit solvent models. *Proteins* **2004**, *57*, 645–650.

52. Brown, S. P.; Muchmore, S. W. High-throughput calculation of protein-ligand binding affinities: modification and adaptation of the MM-PBSA protocol to enterprise grid computing. *J. Chem. Inf. Model.* **2006**, *46*, 999–1005.

53. Bashford, D.; Case, D. A. Generalized born models of macromolecular solvation effects. *Annu. Rev. Phys. Chem.* **2000**, *51*, 129–152.

54. Onufriev, A.; Bashford, D.; Case, D. A. Modification of the generalized Born model suitable for macromolecules. *J. Phys. Chem. B* **2000**, *104*, 3712–3720.

55. Onufriev, A.; Case, D. A.; Bashford, D. Effective Born radii in the generalized Born approximation: the importance of being perfect. *J. Comput. Chem.* **2002**, *23*, 1297–1304.

56. Feig, M.; Onufriev, A.; Lee, M. S.; Im, W.; Case, D. A.; Brooks, C. L., III. Performance comparison of generalized Born and Poisson methods in the calculation of electrostatic solvation energies for protein structures. *J. Comput. Chem.* **2004**, *25*, 265–284.

57. Geney, R.; Layten, M.; Gomperts, R.; Hornak, V.; Simmerling, C. Investigation of salt bridge stability in a generalized born solvent model. *J. Chem. Theory Comput.* **2006**, *2*, 115–127.

58. Nymeyer, H.; Garcia, A. E. Simulation of the folding equilibrium of alpha-helical peptides: a comparison of the generalized born approximation with explicit solvent. *Proc. Natl. Acad. Sci. U.S.A.* **2003**, *100*, 13934–13939.

59. Gilson, M. K.; Honig, B. H. The inclusion of electrostatic hydration energies in molecular mechanics calculations. *J. Comput. Aid. Mol. Des.* **1991**, *5*, 5–20.

60. Head, M. S.; Given, J. A.; Gilson, M. K. "Mining Minima": direct computation of conformational free energy. *J. Phys. Chem. A* **1997**, *101*, 1609–1618.

61. Kolossváry, I. Evaluation of the molecular configuration integral in all degrees of freedom for the direct calculation of conformational free energies: prediction of the anomeric free energy of monosaccharides. *J. Phys. Chem. A* **1997**, *101*(51), 9900–9905.

62. Ragusa, A.; Hayes, J. M.; Light, M. E.; Kilburn, J. D. Predicting enantioselectivity: computation as an efficient experimental tool for probing enantioselectivity. *Eur. J. Org. Chem.* **2006**, *2006*(9), 3545–3549.

63. Ragusa, A.; Hayes, J. M.; Light, M. E.; Kilburn, J. D. A combined computational and experimental approach for the analysis of the enantioselective potential of a new macrocyclic receptor for n-protected α-amino acids. *Chem. Eur. J.* **2007**, *13*(9), 2717–2728.

64. Potter, M. J.; Gilson, M. K. Coordinate systems and the calculation of molecular properties. *J. Phys. Chem. A* **2002**, *106*(3), 563–566.

65. Chang, C.-E. A.; Gilson, M. K. Free energy, entropy, and induced fit in host-guest recognition: calculations with the second-generation mining minima algorithm. *J. Am. Chem. Soc.* **2004**, *126*(40), 13156–13164.

66. Chang, C.-E.; Chen, W.; Gilson, M. K. Calculation of cyclodextrin binding affinities: energy, entropy, and implications for drug design. *Biophys. J.* **2004**, *87*, 3035–3049.

67. Chen, W.; Chang, C.-E. A.; Gilson, M. K. Concepts in receptor optimization: Targeting the rgd peptide. *J. Am. Chem. Soc.* **2006**, *128*(14), 4675–4684.

68. Chang, C.-E. A.; Chen, W.; Gilson, M. K. Ligand configurational entropy and protein binding. *Proc. Natl. Acad. Sci. U.S.A.* **2007**, *104*(5), 1534–1539.

69. Killian, B. J.; Yundenfreund Kravitz, J.; Gilson, M. K. Extraction of configurational entropy from molecular simulations via an expansion approximation. *J. Chem. Phys.* **2007**, *127*(2), 024107.

70. Chang, C.-E. A.; Chen, W.; Gilson, M. K. Evaluating the accuracy of the quasiharmonic approximation. *J. Chem. Theory Comput.* **2005**, *1*(5), 1017–1028.

71. Young, T.; Abel, R.; Kim, B.; Berne, B. J.; Friesner, R. A. Motifs for molecular recognition exploiting hydrophobic enclosure in protein-ligand binding. *Proc. Natl. Acad. Sci. U.S.A.* **2007**, *104*, 808–813.

72. Zwanzig, R. W. High-temperature equation of state by a perturbation method. I. Nonpolar gases. *J. Chem. Phys.* **1954**, *22*(8), 1420–1426.

73. Shirts, M. R.; Pande, V. S. Comparison of efficiency and bias of free energies computed by exponential averaging, the bennett acceptance ratio, and thermodynamic integration. *J. Chem. Phys.* **2005**, *122*, 144107.

74. Lu, N. D.; Singh, J. K.; Kofke, D. A. Appropriate methods to combine forward and reverse free-energy perturbation averages. *J. Chem. Phys.* **2003**, *118*(7), 2977–2984.

75. Wu, D.; Kofke, D. A. Asymmetric bias in free-energy perturbation measurements using two Hamiltonian-based models. *Phys. Rev. E* **2005**, *70*, 066702.

76. Jarzynski, C. Rare events and the convergence of exponentially averaged work values. *Phys. Rev. E* **2006**, *73*, 046105.

77. Widom, B. Some topics in the theory of fluids. *J. Chem. Phys.* **1963**, *39*(11), 2808–2812.

78. Jorgensen, W. L.; Ravimohan, C. Monte Carlo simulation of differences in free energies of hydration. *J. Chem. Phys.* **1985**, *83*(6), 3050–3054.

79. Resat, H.; Mezei, M. Studies on free energy calculations. I. Thermodynamic integration using a polynomial path. *J. Chem. Phys.* **1993**, *99*(8), 6052–6061.

80. Pitera, J. W.; van Gunsteren, W. F. A comparison of non-bonded scaling approaches for free energy calculations. *Mol. Simulat.* **2002**, *28*(1–2), 45–65.

81. Shirts, M. R.; Pitera, J. W.; Swope, W. C.; Pande, V. S. Extremely precise free energy calculations of amino acid side chain analogs: comparison of common molecular mechanics force fields for proteins. *J. Chem. Phys.* **2003**, *119*(11), 5740–5761.

82. Beutler, T. C.; Mark, A. E.; van Schaik, R. C.; Gerber, P. R.; van Gunsteren, W. F. Avoiding singularities and numerical instabilities in free energy calculations based on molecular simulations. *Chem. Phys. Lett.* **1994**, *222*, 529–539.

83. Mobley, D. L. Unpublished data.

84. Pearlman, D. A.; Kollman, P. A. The lag between the Hamiltonian and the system configuration in free-energy perturbation calculations. *J. Chem. Phys.* **1989**, *91*(12), 7831–7839.

85. Hendrix, D. A.; Jarzynski, C. A "fast growth" method of computing free energy differences. *J. Chem. Phys.* **2001**, *114*(14), 5974–5961.

86. Oostenbrink, C.; van Gunsteren, W. F. Calculating zeros: nonequilibrium free energy calculations. *Chem. Phys.* **2006**, *323*, 102–108.

87. Oostenbrink, C.; van Gunsteren, W. F. Free energies of ligand binding for structurally diverse compounds. *Proc. Natl. Acad. Sci. U.S.A.* **2005**, *102*(19), 6750–6754.

88. Crooks, G. E. Path-ensemble averages in systems driven far from equilibrium. *Phys. Rev. E* **2000**, *61*(3), 2361–2366.

89. Bennett, C. H. Efficient estimation of free energy differences from Monte Carlo data. *J. Comput. Phys.* **1976**, *22*, 245–268.

90. Shirts, M. R.; Bair, E.; Hooker, G.; Pande, V. S. Equilibrium free energies from nonequilibrium measurements using maximum-likelihood methods. *Phys. Rev. Lett.* **2003**, *91*(14), 140601.

91. Rick, S. W. Increasing the efficiency of free energy calculations using parallel tempering and histogram reweighting. *J. Chem. Theory Comput.* **2006**, *2*, 939–946.

92. Ferrenberg, A. M.; Swendsen, R. H. Optimized Monte Carlo data analysis. *Phys. Rev. Lett.* **1989**, *63*(12), 1195–1198.

93. Kumar, S.; Bouzida, D.; Swendsen, R. H.; Kollman, P. A.; Rosenberg, J. M. The weighted histogram analysis method for free-energy calculations on biomolecules. I. The method. *J. Comput. Chem.* **1992**, *13*(8), 1011–1021.

94. Bartels, C.; Karplus, M. Multidimensional adaptive umbrella sampling: applications to main chain and side chain peptide conformations. *J. Comput. Chem.* **1997**, *18*(12), 1450–1462.

95. Gallicchio, E.; Andrec, M.; Felts, A. K.; Levy, R. M. Temperature weighted histogram analysis method, replica exchange, and transition paths. *J. Phys. Chem. B* **2005**, *109*, 6722–6731.

96. Souaille, M.; Roux, B. Extension to the weighted histogram analysis method: combining umbrella sampling with free energy calculations. *Comput. Phys. Commun.* **2001**, *135*(1), 40–57.

97. Wang, J.; Deng, Y.; Roux, B. Absolute binding free energy calculations using molecular dynamics simulations with restraining potentials. *Biophys. J.* **2006**, *91*, 2798–2814.

98. Shirts, M. R.; Chodera, J. D. Statistically optimal analysis of samples from multiple equilibrium states. *J. Chem. Phys.* **2008**, *129*, 129105.

99. Steinbrecher, T.; Mobley, D. L.; Case, D. A. Nonlinear scaling schemes for Lennard-Jones interactions in free energy calculations. *J. Chem. Phys.* **2007**, *127*(21).

100. Pearlman, D. A.; Connelly, P. R. Determination of the differential effects of hydrogen bonding and water release on the binding of FK506 to native and TYR82 → PHE82 FKBP-12 proteins using free energy simulations. *J. Mol. Biol.* **1995**, *248*(3), 696–717.

101. Wang, L.; Hermans, J. Change of bond length in free-energy simulations: algorithmic improvements, but when is it necessary? *J. Chem. Phys.* **1994**, *100*(12), 9129–9139.

102. Boresch, S.; Karplus, M. The Jacobian factor in free energy simulations. *J. Chem. Phys.* **1996**, *105*(12), 5145–5154.

103. Zacharias, M.; Straatsma, T. P.; McCammon, J. A. Separation-shifted scaling, a new scaling method for lennard-jones interactions in thermodynamic integration. *J. Phys. Chem.* **1994**, *100*(12), 9025–9031.

104. Shirts, M. R.; Pande, V. S. Solvation free energies of amino acid side chains for common molecular mechanics water models. *J. Chem. Phys.* **2005**, *122*, 134508.

105. Blondel, A. Ensemble variance in free energy calculations by thermodynamic integration: theory, optimal alchemical path, and practical solutions. *J. Comput. Chem.* **2004**, *25*(7), 985–993.

106. Rodinger, T.; Howell, P. L.; Pomès, R. Absolute free energy calcualtions by thermodynamic integration in four spatial dimensions. *J. Chem. Phys.* **2005**, *123*, 034104.

107. Lee, M. S.; Olson, M. A. Calculation of absolute protein-ligand binding affinity using path and endpoint approaches. *Biophys. J.* **2006**, *90*, 864–877.

108. Woo, H.-J.; Roux, B. Calculation of absolute protein-ligand binding free energy from computer simulation. *Proc. Natl. Acad. Sci. U.S.A.* **2005**, *102*, 6825–6830.

109. Ytreberg, F. M. Absolute FKBP binding affinities obtained by nonequilibrium unbinding simulations. *J. Chem. Phys.* **2009**, *130*, 164906-8.

110. Gan, W.; Roux, B. Binding specificity of SH2 domains: insight from free energy simulations. *Proteins* **2008**, *74*, 996–1007.

111. Torrie, G. M.; Valleau, J. P. Non-physical sampling distributions in Monte-Carlo free-energy estimation: umbrella sampling. *J. Comput. Phys.* **1977**, *23*(2), 187–199.

112. Mobley, D. L.; Chodera, J. D.; Dill, K. A. Confine-and-release method: obtaining correct binding free energies in the presence of protein conformational change. *J. Chem. Theory Comput.* **2007**, *3*(4), 1231–1235.

113. Mobley, D. L.; Graves, A. P.; Chodera, J. D.; McReynolds, A. C.; Shoichet, B. K.; Dill, K. A. Predicting absolute ligand binding free energies to a simple model site. *J. Mol. Biol.* **2007**, *371*(4), 1118–1134.

114. Okamoto, Y. Generalized-ensemble algorithms: enhanced sampling techniques for Monte Carlo and molecular dynamics simulations. *J. Mol. Graph. Model.* **2004**, *22*, 425–439.

115. Pitera, J. W.; Kollman, P. A. Exhaustive mutagenesis in silico: multicoordinate free energy calculations in proteins and peptides. *Proteins* **2000**, *41*, 385–397.

116. Roux, B.; Faraldo-Gómez, J. D. Characterization of conformational equilibria through hamiltonian and temperature replica-exchange simulations: assessing entropic and environmental effects. *J. Comput. Chem.* **2007**, *28*(10), 1634–1647.

117. Woods, C. J.; Essex, J. W.; King, M. A. Enhanced configurational sampling in binding free energy calculations. *J. Phys. Chem. B* **2003**, *107*, 13711–13718.

118. Banba, S.; Guo, Z.; Brooks, C. L., III. Efficient sampling of ligand orientations and conformations in free energy calculations using the lambda-dynamics method. *J. Phys. Chem. B*, **2000**, *104*(29), 6903–6910.

119. Bitetti-Putzer, R.; Yang, W.; Karplus, M. Generalized ensembles serve to improve the convergence of free energy simulations. *Chem. Phys. Lett.* **2003**, *377*, 633–641.

120. Hritz, J.; Oostenbrink, C. Hamiltonian replica exchange molecular dynamics using soft-core interactions. *J. Chem. Phys.* **2008**, *128*(14), 144121.

121. Guo, Z.; Brooks, C. L., III, Kong, X. Efficient and flexible algorithm for free energy calculations using the λ-dynamics approach. *J. Phys. Chem. B* **1998**, *102*, 2032–2036.

122. Kong, X.; Brooks, C. L., III. λ-dynamics: a new approach to free energy calculations. *J. Chem. Phys.* **1996**, *105*(6), 2414–2423.

123. Li, H.; Fajer, M.; Yang, W. Simulated scaling method for localized enhanced sampling and simultaneous "alchemical" free energy simulations: a general method for molecular mechanical, quantum mechanical, and quantum mechanical/molecular mechanical simulations. *J. Chem. Phys.* **2007**, *126*, 024106.

124. Zheng, L.; Carbone, I. O.; Lugovskoy, A.; Berg, B. A.; Yang, W. A hybrid recursion method to robustly ensure convergence efficiencies in the simulated scaling based free energy simulations. *J. Chem. Phys.* **2008**, *129*(3), 034105.

125. Zheng, L.; Yang, W. Essential energy space random walks to accelerate molecular dynamics simulations: convergence improvements via an adaptive-length self-healing strategy. *J. Chem. Phys.* **2008**, *129*(1), 014105.

126. Min, D.; Yang, W. Energy difference space random walk to achieve fast free energy calculations. *J. Chem. Phys.* **2008**, *128*(19).

127. Li, H.; Yang, W. Forging the missing link in free energy estimations: lambda-WHAM in thermodynamic integration, overlap histogramming, and free energy perturbation. *Chem. Phys. Lett.* **2007**, *440*(1–3), 155–159.

128. Min, D.; Li, H.; Li, G.; Bitetti-Putzer, R.; Yang, W. Synergistic approach to improve "alchemical" free energy calculation in rugged energy surface. *J. Chem. Phys.* **2007**, *126*(14), 144109.

129. Oostenbrink, C.; van Gunsteren, W. F. Free energies of binding of polychlorinated biphenyls to the estrogen receptor from a single simulation. *Proteins* **2004**, *54*(2), 237–246.

130. Oostenbrink, C.; van Gunsteren, W. F. Single-step perturbations to calculate free energy differences from unphysical reference states: limits on size, flexibility, and character. *J. Comput. Chem.* **2003**, *24*(14), 1730–1739.

131. Schwab, F.; van Gunsteren, W. F.; Zagrovic, B. Computational study of the mechanism and the relative free energies of binding of anticholesteremic inhibitors to squalene-hopene cyclase. *Biochemistry* **2008**, *47*(9), 2945–2951.

132. Srinivasan, J. III; Cheatham, T. E.; Cieplak, P.; Kollman, P. A.; Case, D. A. Continuum solvent studies of the stability of DNA, RNA, and phosphoramidate-DNA helices. *J. Am. Chem. Soc.* **1998**, *120*, 9401–9409.

133. Cheatham, T. E.; Srinivasan, J.; Case, D. A.; Kollman, P. A. Molecular dynamics and continuum solvent studies of the stability of polyG-polyC and polyA-polyT DNA duplexes in solution. *J. Biomol. Struct. Dyn.* **1998**, *16*, 265–280.

134. Chong, L.; Duan, Y.; Wang, L.; Massova, I.; Kollman, P. A. Molecular dynamics and free-energy calculations applied to affinity maturation in antibody 48g7. *Proc. Natl. Acad. Sci. U.S.A.* **1995**, *96*, 14330–14335.

135. Foloppe, N.; Fisher, L. M.; Howes, R.; Kierstan, P.; Potter, A.; Robertson, A. G.; Surgenor, A. E. Structure-based design of novel CHK1 inhibitors: insights into hydrogen bonding and protein-ligand affinity. *J. Med. Chem.* **2005**, *48*, 4332–4345.

136. Bryce, R. A.; Hillier, I. H.; Naismith, J. H. Carbohydrate-protein recognition: molecular dynamics simulations and free energy analysis of oligosaccharide binding to concanavalin a. *Biophys J.*, **2001**, *81*, 1373–1388.

137. Kuhn, B.; Kollman, P. A.; Stahl, M. Prediction of pka shifts in proteins using a combination of molecular mechanical and continuum solvent calculations. *J. Comput. Chem.* **2004**, *25*, 1865–1872.

138. Ferrara, P.; Gohlke, H.; Price, D. J.; Klebe, G.; Brooks, C. L., III. Assessing scoring functions for protein-ligand interactions. *J. Med. Chem.* **2004**, *47*, 3032–3047.

139. Massova, I.; Kollman, P. A. Computational alanine scanning to probe protein-protein interactions: a novel approach to evaluate binding free energies. *J. Am. Chem. Soc.* **1999**, *121*, 8133–8143.

140. Kuhn, B.; Kollman, P. A. A ligand that is predicted to bind better to avidin than biotin: insights from computational fluorine scanning. *J. Am. Chem. Soc.* **2000**, *122*, 3909–3916.

141. Kuhn, B.; Kollman, P. A. Binding of a diverse set of ligands to avidin and streptavidin: an accurate quantitative prediction of their relative affinities by a combination of molecular mechanics and continuum solvent models. *J. Med. Chem.* **2000**, *43*, 3786–3791.

142. Huo, S.; Wang, J.; Cieplak, P.; Kollman, P. A.; Kuntz, I. D. Molecular dynamics and free energy analyses of cathepsin d-inhibitor interactions: insight into structure-based ligand design. *J. Med. Chem.* **2002**, *45*, 1412–1419.

143. Mardis, K. L.; Luo, R.; Gilson, M. K. Interpreting trends in the binding of cyclic ureas to HIV-1 protease. *J. Mol. Biol.* **2001**, *309*, 507–517.

144. Schwarzl, S. M.; Tschopp, T. B.; Smith, J. C.; Fischer, S. Can the calculation of ligand binding free energies be improved with continuum solvent electrostatics and an ideal-gas entropy correction? *J. Comput. Chem.* **2002**, *23*, 1143–1149.

145. Rizzo, R. C.; Toba, S; Kuntz, I. D. A molecular basis for the selectivity of thiadiazole urea inhibitors with stromelysin-1 and gelatinase-A from generalized born molecular dynamics simulations. *J. Med. Chem.* **2004**, *47*, 3065–3074.

146. Brown, S. P.; Muchmore, S. W. Rapid estimation of relative protein-ligand binding affinities using a high-throughput version of MM-PBSA. *J. Chem. Inf. Model.* **2007**, *47*, 1493–1503.

147. Kuhn, B.; Gerber, P. R.; Schulz-Gasch, T.; Stahl, M. Validation and use of the MM-PBSA approach for drug discovery. *J. Med. Chem.* **2005**, *48*, 4040–4048.

148. Pearlman, D. A. Evaluating the molecular mechanics Poisson-Boltzmann surface area free energy method using a congeneric series of ligands to p38 map kinase. *J. Med. Chem.* **2005**, *48*, 7796–7807.

149. Weis, A.; Katebzadeh, K.; Söderhjelm, P.; Nilsson, I.; Ryde, U. Ligand affinities predicted with the MM/PBSA method: dependence on the simulation method and the force field. *J. Med. Chem.* **2006**, *49*, 6596–6606.

150. Rafi, S. B.; Cui, G; Song, K; Cheng, X; Tonge, P. J.; Simmerling, C. Insight through molecular mechanics Poisson-Boltzmann surface area calculations into the binding affinity of triclosan and three analogues for FabI, the *E. Coli* enoyl reductase. *J. Med. Chem.* **2006**, *49*, 4574–4580.

151. Donini, O.; Kollman, P. A. Calculation and prediction of binding free energies for the matrix metalloproteinases. *J. Med. Chem.* **2000**, *43*, 4180–4188.

152. Tembe, B. L.; McCammon, J. A. Ligand-receptor interactions. *Comput. Chem.* **1984**, *8*(4), 281–284.

153. Wong, C. F.; McCammon, J. A. Dynamics and design of enzymes and inhibitors. *J. Am. Chem. Soc.* **1986**, *108*(13), 3830–3832.

154. Hermans, J.; Subramaniam, S. The free energy of xenon binding to myoglobin from molecular dynamics simulation. *Israel J. Chem.* **1986**, *27*, 225–227.

155. Pearlman, D. A. Free energy calculations: methods for estimating ligand binding affinities. In: *Free Energy Calculations in Rational Drug Design*, Rami Reddy, M.; Erion, M. D.; Eds. Academic/Plenum; New York, NY: Kluwer, **2001**.

156. Chipot, C. Free energy calculations in biomolecular simulations: how useful are they in practice? In: *Lecture Notes in Computational Science and Engineering: New Algorithms for Molecular Simulation*, Leimkuhler, B.; Chipot, C.; Elber, R.; Laaksonen, A.; Mark, A. E.; Schlick, T.; Schütte, C.; Skeel, R.; Eds. Vol. 49. New York: Springer, **2005**, 183–209.

157. Rizzo, R. C.; Wang, D. P.; Tirado-Rives, J.; Jorgensen, W. L. Validation of a model for the complex of HIV-1 reverse transcriptase with sustiva through computation of resistance profiles. *J. Am. Chem. Soc.* **2000**, *122*(51), 12898–12900.

158. Wang, D.-P.; Rizzo, R. C.; Tirado-Rives, J.; Jorgensen, W. L. Antiviral drug design: computational analyses of the effects of the l100i mutation for HIV-RT on the binding of nnrtis. *Bioorgan. Med. Chem. Lett.* **2001**, *11*(21), 2799–2802.

159. Udier-Blagovic, M.; Tirado-Rives, J.; Jorgensen, W. L. Structural and energetic analyses of the effects of the K103N mutation of HIV-1 reverse transcriptase on efavirenz analogues. *J. Med. Chem.* **2004**, *47*(9), 2389–2392.

160. Kim, J. T.; Hamilton, A. D.; Bailey, C. M.; Domoal, R. A.; Wang, L.; Anderson, K. S.; Jorgensen, W. L. Fep-guided selection of bicyclic heterocycles in lead optimization for non-nucleoside inhibitors of HIV-1 reverse transcriptase. *J. Am. Chem. Soc.* **2006**, *128*(48), 15372–15373.

161. Jorgensen, W. L.; Ruiz-Caro, J.; Tirado-Rives, J.; Basavapathruni, A.; Anderson, K. S.; Hamilton, A. D. Computer-aided design of non-nucleoside inhibitors of HIV-1 reverse transcriptase. *Bioorg. Med. Chem. Lett.* **2006**, *16*(3), 663–667.

162. Kroeger Smith, M. B.; Rader, L. H.; Franklin, A. M.; Taylor, E. V.; Smith, K. D.; Tirado-Rives, J.; Jorgensen, W. L. Energetic effects for observed and unobserved HIV-1 reverse transcriptase mutations of residues l100, v106, and y181 in the presence of nevirapine and efavirenz. *Bioorg. Med. Chem. Lett.* **2008**, *18*(3), 969–972.

163. Zeevaart, J. G.; Wang, L.; Thakur, V. V.; Leung, C. S.; Tirado-Rives, J.; Bailey, C. M.; Domoal, R. A.; Anderson, K. S.; Jorgensen, W. L. Optimization of azoles as anti-human immunodeficiency virus agents guided by free-energy calculations. *J. Am. Chem. Soc.* **2008**, *120*, 9492–9499.

164. Henin, J.; Maigret, B.; Tarek, M.; Escrieut, C.; Fourmy, D.; Chipot, C. Probing a model of a GPCR/ligand complex in an explicit membrane environment: the human cholecystokinin-1 receptor. *Biophys. J.* **2006**, *90*(4), 1232–1240.

165. Yang, W.; Gao, Y. Q.; Cui, Q.; Ma, J.; Karplus, M. The missing link between thermodynamics and structure in f1-atpase. *Proc. Natl. Acad. Sci. U.S.A.* **2003**, *100*(3), 874–879.

166. Banerjee, A.; Yang, W.; Karplus, M.; Verdine, G. L. Structure of a repair enzyme interrogating undamaged DNA elucidates recognition of damaged DNA. *Nature* **2005** *434*, 612–618.

167. Oostenbrink, C.; Pitera, J. W.; van Lipzig, M. M. H.; Meerman, J. H. N.; van Gunsteren, W. F. Simulations of the estrogen receptor ligand-binding domain: affinity of natural ligands and xenoestrogens. *J. Med. Chem.* **2000**, *43*(24), 4594–4605.

168. Rami Reddy, M.; Erion, M. D. Calculation of relative binding free energy differences for fructose 1,6-bisphosphatase inhibitors using the thermodynamic cycle perturbation approach. *J. Am. Chem. Soc.* **2001**, *123*, 6246–6252.

169. Steinbrecher, T.; Case, D. A.; Labahn, A. A multistep approach to structure-based drug design: studying ligand binding at the human neutrophil elastase. *J. Med. Chem.* **2006**, *49*, 1837–1844.

170. Gouda, H.; Kuntz, I. D.; Case, D. A.; Kollman, P. A. Free energy calculations for theophylline binding to an RNA aptamer: comparison of MM-PBSA and thermodynamic integration methods. *Biopolymers* **2003**, *68*, 16–34.

171. Tanida, Y.; Ito, M.; Fujitani, H. Calculation of absolute free energy of binding for theophylline and its analogs to RNA aptamer using nonequilibrium work values. *Chem. Phys.* **2007**, *337*(1–3), 135–143.

172. Jiao, D.; Golubkov, P. A.; Darden, T. A.; Ren, P. Calculation of protein-ligand binding free energy using a polarizable potential. *Proc. Natl. Acad. Sci. U.S.A.* **2008**, *105*(17), 6290–6295.

173. Khoruzhii, O.; Donchev, A. G.; Galkin, N.; Illarionov, A.; Olevanov, M.; Ozrin, V.; Queen, C.; Tarasov, V. Application of a polarizable force field to calculations of relative protein-ligand binding affinities. *Proc. Natl. Acad. Sci. U.S.A.* **2008**, *105*(30), 10378–10383.

174. Price, D. J.; Jorgensen, W. L. Improved convergence of binding affinities with free energy perturbation: application to non-peptide ligands with pp60src SH2 domain. *J. Comput. Aided. Mol. Des.* **2001**, *15*, 681–695.

175. Fowler, P. W.; Jha, S.; Coveney, P. V. Grid-based steered thermodynamic integration accelerates the calculation of binding free energies. *Philos. T. R. Soc. B.*, **2005**, *363*, 1999–2015.

176. Chipot, C.; Rozanska, X.; Dixit, S. B. Can free energy calculations be fast and accurate at the same time? Binding of low-affinity, non-peptide inhibitors to the SH2 domain of the src protein. *J. Comput. Aided Mol. Des.* **2005**, *19*, 765–770.

177. Fowler, P. W.; Geroult, S.; Jha, S.; Waksman, G.; Coveney, P. V. Rapid, accurate, and precise calculation of relative binding affinities for the SH2 domain using a computational grid. *J. Chem. Theory Comput.* **2007**, *3*(3), 1193–1202.

178. Pearlman, D. A.; Charifson, P. S. Are free energy calculations useful in practice? A comparison with rapid scoring functions for the p38 map kinase protein system. *J. Med. Chem.* **2001**, *44*, 3417–3423.

179. Mobley, D. L.; Chodera, J. D.; Dill, K. A. On the use of orientational restraints and symmetry corrections in alchemical free energy calculations. *J. Chem. Phys.* **2006**, *125*, 084902.

180. Gilson, M. K.; Given, J. A.; Bush, B. L., McCammon, J. A. A statistical-thermodynamic basis for computation of binding affinities: a critical review. *Biophys. J.* **1997**, *72*(3), 1047–1069.

181. Deng, Y.; Roux, B. Computations of standard binding free energies with molecular dynamics simulations. *J. Phys. Chem. B* **2008**, in press.

182. Helms, V.; Wade, R. C. Hydration energy landscape of the active site cavity in cytochrome P450cam. *Proteins* **1998**, *32*(3), 381–396.

183. Helms, V.; Wade, R. C. Computational alchemy to calculate absolute protein-ligand binding free energy. *J. Am. Chem. Soc.* **1998**, *120*(12), 2710–2713.

184. Deng Y.; Roux, B. Computation of binding free energy with molecular dynamics and grand canonical Monte Carlo simulations. *J. Chem. Phys.* **2008**, *128*(11).

185. Zhang, L.; Hermans, J. Hydrophilicity of cavities in proteins. *Proteins* **1996**, *24*(4), 433–438.

186. Olano, L. R.; Rick, S. W. Hydration free energies and entropies for water in protein interiors. *J. Am. Chem. Soc.* **2004**, *126*(25), 7991–8000.

187. Barillari, C.; Taylor, J.; Viner, R.; Essex, J. W. Classification of water molecules in protein binding sites. *J. Am. Chem. Soc.* **2007**, *129*(9), 2577–2587.

188. Hamelberg, D.; McCammon, J. A. Standard free energy of releasing a localized water molecule from the binding pockets of proteins: double-decoupling method. *J. Am. Chem. Soc.* **2004**, *126*, 7683–7689.

189. Lu, Y.; Wang, C.-Y.; Wang, S. Binding free energy contributions of interfacial waters in HIV-1 protease/inhibitor complexes. *J. Am. Chem. Soc.* **2006**, *128*, 11830–11839.

190. Roux, B.; Nina, M.; Pomès, R.; Smith, J. C. Thermodynamic stability of water molecules in the bacteriorhodopsin proton channel: a molecular dynamics free energy perturbation study. *Biophys. J.* **1996**, *71*(2), 670–681.

191. De Simone, A.; Dobson, G. G.; Verma, C. S.; Zagari, A.; Fraternali, F. Prion and water: tight and dynamical hydration sites have a key role in structural stability. *Proc. Natl. Acad. Sci. U.S.A.* **2005**, *102*(21), 7535–7540.

192. Pan, C.; Mezei, M.; Mujtaba, S.; Muller, M.; Zeng, L.; Li, J.; Wang, Z.; Zhou, M. M. Structure-guided optimization of small molecules inhibiting human immunodeficiency virus 1 tat association with the human coactivator p300/CREB binding protein-associated factor. *J. Med. Chem.* **2007**, *50*(10), 2285–2288.

193. Eriksson, A. E.; Baase, W. A.; Zhang, X. J.; Heinz, D. W.; Blaber, M.; Baldwin; E. P.; Matthews, B. W. Response of a protein structure to cavity-creating mutations and its relation to the hydrophobic effect. *Science* **1992**, *255*, 178–183.

194. Eriksson, A. E.; Baase, W. A.; Matthews, B. W. Similar hydrophobic replacements of leu99 and phe153 within the core of T4 lysozyme have different structural and thermodynamic consequences. *J. Mol. Biol.* **1993**, *229*, 747–769.

195. Morton, A.; Matthews, B. W. Specificity of ligand binding in a buried nonpolar cavity of T4 lysozyme: linkage of dynamics and structural plasticity. *Biochemistry* **1995**, *34*, 8576–8588.

196. Morton, A.; Baase, W. A.; Matthews, B. W. Energetic origins of specificity of ligand binding in an interior nonpolar cavity of T4 lysozyme. *Biochemistry* **1995**, *34*, 8564–8575.

197. Wei, B. Q.; Baase, W. A.; Weaver, L. H.; Matthews, B. W.; Shoichet, B. K. A model binding site for testing scoring functions in molecular docking. *J. Mol. Biol.* **2002**, *322*, 339–355.

198. Wei, B. Q.; Weaver, L. H.; Ferrari, A. M.; Matthews, B. W.; Shoichet, B. K. Testing a flexible-receptor docking algorithm in a model binding site. *J. Mol. Biol.* **2004**, *337*, 1161–1182.

199. Graves, A. P.; Brenk, R.; Shoichet, B. K. Decoys for docking. *J. Med. Chem.* **2005**, *48*, 3714–3728.

200. Hermans, J.; Wang, L. Inclusion of the loss of translational and rotational freedom in theoretical estimates of free energies of binding. Application to a complex of benzene and mutant T4 lysozyme. *J. Am. Chem. Soc.* **1997**, *119*, 2707–2714.

201. Mann, G.; Hermans, J. Modeling protein-small molecule interactions: structure and thermodynamics of noble gases binding in a cavity in mutant phage T4 lysozyme L99A. *J. Mol. Biol.* **2000**, *302*, 979–989.

202. Boresch, S.; Tettinger, F.; Leitgeb, M.; Karplus, M. Absolute binding free energies: a quantitative approach for their calculation. *J. Phys. Chem. A* **2003**, *107*(35), 9535–9551.

203. Deng, Y.; Roux B. Calculation of standard binding free energies: aromatic molecules in the T4 lysozyme l99A mutant. *J. Chem. Theory Comput.* **2006**, *2*, 1255–1273.

204. Clark, M.; Guarnieri, F.; Shkurko, I.; Wiseman, J. Grand canonical Monte Carlo simulation of ligand-protein binding. *J. Chem. Info. Model.* **2006**, *46*(1), 231–242.

205. Mobley, D. L.; Dumont, È.; Chodera, J. D.; Dill, K. A. Comparison of charge models for fixed-charge force fields: small-molecule hydration free energies in explicit solvent. *J. Phys. Chem. B* **2007**, *111*(9), 2242–2254.

206. Holt, D. A.; Luengo, J. I.; Yamashita, D. S.; Oh, H. J.; Konialian, A. L.; Yen, H. K.; Rozamus, L. W.; Brandt, M.; Bossard, M. J.; Levy, M. A.; Eggleston, D. S.; Liang, J.; Schultz, L. W.; Stout, T. J.; Clardy, J. Design, synthesis, and kinetic evaluation of high-affinity FKBP ligands and the x-ray crystal structures of their complexes with FKBP12. *J. Am. Chem. Soc.* **1993**, *115*(22), 9925–9938.

207. Shirts, M. R. *Calculating precise and accurate free energies in biomolecular systems.* Ph.D. dissertation, Stanford, January **2005**.

208. Fujitani, H.; Tanida, Y.; Ito, M.; Shirts, M. R.; Jayachandran, G.; Snow, C. D.; Sorin E. J.; Pande, V. S. Direct calculation of the binding free energies of FKBP ligands. *J. Chem. Phys.* **2005**, *123*, 84–108.

209. Jayachandran, G.; Shirts, M. R.; Park, S.; Pande, V. S. Parallelized-over-parts computation of absolute binding free energy with docking and molecular dynamics. *J. Chem. Phys.* **2006**, *125*, 084901.

210. Dixit, S. B.; Chipot, C. Can absolute free energies of association be estimated from molecular mechanical simulations? The biotin-streptavidin system revisited. *J. Phys. Chem. A* **2001**, *105*(42), 9795–9799.

211. Hess, B.; van der Vegt, N. F. A. Hydration thermodynamic properties of amino acid analogues: a comparison of biomolecular force fields and water models. *J. Phys. Chem. B* **2006**, *110*, 17616–17626.

212. Nicholls, A.; Mobley, D. L.; Guthrie, P. J.; Chodera, J. D.; Pande, V. S. Predicting small-molecule solvation free energies: an informal blind test for computational chemistry. *J. Med. Chem.* **2008**, *51*, 769–779.

213. Steinbrecher, T.; Hrenn, A.; Dormann, K. L.; Merfort, I.; Labahn, A. Bornyl (3,4,5-trihydroxy)-cinnamate: an optimized human neutrophil elastase inhibitor designed by free energy calculations. *Bioorgan. Med. Chem.* **2008**, *16*(5), 2385–2390.

214. Talhout, R.; Villa, A.; Mark, A. E.; Engberts, J. B. Understanding binding affinity: a combined isothermal titration calorimetry/molecular dynamics study of the binding of a series of hydrophobically modified benzamidinium chloride inhibitors to trypsin. *J. Am. Chem. Soc.* **2003**, *125*(35), 10570–10579.

215. Mao, H. Z.; Weber, J. Identification of the betatp site in the x-ray structure of f1-atpase as the high-affinity catalytic site. *Proc. Natl. Acad. Sci. U.S.A.* **2007**, *104*(47), 18478–18483.

216. Zagrovic, B.; van Gunsteren, W. F. Computational analysis of the mechanism and thermodynamics of inhibition of phosphodiesterase 5a by synthetic ligands. *J. Chem. Theory Comput.* **2007**, *3*, 301–311.

217. Leitgeb, M.; Schröder, C.; Boresch, S. Alchemical free energy calculations and multiple conformational substates. *J. Chem. Phys.* **2005**, *122*, 084109.

218. de Graaf, C.; Oostenbrink, C.; Keizers, P. H. J.; van Vugt-Lussenburg, B. M. A.; Commandeur, J. N. M.; Vermeulen, N. P. E. Free energies of binding of R- and S- propranolol to wild-type and f483a mutant cytochrome p450 d26 from molecular dynamics simulations. *Eur. Biophys. J.* **2007**, *36*(6), 589–599.

219. van den Bosch, M.; Swart, M.; Snijders, J. G.; Berendsen, H. J. C.; Mark, A. E.; Oostenbrink, C.; van Gunsteren, W. F.; Canters, G. W. Calculation of the redox potential of the protein azurin and some mutants. *ChemBioChem* **2005**, *6*(4), 738–746.

220. Dolenc, J.; Oostenbrink, C.; Koller, J.; van Gunsteren, W. F. Molecular dynamics simulations and free energy calculations of netropsin and distamycin binding to an aaaaa DNA binding site. *Nucleic Acids Res.* **2005**, *33*(2), 725–733.

221. Donnini, S.; Juffer, A. H. Calculations of affinities of peptides for proteins. *J. Comput. Chem.* **2004**, *25*, 393–411.

222. Oostenbrink, C.; Villa, A.; Mark, A. E.; van Gunsteren, W. F. A biomolecular force field based on the free enthalpy of hydration and solvation: the GROMOS force-field parameter sets 53a5 and 53a6. *J. Comput. Chem.* **2004**, *25*(13), 1656–1676.

223. Hornak, V.; Abel, R.; Okur, A.; Strockbine, B.; Roitberg, A. E.; Simmerling, C. Comparison of multiple amber force fields and development of improved protein backbone parameters. *Proteins* **2006**, *65*(3), 712–725.

224. Kaminski, G.; Friesner, R. A.; Rives, J.; Jorgensen, W. L. Evaluation and reparametrization of the opls-aa force field for proteins via comparison with accurate quantum chemical calculations on peptides. *J. Phys. Chem. B* **2001**, *105*(28), 6474–6487.

225. Wang, J.; Wolf, R. M.; Caldwell, J. W.; Kollman, P. A.; Case, D. A. Development and testing of a general amber force field. *J. Comput. Chem.* **2004**, *25*(9), 1157–1174.

226. Jakalian, A.; Bush, B. L.; Jack, D. B.; Bayly, C. I. Fast, efficient generation of high-quality atomic charges, AM1-BCC model. I. Method. *J. Comput. Chem.* **2000**, *21*(2), 132–146.

227. Jakalian, A.; Jack, D. B.; Bayly, C. I. Fast, efficient generation of high-quality atomic charges, AM1-BCC model. II. Parameterization and validation. *J. Comput. Chem.* **2002**, *23*(16), 1623–1641.

228. Ponder, J. W.; Case, D. A. Force fields for protein simulations, in *Advances in Protein Chemistry*, Dagget, V.; Ed. San Diego, CA: Academic Press **2003**, *66*, 27–86.

229. Michel, J.; Verdonk, M. L.; Essex, J. W. Protein-ligand binding free energy predictions by implicit solvent simulation: a tool for lead optimization? *J. Med. Chem.* **2006**, *49*, 7427–7439.

230. Li, L.; Dantzer, J. J.; Nowacki, J.; O'Callaghan, B. J.; Meroueh, S. O. PDBCAL: a comprehensive dataset for receptor-ligand interactions with three-dimensional structures and binding thermodynamics from isothermal titration calorimetry. *Chem. Bio. Drug Des.* **2008**, *71*(6), 529–532.

231. Rami Reddy, M.; Erion, M. D., Eds. *Free Energy Calculations in Rational Drug Design.* Amsterdam: Kluwer Academic, **2001**.

232. Marti-Renom, M. A.; Madhusudhan, M. S.; Fiser, A.; Rost, B.; Sali, A. Reliability of assessment of protein structure prediction methods. *Structure* **2002**, *10*(3), 435–440.

233. Méndez, R.; Leplae, R.; Lesink, M. F.; Wodak, S. J. Assessment of CAPRI predictions in rounds 3-5 shows progress in docking procedures. *Proteins* **2005**, *60*(2), 150–169.

234. Day, G.M.; Motherwell, W. D. S.; Ammon, H. L.; Boerrigter, S. X. M.; Della Valle, R. G.; Venuti, E.; Dzyabchenko, A.; Dunitz, J. D.; Schweizer, B.; van Eijck, B. P.; Erk, P.; Facelli, J. C.; Bazterra, V. E.; Ferraro, M. B.; Hofmann, D. W. M.; Leusen, F. J. J.; Liang, C.; Pantelides, C. C.; Karamertzanis, P. G.; Price, S. L.; Lewis, T. C.; Nowell, H.;Torrisi, A.; Scheraga, H. A.; Arnautova, Y. A., Schmidt, M. U.; and Verwer, P. A third blind test of crystal structure prediction. *Acta Crystall. B-Struc.*, **2005**, *61*(5), 511–527.

235. Parker, C. N. McMaster University data-mining and docking competition: computational models on the catwalk. *J. Biomol. Screen.* **2005**, *10*(7), 647–648.

236. Villa, A.; Zangi, R.; Pieffet, G.; Mark, A. E. Sampling and convergence in free energy calculations of protein-ligand interactions: the binding of triphenoxypyridine derivatives to factor xa and trypsin. *J. Comput. Aided Mol. Des.* **2003**, *17*(10), 673–686.

237. Naim, M.; Bhat, S.; Rankin, K. N.; Dennis, S.; Chowdhury, S. F.; Siddiqi, I.; Drabik, P.; Sulea, T.; Bayly, C. I.; Jakalian, A.; Purisima, E. O. Solvated interaction energy (sie) for scoring protein-ligand binding affinities. 1. Exploring the parameter space. *J. Chem. Info. Model.* **2007**, *47*(1), 122–133.

238. Jorgensen, W. L. The many roles of computation in drug discovery. *Science* **2004**, *303*(5665), 1813–1818.

239. Chipot, C.; Pearlman, D. A. Free energy calculations: the long and winding gilded road. *Mol. Simulat.* **2002**, *28*(1–2), 1–12.

240. Mobley, D. L.; Dill, K. A. Binding of small-molcule ligand to proteins. "What you see" is not always "what you get." *Structure* **2009**, *17*, 489–498.

241. Kollman, P. A. Free energy calculations: applications to chemical and biochemical phenomena. *Chem. Rev.* **1993**, *7*, 2395–2417.

242. Jorgensen, W. L. Free energy calculations: a breakthrough for modeling organic chemistry in solution. *Accounts Chem. Res.* **1989**, *22*(5), 184–189.

6

Studies of drug resistance and the dynamic behavior of HIV-1 protease through molecular dynamics simulations

Fangyu Ding and Carlos Simmerling

INTRODUCTION

The human immunodeficiency virus (HIV) was first discovered to be the causative agent of acquired immunodeficiency syndrome (AIDS) in the early 1980s.[1,2] There are currently three main avenues for preventing virus replication. The first is to block attachment of virus to the host cell surface by inhibitors of binding to coreceptors, such as CCR5.[3,4] The second is to block the process of reverse transcription,[5] an approach taken by a major class of anti-AIDS drugs, including, for example, azidothymidine (AZT), delavirdine, nevirapin, and so on. The third way is to disrupt the function of the viral protease (HIV-PR) that cleaves the gag-pol polyproteins required to assemble an active virus by binding an inhibitor to the center of the protease and freezing it closed; this is described in more detail in this review. At present there are eleven FDA-approved protease inhibitors in clinical use: Agenerase (amprenavir), Aptivus (tipranavir), Crixivan (indinavir), Fortovase (saquinavir soft gel), Invirase (saquinavir hard gel), Kaletra (lopinavir-ritonavir), Lexiva (Fosamprenavir), Norvir (ritonavir), Prezista (darunavir), Reyataz (atazanavir), and Viracept.[6] All these inhibitors can lose most of their potency when confronted with mutations associated with drug resistance.[7] Therefore, a thorough understanding of the mechanistic events associated with binding of HIV-PR substrates and inhibitors is pharmacologically critical for the design of novel inhibitors of the enzyme. There is evidence that flexibility of the enzyme plays an important role in inhibitor binding and resistance.[8,9]

This chapter focuses on recent advances and challenges in understanding protease dynamics and its potential for revealing new approaches to HIV-PR drug design. A particular focus is the application of computational techniques that can provide detailed insight into the dynamic aspects of HIV-PR behavior. Because recent molecular dynamics simulations of HIV-PR have suggested that the dynamics of this enzyme is crucial for its function, affecting flexibility of the protease by, for example, allosteric inhibitors could provide new opportunities to design a more potent inhibitor.

Experimental data on structure of HIV-1 protease: Large structural rearrangement on binding

An extensive set of x-ray crystal structures of HIV-1 protease in both bound and unbound forms has been solved,[10] revealing a C_2 symmetric homodimer with a large substrate binding pocket covered by two glycine-rich beta-hairpins or flaps.[11–13] In almost all of the liganded forms, both flaps are pulled in toward the bottom of the active site ["closed" form, Figure 6.1(a)]. However, there are several crystal structures that have been resolved in an unusual "flap-intermediate" conformation with one flap partly and the other flap fully closed.[14,15] These observations provide experimental supports to the hypothesis that the substrate enters the protease binding site through the flaps and the subsequent flap motion is asynchronous with one flap closing first. In contrast to the bound structures, crystal structures of the ligand-free protease are more heterogeneous[16]; three conformations of the flap domains have been captured: "closed," "semiopen," and "wide-open" forms. Although the relationship between the conformational flexibility and catalytic activity is still unclear, it has been suggested that mutations might affect the flexibility of the unbound enzyme; for example, the M46I mutation appears to stabilize the closed form of the flaps.[17] Most ligand-free HIV-PR adopt the semiopen form [Figure 6.1(b)], in which the flaps are pulled up and shifted away from the active site, but still substantially cover the active site. A more striking difference between the semiopen and closed form of unbound enzyme is that the relative orientation of the flaps is reversed (top views in Figure 6.1). Despite the observation of semiopen conformation in five of the nine available crystal structures of unbound HIV-PR,[11–13,18–23] it was not entirely clear whether this reflects the preferred flap conformation in solution or is a result of crystal-packing effects.[24–26] Although a large-scale flap opening is presumably required for normal substrate access to the active site [Figure 6.1(c)], a transient open form was observed only in molecular dynamics (MD) studies[27,28] [Figure 6.1(c)], and an x-ray "wide-open" structure[18,21,22] is more likely an artifact due to the crystal-packing contact,[29] in which each flap

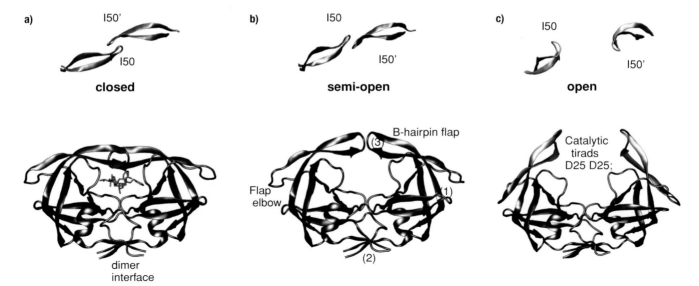

Figure 6.1. Top and side views of the three important conformations of HIV-1 protease. (a) The "closed" form is observed in crystal structures with substrate bound (structure with pdb code 1TSU is shown). (b) The flaps of the free protease assume a "semiopen" conformation in crystal structures (1HHP is shown). (c) The fully "open" form in which the active site becomes accessible to substrate or inhibitors was not observed in crystal structures but was implied from NMR experiments. The structure shown is from molecular dynamics simulations. The top views of flaps highlight the change in flap handedness between "closed" and "semiopen" structures. The flaps in the fully "open" form captured in our MD simulations adopt the semiopen handedness that is distinct from the x-ray "wide-open" structure, 1TW7.[21]

tip is buried between the elbow and fulcrum regions of a neighbor dimer (Figure 6.5), with the unusual P81':I50 contact enclosed by five residues from the symmetry-related neighbor (P39, R41, D60, Q61, I72). Because the conformations of the elbow and fulcrum regions have been shown to be correlated with flap opening,[13,14] wedging a flap tip between the fulcrum and elbow could further stabilize the open conformation observed in the crystal. We note that the heterogeneity of those x-ray crystal structures of ligand-free enzymes might be attributed to the crystal packing effect, because the glycine-rich flaps often are in direct contacts with symmetry-related neighbors; however, another possible explanation is that the unbound form of HIV-PR is more flexible than the bound form, especially the flap regions. This explanation is consistent with experimental results obtained from nuclear magnetic resonance (NMR)[30-32] and pulsed electron paramagnetic resonance (EPR) spectroscopy.[33] Solution NMR data for the free protease obtained from Torchia's group have suggested[31,34,35] that the ensemble of unbound structures is dominated by the "semiopen" family with subnanosecond time-scale fluctuation in the flap tips, and with "closed" structures possibly being a minor component of the ensemble. The semiopen form is in slow equilibrium ($\sim$100 μs) with a less structured, open form that exposes the binding site cavity. Ishima and Louis investigated the possible conformations of the flaps of the dimer by comparison of the NMR chemical shifts and relaxation data of the monomer and dimer.[32] For the first time, they demonstrated that the

tips of the flaps in the unliganded protease dimer interact with each other in solution. Recently, Fanucci's group used EPR spectroscopy to investigate dipolar coupling of the unpaired nitroxide electrons in spin labels attached to K55C/K55'C on each flap. A different flexibility of the flaps in the bound and unbound forms was clearly identified, and the data suggested that the unbound flaps sampled a much larger degree of separation than those in the bound form, with the distance between two spin labels ranging from 26Å to 48Å. These data provide strong support for the hypothesis that the flaps in the unbound state exist in a diverse ensemble of conformations fluctuating between semiopen, closed, and open, and exhibit considerable flexibility which allows substrate entry and product exit. Despite these findings, many aspects of both the structure and dynamics of HIV-PR in aqueous solution remain unresolved as the experiments provide only indirect evidence of flap structures in solution.

Simulations of HIV-1 protease: Exploring flap flexibility

Although x-ray crystallography provides invaluable high-resolution structures, they primarily reflect an average structure of a single low-energy conformation under low-temperature, crystalline conditions; therefore, a crystal structure might not represent the most stable state in solution. NMR experiments provide a more realistic view of the dynamic behavior in solution and at more biologically relevant temperatures. Although several HIV-PR structures with bound inhibitors were fully solved by solution NMR, thus far this technique has not provided structural data for the unbound protease in solution, because of difficulties related to protease autocleavage, as well as its high flexibility in solution. As discussed above, site-directed spin labeling (SDSL) double electron-electron resonance (DEER) has also been applied to study the conformations of the flaps of HIV-1 PR in the bound and unbound forms. However, the distance measured by this EPR method is based on the dipolar coupling between the unpaired nitroxide electrons, which are located ~7Å from the Cα atom of the protein backbone. It is likely that the observed label distributions report on flap dynamics, rather than changes in the labels, but a lack of clear structural data prevents detailed interpretation of the EPR data in terms of specific changes to flap conformations on ligand binding. The shift in the label distribution in the presence of inhibitor could reflect the rearrangement of the flaps from semiopen to closed handedness or could arise from decreased flap motion due to direct interactions between flaps and inhibitor. However, the successful interpretation of SDSL-EPR data and potential application to drug-resistant HIV-PR requires additional data concerning that specific flap conformations give rise to particular ranges of spin label distances and how these ensembles are affected by inhibitor binding. Importantly, it is unclear whether the observed interspin distance distribution can be explained solely by an ensemble consisting of conformations seen in the various crystal structures or whether other conformations contribute significantly to the ensemble in solution. Therefore, establishing a correlation between EPR-measured interspin distances and structural dynamic features of the flaps is essential in the interpretation of the current and future EPR data for this system and use of EPR to explore drug resistance. Computational methods such as molecular dynamics simulations can provide a detailed, atomic resolution model for time-dependent structural variation and insight into thermodynamic aspects involved not only in binding but also in conversion between different protease conformations. Unfortunately, until recently, realistic simulations have been hampered by limitations in the model description and time scales that could be reached.

Numerous prior computational studies have aimed at understanding flap-opening dynamics. Collins et al. reported flap opening resulting from MD simulations in the gas phase that involved forcing the atomic coordinates for nonflap regions of a closed structure to the semiopen state.[36] Scott and Schiffer[37] also observed irreversible flap opening, but the extent of opening was not quantitatively described. Instead the authors focused on the flap tip regions, which "curled" back into the protein structure prior to the opening event, burying several hydrophobic residues. This flap curling was hypothesized to provide a key conformational trigger necessary for the subsequent large-scale flap opening. However, a more recent study[38] by Carlson et al. highlighted the challenges in obtaining accurate simulation data by demonstrating that similar irreversible flap opening could arise from insufficient equilibration during system setup; these events were not observed when more extensive solvent equilibration was performed. More recently, Hamelberg and McCammon[39] applied activated dynamics to produce flap opening in HIV-PR. In this case, a *trans→cis* isomerization of the Gly-Gly peptide bond was hypothesized to trigger the flap opening. Perryman et al. reported dynamics of unbound wild-type and V82F/I84V mutant in which the closed form opened somewhat, but the authors did not report whether the flaps in these unbound mutant simulations actually adopted the semiopen flap handedness as observed in crystal structures of unbound proteases.[40,41] Nevertheless, the high flexibility of the flaps, particularly for the mutant, was demonstrated and used for active site inhibitor design for the drug-resistant mutant.[42] Notably, none of these prior computational studies of the free protease reported that the flaps were able to adopt the semiopen conformation from either the open structures that were sampled or in other cases from the initial closed conformation. Therefore it is uncertain if the behavior in these simulations is relevant to the true dynamics of the HIV protease; it might simply represent an inability of the simulation models to reproduce experimental observations, or perhaps suggest that the semiopen form is an artifact of crystal packing and does not contribute to the solution ensemble probed by the simulations.

Recently, several reports were published where multiple and, most importantly, reversible opening of the protease flaps was observed. These works serve as a testimony that simulation methods have finally reached a state where they can provide valuable insights into enzyme function on biologically relevant time scales. McCammon and coworkers[43,44] developed a coarse-grain model of HIV protease in which each residue is modeled using a single bead at the position of the Cα carbon. This treatment substantially reduces the complexity of the system, permitting the simulations to model behavior on the microsecond time scale. Numerous opening and closing events were seen; these were realized primarily by large lateral movements of the flaps that exposed the binding cavity. With the current coarse-grain model, however, the long time scales are enabled through neglect of atomic detail, which comes at the cost of not being able to describe more subtle differences, such as those observed between closed and semiopen crystal structures. There is also no straightforward way to determine how flap behavior is influenced by dynamics on the atomic level in terms of specific side-chain interactions or to gain an understanding of how solvation is coupled to dynamics.

More recently, our group simulated a multiscale model of HIV-PR dynamics, in which full atomic detail was maintained for the protease, and aqueous solvent was modeled using a continuum approach.[45] These simulations showed spontaneous conversion between the bound and unbound

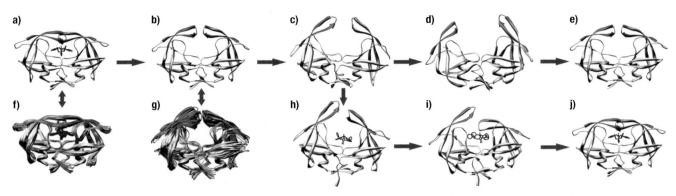

Figure 6.2. Snapshots from molecular dynamics simulations of inhibitor bound and free protease, and from simulations following the manual docking of the inhibitor into the binding site. The "closed" conformation (a) is represented by ensemble of closed structures with high similarity (f). In contrast, the "semiopen" conformation (b) represents a much more flexible ensemble (g) with larger fluctuations of the flaps. Those eventually lead to full opening of flaps (c and d); the open form is transient and returns to semiopen conformation (e). When the inhibitor is manually placed into a binding site (h), it induces an asymmetric flap closure with initial closing of one of the flaps (i) and finally converting to fully closed form (j) with flaps pulled into the binding site and flap handedness appropriate for the closed state.

crystal forms on removal of an inhibitor and reversible opening of the flaps. Although the simulations of inhibitor bound form were very stable with no substantial conformational changes [Figures 6.2(a) and (f)], the behavior of the system changed dramatically if the ligand was not present. Removal of the ligand from the protease resulted in spontaneous conversion of the closed flap conformation to the semiopen form [Figure 6.2(b)], similar to that observed in ligand-free protease crystal structures. Notably, this conversion in the simulations is accompanied by the change in flap handedness that is in excellent agreement with crystal structures (Figure 6.1).

Another characteristic feature of the semiopen ensemble generated in these molecular dynamics simulations was that it exhibited much higher flexibility, particularly in the flaps region [Figures 6.2(b) and (g)], as compared to the closed ensemble. Simulations initiated from the free protease crystal structures showed the same behavior. When these simulations were extended to longer times, flexibility of the flaps produced transient openings with large-scale rearrangements of the flaps and flap-tip distances over 20Å [Figures 6.2(c) and (d)], which can easily accommodate entry of substrates. Importantly, these fully open conformations were only transiently populated and reproducibly returned to the semiopen state [Figure 6.2(e)], providing evidence that the opening events were not artifacts caused by instability of the system or a poor quality model. Full flap opening in the simulations occurred through a concerted downward rotation around the center in the vicinity of the dimer interface and resulted in noticeable mutual rotation of the two monomers accompanied by large upward motions of the flaps, in contrast to opening via lateral movements of the flaps as observed in the coarse-grain model.[44]

Although implicit solvent models have been reported to provide results that are in good qualitative agreement with the explicit solvent simulations and experimental data, some discrepancies, in particular with respect to inadequate hydrophobic interactions, the stability of salt bridges and biasing the secondary structure have also been reported.[46–50] Therefore, exploring dynamics with explicit solvent model is essential to resolve many fundamental questions associated with the quantitative details of the enzyme dynamics. Most recently, our group performed one microsecond MD simulations with explicit solvation model (unpublished data). For the first time, spontaneous and multiple interconversions among different flap conformations of ligand-free HIV-PR were obtained in explicit solvent simulations. Consistent with our previous implicit solvent simulations, in the absence of the ligand the protease spontaneously and reversibly converted between the closed and semiopen states with the appropriate reversal of the flap handedness. This observation provides further evidence that the closed and semiopen crystal forms are both sampled in the ensemble of the apo protease in solution and that the conformational change associated with ligand binding involves conformational selection rather than induced fit. Detailed structural analysis revealed that the rearrangement of Ile50 between intramonomer and intermonomer hydrophobic clusters, defined by Ile50 and several hydrophobic residues in the core domain from the same monomer or its symmetry-related monomer, respectively, is coupled to the transition between the semiopen and closed form; thus the dynamics of those two hydrophobic clusters is critical in the mechanism of the conformational change and its function. Consistent with this view, a new class of inhibitor just made its debut, which targets the hydrophobic pocket (or so-called flap-recognition site)[51] in the semiopen state and prevents the flaps from assuming the proper closed conformation. The experimentally confirmed activity of this novel inhibitor not only provides a testimonial for the transition mechanism revealed by our MD simulations, but suggests that modulating the conformational behavior of HIV-PR could be achieved by disrupting the dynamics of intramonomer and intermonomer hydrophobic clusters. In the same simulation, a spontaneous and large-scale opening of the flaps was also captured, which took place in the similar fashion as observed in implicit solvent simulations.[52] The flap opening dynamics explored by this MD simulation suggested that the flap opening form is likely an intermediate state along the path of the dissociation of the dimer, and may therefore be a manifestation of the dissociative propensity of the dimer exhibited in experiments[1]. We proposed that the disruption of the dimer interfaces decreases the binding stability, which in turn results in large rearrangements of the protein, including the flap opening. This proposed mechanism is in accord with experimental observations of the importance of the dimer interactions, such as intra- and intermonomer salt bridges involving R87, D29A and intermolecular interactions involving Thr26 in the stabilization of the dimer[2].

Even though the direct observation of the fully open structures and conversion between different flap conformations in atomic detail simulations were very encouraging, the question of how relevant the open state was for ligand binding remained open. We carried out a study to address these questions by performing unrestrained, all-atom MD simulations following manual placement of a cyclic urea inhibitor into the substrate binding site of the open protease [Figure 6.2(h)].[52] In those simulations, the inhibitor reproducibly induced the protease to undergo spontaneous conversion to the closed form [Figure 6.2(j)], as seen in all inhibitor-bound HIV-PR crystal structures. In control simulations without the inhibitor, the open flaps always returned to the semiopen form. In a typical trajectory, the inhibitor formed specific hydrogen bonds with one of the catalytic aspartic acids and one flap [Figure 6.2(i)], accelerating the closing process. Subsequently, the other flap closed and helped to pack bulky napthyl groups of the inhibitor into the binding pockets [Figure 6.2(j)]. Significantly, the asynchronous closing of two flaps observed in this MD simulation is consistent with the x-ray crystallographic study,[14] which captured a novel intermediate conformation in both the wild-type and drug-resistant variant complexes, with one flap intermediate and the other flap closed. In addition, our simulations reproduced not only the greater degree of flap closure but also the striking difference in the flap handedness between bound and unbound proteases. The transitions between the three forms are summarized in Figure 6.3. These simulations provide further evidence that a rearrangement of the ensemble of conformations sampled by the protease-binding pocket indeed occurs on ligand binding.

Another report used molecular dynamics constrained to dihedral angle space to speed up the sampling.[57] The authors also observed transitions between semiopen and

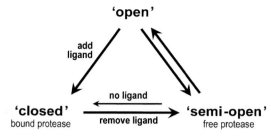

Figure 6.3. Schematic representation of simulated transitions between the three protease forms. The closed flap conformation converts to semiopen on removal of ligand. Ligand induces the closure of the open form. Free protease exists primarily in semiopen form but transiently changes to fully open and, occasionally, even to the closed form that is only weakly populated in the absence of a ligand.

open conformations, although the semiopen structure following the opening event did not show close agreement with the crystallographic form, which might have resulted from simplifications used in internal coordinate space dynamics. The same authors followed this report with another study reporting protease flap closing induced by substrate binding.[58] Once again, flap closing was observed to follow an asymmetric path, in accord with our observations.

In summary, the recent molecular dynamics simulations coming from different groups and using different simulation methodologies and force fields provide compelling evidence that the major features of protease dynamics are generally reproduced and are independent of specific system setup details. These studies also serve as a clear indication that the flexibility and the dynamic behavior of HIV-1 protease are amenable to computational analysis, and the resulting data may form the foundation of a flexibility-based drug design process.

The ensemble of HIV-PR unbound structures in solution

Both simulations and NMR results agree that a wide-open flap conformation is a rare event. However, there is no consensus about the predominant flap conformation of the free protease in solution; that is, is it an ensemble of semiopen forms, closed, or the curled conformation? Although a semiopen flap conformation was most often observed in crystal structures of the dimer, the free enzyme might adopt a different conformation in solution, because crystal packing contacts and crystallization conditions may alter the conformations of the flaps in crystal structures of HIV proteases.[59–61] To address this question, we carried out a series of simulations of the HIV-PR (PDB code:2G69) with or without the inclusion of the crystal-packing environment and observed that without the surrounding crystal packing contacts, the semiopen x-ray structure in solution rapidly adopts a variety of conformations, including the closed conformation (unpublished data). When crystallographic neighbors were included in the simulation, the semiopen form was stable throughout and did not undergo

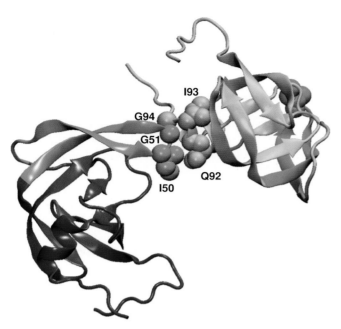

Figure 6.4 Detailed view of 2G69 crystal packing interactions involving HIV-PR flaps (shown in green). Ile50 and Gly51 on the flap tip of one monomer (purple) interact with Gln92 and Ile93 on the helical region of a monomer in a neighboring dimer (yellow).

conformational changes due to the interactions between Ile50, Gly51 on the flap (loop), and Gln92/Ile93 from the surrounding lattice molecule (shown in Figure 6.4). Thus crystallographic contacts likely play a role in the observed flap conformations, but it remains unclear to what extent this relatively small energetic influence can affect the overall ensemble.

On the basis of nuclear Overhauser effect spectroscopy (NOESY) spectra, NMR relaxation data of the dimer,[34,62] and available crystal structures, Ishima et al. have proposed that the flaps are best described as an ensemble of semiopen conformations that are mostly hydrogen-bonded beta-hairpin structures but undergo rapid conformational exchange in the tips of the flaps (residues 49–52). In addition, other simulations[38,52,55] and our comparison study of MD simulation ensembles and EPR experiments[28] have predicted that the predominant flap conformation of the dimer in solution is likely to be represented by an ensemble of semiopen forms. However, several recent simulations also predicted that the flaps could adopt diverse curled conformations,[37] with or without the exposure of the active site to solvent. Although there is no direct experimental evidence to support curled conformations, the existence of a curled conformation as a minor conformer should not be ruled out, because the generalized order parameters derived from simulations that predicted both semiopen and curled conformations qualitatively reproduce those derived from NMR relaxation data.[52,63] Additionally, curled and semiopen models both qualitatively satisfy the characteristic beta-hairpin ^{1}H-^{1}H intrasubunit NOEs,[34] because the flaps mostly adopt a beta-hairpin conformation in both

models. One possible explanation for the structural heterogeneity of apo HIV-PR is that it has evolved to be as rigid as possible while remaining flexible enough to recognize its diverse substrates and adapt their structures to different binding partners as observed in other proteins;[64–66] thus, it is possible that the true ensemble of apo HIV-PR might cover the complete structural heterogeneity observed in both crystals and MD simulations. In addition, it is assumed that the conformational selection might be responsible for the binding of the ligand rather than the induced fit; this selection scheme might account for the "sloppy" recognition of HIV-PR,[67,68] which still remains incompletely understood.

Proposed molecular mechanisms of resistance

Classical and ab initio MD simulations reveal[69,70] that protease flexibility modulates the activation free-energy barrier of the enzymatic cleavage reaction. In drug-resistant mutants, the active site mutations are often associated with mutations that partially restore the enzymatic function ("compensatory mutations") and frequently occur in regions distant from the active site. The mutations in these positions may enhance the catalytic rate of the protease mutants by affecting the flexibility of the protein. Although the authors provide a plausible explanation of how compensatory mutations work, they do not suggest how this understanding could be extended to the design of drugs that escape protease mutations.

Schiffer, in her earlier MD simulation study,[37] proposes a model for overcoming resistance based on an observation of HIV-1 protease conformation with flaps "curled" such that they allow substrate access to the active site. The authors suggest that this "open" conformation is crucial and the inhibitors should be designed to lock the flaps in their "open" conformation and believe that such inhibitors would be less susceptible to the development of drug-resistant variants. Along this line, three crystal structures of apo wild-type HIV-PR (PDB code 2PC0) and multiple drug resistance (PDB code 1RPI and 1TW7) in a "wide-open" conformation were reported recently.[18,21,22] These observations provide insight into the flexibility of the flap regions, the nature of their motions, and their critical role in binding substrates and inhibitors. Nevertheless, unlike all previous apo HIV-PR crystal structures, the binding pockets in all three "wide-open" x-ray crystal sturctures are more exposed because of much further separation of the flaps. Even though the structure differs from the "open" structure proposed by Schiffer, the idea of resistance remains roughly the same. The authors indicate that the structural flexibility with respect to flap dynamics and induced-fit recognition of substrates and inhibitors might account for the emergence of drug resistance. However, in a recent report, molecular dynamics simulations were performed for the MDR isolate, starting from the open crystal structure (PDB code 1TW7). Although simulations including crystal packing contacts

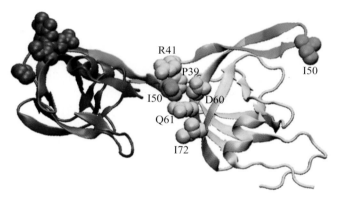

Figure 6.5. Detailed view of 1TW7 crystal packing interactions involving HIV-PR flaps (shown in green). The flap tip of one monomer (purple) is wedged into the elbow region of a monomer in a neighboring dimer (yellow).

reproduced the crystal structure, simulations without crystal packing contacts reproducibly reverted to the closed form observed in crystal structures of the bound wild-type protease.[71] Further analysis suggests that the wide-open structure observed for MDR 769 arises not from sequence variation but instead is an artifact from crystal packing (Figure 6.5) at the elbow region. Therefore, whether the "wide-open" conformation is relevant to the flap dynamics and drug resistant remains an open question.

Kollman and coworkers used free-energy calculations for HIV-PR inhibitors to study drug resistance.[72] They decomposed binding affinities into contributions from different side chains in the active site. Based on the results, they suggested that inhibitors deriving significant fractions of their binding affinity from interactions with side chains that were not correspondingly important for substrate affinity would be more susceptible to mutation. The authors suggested that drugs should be designed to fall within the free-energy "recognition profile" and not gain a large amount of their affinity through interaction with nonconserved residues. Recently, Schiffer's group proposed an interesting variation on this approach, the substrate envelope hypothesis.[73] They suggest that the recognition of an asymmetric substrate is based on its complementary shape (i.e., whether it fits well to the cleavage site). By analyzing the steric region occupied by a variety of substrates and inhibitors, they showed that resistance often arises when inhibitors venture beyond this "permitted" volume. Therefore, inhibitors that fit within the steric envelope of HIV-1 protease might be more effective and less susceptible to drug resistance mutations. The same group suggested another possible mechanism for drug resistance,[74] based on observation of the importance of the nineteen core hydrophobic residues in facilitating conformational changes of HIV-1 protease. They suggested that sliding of those hydrophobic core residues by each other enables them to exchange the partner of hydrophobic contacts, while maintaining many structurally important hydrogen bonds. Mutations of these residues in HIV-1 protease would alter the packing of the hydrophobic

core, thus affecting the conformational dynamics of the protease.

Another appealing explanation of resistance was provided by Freire based on microcalorimetric measurements of protease-binding thermodynamics.[75,76] In solution the peptide substrate has a higher flexibility than the synthetic inhibitors and therefore suffers a higher conformational entropy loss on binding. However, because of its higher flexibility, the peptide substrate is more amenable to adapt to backbone rearrangements or subtle conformational changes induced by mutations in the protease. The synthetic inhibitors are less flexible, and their capacity to adapt to changes in the geometry of the binding pocket is more restricted.

Both computational and experimental studies showed that, in case of HIV-1 protease, there are differences in thermodynamic stability among the alternate protease forms that should be included when considering ligand-binding affinity. Because the structure of the transient open form was suggested in only recent molecular dynamics studies, the description thus far has focused on thermodynamic differences between closed and semiopen forms. For example, the free energy change ΔG calculated by reaction path method estimated that the semiopen form is more favorable than closed, with stabilization contribution coming primarily from the entropic term.[77] This analysis is consistent with NMR relaxation data and is very reasonable given the high glycine content of the flap tips. As was shown by calorimetric experiments, a large favorable entropy change is also the major driving force for high binding affinity of current HIV-1 PR inhibitors.[78,79] However, in this case it is the favorable solvation entropy associated with the burial of a large hydrophobic surface on inhibitor binding. Detailed thermodynamic analysis[78] of wild-type and active site resistant mutant (V82F/I84V) suggests that the mutation lowers the binding affinity in two ways: first, directly by altering the interaction between inhibitors and the protease (binding enthalpy and entropy), and second, indirectly by altering the relative stability of free (semiopen) and bound (closed) form on inhibitor binding. Importantly, mutations that stabilize the semiopen flap conformation will lower binding affinity due to the increased energy penalty required for flap reorganization on substrate/inhibitor binding. Therefore, the free-energy penalty associated with shifting the ensemble of conformations sampled by the protease should be included in any accurate calculation of binding affinity.

These few examples of proposed mechanism of resistance raise several important points. To preserve the function of the mutant protease (i.e., still efficiently cleave the viral polyprotein) the enzyme can introduce alterations in the active site but the correct dynamics or flexibility must be preserved and/or the active site changes must be compensated by the flexibility of the substrate. Because the competitive advantage of the synthetic inhibitors' strong binding likely arises from their rigidity, it has been rather challenging to design flexible inhibitors that bind stronger than the natural substrate while retaining the ability to adapt to a binding pocket that varies in shape. An example of such a flexible inhibitor is KNI-764 (also known as JE-2147), which was shown to remain potent against MDR protease strains.[80] It was again demonstrated by calorimetric measurements[81,82] that, in contrast to previous inhibitors, these second-generation inhibitors bind strongly mainly due to favorable enthalpy change.

Another strategy to evade mutations in the active site is to design inhibitors that primarily form interactions with the backbone rather than side chains of the active site[83,84] such that mutations in the binding site may not effect the inhibitor binding. A conceptually different strategy arises from consideration of HIV-PR flexibility. Rather than accommodating changes in shape or affinity of the binding site, one may try to interfere with the dynamics of the protein. Assuming that enzyme dynamics must remain conserved, the virus may have a more difficult time evolving mutations that would restore functional dynamics of the protease.

Drug design targeting protein flexibility: New allosteric inhibitors

In light of the discussion above, an attractive alternative approach to designing protease inhibitors would target the thermodynamic balance of the closed, semiopen, and open ensembles. This might be achieved by designing allosteric inhibitors that do not directly compete with substrate for the same binding site but indirectly change the flexibility of the protease such that the balance of the three states is shifted.

The possibility of allosteric inhibitors of HIV protease was suggested previously.[40,41] Based on molecular dynamics simulations that showed anticorrelated behavior between the flap opening and the compression of the elbow region, the authors suggested targeting the protease elbow region [see Figure 6.1(b)] as an allosteric site. However, no experimental evidence to support this hypothesis is yet available. It is interesting to note, however, that the only experimentally determined structure with an open binding pocket[85] (the crystal structure of the MDR isolate discussed above and shown in Figure 6.5) indeed has a crystal packing contact involving insertion of residues from a symmetry-related neighbor into the elbow region.[71] This observation provides strong experimental support that this site may be a promising candidate for allosteric inhibition.

Another potential target for allosteric inhibition is the protease dimer interface [see Figure 6.1(b)]. NMR experiments measuring backbone amide chemical exchange transverse relaxation rates[34] indicated that the flexibility in the four-stranded beta-sheet dimer interface increases on inhibitor binding. This suggests a coupling between the ligand-binding site and the dimer interface. This coupling (even though in the opposite direction) is also observed in the crystal structure of a free HIV-1 protease in which

the N- and C-termini of the two protease monomers were tethered.[86] Unlike all other crystal structures of the free protease, this "monomeric" protease exhibits the closed flap conformation. Last but not least, there has been a continuing effort to design inhibitors of protease dimerization.[87,88] An interesting recent report[89] demonstrated that some of the inhibitors initially designed to prevent dimerization actually did not disrupt the dimer interface and yet showed substantial protease inhibition. The authors thus concluded that these compounds acted as allosteric inhibitors binding at the dimer interface, indirectly reducing the binding affinity of the substrate.

Further evidence that these sites may provide useful targets for allosteric inhibitors has been shown by Rezacova et al.,[90] who developed monoclonal antibodies with potent inhibition of the protease function. These targeted two non-binding site regions of the enzyme: one corresponds to residues 36–46 (flap elbow) and the other to residues 1–6 at the dimer interface. Significantly, the inhibition mechanism of this new class of inhibitor is revealed by the observation of anticorrelation behavior between the compression of the same exo site and the flap opening during our simulation (unpublished data). Therefore, those inhibitors may function as an allosteric inhibitor by disrupting the native fold or even dimerization interface. Yet another example of potentially exploitable allosteric inhibition was reported for β-lactam compounds.[91] The authors demonstrated that the inhibitors are noncompetitive and that they only interact with ligand-bound enzyme and suggested the mechanism of inhibition through interaction of β-lactam compounds with the closed flap region of the enzyme-substrate complex.

A novel class inhibitor targeting the hydrophobic core of one monomer (or so-called flap-recognition pocket) has recently been proposed.[51] It suggests that the presence of a ligand in the core hydrophobic pocket might alter the conformational behavior of the flap region and prevents the substrate's access to the active site or disrupts substrate cleavage due to the inappropriate or incomplete flap closure. This class of inhibitor highlights the importance of hydrophobic contacts between the flap and core domain in the stability of different conformations and thus provides further evidence of the transition mechanism the flaps suggested by MD simulations.

Even though the existence of HIV-PR allosteric sites has not yet been shown experimentally, it has been argued that their presence is very likely for all dynamic proteins.[92] The allosteric inhibitors do not compete with natural substrate and thus their effect is not decreased by higher concentration of the substrate. They also have a potential for better selectivity.[92] Moreover, the hydrophobic character of the HIV-PR active site leads to hydrophobic protease inhibitors and therefore results in their undesirable poor water solubility.[93,94] Thus an additional advantage of the three allosteric sites discussed above stems from their polar character, which could improve bioavailability.

CONCLUSIONS

The pronounced differences in bound and unbound protease crystal structures and NMR studies provide experimental evidence that HIV-1 protease flexibility plays a crucial role in its function. Numerous computational studies reviewed here emphasized the importance of protease dynamics in substrate and inhibitor binding. Taken together, this opens new opportunities for developing protease inhibitors in which protease dynamics and flexibility, as determined through computer simulation, are explicitly targeted in the inhibitor design process. Specifically, influencing the thermodynamics of the three protease states (closed, semiopen, and open) might disrupt its function. It remains to be seen whether this approach makes it more difficult for the enzyme to evolve resistant mutations.

Computer simulations aimed at accurate quantitative description of protease dynamics still face challenges, even though atomic-level and coarse-grain simulations complement each other in their predictive abilities. All-atom simulations provide a model that is able to reproduce experimentally observed structural changes, predict a new open structure inferred from experiments, and show transitions between all these forms. However, coarse-grain models could provide a more statistically valid thermodynamic description of the flap opening and thereby provide quantitative estimates for the shift in equilibrium arising from protease mutations. Thus far, the accuracy of the coarse-grain model does not appear to be sufficient to reproduce the detailed conformational changes that accompany binding (i.e., changes between closed and semiopen forms). Full atomistic models may therefore serve as an important reference for calibrating and improving the coarse-grain models.

In summary, because of improved quality of the computational models and the ability to extend simulations to biologically relevant time scales, computational techniques have finally reached the stage where they can reproduce experimental observations. Perhaps more important, however, is that simulations can now complement experiments by providing valuable insights into dynamic events as well as energetic aspects of ligand binding and drug resistance.

REFERENCES

1. Barresinoussi, F.; et al. Isolation of a T-lymphotropic retrovirus from a patient at risk for acquired immune-deficiency syndrome (AIDS). *Science* **1983**, *220*(4599), 868–871.
2. Gallo, R. C.; et al. Isolation of human T-cell leukemia-virus in acquired immune-deficiency syndrome (AIDS). *Science* **1983**, *220*(4599), 865–867.
3. Blair, W. S.; et al. HIV-1 entry – an expanding portal for drug discovery. *Drug Discov. Today* **2000**, *5*(5), p. 183–194.
4. Moore, J. P.; Stevenson, M. New targets for inhibitors of HIV-1 replication. *Nat. Rev. Mol. Cell Biol.* **2000**, *1*(1), 40–49.
5. Ren, J. S.; et al. High-resolution structures of HIV-1 RT from 4 RT-inhibitor complexes. *Nat. Struct. Biol.* **1995**, *2*(4), 293–302.
6. Rhee, S. Y.; et al. Human immunodeficiency virus reverse transcriptase and protease sequence database. *Nucleic Acids Res.* **2003**, *31*(1), 298–303.
7. Condra, J. H.; et al. In-vivo emergence of HIV-1 variants resistant to multiple protease inhibitors. *Nature* **1995**, *374*(6522), 569–571.
8. Teague, S. J. Implications of protein flexibility for drug discovery. *Nat. Rev. Drug Discov.* **2003**, *2*(7), 527–541.
9. McCammon, J. A. Target flexibility in molecular recognition. *Biochim. Biophys. Acta* **2005**, *1754*(1–2), 221–224.
10. Vondrasek, J.; Wlodawer, A. HIVdb: a database of the structures of human immunodeficiency virus protease. *Proteins* **2002**, *49*(4), 429–431.
11. Navia, M. A.; et al. 3-dimensional structure of aspartyl protease from human immunodeficiency virus HIV-1. *Nature* **1989**, *337*(6208), 615–620.
12. Wlodawer, A.; et al. Conserved folding in retroviral proteases – crystal-structure of a synthetic HIV-1 protease. *Science* **1989**, *245*(4918), 616–621.
13. Lapatto, R.; et al. X-ray-analysis of HIV-1 proteinase at 2.7 a resolution confirms structural homology among retroviral enzymes. *Nature* **1989**, *342*(6247), 299–302.
14. Prabu-Jeyabalan, M.; et al. Mechanism of substrate recognition by drug-resistant human immunodeficiency virus type 1 protease variants revealed by a novel structural intermediate. *J. Virol.* **2006**, *80*(7), 3607–3616.
15. Prabu-Jeyabalan, M.; et al. Mechanism of substrate recognition by drug-resistant human immunodeficiency virus type 1 protease variants revealed by a novel structural intermediate. *J. Virol.* **2006**, 3607–3616.
16. Heaslet, H.; et al. Conformational flexibility in the flap domains of ligand-free HIV protease. *Acta Crystallogr. D Biol. Crystallogr.* **2007**, *63*(Pt 8), 866–875.
17. Collins, J. R.; Burt, S. K.; Erickson, J. W. Flap opening in HIV-1 protease simulated by 'activated' molecular dynamics. *Nat. Struct. Mol. Biol.* **1995**, *2*(4), 334–338.
18. Heaslet, H.; et al. Conformational flexibility in the flap domains of ligand-free HIV protease. *Acta Crystallogr. D Biol. Crystallogr.* **2007**, 866–875.
19. Spinelli, S.; et al. The 3-dimensional structure of the aspartyl protease from the HIV-1 isolate Bru. *Biochimie* **1991**, *73*(11), 1391–1396.
20. Liu, F. L.; et al. Mechanism of drug resistance revealed by the crystal structure of the unliganded HIV-1 protease with F53L mutation. *J. Mol. Biol.* **2006**, *358*(5), 1191–1199.
21. Martin, P.; et al. "Wide-open" 1.3 A structure of a multidrug-resistant HIV-1 protease as a drug target. *Structure* **2005**, *13*(12), 1887–1895.
22. Logsdon, B. C.; et al. Crystal structures of a multidrug-resistant human immunodeficiency virus type 1 protease reveal an expanded active-site cavity. *J. Virol.* **2004**, *78*(6), 3123–3132.
23. Panchal, S. C.; et al. HIV-1 protease tethered heterodimer-pepstatin-A complex: NMR characterization. *Curr. Sci.* **2000**, *79*(12), 1684–1695.
24. LangeSavage, G.; et al. Structure of HOE/BAY 793 complexed to human immunodeficiency virus (HIV-1) protease in two different crystal forms – structure/function relationship and influence of crystal packing. *Eur. J. Biochem.* **1997**, *248*(2), 313–322.
25. Miller, M.; et al. Structure of complex of synthetic HIV-1 protease with a substrate-based inhibitor at 2.3-a resolution. *Science* **1989**, *246*(4934), 1149–1152.

26. Wlodawer, A.; Vondrasek, J. Inhibitors of HIV-1 protease: a major success of structure-assisted drug design. *Annu. Rev. Biophys. Biomol. Struct.* **1998**, *27*, 249–284.

27. Hornak, V.; et al. HIV-1 protease flaps spontaneously open and reclose in molecular dynamics simulations. *Proc. Natl. Acad. Sci. U.S.A.* **2006**, *103*(4), 915–920.

28. Ding, F.; Layten, M.; Simmerling, C. Solution structure of HIV-1 protease flaps probed by comparison of molecular dynamics simulation ensembles and EPR experiments. *J. Am. Chem. Soc.* **2008**, *130*(23), 7184–7185.

29. Layten, M.; Hornak, V.; Simmerling, C. The open structure of a multi-drug-resistant HIV-1 protease is stabilized by crystal packing contacts. *J. Am. Chem. Soc.* **2006**, *128*(41), 13360–13361.

30. Nicholson, L. K.; et al. Flexibility and function in HIV-1 protease. *Nat. Struct. Biol.* **1995**, *2*(4), 274–280.

31. Freedberg, D. I.; et al. Rapid structural fluctuations of the free HIV protease flaps in solution: relationship to crystal structures and comparison with predictions of dynamics calculations. *Protein Sci.* **2002**, *11*(2), 221–232.

32. Ishima, R.; Louis, J. M. A diverse view of protein dynamics from NMR studies of HIV-1 protease flaps. *Proteins* **2007**, *70*, 1408–1415.

33. Galiano, L.; Bonora, M.; Fanucci, G. E. Interflap distances in HIV-1 protease determined by pulsed EPR measurements. *J. Am. Chem. Soc.* **2007**, *129*(36), 11004–11005.

34. Ishima, R.; et al. Flap opening and dimer-interface flexibility in the free and inhibitor-bound HIV protease, and their implications for function. *Structure* **1999**, *7*(9), 1047–1055.

35. Katoh, E.; et al. A solution NMR study of the binding kinetics and the internal dynamics of an HIV-1 protease-substrate complex. *Protein Sci.* **2003**, *12*(7), 1376–1385.

36. Collins, J. R.; Burt, S. K.; Erickson, J. W. Flap opening in HIV-1 protease simulated by activated molecular dynamics. *Nat. Struct. Biol.* **1995**, *2*(4), 334–338.

37. Scott, W. R. P.; Schiffer, C. A. Curling of flap tips in HIV-1 protease as a mechanism for substrate entry and tolerance of drug resistance. *Structure* **2000**, *8*(12), 1259–1265.

38. Meagher, K. L.; Carlson, H. A. Solvation influences flap collapse in HIV-1 protease. *Proteins* **2005**, *58*(1), 119–125.

39. Hamelberg, D.; McCammon, J. A. Fast peptidyl *cis-trans* isomerization within the flexible Gly-Rich flaps of HIV-1 protease. *J. Am. Chem. Soc.* **2005**, *127*(40), 13778–13779.

40. Perryman, A. L.; Lin, J. H.; McCammon, J. A. HIV-1 protease molecular dynamics of a wild-type and of the V82F/I84V mutant: possible contributions to drug resistance and a potential new target site for drugs. *Protein Sci.* **2004**, *13*(4), 1108–1123.

41. Perryman, A. L.; Lin, J. H.; McCammon, J. A. Restrained molecular dynamics simulations of HIV-1 protease: the first step in validating a new target for drug design. *Biopolymers* **2006**, *82*(3), 272–284.

42. Perryman, A. L.; Lin, J. H.; McCammon, J. A. Optimization and computational evaluation of a series of potential active site inhibitors of the V82F/I84V drug-resistant mutant of HIV-1 protease: an application of the relaxed complex method of structure-based drug design. *Chem. Biol. Drug Des.* **2006**, *67*(5), 336–345.

43. Chang, C. E.; et al. Gated binding of ligands to HIV-1 protease: Brownian dynamics simulations in a coarse-grained model. *Biophys. J.* **2006**, *90*(11), 3880–3885.

44. Tozzini, V.; McCammon, J. A. A coarse grained model for the dynamics of flap opening in HIV-1 protease. *Chem. Phys. Lett.* **2005**, *413*(1–3), 123–128.

45. Hornak, V.; et al. HIV-1 protease flaps spontaneously open and reclose in molecular dynamics simulations. *Proc. Natl. Acad. Sci. U.S.A.* **2006**, *103*(4), 915–920.

46. Pitera, J. W.; Swope, W. Understanding folding and design: Replica-exchange simulations of "Trp-cage" miniproteins. *Proc. Natl. Acad. Sci. U.S.A.* **2003**, *100*(13), 7587–7592.

47. Zhou, R. Free energy landscape of protein folding in water: explicit vs. implicit solvent. *Proteins* **2003**, *53*(2), 148–161.

48. Zhou, R.; Berne, B. J. Can a continuum solvent model reproduce the free energy landscape of a β-hairpin folding in water? *Proc. Natl. Acad. Sci. U.S.A.* **2002**, *99*, 12777–12782.

49. Roe, D. R.; et al. Secondary structure bias in generalized born solvent models: Comparison of conformational ensembles and free energy of solvent polarization from explicit and implicit solvation. *J. Phys. Chem. B* **2007**, *111*(7), 1846–1857.

50. Geney, R.; et al. Investigation of salt bridge stability in a generalized born solvent model. *J. Chem. Theor. Comput.* **2006**, *2*(1), 115–127.

51. Damm, K. L.; Ung, P. M.; Quintero, J. J.; Gestwicki, J. E.; Carlson, H. A. A poke in the eye: inhibiting HIV-1 protease through its flap-recognition pocket. *Biopolymers* **2008**, *89*, 643–652.

52. Hornak, V.; et al. HIV-1 protease flaps spontaneously close to the correct structure in simulations following manual placement of an inhibitor into the open state. *J. Am. Chem. Soc.* **2006**, *128*(9), 2812–2813.

53. Krausslich, H. G. Human immunodeficiency virus proteinase dimer as component of the viral polyprotein prevents particle assembly and viral infectivity. *Proc. Natl. Acad. Sci. U.S.A.* **1991**, *88*(8), 3213–3217.

54. Sayer, J. M.; Liu, F.; Ishima, R.; Weber, I. T.; Louis, J. M. Effect of the active site D25N mutation on the structure, stability, and ligand binding of the mature HIV-1 protease. *J. Biol. Chem.* **2008**, *283*(19), 13459–13470.

55. Perryman, A. L.; Lin, J.-H.; McCammon, J. A. HIV-1 protease molecular dynamics of a wild-type and of the V82F/I84V mutant: possible contributions to drug resistance and a potential new target site for drugs. *Protein Sci.* **2004**, *13*(4), 1108–1123.

56. Tyndall, J. D. A.; et al. Crystal structures of highly constrained substrate and hydrolysis products bound to HIV-1 protease: implications for the catalytic mechanism. *Biochemistry* **2008**, *47*(12), 3736–3744.

57. Toth, G.; Borics, A. Flap opening mechanism of HIV-1 protease. *J. Mol. Graph. Model.* **2006**, *24*(6), 465–474.

58. Toth, G.; Borics, A. Closing of the flaps of HIV-1 protease induced by substrate binding: a model of a flap closing mechanism in retroviral aspartic proteases. *Biochemistry* **2006**, *45*(21), 6606–6614.

59. Spinelli, S.; et al. The three-dimensional structure of the aspartyl protease from the HIV-1 isolate BRU. *Biochimie* **1991**, *73*(11), 1391–1396.

60. Lapatto, R.; et al. X-ray analysis of HIV-1 proteinase at 2.7 [angst] resolution confirms structural homology among retroviral enzymes. *Nature* **1989**, *342*(6247), 299–302.

61. Marqusee, S.; Robbins, V. H.; Baldwin, R. L. Unusually stable helix formation in short alanine-based peptides. *Proc. Natl. Acad. Sci. U.S.A.* **1989**, *86*(14), 5286–5290.

62. Freedberg, D. I.; et al. Rapid structural fluctuations of the free HIV protease flaps in solution: relationship to crystal structures and comparison with predictions of dynamics calculations. *Protein Sci.* **2002**, *11*(2), 221–232.

63. Dmytro Kovalskyy, Dubyna, V.; Mark, A. E.; Kornelyuk, A. A molecular dynamics study of the structural stability of HIV-1

protease under physiological conditions: the role of Na+ ions in stabilizing the active site. *Proteins* **2005**, *58*(2), 450–458.

64. Eisenmesser, E. Z.; Bosco, D. A.; Akke, M.; Kern, D. Enzyme dynamics during catalysis. *Science* **2002**, *295*(5559), 1520–1523.

65. Huang, Y. J.; Montelione, G. T. Structural biology: proteins flex to function. *Nature* **2005**, *438*(7064), 36–37.

66. Lange, O. F.; Lakomek, N.-A.; Farès, C.; Schröder, G. F.; Walter, K. F. A.; Becker, S.; Meiler, J.; Grubmüller, H.; Griesinger, C.; de Groot, B. L. Recognition dynamics up to microseconds revealed from an RDC-derived ubiquitin ensemble in solution. *Protein*, **2008**, *320*(5882) 1471–1475.

67. Kohl, N. E.; et al. Active human immunodeficiency virus protease is required for viral infectivity. *Proc. Natl. Acad. Sci. U.S.A.* **1988**, *85*(13), 4686–4690.

68. O'Loughlin, T. L.; Greene, D. N.; Matsumura, I. Diversification and specialization of HIV protease function during in vitro evolution. *Mol. Biol. Evol.* **2006**, *23*(4), 764–772.

69. Piana, S.; Carloni, P.; Rothlisberger, U. Drug resistance in HIV-1 protease: flexibility-assisted mechanism of compensatory mutations. *Protein Sci.* **2002**, *11*(10), 2393–2402.

70. Piana, S.; Carloni, P.; Parrinello, M. Role of conformational fluctuations in the enzymatic reaction of HIV-1 protease. *J. Mol. Biol.* **2002**, *319*(2) 567–583.

71. Layten, M.; Hornak, V.; Simmerling, C. The open structure of a multi-drug-resistant HIV-1 protease is stabilized by crystal packing contacts. *J. Am. Chem. Soc.* **2006**, *128*(41), 13360–13361.

72. Wang, W.; Kollman, P. A. Computational study of protein specificity: the molecular basis of HIV-1 protease drug resistance. *Proc. Natl. Acad. Sci. U.S.A.* **2001**, *98*(26), 14937–14942.

73. Prabu-Jeyabalan, M.; Nalivaika, E.; Schiffer, C. A. Substrate shape determines specificity of recognition for HIV-1 protease: analysis of crystal structures of six substrate complexes. *Structure* **2002**; *10*(3), 369–381.

74. Foulkes-Murzycki, J. E.; Scott, W. R. P.; Schiffer, C. A. Hydrophobic sliding: a possible mechanism for drug resistance in human immunodeficiency virus type 1 protease. *Structure* **2007**, *15*(2), 225–233.

75. Luque, I.; et al. Molecular basis of resistance to HIV-1 protease inhibition: a plausible hypothesis. *Biochemistry* **1998**, *37*(17), 5791–5797.

76. Vega, S.; et al. A structural and thermodynamic escape mechanism from a drug resistant mutation of the HIV-1 protease. *Proteins* **2004**, *55*(3), 594–602.

77. Rick, S. W.; Erickson, J. W.; Burt, S. K. Reaction path and free energy calculations of the transition between alternate conformations of HIV-1 protease. *Proteins* **1998**, *32*(1), 7–16.

78. Todd, M. J.; et al. Thermodynamic basis of resistance to HIV-1 protease inhibition: calorimetric analysis of the V82F/I84V active site resistant mutant. *Biochemistry* **2000**, *39*(39) 11876–11883.

79. Ohtaka, H.; et al. Thermodynamic rules for the design of high affinity HIV-1 protease inhibitors with adaptability to mutations and high selectivity towards unwanted targets. *Int. J. Biochem. Cell Biol.* **2004**, *36*(9), 1787–1799.

80. Yoshimura, K.; et al., JE-2147: a dipeptide protease inhibitor (PI) that potently inhibits multi-PI-resistant HIV-1. *Proc. Natl. Acad. Sci. U.S.A.* **1999**, *96*(15), 8675–8680.

81. Velazquez-Campoy, A.; Freire, E. Incorporating target heterogeneity in drug design. *J. Cell. Biochem.* **2001**, *37*, 82–88.

82. Velazquez-Campoy, A.; Kiso, Y.; Freire, E. The binding energetics of first- and second-generation HIV-1 protease inhibitors: implications for drug design. *Arch. Biochem. Biophys.* **2001**, *390*(2), 169–175.

83. Ghosh, A. K.; et al. Structure-based design of novel HIV-1 protease inhibitors to combat drug resistance. *J. Med. Chem.* **2006**, *49*(17), 5252–5261.

84. Tie, Y. F.; et al. High resolution crystal structures of HIV-1 protease with a potent non-peptide inhibitor (UIC-94017) active against multi-drug-resistant clinical strains. *J. Mol. Biol.* **2004**, *338*(2), 341–352.

85. Martin, P.; et al. "Wide-open" 1.3 angstrom structure of a multidrug-resistant HIV-1 protease as a drug target. *Structure* **2005**, *13*(12), 1887–1895.

86. Pillai, B.; Kannan, K. K.; Hosur, M. V. 1.9 angstrom X-ray study shows closed flap conformation in crystals of tethered HIV-1PR. *Proteins* **2001**, *43*(1), 57–64.

87. Hwang, Y. S.; Chmielewski, J. Development of low molecular weight HIV-1 protease dimerization inhibitors. *J. Med. Chem.* **2005**, *48*(6), 2239–2242.

88. Shultz, M. D.; et al. Small-molecule dimerization inhibitors of wild-type and mutant HIV protease: a focused library approach. *J. Am. Chem. Soc.* **2004**, *126*(32), 9886–9887.

89. Bowman, M. J.; Byrne, S.; Chmielewski, J. Switching between allosteric and dimerization inhibition of HIV-1 protease. *Chem. Biol.* **2005**, *12*(4), 439–444.

90. Rezacova, P.; et al. Crystal structure of a cross-reaction complex between an anti-HIV-1 protease antibody and an HIV-2 protease peptide. *J. Struct. Biol.* **2005**, *149*(3), 332–337.

91. Sperka, T.; et al. Beta-lactam compounds as apparently uncompetitive inhibitors of HIV-1 protease. *Bioorg. Med. Chem. Lett.* **2005**, *15*(12), 3086–3090.

92. Gunasekaran, K.; Ma, B. Y.; Nussinov, R. Is allostery an intrinsic property of all dynamic proteins? *Proteins* **2004**, *57*(3), 433–443.

93. Fleisher, D.; Bong, R.; Stewart, B. H. Improved oral drug delivery: solubility limitations overcome by the use of prodrugs. *Adv. Drug Deliv. Rev.* **1996**, *19*(2), 115–130.

94. Sohma, Y.; et al. Development of water-soluble prodrugs of the HIV-1 protease inhibitor KNI-727: importance of the conversion time for higher gastrointestinal absorption of prodrugs based on spontaneous chemical cleavage. *J. Med. Chem.* **2003**, *46*(19), 4124–4135.

7

Docking: a domesday report

Martha S. Head

In 1085, most likely from a desire to audit his tax revenues, William the Conqueror commissioned a survey of the land and resources of the country over which he reigned.[1] The results of that survey come down to us in two tomes, the Little Domesday and the Great Domesday, in which were recorded voluminous amounts of data concerning the land, people, buildings, and chattel throughout England. By no means was this a complete record; large swathes of urban England – London, for example – were not included, nor was there any census of church personnel or property. The Little and Great Domesday books accordingly are an odd mix of completeness and incompleteness, leaving out such large parts of English society yet cataloguing to an excruciating level of detail within the areas surveyed.

Similarly, this chapter is a complete yet incomplete survey of the docking and scoring landscape. We do not review the general principles of docking technologies; a sufficient number of such reviews have been published in peer-reviewed journals alone.[2-20] Nor do we evaluate the state of the art for docking programs and scoring functions; a number of well-regarded and careful evaluations describe the current capabilities and limitations of the technology.[21-26] Instead, under "Comments on the Theory of Docking" we will make explicit the connections between docking and a theory of noncovalent association. Under "Finding New Leads with Docking" we take census of docking virtual screens carried out in this decade, and under "Predicting Bound Poses with Docking" we examine the role of expertise in predicting docked poses of small molecules bound to protein targets. From this mix of general overview and detailed analysis, it is hoped that we will develop a realistic snapshot of how docking is used in the pharmaceutical industry as a tool for drug discovery and design.

COMMENTS ON THE THEORY OF DOCKING

The standard free energy of noncovalent association of a protein and ligand in solution at constant pressure can be written as[27]

$$\Delta G^{\circ}_{\text{sol,PL}} = -RT \ln \left(\frac{C^{\circ}}{8\pi^2} \frac{\sigma_P \sigma_L}{\sigma_{PL}} \right) - RT \ln \left(\frac{Z_{PL}}{Z_P Z_L} \right) + P^{\circ} \Delta \bar{V}, \tag{7.1}$$

where C° is the standard concentration (generally one molar), σ_X are symmetry numbers for each species, P° is the standard pressure (generally one atmosphere), $\Delta \bar{V}$ is the change in equilibrium volume, and Z_X are configuration integrals for each species:

$$Z_X \equiv \int e^{-\beta E(\mathbf{r})} d\mathbf{r}. \tag{7.2}$$

The work $P^{\circ} \Delta \bar{V}$ associated with changes in equilibrium volume due to complex formation is generally negligible, and the first term of Equation (7.1) is fully specified for a given protein/ligand pair at a particular standard concentration; the task of computing the free energy of association accordingly reduces to computation of the configuration integrals Z_P, Z_L, and Z_{PL}. For the rest of the discussion, therefore, equations will be written in a simpler and more compact format, for example:

$$\Delta G^{\circ}_{\text{sol,PL}} = -RT \ln \left(\frac{Z_{PL}}{Z_P Z_L} \right), \tag{7.3}$$

but it should be kept in mind that those missing terms are still implied.

In principle, Equation (7.1) provides an exact expression for the free energy of noncovalent association; putting the theory into practice, however, presents a number of computational challenges. In the previous chapter, Shirts, Mobley, and Brown described several strategies for computing both relative and absolute free energies,[28] many of which tie directly to the theory underlying Equation (7.1). For example, alchemical techniques for computing relative free-energy differences between two related ligands L_1 and L_2 binding to the same protein can be expressed as ratios of configuration integrals[27]:

$$\Delta\Delta G = \Delta G_{PL_2} - \Delta G_{PL_1} = -RT \ln \left(\frac{Z_{PL_2}}{Z_{PL_1}} \right) + RT \ln \left(\frac{Z_{L_2}}{Z_{L_1}} \right), \tag{7.4}$$

while the Zwanzig relationship discussed by Shirts et al. corresponds to replacing those ratios with the average free-energy difference extracted from simulations run under the Hamiltonian of ligand L_1:

$$\frac{Z_{PL_2}}{Z_{PL_1}} = \left\langle \exp^{-\beta[H_{PL_2}(x) - H_{PL_1}(x)]} \right\rangle_{PL_1}$$
$$\frac{Z_{L_2}}{Z_{L_1}} = \left\langle \exp^{-\beta[H_{L_2}(x) - H_{L_1}(x)]} \right\rangle_{L_1}. \tag{7.5}$$

The implicit-solvent predominant-states methods[29-31] mentioned by Shirts et al. replace the full configuration integrals of Equation (7.2) with a summation over configuration integrals for the most favorable minima on the potential energy surface:

$$Z_X = \sum_{i=1}^{M} z_i, \qquad (7.6)$$

where the M individual configuration integrals z_i are computed using techniques such as estimation by harmonic approximation, harmonically biased sampling, or unbiased Monte Carlo integration.

Similar connections can be made between docking and Equation (7.1). As with the relative free-energy methods, the contribution due to the protein in solution is constant across a set of ligands binding to the same protein. For relative free-energy methods the protein configuration integrals cancel in the expression for $\Delta\Delta G$, Equation (7.4); in comparison, for docking Z_P is assumed constant:

$$\Delta G^\circ_{\mathrm{sol,PL}} \approx -RT\ln\left(\frac{Z_{\mathrm{PL}}}{Z_{\mathrm{L}}}\right) + K, \qquad (7.7)$$

where K has been explicitly written to emphasize that the protein configuration integral Z_P has been subsumed into K with the symmetry-number and standard-concentration portions of Equation (7.1). For most but not all docking methods, the contribution due to the ligand free in solution is also treated as constant. Finally, in analogy to an extreme case of the predominant states methods, docking methods generally replace the full configuration integrals of Equation (7.2) with the single energetically most favorable state:

$$\Delta G^\circ_{\mathrm{sol,PL}} \approx -RT\ln\left(\frac{z_{\mathrm{PL,0}}}{z_{\mathrm{L,0}}}\right) + K \qquad (7.8)$$

and the entropic component of the integral is either ignored:

$$z_{X,0} \equiv \int \exp^{-\beta E_X(\mathbf{r_0})}\, d\mathbf{r_0} \approx \exp^{-\beta E_{X,0}} \qquad (7.9)$$

or is approximated by inclusion of terms to account for the entropic penalty of confining the ligand within the protein binding site (Chang, Chen, and Gilson and references therein).[32] On application of all of the approximations that are typically inherent in docking calculations, Equation (7.1) reduces to

$$\Delta G^\circ_{\mathrm{sol,PL}} \approx E_{\mathrm{PL}}, \qquad (7.10)$$

where a docking "score" E_{PL} is computed for a single pose of a ligand docked into a protein binding site. In specific docking implementations, that score might be as simple as a counting of favorable interactions between protein and ligand or as complicated as a force field energy calculation supplemented by estimates of the free energy of the ligand in solution, the solvation differences between uncomplexed and complexed species, and the entropic cost for localizing the ligand to a specific location.

Given the approximations made to the underlying theory, it is no surprise that most studies have shown no correlation between docking score and affinity for closely related analogs.[24,33] There have of course been reports of specific examples where a correlation is seen between affinity and docking score[34,35] or between affinity and interaction energy.[36] As a general practice, therefore, the experienced computational chemist will explore all possible correlations in the hope that one will prove reliable enough to guide design and synthesis. The more typical case, however, is that there will be no reliable signal for decision-making, and the computational chemist must fall back on more computationally expensive methods such as those described by Shirts et al. or on more heuristic strategies – for example, docking large numbers of analogs and assessing emerging patterns of interactions.

FINDING NEW LEADS WITH DOCKING

The availability of large numbers of protein crystal structures (almost 54,000 public structures in the RCSB as of October 2008[37]) strengthens the impetus to make use of that structural information, particularly in those pharmaceutical companies that have made substantial internal investments in structural biology personnel and infrastructure. The intuitive hope has been that protein structures would prove particularly useful for finding novel starting points – leads – for drug discovery efforts, and docking and scoring technologies have seemed particularly relevant tools for virtual screens of large databases of compounds against these protein structures because docking-based virtual screens are in principle not limited by a need for or similarity to known ligands. Indeed, in many recent publications, authors have asserted that docking technologies have improved and that virtual screening successes have become more prevalent. In this section, a survey of the docking landscape will examine whether such assertions are well-founded pragmatism or unwarranted optimism.

Taking census of docking screens, 2000–2008

A census has been carried out for all docking-based virtual screens reported during the period January 2000 through October 2008; the census covered all peer-reviewed scientific journals up through the time of the submission of this chapter to the book editors. Literature searches using terms such as "docking," "virtual screening," and so on, were carried out in SciFinder,[38] PubMed,[39] and Google Scholar.[40] Non-English-language journals were included in the census only if abstracts provided sufficient detail concerning the virtual screening process and results. The initial manuscripts from these literature searches were supplemented to include examples from docking reviews that were not found using simple docking-related search terms. This set of literature searches returned substantially more than 1,000 publications for review and compilation.

From the collection of virtual-screen reports compiled, screens against DNA or RNA targets were removed; the census included only virtual screens to identify small molecules interacting with protein targets. Protein target classes were not categorized for the census, nor was any differentiation made between virtual screens against protein crystal structures or homology models. The collection of reports was further filtered to include only prospective virtual screens to identify small molecules active against a particular protein target; validation studies were included only if they included some prospective lead-identification component. In many examples included in the census, additional techniques were used to prefilter compound databases or postscore docking results – indeed, it was only a rare occurrence when the screen practitioner did not at least postscore the results by visual inspection. Reports in which docking was the primary part of the virtual screening process were retained, but reports in which docking was only a minor adjunct to a virtual screen using pharmacophores, molecular shapes, substructures, or 2D descriptors were excluded. The actual docking programs used were not categorized, and the census represents every major and many minor docking programs.

Virtual screen results were extracted from the collection of reports that survived this filtering process. A surprisingly large number of peer-reviewed manuscripts reported no experimental data and instead reported only computed docking scores without any experimental verification of the proposed inhibition; all such reports were removed from the final tally. For the virtual screens with reported experimental data, scientists performing the docking studies selected a widely varying number of compounds for experimental assays, from as few as two molecules to more than 500. The final tally did not include every experimental result for every selected molecule from any particular virtual screen but instead included only the single best result for any molecule chosen in the virtual screening process. In some studies, hits were followed up by substructure searching or synthesis of related molecules; only the original hits from the virtual screen were included in the tally. In many cases, authors reported experimental results from the primary assay but had not performed orthogonal assays to confirm those results. In these instances I made no attempt to assess the plausibility of any particular result; no reported hits were excluded, even in cases where hit molecules contained features conducive to aggregation or assay interference. The literature search and filtering process described here of course could not produce a complete and exhaustive set of all manuscripts describing a prospective docking-based virtual screen, but the process has generated a sufficiently representative set of publications to allow for the analysis of trends in the real-life use of docking for lead identification.

Analysis of the census results

At the end of this literature search and filtering process, the final census included ninety-eight publications represent-

Table 7.1. Docking-based virtual screens for which experimental results were reported during the period January 2000–October 2008, aggregated into activity bins

Activity range	Count	Reference
<1 μM	18	41–58
1–10 μM	32	59–89
10–100 μM	37	90–126
>100 μM	9	104; 127–134
No hits	3	135–137

ing ninety-nine docking-based virtual screens for which experimental data were reported.[41–137] The best reported activity for each screen has been tabulated and binned into five activity categories: <1 μM, 1–10 μM, 10–100 μM, >100 μM, and no hits; these aggregate affinity results are listed in Table 7.1. The largest number of hits fell in the 10–100 μM range; for this category, the average IC_{50} value was 33 μM and the median value 24 μM. Eighteen virtual screening hits were reported to have experimental activities of <1 μM, which corresponds to two potent hits for each year in the census period. The census compilation contained very few results with affinities >100 μM, presumably due to reporting bias and lowered publication acceptance rates for negative results.

These aggregate data have been broken out by year (Figure 7.1); in this graph, the final two categories, ">100 μM" and "no hits," were combined into a single bin. As expected based on simple averaging, roughly two submicromolar hits per year were reported during the census period, with only two years early in the decade for which no such hits were reported. In 2007, the number of published docking-based virtual screens increased substantially, relative both to the previous year and to the pattern of increases over the period 2000–2005. Albeit with small changes in the actual distribution between the two low-IC_{50} categories, the number

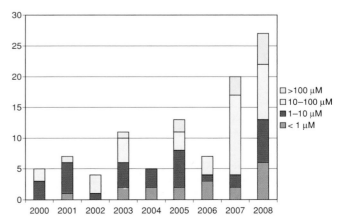

Figure 7.1. Docking-based virtual screens for which experimental results were reported during the period January 2000–July 2008, categorized by year.

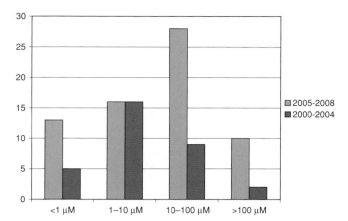

Figure 7.2. Docking-based virtual screens for which experimental results were reported, January 2000–July 2008; distribution of potencies by half-decade.

of compounds with activities less than 10 μM was roughly constant across the census period; the largest increase in number of reports was for compounds with IC_{50} greater than 10 μM. Given the increase in number of hits with poorer activity, it at first blush appears that docking did not improve but instead stagnated or even deteriorated during the census period. Because there were as many as ninety-nine individual reports in the census, a sufficient amount of data was available to more carefully assess whether the apparent trend toward less potent compounds was statistically significant.

The census data were further aggregated by half-decade to smooth out the annual fluctuations in number of reported screens and in distribution of hit activities, particularly for the dips in number of reports in 2002, 2004, and 2006. The binned data for the two half-decades, 2000–2004 and 2005–2008, are shown in Figure 7.2. The distribution for 2000–2004, magenta bars in Figure 7.2, is roughly symmetric with a peak at the 1–10 μM bin, while the 2005–2008 distribution, periwinkle bars, peaks at 10–100 μM but has a substantial tail on the more potent, lower IC_{50} side of the graph. Both the shapes of the distributions and the average activities appear to differ between the first and second half of the decade.

Two statistical tests were applied to assess the significance of the apparent differences in distributions and averages between the two half-decades. Differences in distribution were assessed using the χ^2 test for consistency in $2 \times K$ table.[138] The null hypothesis for this test asserts that the histograms in Figure 7.2 reflect samples drawn from two underlying distributions that are identical; a χ^2 value substantially greater than zero would support the visual impression that the two half-decade distributions differ. Expected frequency distributions for the two half-decades were computed according to Equation (7.11):

$$e_{ij} = \frac{N_i n_{ij}}{N_1 + N_2},$$ (7.11)

Table 7.2. Docking-based virtual screens for which experimental results were reported; average IC_{50} values for each half-decade

Time period	Median activity	95% Confidence interval
2000–2004	5 μM	2–20 μM
2005–2008	13 μM	5–20 μM

where i takes on the values 1 and 2 representing each of the half-decades, j ranges from 1 to 4 representing each activity bin in the histogram, n_{ij} is the number of samples for a specific activity bin in a specific half-decade, N_1 is the total number of samples for 2000–2004, and N_2 is the total number of samples for 2005–2008, resulting in e_{ij}, two new distributions in which the observed frequencies in Figure 7.2 have been normalized by the fraction of all reported virtual screens that occurred during each half-decade. The χ^2_3 statistic for three degrees of freedom was computed from these normalized expected frequencies according to Equation (7.12):

$$\chi^2_3 = \sum_{j=1}^{4} \frac{(n_{1j} - e_{1j})^2}{e_{1j}} + \sum_{j=1}^{4} \frac{(n_{2j} - e_{2j})^2}{e_{2j}}.$$ (7.12)

The computed χ^2_3 statistic for the distributions in Figure 7.2 is 7.17, which corresponds to a cumulative probability of 0.93.[139] We can therefore reject the null hypothesis at the $p < 0.07$ significance level and conclude that the underlying distributions likely differ between the periods 2000–2004 and 2005–2008.

For the 2005–2008 period, an increase was seen for the number of hits in both the high-potency "<1 μM" and the poorer potency "10–100 μM" categories. Therefore, although the shapes of the distributions differ, the null hypothesis that average activities for the half-decades are identical remains plausible. Medians were used to examine average activities because medians are robust to experimental errors (a likely issue with data for many different proteins measured in many different labs), robust to outliers such as the three no-hit examples to which a measured activity value could not be assigned, and robust to nonnormal distributions – we have no reason to expect a Gaussian distribution for these data. Median activity values were computed along with the 95% confidence intervals for those averages (Table 7.2). The median activity for the second half-decade was less potent than that for the first half-decade, but there was significant overlap of the range in which the true average probably lies. The Wilcoxon-Mann–Whitney nonparametric rank-order test was therefore used to assess the statistical significance of the differences in average affinity[140]:

$$Z = \frac{|\mu - T| - 0.5}{\sigma},$$ (7.13)

where

$$\mu = \frac{N_1(N_1 + N_2 + 1)}{2}$$

$$\sigma = \sqrt{\frac{N_2\mu}{6}}$$

and T is the smaller sum of ranks in an ordered list of the merged set of activities for the two half-decades. For these census data, $T = 1468$, $N_1 = 32$, $N_2 = 67$, and Z was therefore 0.98. By reference to a normal distribution table, this corresponds to a 68% confidence that the average affinities are different. Note that there were three virtual screens for which the reported high-potency hits were not sufficiently well characterized (vide infra); if these three values are removed, it is 84% likely that the average affinities for 2005–2008 are less potent than for 2000–2004.

Recommendations from census results

In the previous section, we saw that distributions of hit activities differed between the periods 2000–2004 and 2005–2008 and that there was a 68% probability that the average potency decreased for the latter half-decade. One hypothesis that might explain these statistically significant differences is that docking algorithms have gotten worse over the decade; however, the number of hits <10 μM has remained relatively constant across the years, an observation that is more consistent with the hypothesis that docking algorithms as a class have performed at a consistent level across the decade. Although there have almost certainly been modifications and improvements to specific docking algorithms, the census data for prospective virtual screens suggest that those improvements have been incremental at best. A second hypothesis to explain increased average hit IC$_{50}$s is that docking has been applied to harder targets during the second half-decade. Although I have not painstakingly catalogued the target classes in all ninety-nine virtual screens, a quick scan of the specific targets in these screens suggests that differences in target class do not explain differences in average activity. Enzymes are the most represented class of targets, with kinases, proteases, transferases, phosphatases, and so forth having been screened regularly during the years in this survey. If anything, targets were more difficult earlier in the decade, with a few brave (foolhardy?) researchers applying docking to lead identification for ion channels, protein/protein interactions, and even G-protein-coupled receptors (GPCRs). It is also plausible to hypothesize that the pattern of activities, especially in 2007 and 2008, is due to a greater willingness to publish computational studies with less positive results. If so, that would be a valuable practice for the field as it would allow a more accurate assessment of how docking algorithms perform in the real world of prospective screens rather than in retrospective tests. And one final hypothesis must be that docking has become a tool for the unwary; docking programs have gotten easier to use, performance improvements have been made to individual docking programs, more structural

data and larger collections of purchasable compounds have become available, and all of these factors have led to more opportunities for less experienced users to give it a try. No matter what the underlying explanation for differing distributions, a closer examination of the eighteen most potent hits in the census, listed in Table 7.3, suggests strategies that might improve the chances for identifying submicromolar hits from docking-based virtual screens.

To identify docking strategies that might have been conducive to the identification of submicromolar hits, all ninety-eight references were read but the eighteen references in Table 7.3 were examined much more carefully. Of the eighteen virtual screens represented in Table 7.3, the vast majority sought enzyme inhibitors; of the three nonenzyme protein targets, two virtual screens sought competitive binders to the estrogen receptor and the third sought ATP-competitive antagonists of the chaperone Hsp90; none of the eighteen virtual screens targeted the much more challenging ion-channel, protein/protein interaction, or GPCR target classes. Of the enzyme targets in these eighteen virtual screens, the most highly populated classes were kinases (4) or oxidoreductases (3). One might therefore hypothesize that the secret to success would be to carry out a docking-based virtual screen against a protein kinase. Assessing that hypothesis more closely, 22% of the targets in the <1 μM activity bin are kinases; in contrast, 20% of the targets in the combined 1–10 μM and 10–100 μM bins are kinases, while there are no kinases among the nine virtual screens with hits >100 μM. The more likely hypothesis, then, is that a virtual screen of a protein kinase is likely to produce hits with measurable experimental activity, but those hits are as likely to be 10 μM as 10 nM. Instead, exact methodological details of how a virtual screen was run seems a more important factor in success rates for identifying the more potent hits:

- Of the virtual screens in Table 7.3, only four used any variant of the NCI database as a source for searchable compounds, while a higher proportion of screens with less potent hits searched databases from that source. Instead, the virtual screens with submicromolar hits were more likely to search in-house or corporate collections for which care had been taken in choosing the compounds that populate the search database. Given the 2005 publication of the ZINC virtual screening database,[141] there is no longer any reason for even those researchers without access to large corporate collections to not search a carefully chosen and curated database.
- Once a database for searching had been selected, the virtual screeners of Table 7.3 generally prefiltered that database to remove unappealing molecules. In some cases, this filtering was as simple as the removal of reactive or non-drug-like molecules. In other cases, search databases were filtered to remove compounds incompatible with chemical features of the protein binding site – for example, removing anionic compounds before

Table 7.3. Structures and activities for most potent hits

Compound	IC$_{50}$	Target	Compound	IC$_{50}$	Target
1	0.5 nM[a]	CatD[44]	**10**	450 nM[d]	Chk1[55]
2	19 nM	ERβ[53]	**11**	590 nM	AChE[54]
3	40 nM[b]	CK2[49]	**12**	600 nM	hLigI[43]
4	54 nM	ERα[48]	**13**	600 nM	Hsp90[90]
5	80 nM	CK2[57]	**14**	700 nM	HIV RT-1[41]
6	91 nM	Pim-1k[45]	**15**	700 nM	NQO1[51]
7	99 nM[b]	20α-HSD[47]	**16**	820 nM	Cdc25A[42]
8	260 nM	11β-HSD[46]	**17**	900 nM	DHFR[56]
9	400 nM[c]	DNMT1[50]	**18**	924 nM	MTSP1[58]

[a] Data do not preclude interference with FRET assay.
[b] Data do not preclude inhibition due to aggregation.
[c] Estimate based on gel readout for assay.
[d] Structure of 110 nM hit not disclosed.

screening against a binding site with a high proportion of negatively charged amino acids. Moreover, in a few cases, prescreen filtering used more sophisticated pharmacophores or SMARTS patterns to enrich the database in compounds with desired interacting features, for example, features that could provide hydrogen bonds to a kinase hinge region or electrostatic interactions with catalytic residues of an oxidoreductase.

- Before commencing the actual prospective screen, several of the virtual screeners of Table 7.3 carried out validation docking runs. For two of these, the validation involved confirming that the chosen docking protocol could successfully recapitulate the docking mode for a known protein/ligand crystal structure. A larger number of the virtual screeners salted a small number of known actives into the search database and carried out test docking runs; parameters of the docking protocols and score cutoffs for hit selections were fine-tuned to ensure that these known hits were recovered high in the docking hit list.

- Once the prospective screens were completed and potential hit lists compiled, all of the virtual screeners of Table 7.3 used alternative means for winnowing the lists to remove potential false positives. At the very least, in virtual screens across all of the activity bins in Table 7.1, the top docking hits were visually inspected in the protein environment, keeping only those compounds that were predicted to make interesting interactions with the protein. For those screens that produced submicromolar hits, most of the screeners used either alternative scoring strategies (e.g., consensus scoring, quantification of specific desired protein/ligand interactions, removal of compounds with high strain energy), subsequent more computationally intensive virtual screening protocols (e.g., fast rigid docking followed by slower flexible docking, docking followed by energy-based refinement), or some combination of both.

- Not all of the methodological details for these screens were conducive to true success; at least three compounds in Table 7.3 exhibit properties that would warrant orthogonal confirmatory assays to ensure that inhibition was due to the desired mechanism. For example, compound **1** and a close analog were reported as extremely potent inhibitors of the aspartyl proteases cathepsin D and plasmepsin; these acridine-containing compounds were identified by fluorescence resonance energy transfer (FRET) assay.[44] However, no data were provided that would allow assessment of any intrinsic fluorescence of the putative inhibitors nor of any possible interference with the FRET signal, even though acridine itself fluoresces[142] as do substituted versions of acridine such as quinacrine.[143] Compound **3**, ellagic acid, was reported to be a 40 nM, ATP-competitive inhibitor of protein kinase CK2 based on a phosphorylation inhibition assay using ^{33}P-labeled ATP[49]; virtual and experimental screening results were reported for only

this single compound. This same compound has also been reported to be an inhibitor of AmpC β-lactamase under detergent-free assay conditions[94,144]; after further mechanistic characterization, these authors concluded that ellagic acid was a detergent-resistant promiscuous aggregator and that this aggregation behavior was responsible for inhibition in assays of β-lactamase, chymotrypsin, malate dehydrogenase, and cruzain. At a reported IC$_{50}$ of 40 nM, ellagic acid may well be inhibiting through some mechanism other than aggregation, but the data reported[49] do not allow for assessment one way or the other. Finally, compound **7**, diiodosalicylic acid, was reported as a 99 nM inhibitor of 20α-HSD; activities for the related compounds aspirin and salicylic acid were reported to be 21 and 7.8 μM, respectively.[47] All three analogs are known metal chelators,[145,146] and the apparent SAR for inhibition of 20α-HSD is in line with pK_a trends for acetylsalicylic acid, salicylic acid, and diiodosalicylic acid. In the absence of additional data to the contrary, it is therefore equally plausible to hypothesize that either metal-chelate forms of each analog or the pure compounds themselves were responsible for inhibition.

Of course, one might follow absolute best practice for docking-based virtual screening – targeting a well-characterized protein system, searching a database of chemically reasonable molecules, carrying out detailed validation studies, postscoring docking hits at a higher level of theory – and still not be successful in experimentally identifying compounds with submicromolar activity. As a specific case in point, Barriero et al.[136] report virtual screening efforts directed at the identification of novel nonnucleoside inhibitors of HIV-1 reverse transcriptase, a target represented in Table 7.3. These researchers first carried out a similarity search to identify compounds similar to known NNRTIs, and then docked these similarity hits and the known actives into the NNRTI binding site. Docking hits were rescored using molecular mechanics and an implicit solvation model; six of the twenty top-scoring hits were purchased and assayed, but no active compounds resulted from that experimental assay. Visual inspection of the six docking hits gave these researchers some confidence that one of those six hits represented a promising scaffold and that the predicted interactions between protein and putative ligand were favorable for activity. Barriero et al. therefore committed synthetic resource to follow up on that scaffold through synthesis of a small number of analogs that differed in substitution pattern on two phenyl rings. That at-risk gamble based on a gut-instinct assessment of prediction reliability paid off in this particular instance; of the newly synthesized analogs, at least one was a submicromolar anti-HIV agent with an EC$_{50}$ of 310 nM. Although in this particular case the original virtual screen produced no active inhibitors, in general following best practice and carrying out one's screens carefully is likely to at least marginally improve the chances of finding more potent active compounds from docking-based virtual screens.

PREDICTING BOUND POSES WITH DOCKING

In the preceding sections, we have presented a theoretical framework underpinning docking algorithms and have examined the real-world performance of docking as a prospective virtual screening tool. In the pharmaceutical industry, however, it is generally the case that the primary use of docking is predicting the bound pose of a specific molecule to a suitable degree of reliability. One may have a known active compound from a high-throughput screen or ongoing drug discovery effort and want to understand how that compound interacts with the protein target. Or one may have a collection of known actives and want to examine protein/ligand complementarity to rationalize differences in activity or selectivity. Or one might have multiple active series and want to design novel hybrid molecules using the best possible three-dimensional overlay. Or one might have synthesis proposals from medicinal or computational chemists and want to assess the likelihood for maintaining potency or to propose modifications to increase the likelihood of success. In all of these examples, the first steps would be the prediction of a bound pose for one or more molecules and the estimation of the reliability of that prediction.

It is particularly important for successful lead optimization that the computational and medicinal chemists have an understanding of the level of confidence in their docking mode predictions. Is a prediction expected to be accurate enough that I can make design and synthesis decisions at an atomic level of detail? Is the prediction accuracy such that I can draw only general conclusions about types and locations of substitutions on the core scaffold? Or is the confidence level low enough that the prediction can at best provide multiple testable hypotheses, and I should therefore design molecules to probe those hypotheses? Numerous evaluations of the ability to predict docked poses have been published,[24,147] and these evaluations support one general conclusion: Many docking programs can generate poses near the crystal conformation, but no scoring function can consistently score the correct pose at the top of the list. Therefore, in everyday practice, a computational chemist uses a docking program to generate poses for visual inspection and then selects the pose thought to be "best" based on chemical intuition and compatibility with any available SAR data. And in practice we can all point to examples of successful predictions, so it is our instinct that human experience and expertise in combination with computational tools is sufficiently predictive. This assertion, however, has not been validated through analysis of success rates for blind predictions. In this section preliminary results for both manual and automated docking mode predictions from SAMPL-1, a blind prediction challenge, are described.[148] The full results and crystallographic data from SAMPL-1 are not yet public, so the results for automated procedures are not discussed in any detail but instead results for the single manual predictor to the aggregate performance of automated docking procedures.

The SAMPL challenge

The SAMPL challenge was made possible by the generous contribution of two protein/ligand data sets, urokinase plasminogen activator provided by Abbott Laboratories and JNK3 protein kinase provided by Vertex Pharmaceuticals. The challenge proceeded in three phases corresponding to three typical drug discovery activities: (1) identification of active compounds from a background pool of inactive compounds, (2) prediction of the bound poses of active compounds, and (3) rank-ordering of active compounds by affinity. Data for the challenge were released to individual predictors in a correspondingly phased manner: if a predictor requested and received data for phase 2 or 3, that predictor could not subsequently obtain data or make predictions for phase 1. Only the results for phase 2, docking mode prediction, will be discussed here.

Details of the docking mode challenge. The docking mode prediction portion of the challenge also proceeded in phases, an initial "cross-docking" phase followed by a second "self-docking" phase. The cross-docking exercise more closely mimics the real-life situation in drug discovery while the second self-docking exercise allows for assessment of the importance of protein flexibility for successful prediction. Manual docking was applied only to the cross-docking exercise so details for the self-docking exercise are not discussed. For the cross-docking exercise, the SAMPL-1 organizers provided one urokinase and two JNK3 protein structures; the primary difference between the two JNK3 structures was in the side-chain conformation of the "gatekeeper" methionine. None of the three docking structures contained a bound ligand. In addition, during the previous virtual screening portion of the challenge, the organizers had provided two urokinase and two JNK3 structures, each with a ligand bound. SAMPL-1 organizers further provided SD files containing thirty-four compounds for docking to urokinase and sixty-two compounds for docking to JNK3. The small molecule conformations contained in the provided SD files had been generated from 2D representations and so differed from the conformation in any crystal structure. Some inactive compounds were included in those two lists, but the organizers did not reveal which compounds were inactive until after the completion of the full challenge. After the cross-docking challenge closed, SAMPL-1 organizers provided the raw results to me; none of the automated predictors – neither the names of the predictors nor the programs used – were identified in this output. Results were reported as follows:

$$rmsd - DPI; \quad rmsd > DPI$$
$$0; \quad rmsd \leq DPI,$$

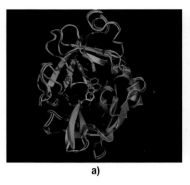
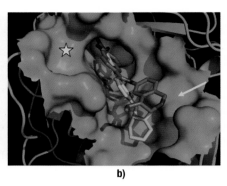

a)   b)

Figure 7.3. (a) Overlay of urokinase crystal structures provided for virtual screening (cyan and magenta ribbons) and cross-docking challenges (green ribbons and surface); **(b)** ligands in crystal structures 1o5c (cyan carbons) and 1owd (magenta carbons) in cross-docking structure.

where rmsd is the root-mean-squared deviation between docked pose and crystallographically identified conformation and DPI is the coordinate precision error of the crystal structure.[149-151] For urokinase twenty-seven of the thirty-four compounds were active and had been crystallized in the protein; for JNK3 fifty-two of the sixty-two compounds were active and had been crystallized in the protein. Results are presented here for only the seventy-nine compounds with protein/ligand crystal structures.

Manual docking process. Although other practitioners might use other specific computational tools at each stage of the process, in broad outline the manual docking protocol used here matches standard practice for supporting a drug discovery team. Before beginning any actual docking, all available structural data were examined closely. For the SAMPL-1 challenge, available data included the four ligand-bound structures from the virtual screening challenge along with the three ligand-free structures provided for the cross-docking exercise; no structural information from the public domain or from in-house drug discovery efforts was sought or used. Structures for each individual protein target were aligned and compared to assess the degree of protein flexibility, to identify protein features likely to be important for interactions with ligands, and to contemplate protonation states and side-chain conformations within the binding site. Before any docking began, 2D representations of the ligands to be docked were also closely examined. The goal here was to divide the ligands into related classes that would be expected to bind similarly, to identify ligand features likely to be important for interactions with the protein, and to identify ligand features – for

example, unusual functional groups, possible tautomers, protonation states – that might cause difficulties or require special treatment during docking.

In preparation for semiautomated docking, 3D conformations for all ligands were generated with OMEGA 2.1.0[152] using default parameters, the standard omega fragment library, and provided SD files as input. To generate a good starting point for docking, Rocs 2.2[153] was used to overlay the omega ligand conformers to each ligand in the ligand-bound protein structures from the virtual screening challenge; overlays were optimized using the Implicit Mills–Dean color force field provided with Rocs, and overlays were ranked using the combo shape-and-color score. All overlays were visually inspected to select one or more starting points for docking and to decide which molecules would need to be built by hand. For JNK3, overlays were visually inspected in the context of the provided protein structures to decide into which structure each ligand should be docked.

Starting from the selected Rocs overlays, the February 2003 version of Flo/qxp[154] was used to explore pose space for each of the ninety-six ligands in the cross-docking challenge. For some of the ligands, the initial overlay was considered sufficiently likely, and the ligand was therefore merely minimized in the binding-site environment. For most of the other ligands, the central scaffold was allowed to minimize and the mcdock algorithm in Flo was used to search conformation space for substituents on that scaffold. For a very few molecules for which no good starting alignment was identified, a full docking run was carried out using mcdock with 1,000 or 2,000 search cycles. And a final few molecules were hand built; the core scaffold was manually placed at a desired location in the protein and conformations explored as substituents were added to that core. For JNK3, constraints were included during docking and minimization to enforce expected interactions between ligands and backbone atoms in the hinge region of the kinase.

The final computational step was to clean the small-molecule conformations for the selected docked pose for each ligand by minimization in MOE. All hydrogen atoms were added to the protein and to each ligand in turn. For JNK3, constraints were imposed on the hinge-binding interactions; for both JNK3 and urokinase, the protein was kept rigid during minimization using the MMFF. In those few cases where it appeared necessary to do so, ligand atoms were held rigid and selected portions of the protein were allowed to minimize or side-chain conformations were optimized using the CHARMM force field.

At the end of this semiautomated, semimanual docking process, a single docked

Figure 7.4. Small molecules from urokinase crystal structures provided for the virtual screening challenge.

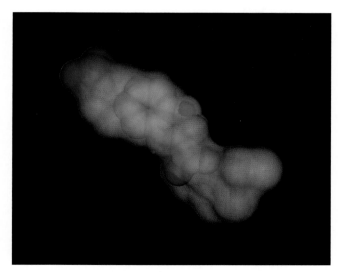

Figure 7.5. Rocs overlay to 1o5c ligand does not place small fragment in S1 binding pocket. Transparent surface with gray carbons represents the molecular shape of the 1o5c ligand; solid surface with green carbons represents the molecular shape of compound uk.1-14.

pose had been selected and refined for each ligand in the urokinase and JNK3 data sets. These final docked poses were collated and shown to a local medicinal chemist who has not worked on urokinase or JNK3 program teams. That medicinal chemist visually inspected each docked pose within the context of the binding site environment and offered comments and critiques of the predicted poses; a limited number of docked poses were further refined based on those comments before submitting the predictions to the SAMPL-1 organizers.

Urokinase plasminogen activator

Urokinase is a serine protease that converts plasminogen to plasmin. I personally have neither worked with nor done computational design for this or any other serine protease, although other members of GSK Computational Chemistry US have supported other serine protease programs. Two public urokinase structures (PDB codes 1o5c and 1owd) were provided as part of the virtual screening challenge and a third structure provided as part of the cross-docking challenge; a sequence- and structure-based overlay of those structures is shown in Figure 7.3. Among the three structures, there was little variation in backbone conformation in the binding-site region [Figure 7.3(a)]; there were small differences in the orientations of some sides chains (not shown), and three residues near the binding pocket were seen in different rotamer states (not shown) – only one of these three was expected to have an appreciable effect on the docking of ligands to the urokinase binding site. Structures 1o5c and 1owd each contained a ligand bound in the protease active site [Figure 7.3(b), 2D structures shown in Figure 7.4]. In both structures the arylamidine arginine mimic binds in the deep S1 pocket, while the bulk of each inhibitor fills the length of the solvent-exposed binding

cavity. The amine in the 1owd interacts with an aspartic acid on the protein surface [indicated by a yellow arrow in Figure 7.3(b)]. In both structures, the subpocket marked by a yellow star in Figure 7.3(b) is not filled by any portion of the ligand. When assessing docked poses for any ligands with branched substituents near the arginine mimic, poses that filled this subpocket were manually selected over those that did not fill this region of the binding site.

All of the urokinase ligands to be docked contained some sort of arginine mimic, generally a guanidine or arylamidine although there were two ligands that contained heteroaryl-amine arginine mimics. Most of the ligands to be docked were large enough to be expected to dock across the entire binding cavity; there were, however, six fragment-sized molecules with molecular weight ≤ 250. The Rocs overlay procedure did not work well for these six molecules, tending to place them in the center of the binding pocket rather than in the S1 pocket (example Rocs overlay shown in Figure 7.5). Docking poses for these six small molecules were generated from a docked pose for a larger molecule containing the relevant S1-binding scaffold; extraneous substituents were removed from the larger docked molecule, and the smaller fragment minimized within the binding site.

For each ligand for which there was a protein/ligand structure, the average rmsd-DPI was computed for all automated predictions; this average is graphed in bold black in Figure 7.6, with 95% confidence intervals shown in dashed black lines; rmsd-DPI values for the manual predictions are shown in bold magenta. The graphed results have been sorted in order of increasing rmsd-DPI for the manual predictions, which has the effect of overemphasizing the manual prediction results; the apparent jaggedness of the automated prediction average is a result of this ordering and has no meaning.

For this serine protease target for which I have no special expertise, the performance for manual and automated predictions is similar. The manual predictions fall inside or

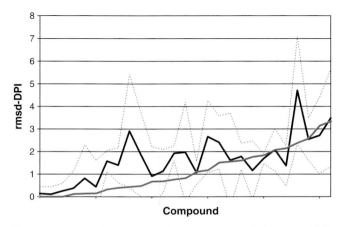

Figure 7.6. Results for urokinase docking mode predictions: rmsd-DPI values for manual predictions are shown in bold magenta; mean rmsd-DPI values for automated predictions are shown in bold black with $\pm 1\sigma$ in dashed black lines.

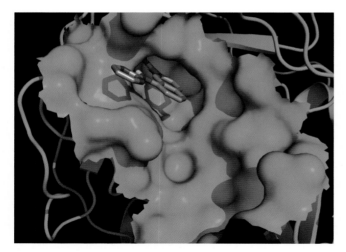

Figure 7.7. Docked pose for compound uk.1-7 fills extra subpocket near S1.

below the 95% confidence interval for all docked ligands, and the manual predictions are at or below the average automated prediction for all but three molecules. Of these three less-well-docked molecules, one was a small, fragmentlike compound with an acylguanidine arginine mimic; none of the larger acylguanidine-containing molecules were particularly well docked so there was no good starting point in the S1 pocket for this small fragment. For the second of the less-well-docked compounds, the predicted pose for the solvent-exposed portion of the molecule is tilted to the left of the binding site when compared to the crystallographically determined poses illustrated in Figure 7.3(b); in this case, a more careful comparison of this docked pose to others in the set of ligands would almost certainly have resulted in a better prediction. The third of the less-well-docked compounds contained a positively charged nitrogen; the lack of electrostatic screening in the Flo/qxp scoring function dominated the bound conformations, resulting in the arginine mimic being pulled slightly out of the S1 pocket. In this instance, I would likely have found a better docked pose if I had not protonated the basic nitrogen when docking using Flo/qxp.

Conversely, there were three molecules for which the manual prediction was better than one σ below the mean automated prediction. One of these three, shown in Figure 7.7, is a branched molecule that fills the extra pocket highlighted in Figure 7.3(b). The final two of the well-docked molecules (uk.1-2 and uk.1-19) are similar to the 1owd ligand, and so the starting conformations generated by Rocs overlay are likely to be close to the correct answers. Strangely, however, the 1owd ligand itself was contained in the set to be docked, but the prediction for that molecule was worse than the predictions for uk.1-2 and uk.1-19. The 1owd ligand also contains a basic nitrogen; it is therefore my expectation that the lack of electrostatic screening in the Flo/qxp scoring function is again the culprit and has again resulted in the arginine mimic being pulled slightly out of the S1 pocket.

JNK3 protein kinase

JNK3 is a serine/threonine protein kinase that phosphorylates Ser63 and Ser73 in the transcriptional activation domain of c-Jun. I personally have not supported a JNK3 drug discovery effort, but I have directly carried out computational design for more than five kinase programs, and members of GSK Computational Chemistry US have supported more than twenty-five kinase programs. I therefore have a substantial amount of kinase drug discovery experience and have closely examined hundreds if not thousands of kinase-ligand crystal structures and docking models.

Two public JNK3 structures (PDB codes 1jnk and 1pmq) were provided as part of the virtual screening challenge and an additional two structures provided as part of the cross-docking challenge. A sequence- and structure-based alignment of the four structures is shown in Figure 7.8(a); the structures were aligned to emphasize the overlay of backbone atoms for the hinge residues, the catalytic lysine, and the DFG motif. As would be expected for most kinases, there was a substantial amount of variation in backbone conformation among the four structures. The activation loop in particular exhibited a wide conformational variance; for the virtual screening structures the activation loop packed against the glycine-rich loop and closed off the right side of the ATP binding site, while for the cross-docking structures there was missing density and therefore an undefined conformation of the activation loop. The glycine-rich loop itself exhibited a span of conformations; in the virtual screening structures these two beta strands were lifted away from the ATP binding site relative to the cross-docking structures. Structures 1jnk and 1pmq each contained a ligand bound in the ATP binding site [Figure 7.8(b), 2D structures shown in Figure 7.9]. Both the nonhydrolyzable ATP mimetic AMPPNP of 1jnk and the aminopyrimidine of 1pmq fill the binding site and make hydrogen bonds

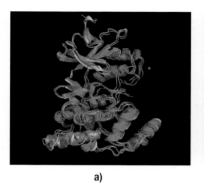
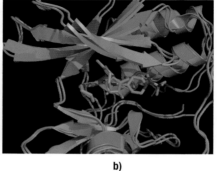

a)   b)

Figure 7.8. (a) Overlay of JNK3 crystal structures provided for virtual screening (in green and cyan) and cross-docking challenges (in magenta and yellow); **(b)** ligands from structures 1jnk (green carbons) and 1pmq (cyan carbons) in cognate crystal structures.

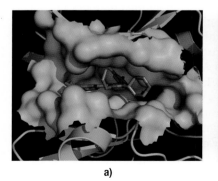

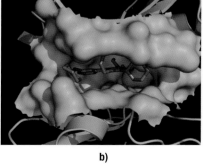

Figure 7.9. Ligands in structures.

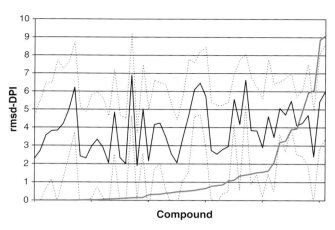

Figure 7.11. Results for JNK3 docking mode predictions: rmsd-DPI values for manual predictions are shown in bold magenta; mean rmsd-DPI values for automated predictions are shown in bold black with ±1σ in dashed black lines.

to the hinge backbone atoms. Structure 1pmq also contains a molecule of AMPPNP in a ternary complex with JNK3 and the aminopyrimidine inhibitor; this location of the AMPPNP was likely an artifact of crystallization so it was ignored during structural analysis and Rocs overlay of JNK3 inhibitors.

Two structures were provided for the cross-docking challenge. I was particularly happy to see that the SAMPL-1 organizers had provided one structure with an open "back pocket" [Figure 7.10(a)] and one with a closed back pocket [Figure 7.10(b)]; in these figures the ligand from structure 1pmq is shown in the binding-site cavity for reference. Rotamer differences in the methionine gatekeeper residue along with other conformational differences near the binding pocket resulted in a well-defined subpocket on the back face of the ATP binding site. As seen in Figure 7.10(a), the *m,p*-dichlorophenyl group of the 1pmq and related ligands filled this open back pocket, while there was no room in the closed-pocket structure to accommodate this functional group. During the generation of docked poses, therefore, I chose the protein structures into which to dock based on the presence or absence of groups expected to access the open back pocket.

The set of ligands to be docked encompassed at least seven distinct compound classes, with an additional few singleton compounds that did not fit into any of these classes. Most of the compounds contained features that would be expected to interact with backbone atoms in the hinge region of JNK3, and a large number of compounds contained aryl substituents that I expected would bind

in the open-pocket structure. Potential starting conformations were generated by Rocs overlay to the AMPPNP of 1jnk and the aminopyrimidine of 1pmq. None of the overlays to AMPPNP produced starting points for docking that made sense in the context of the ATP binding-site environment; therefore, for all but the hand-built molecules, the starting point for docking was selected from the 1pmq overlay.

The prediction results for all compounds with a crystal structure are shown in Figure 7.11; the mean rmsd-DPI values for automated predictions are again graphed in bold black with 95% confidence intervals shown in dashed black lines; rmsd-DPI values for the manual predictions are shown in bold magenta. For this protein target class for which I have a substantial amount of experience, almost all of the manual predictions are better than the average automated predictions. The manual predictions are often well below the 95% confidence interval for the automated predictions, with only three manual predictions above the mean plus one σ boundary.

Aminopyrimidines were by far the largest class of JNK3 inhibitors, encompassing thirty of the sixty-two to be docked; twenty-five of the thirty aminopyrimidines can be described by the reference structures shown in Figure 7.12, while the other five examples were singletons incorporating different nitrogen-containing five-membered or six-membered aromatic rings at the pyrimidine 4-position. There was a strong similarity between this compound class and the 1pmq ligand; the Rocs overlay was therefore expected to generate good starting points for the core scaffold. All but one of the thirty aminopyrimidines contained an aromatic back-pocket binder so the open-pocket structure was used for these twenty-nine docking calculations; the one outlier had a methyl group in this region of the

Figure 7.10. JNK3 structures for cross-docking challenge. **(a)** Structure with open "back pocket." **(b)** Structure with closed "back pocket"; ligand from structure 1PMQ included for reference.

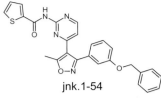

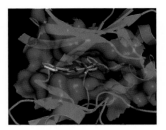

Figure 7.12. Aminopyrimidine class of JNK3 inhibitors.

Figure 7.14. Manual docking mode prediction for compound jnk.1-54.

ligand structure and was therefore docked into the closed-pocket structure. The primary computational effort for this compound class was in optimizing the orientation of the R1 substituent at the solvent front of the binding pocket. The mcdock algorithm in Flo/qxp was used to extensively search R1 conformational space, with simultaneous searching for R2 substituents larger than ethyl; the aminopyrimidine core was allowed to minimize during each search cycle. An Asn side chain with multiple rotameric states is located near where R1 and R2 bind; this side chain was accordingly left flexible during docking calculations, and careful attention was paid to the side-chain conformation when selecting docked poses.

The subset of results for this compound class are shown in Figure 7.13; in addition to the manual and mean automated rmsd-DPI values, the best automated prediction is graphed in bold cyan. For this compound class, the best automated predictor was E220, although no information is available concerning what program was used by that predictor. For the aminopyrimidines, the manual predictions are always better than mean automated prediction, but this specific predictor did very well, with only four blips where the automated prediction was worse than the manual. One of those blips in particular is worth commenting on. For compound jnk.1-54, the back-pocket binder can extend even further than the dichlorophenyl of 1pmq; because I

built this substituent conformation by hand it was relatively easy to thread the flexible R group into and beyond the back pocket (Figure 7.14), while an automated procedure must search conformational space sufficiently well to explore the necessary substituent conformation.

A second class of molecules bore a striking resemblance to SB-203580 (Figure 7.15). SB-203580 is a p38 inhibitor synthesized by the first chemistry team with which I worked after joining SmithKline Beecham (SB) in 1997. The protein/ligand structure of this compound in p38 was solved in 1997[155]; being one of the early kinase/ligand complexes solved, this structure was much discussed during my first years at SB. Therefore, even though I did not go out of my way to look up the exact bound conformation of compounds like SB-203580, I have known for more than a decade how these compounds sit in the ATP binding site of a protein kinase, and it would be reprehensible for me to not be able to generate a good prediction. My docking models for jnk.1-7, jnk.1-14, and jnk.1-48 were generated by constrained docking of the pyridine core followed by building of the rest of the molecule by hand, placing the fluorophenyl group into the back pocket.

The subset of results for these three predictions are shown in Figure 7.16. Two automated predictors (E252 and E302) did extraordinarily well, with equivalent predictions that were within the coordinate precision error of the crystal structures. Although there is again no identifying information concerning who these predictors were or what program they used for docking, it is the case that p38 inhibitors were included in the training sets for several popular docking programs. It is therefore reasonable to wonder whether these predictors used one of those programs for which SB-203580 was part of the training set on which docking parameters and algorithmic details were optimized.

The oximes, Figure 7.17, were the second largest class in this data set, with nine of the sixty-two to be docked. Neither the Rocs overlay nor a 1,000-cycle Flo/qxp docking search was able to identify a credible docking pose for even the smallest of these molecules, so the scaffold for this class was manually docked and substituents for the nine molecules were built by hand. Manual docking began by first examining the small-molecule crystal structure of a compound containing the oxime core (CCDC code EOISOX, Figure 7.17) to check my assumptions about small-molecule geometries. I assumed that the oxime OH donated a hydrogen bond to a hinge backbone carbonyl while one or

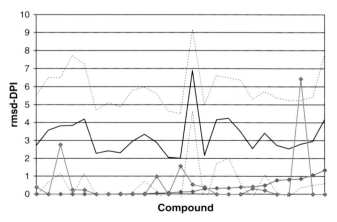

Figure 7.13. Results for aminopyrimidine docking mode predictions: rmsd-DPI values for manual predictions are shown in bold magenta; mean rmsd-DPI values for automated predictions are shown in bold black with $\pm 1\sigma$ in dashed black lines; the best overall automated prediction for this class (predictor E220) is shown in bold cyan.

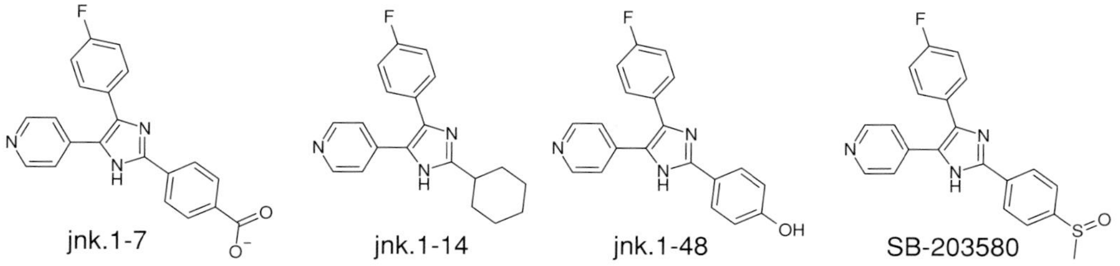

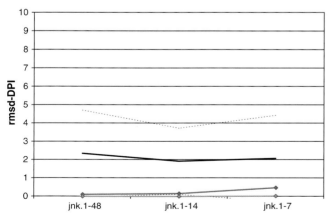

Figure 7.15. Pyrimidinyl-imidazole class of JNK3 inhibitors; the structure of SB-203580 is shown for reference.

both of the oxime nitrogen and carbonyl oxygen accepted a hydrogen bond from a hinge backbone NH. I therefore imposed constraints in Flo/qxp to force these hydrogen bond interactions and then carried out multiple rounds of short docking searches and minimizations to force the oxime core into a docked orientation that matched my prejudices and that allowed me to build the benzodioxin substituent at the solvent front of the binding pocket. Most of the oxime compounds were built into the closed-pocket structure; compounds jnk.1-13, jnk.1-16, and jnk.1-53 were docked into the open-pocket structure.

The docked conformation of the oxime core made good interactions with the hinge [Figure 7.18(a)], and there was an extremely appealing shape complementarity between the benzodioxin and the protein surface [Figure 7.18(b)]. For the full oxime set, all of the cores were well placed; compounds jnk.1-46 and jnk.1-62 made favorable interactions with the catalytic lysine or the backbone of the glycine-rich loop, the long substituent of jnk.1-53 threaded through the back pocket in a manner similar to the predicted pose for jnk.1-54, and the resident medicinal chemist agreed completely with my predicted orientation of the oxime scaffold. I therefore felt quite confident in my predictions for all nine of the molecules in this class.

The subset of results for these oxime predictions are shown in Figure 7.19; the best overall automated prediction (E219) is shown in bold cyan. All of the manual predictions were substantially better than the performance of any automated predictor; this is an example where, given a good prediction for the scaffold, manual building of substituents presents large benefits over an automated docking procedure that has to start from outside the binding pocket for every prediction. The rmsd-DPI values for the manual predictions are less good for jnk.1-46 and jnk.1-62, longer molecules with polar substituents; the falloff in prediction accuracy may have been due both to the lack of electrostatic screening in Flo/qxp and to magnification along the molecule of small errors in scaffold placement.

The four molecules for which manual predictions were particularly atrocious all contained a pyrazole core (Figure 7.20). The subset of results for these oxime predictions is shown in Figure 7.21; the best automated prediction (E218) is shown in bold cyan. All of the manual predictions are above the 95% confidence interval for automated predictions; in comparison, automated predictor E218 did well across all four molecules, with two of those predictions at or near the coordinate precision of the crystal structures.

Manual docking proceeded by placing the pyrazole core in the binding site and applying constraints to enforce hydrogen bonding interactions with the hinge (Figure 7.22). After the cross-docking challenge was over and preliminary results released, I compared the docked pose of the pyrazole core to the crystallographically determined location of that core; there was a good overlap of the pyrazole core in this initial placement and in the crystal structure. Starting from this pyrazole placement, substituents were manually built off the core based on my assumptions on how the compounds would interact with the protein; those assumptions were formed from years of closely examining kinase/ligand protein structures. For compound jnk.1-57, I reasoned by analogy to the aminopyrimidines and assumed that the phenyl group would dock into the open back pocket and that the nitrile nitrogen would interact with the side chain of the catalytic lysine. For compounds jnk.1-47 and jnk.1-61, I assumed that the amide carbonyl would interact with the catalytic lysine and that the pendant benzyl substituent would curl back up to tuck into the inward face of the glycine-rich loop.

Figure 7.16. Results for pyridine docking mode predictions: rmsd-DPI values for manual predictions are shown in bold magenta; mean rmsd-DPI values for automated predictions are shown in bold black with ±1σ in dashed black lines; the best overall automated prediction for this class (predictors E252 and E302) is shown in bold cyan.

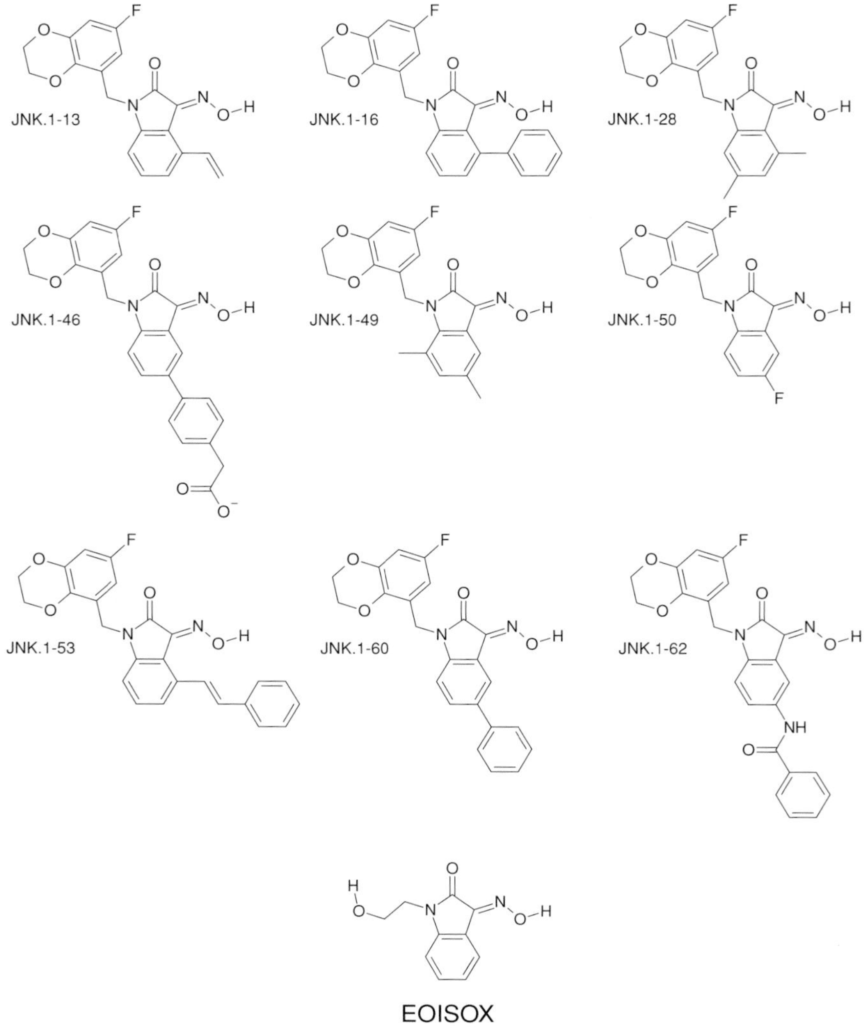

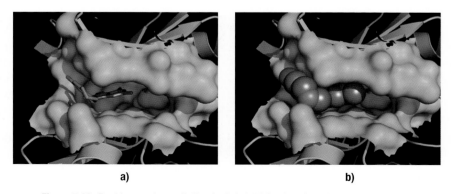

Figure 7.17. Oxime class of JNK3 inhibitors; EOISOX is shown for a reference.

If I had been docking into ERK kinase, this would have been a good but not perfect prediction [Figure 7.23(a)]; some details of the docking mode needed to be refined more carefully, but there was a reasonable correspondence of the intended docking features to what is seen in a public

ERK structure. However, the cross-docking challenge was for JNK3, and in that protein this class of compounds interacts with the hinge through the alternative tautomer of the pyrazole core. The molecule is flipped relative to the orientation in ERK [Figure 7.23(b)], the fluorophenyl interacts

Figure 7.18. Docking mode prediction for jnk.1-28 in closed-pocket JNK3 structure.

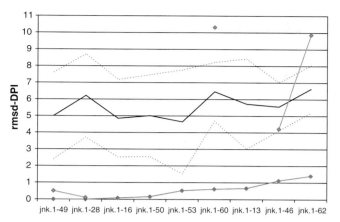

Figure 7.19. Results for oxime docking mode predictions: rmsd-DPI values for manual predictions are shown in bold magenta; mean rmsd-DPI values for automated predictions are shown in bold black with ±1σ in dashed black lines; the best overall automated prediction for this class – predictor E219 – is shown in bold cyan.

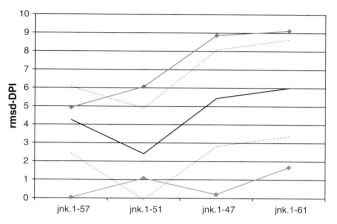

Figure 7.21. Results for pyrazole docking mode predictions: rmsd-DPI values for manual predictions are shown in bold magenta; mean rmsd-DPI values for automated predictions are shown in bold black with ±1σ in dashed black lines; the best overall automated prediction for this class – predictor E219 – is shown in bold cyan.

with the catalytic lysine, and the benzyl group packs up against the protein surface along a solvent-exposed edge of the binding site. The comparison to an ERK protein/ligand crystal structure affirms that the prediction was not unreasonable; I would not have a priori selected a docked pose in which the benzyl group was not buried in the binding site without substantial SAR information that ruled out the pose predicted manually for compounds jnk.1-47 and jnk.1-61.

Comments concerning manual versus automated binding mode prediction

The work described here compared a single manual docking strategy to multiple automated methods, all applied to the blind prediction of binding modes for inhibitors of urokinase plasminogen activator and JNK3 protein kinase. I do not claim for myself any special ability in docking small molecules into proteins; I would expect that any experienced computational chemist would be equally likely to

generate predictions as good as or better than the results presented here. In this particular blind study, the best overall manual prediction success was seen for the protein kinase target class with which I have a substantial amount of experience, while my prediction success rate was comparable only with that of the automated predictions for the serine protease system with which I have only limited experience. I therefore would contend that the results for the SAMPL-1 cross-docking challenge support a hypothesis that expertise in combination with standard docking technologies leads to generally successful prediction rates. One might therefore suggest that mimicking features of the manual process might improve the predictiveness of automated methods, and indeed, one such docking methodology has been previously described in which docked poses for kinase inhibitors are generated by overlaying related scaffolds onto known ligand poses from kinase/ligand crystal structures.[156] Such an automated technique is likely to be generally predictive, particularly for protein targets

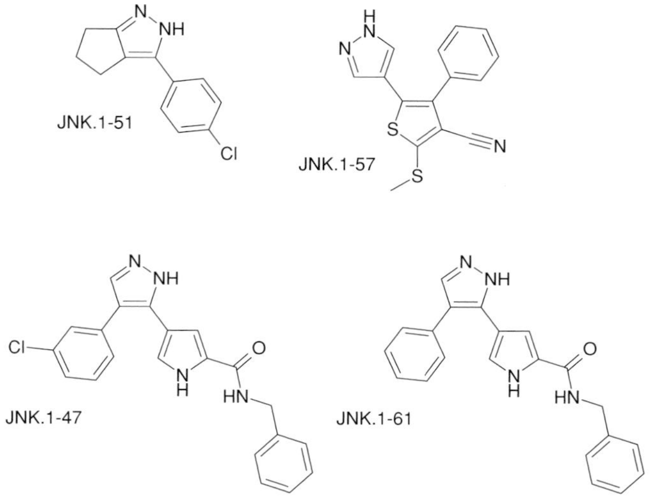

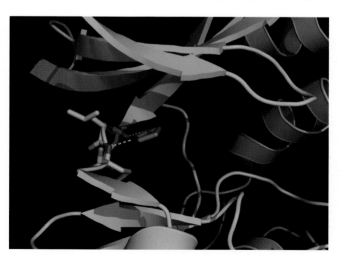

Figure 7.20. Pyrazole class of JNK3 inhibitors.

Figure 7.22. Docking mode prediction for pyrazole core.

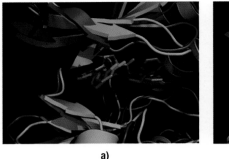 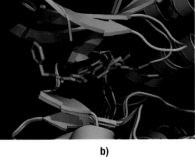

a)   b)

Figure 7.23. Docking mode prediction for jnk.1-47 in open-pocket JNK3 structure. **(a)** Comparison to ERK crystal structure for this molecule; **(b)** comparison to JNK3 crystal structure. In both comparisons the carbons of the predicted pose are colored gray.

where inhibitors make specific conserved interactions with binding site residues; it is not known whether a scaffold-matching automated procedure was one of the automated techniques used here, so it is not possible to comment on the performance of such an algorithm in blind prediction. However, the docking results for the pyrazole class of compounds highlight an important caveat for automated methods that rely heavily on known crystal structures; if one had had only a single crystal example for either ERK or JNK3, in this case one might have been led astray when predicting a bound pose in the other protein kinase. For short-term progress in docking mode prediction, a scaffold-matching or similar automated approach is consistent with standard manual docking practices and is likely to prove pragmatically useful but is not likely to be the complete answer for long-term progress in improving our understanding of the physical basis for docking of small molecules to protein binding sites.

A FEW FINAL REMARKS

In this domesday report on docking, we have explored the connection between docking and a theory of noncovalent association, have carried out a rather detailed census of docking-based virtual screens during this decade, and have examined the relative performance of manual and automated procedures for blind prediction of protein-bound ligand poses. The news from this report is not all doom and gloom; there clearly have been virtual screens that identified compounds with micromolar and better activity, and both manual and automated predictors were able to identify docked poses correctly enough to support decision-making in the optimization of lead compounds. The reality is that docking is an integral part of structure-based design when used with care and pragmatism but is also not a "black-box" technology with well-characterized error bars around docking predictions; successful use of docking technology requires human intervention based on experience and expertise.

To move forward, we need a strategy that allows us to incorporate parts of the underlying theory that are currently missing in a manner that also allows us to test how each new theoretical or algorithmic modification affects success, validating technologies both retrospectively and prospectively. Some of the features plausibly missing from current docking algorithms relate to questions such as: We assume that a single conformation predominates in the docking of a molecule to a protein binding site; is this indeed a good approximation? If not, how might we include additional conformations, protonation states, tautomer forms, and so on? We generally neglect the entropic cost for localizing a ligand into a protein binding site or at best treat such effects with back-of-the-envelope estimates; how can we do better? We hope that the scoring functions used in docking recapitulate physical reality; what changes are required to our scoring functions and force fields so that our calculations are more predictive? As we seek to address these and related questions, algorithmic progress is likely to require access to even more data sets such as those provided by Abbott and Vertex for the SAMPL-1 challenge. We are therefore encouraged by the recent announcement of the awarding of a grant for the Community Structure-Activity Resource[157]; this government/academic/industrial partnership will over time provide access to sufficient amounts of data that will both enable us to assess prediction error bars for current docking technologies and underpin new methodological developments.

ACKNOWLEDGMENTS

I thank the members of the Computational Chemistry US group at GSK for on going helpful discussions about this manuscript and many other topics; CC US is a collection of extraordinary scientists from whom I learn something new every day. I also thank Christopher Bayly, Ajay Jain, Anthony Nicholls, Carleton Sage, and Michael Shirts for useful conversations during the writing of this chapter. I thank Dennis Yamashita for critically assessing my docking mode predictions for the SAMPL-1 challenge. I especially thank Geoff Skillman of OpenEye Scientific for organizing and running SAMPL-1; these kinds of blind challenges are extraordinarily useful but require a huge amount of work and effort for the organizers. I am particularly grateful to Geoff for providing me with raw results from the cross-docking exercise and for incredibly useful discussions about the performance of various predictors.

REFERENCES

1. http://www.nationalarchives.gov.uk/domesday/.
2. Kontoyianni, M.; Madhav, P.; Suchanek, E.; Seibel, W. Theoretical and practical considerations in virtual screening: a beaten field? *Curr. Med. Chem.* **2008,** *15,* 107–116.

3. Cavasotto, C. N.; Orry, A. J. W. Ligand docking and structure-based virtual screening in drug discovery. *Curr. Top. Med. Chem.* **2007**, *7*, 1006–1014.

4. Zhong, S.; Macias, A. T.; MacKerell, A. D., Jr. Computational identification of inhibitors of protein-protein interactions. *Curr. Top. Med. Chem.* **2007**, *7*, 63–82.

5. Sousa, S. F.; Fernandes, P. A.; Ramos, M. J. Protein-ligand docking: current status and future challenges. *Proteins* **2006**, *65*, 15–26.

6. Rester, U. Dock around the clock: current status of small molecule docking and scoring. *QSAR Comb. Sci.* **2006**, *25*, 605–615.

7. Coupez, B.; Lewis, R. A. Docking and scoring: theoretically easy, practically impossible? *Curr. Med. Chem.* **2006**, *13*, 2995–3003.

8. Mohan, V.; Gibbs, A. C.; Cummings, M. D.; Jaeger, E. P.; DesJarlais, R. L. Docking: successes and challenges. *Curr. Pharm. Des.* **2005**, *11*, 323–333.

9. Schulz-Gasch, T.; Stahl, M. Scoring functions for protein-ligand interactions: a critical perspective. *Drug Disc. Today* **2004**, *1*, 231–239.

10. Kitchen, D. B.; Decornez, H.; Furr, J. R.; Bajorath, J. Docking and scoring in virtual screening for drug discovery: methods and applications. *Nat. Rev. Drug Discov.* **2004**, *3*, 935–949.

11. Alvarez, J. C. High-throughput docking as a source of novel drug leads. *Curr. Opin. Chem. Biol.* **2004**, *8*, 365–370.

12. Muegge, I.; Enyedy, I. J. Virtual screening for kinase targets. *Curr. Med. Chem.* **2004**, *11*, 693–707.

13. Brooijmans, N.; Kuntz, I. D. Molecular recognition and docking algorithms. *Annu. Rev. Biophys. Biomol. Struct.* **2003**, 335–373.

14. Glen, R. C.; Allen, S. C. Ligand-protein docking: cancer research at the interface between biology and chemistry. *Curr. Med. Chem.* **2003**, *10*, 763–777.

15. Taylor, R. D.; Jewsbury, P. J.; Essex, J. W. A review of protein-small molecule docking methods. *J. Comput. Aided Mol. Des.* **2002**, *16*, 151–166.

16. Lyne, P. D. Structure-based virtual screening: an overview. *Drug Disc. Today* **2002**, *7*, 1047–1055.

17. Shoichet, B. K.; McGovern, S. L.; Wei, B.; Irwin, J. J. Lead discovery using molecular docking. *Curr. Opin. Chem. Biol.* **2002**, *6*, 439–446.

18. Halperin, I.; Ma, B.; Wolfson, H.; Nussinov, R. Principles of docking: an overview of search algorithms and a guide to scoring functions. *Proteins* **2002**, *47*, 409–443.

19. Schneider, G.; Bohm, H. J. Virtual screening and fast automated docking methods. *Drug Disc. Today* **2002**, *7*, 64–70.

20. Abagyan, R.; Totrov, M. High-throughput docking for lead generation. *Curr. Opin. Chem. Biol.* **2001**, *5*, 375–382.

21. Sheridan, R. P.; McGaughey, G. B.; Cornell, W. D. Multiple protein structures and multiple ligands: effects on the apparent goodness of virtual screening results. *J. Comput. Aided Mol. Des.* **2008**, *22*, 257–265.

22. McGaughey, G. B.; Sheridan, R. P.; Bayly, C. I.; Culberson, J. C.; Kreatsoulas, C.; Lindsley, S.; Maiorov, V.; Truchon, J. F.; Cornell, W. D. Comparison of topological, shape, and docking methods in virtual screening. *J. Chem. Inf. Model.* **2007**, *47*, 1504–1519.

23. Cornell, W. D. Recent evaluations of high throughput docking methods for pharmaceutical lead finding: consensus and caveats. *Annu. Rep. Comp. Chem.* **2006**, *2*, 297–323.

24. Warren, G. L.; Andrews, C. W.; Capelli, A. M.; Clarke, B.; LaLonde, J.; Lambert, M. H.; Lindvall, M.; Nevins, N.; Semus, S. F.; Senger, S.; Tedesco, G.; Wall, I. D.; Woolven, J. M.; Peishoff, C. E.; Head, M. S. A critical assessment of docking programs and scoring functions. *J. Med. Chem.* **2006**, *49*, 5912–5931.

25. Cummings, M. D.; DesJarlais, R. L.; Gibbs, A. C.; Mohan, V.; Jaeger, E. P. Comparison of automated docking programs as virtual screening tools. *J. Med. Chem.* **2005**, *48*, 962–976.

26. Perola, E.; Walters, W. P.; Charifson, P. S. A detailed comparison of current docking and scoring methods on systems of pharmaceutical relevance. *Proteins* **2004**, *56*, 235–249.

27. Gilson, M. K.; Given, J. A.; Bush, B. L.; McCammon, J. A. The statistical-thermodynamic basis for computation of binding affinities: a critical review. *Biophys. J.* **1997**, *72*, 1047–1069.

28. Shirts, M. R.; Mobley, D. L.; Brown, S. P. Free energy calculations. In: *Structure-Based Drug Design*, Merz, K. M.; Ringe, D.; Reynolds, C. H., Eds. **2008**, in press.

29. Chang, C. E.; Potter, M. J.; Gilson, M. K. Calculation of molecular configuration integrals. *J. Phys. Chem. B* **2003**, *107*, 1048–1055.

30. Kolossváry, I. Evaluation of the molecular configuration integral in all degrees of freedom for the direct calculation of conformational free energies: prediction of the anomeric free energy of monosaccharides. *J. Phys. Chem. A* **1997**, *101*(51), 9900–9905.

31. Head, M. S.; Given, J. A.; Gilson, M. K. Mining minima: direct computation of conformational free energy. *J. Phys. Chem. A* **1997**, *101*, 1609–1618.

32. Chang, C.-E.; Chen, W.; Gilson, M. K. Ligand configurational entropy and protein binding. *Proc. Natl. Acad. Sci. U.S.A.* **2007**, *104*, 1534–1539.

33. Kim, R.; Skolnick, J. Assessment of programs for ligand binding affinity prediction. *J. Comp. Chem.* **2008**, *29*, 1316–1331.

34. Manetti, F.; Falchi, F.; Crespan, E.; Schenone, S.; Maga, G.; Botta, M. *N*-(thiazol-2-yl)-2-thiophene carboxamide derivatives as Abl inhibitors identified by a pharmacophore-based database screening of commercially available compounds. *Bioorg. Med. Chem. Lett.* **2008**, *18*, 4328–4331.

35. Olsen, L.; Pettersson, I.; Hemmingsen, L.; Adolph, H.-W.; Jørgensen, F. S. Docking and scoring of metallo-β-lactamase inhibitors. *J. Comput. Aided Mol. Des.* **2004**, *18*, 287–302.

36. Holloway, M. K.; Wai, J. M.; Halgren, T. A.; Fitzgerald, P. M. D.; Vacca, J. P.; Dorsey, B. D.; Levin, R. B.; Thompson, W. J.; Chen, J.; deSolms, J.; Gaffin, N.; Ghosh, A. K.; Giuliani, E. A.; Graham, S. L.; Guare, J. P.; Hungate, R. W.; Lyle, T. A.; Sanders, W. M.; Tucker, T. J.; Wiggins, M.; Wiscount, C. M.; Woltersdorf, O. W.; Young, S. D.; Darke, P. L.; Zugay, J. A. *A priori* prediction of activity for HIV-1 protease inhibitors employing energy minimization in the active site. *J. Med. Chem.* **1995**, *38*, 305–317.

37. http://www.rcsb.org/pdb/.

38. http://www.cas.org/products/scifindr/index.html.

39. http://www.ncbi.nlm.nih.gov/sites/entrez?db=pubmed.

40. http://scholar.google.com/.

41. Herschhorn, A.; Hizi, A. Virtual screening, identification, and biochemical characterization of novel inhibitors of the reverse transcriptase of human immunodeficiency virus type-1. *J. Med. Chem.* **2008**, *51*, 5702–5713.

42. Park, H.; Bahn, Y. J.; Jung, S. K.; Jeong, D. G.; Lee, S.-H.; Seo, I.; Yoon, T.-S.; Kim, S. J.; Ryu, S. E. Discovery of novel Cdc25 phosphatase inhibitors with micromolar activity based on the structure-based virtual screening. *J. Med. Chem.* **2008**, *51*, 5533–5541.

43. Zhong, S.; Chen, X.; Zhu, X.; Dziegielewska, B.; Bachman, K. E.; Ellenberger, T.; Ballin, J. D.; Wilson, G. M.; Tomkinson, A. E.; MacKerell, A. D., Jr. Identification and validation of human DNA ligase inhibitors using computer-aided drug design. *J. Med. Chem.* **2008**, *51*, 4553–4562.

44. Azim, M. K.; Ahmed, W.; Khan, I. A.; Rao, N. A.; Khan, K. M. Identification of acridinyl hydrazides as potent aspartic protease inhibitors. *Bioorg. Med. Chem. Lett.* **2008**, *18*, 3011–3015.

45. Pierce, A. C.; Jacobs, M.; Stuver-Moody, C. Docking study yields four novel inhibitors of the protooncogene Pim-1 kinase. *J. Med. Chem.* **2008**, *51*, 1972–1975.

46. Yang, H.; Dou, W.; Lou, J.; Leng, Y.; Shen, J. Discovery of novel inhibitors of 11β-hydroxysteroid dehydrogenase type 1 by docking and pharmacophore modeling. *Bioorg. Med. Chem. Lett.* **2008**, *18*, 1340–1345.

47. Dhagat, U.; Carbone, V.; Chung, R. P.-T.; Matsunaga, T.; Endo, S.; Hara, A.; El-Kabbani, O. A salicylic acid-based analogue discovered from virtual screening as a potent inhibitor of human 20α-hydroxysteroid dehydrogenase. *Med. Chem.* **2007**, *3*, 546–550.

48. Knox, A. J. S.; Meegan, M. J.; Sobolev, V.; Frost, D.; Zisterer, D. M.; Williams, D. C.; Lloyd, D. G. Target specific virtual screening: optimization of an estrogen receptor screening platform. *J. Med. Chem.* **2007**, *50*, 5301–5310.

49. Cozza, G.; Bonvini, P.; Zorzi, E.; Poletto, G.; Pagano, M. A.; Sarno, S.; Donella-Deana, A.; Zagotto, G.; Rosolen, A.; Pinna, L. A.; Meggio, F.; Moro, S. Identification of ellagic acid as potent inhibitor of protein kinase CK2: a successful example of a virtual screening application. *J. Med. Chem.* **2006**, *49*, 2363–2366.

50. Siedlecki, P.; Garcia Boy, R.; Musch, T.; Brueckner, B.; Suhai, S.; Lyko, F.; Zielenkiewicz, P. Discovery of two novel, small-molecule inhibitors of DNA methylation. *J. Med. Chem.* **2006**, *49*, 678–683.

51. Nolan, K. A.; Timson, D. J.; Stratford, I. J.; Bryce, R. A. In silico identification and biochemical characterization of novel inhibitors of NQO1. *Bioorg. Med. Chem. Lett.* **2006**, *16*, 6246–6254.

52. Barril, X.; Brough, P.; Drysdale, M.; Hubbard, R. E.; Massey, A.; Surgenor, A.; Wright, L. Structure-based discovery of a new class of Hsp90 inhibitors. *Bioorg. Med. Chem. Lett.* **2005**, *15*, 5187–5191.

53. Zhao, L.; Brinton, R. D. Structure-based virtual screening for plant-based ERβ-selective ligands as potential preventative therapy against age-related neurodegenerative diseases. *J. Med. Chem.* **2005**, *48*, 3463–3466.

54. Mizutani, M. Y.; Itai, A. Efficient method for high-throughput virtual screening based on flexible docking: discovery of novel acetylcholinesterase inhibitors. *J. Med. Chem.* **2004**, *47*, 4818–4828.

55. Lyne, P. D.; Kenny, P. W.; Cosgrove, D. A.; Deng, C.; Zabludoff, S.; Wendoloski, J. J.; Ashwell, S. Identification of compounds with nanomolar binding affinity for checkpoint kinase-1 using knowledge-based virtual screening. *J. Med. Chem.* **2004**, *47*, 1962–1968.

56. Rastelli, G.; Pacchioni, S.; Sirawaraporn, W.; Sirawaraporn, R.; Parenti, M. D.; Ferrari, A. M. Docking and database screening reveal new classes of *Plasmodium falciparum* dihydrofolate reductase inhibitors. *J. Med. Chem.* **2003**, *46*, 2834–2845.

57. Vangrevelinghe, E.; Zimmermann, K.; Schoepfer, J.; Portmann, R.; Fabbro, D.; Furet, P. Discovery of a potent and selective protein kinase CK2 inhibitor by high-throughput docking. *J. Med. Chem.* **2003**, *46*, 2656–2662.

58. Enyedy, I. J.; Lee, S.-L.; Kuo, A. H.; Dickson, R. B.; Lin, C.-L.; Wang, S. Structure-based approach for the discovery of bis-benzamidines as novel inhibitors of matriptase. *J. Med. Chem.* **2001**, *44*, 1349–1355.

59. Park, H.; Bahn, Y. J.; Jeong, D. G.; Woob, E. J.; Kwon, J. S.; Ryu, S. E. Identification of novel inhibitors of extracellular signal-regulated kinase 2 based on the structure-based virtual screening. *Bioorg. Med. Chem. Lett.* **2008**, *18*, 5372–5376.

60. Identification of BRAF inhibitors through in silico screening. *J. Med. Chem.* **2008**, *51*, 6121–6127.

61. Schlicker, C.; Rauch, A.; Hess, K. C.; Kachholz, B.; Levin, L. R.; Buck, J.; Steegborn, C. Structure-based development of novel adenylyl cyclase inhibitors. *J. Med. Chem.* **2008**, *51*, 4456–4464.

62. Park, H.; Jung, S.-K.; Jeong, D. G.; Ryu, S. E.; Kim, S. J. Discovery of VHR phosphatase inhibitors with micromolar activity based on structure-based virtual screening. *ChemMedChem* **2008**, *3*, 880–887.

63. Corbeil, C. R.; Englebienne, P.; Yannopoulos, C. G.; Chan, L.; Das, S. K.; Bilimoria, D.; L'Heureux, L.; Moitessier, N. Docking ligands into flexible and solvated macromolecules. 2. Development and application of FITTED 1.5 to the virtual screening of potential HCV polymerase inhibitors. *J. Chem. Inf. Model.* **2008**, *48*, 902–909.

64. Kolb, P.; Huang, D.; Dey, F.; Caflisch, A. Discovery of kinase inhibitors by high-throughput docking and scoring based on a transferable linear interaction energy model. *J. Med. Chem.* **2008**, *51*, 1179–1188.

65. Salam, N. K.; Huang, T. H-W.; Kota, B. P.; Kim, M. S.; Li, Y.; Hibbs, D. E. Novel PPAR-gamma agonists identified from a natural product library: a virtual screening, induced-fit docking and biological assay study. *Chem. Biol. Drug Des.* **2008**, *71*, 57–70.

66. Katritch, V.; Byrd, C. M.; Tseitin, V.; Dai, D.; Raush, E.; Totrov, M.; Abagyan, R.; Jordan, R.; Hruby, D. E. Discovery of small molecule inhibitors of ubiquitin-like poxvirus proteinase I7L using homology modeling and covalent docking approaches. *J. Comput. Aided Mol. Des.* **2007**, *21*, 549–558.

67. Hu, X.; Prehna, G.; Stebbins, C. E. Targeting plague virulence factors: a combined machine learning method and multiple conformational virtual screening for the discovery of Yersinia protein kinase A inhibitors. *J. Med. Chem.* **2007**, *50*, 3980–3983.

68. Rummey, C.; Nordhoff, S.; Thiemannc, M.; Metz, G. In silico fragment-based discovery of DPP-IV S1 pocket binders. *Bioorg. Med. Chem. Lett.* **2006**, *16*, 1405–1409.

69. Irwin, J. J.; Raushel, F. M.; Shoichet, B. K. Virtual screening against metalloenzymes for inhibitors and substrates. *Biochemistry* **2005**, *44*, 12316–12328.

70. Hancock, C. N.; Macias, A.; Lee, E. K.; Yu, S. Y., Jr.; MacKerell, A. D.; Shapiro, P. Identification of novel extracellular signal-regulated kinase docking domain inhibitors. *J. Med. Chem.* **2005**, *48*, 4586–4595.

71. Toledo-Sherman, L.; Deretey, E.; Slon-Usakiewicz, J. J.; Ng, W.; Dai, J.-R.; Estelle Foster, J.; Redden, P. R.; Uger, M. D.; Liao, L. C.; Pasternak, A.; Reid, N. Frontal affinity chromatography with MS detection of EphB2 tyrosine kinase receptor. 2. Identification of small-molecule inhibitors via coupling with virtual screening. *J. Med. Chem.* **2005**, *48*, 3221–3230.

72. Forino, M.; Jung, D.; Easton, J. B.; Houghton, P. J.; Pellecchia, M. Virtual docking approaches to protein kinase B inhibition. *J. Med. Chem.* **2005**, *48*, 2278–2281.

73. Mozziconacci, J.-C.; Arnoult, E.; Bernard, P.; Do, Q. T.; Marot, C.; Morin-Allory, L. Optimization and validation of a docking-scoring protocol and application to virtual screening for COX-2 inhibitors. *J. Med. Chem.* **2005**, *48*, 1055–1068.

74. Chen, L.; Gui, C.; Luo, X.; Yang, Q.; Guenther, S.; Scandella, E.; Drosten, C.; Bai, D.; He, X.; Ludewig, B.; Chen, J.; Luo, H.; Yang, Y.; Yang, Y.; Zou, J.; Thiel, V.; Chen, K.; Shen, J.; Shen, X.; Jiang, H. Cinanserin is an inhibitor of the 3C-like proteinase of

severe acute respiratory syndrome coronavirus and strongly reduces virus replication in vitro. *J. Virol.* **2005**, *79*, 7095–7103.

75. Li, C.; Xu, L.; Wolan, D. W.; Wilson, I. A.; Olson, A. J. Virtual screening of human 5-aminoimidazole-4-carboxamide ribonucleotide transformylase against the NCI diversity set by use of Autodock to identify novel nonfolate inhibitors. *J. Med. Chem.* **2004**, *47*, 6681–6690.

76. Ferrari, A. M.; Wei, B. Q.; Costantino, L.; Shoichet, B. K. Soft docking and multiple receptor conformations in virtual screening. *J. Med. Chem.* **2004**, *47*, 5076–5084.

77. Thurmond, R. L.; Beavers, M. P.; Cai, H.; Meduna, S. P.; Gustin, D. J.; Sun, S.; Almond, H. J.; Karlsson, L.; Edwards, J. P. Nonpeptidic, noncovalent inhibitors of the cysteine protease cathepsin S. *J. Med. Chem.* **2004**, *47*, 4799–4801.

78. Schapira, M.; Raaka, B. M.; Das, S.; Fan, L.; Totrov, M.; Zhou, Z.; Wilson, S. R.; Abagyan, R.; Samuels, H. H. Discovery of diverse thyroid hormone receptor anagonists by high-throughput docking. *Proc. Natl. Acad. Sci. USA* **2003**, *100*, 7354–7359.

79. Wu, S. Y.; McNae, I.; Kontopidis, G.; McClue, S. J.; McInnes, C.; Stewart, K. J.; Wang, S.; Zheleva, D. I.; Marriage, H.; Lane, D. P.; Taylor, P.; Fischer, P. M.; Walkinshaw, M. D. Discovery of a novel family of CDK inhibitors with the program LIDAEUS structural basis for ligand-induced disordering of the activation loop. *Structure* **2003**, *11*, 399–410.

80. Liu, H.; Li, Y.; Song, M.; Tan, X.; Cheng, F.; Zheng, S.; Shen, J.; Luo, X.; Ji, R.; Yue, J.; Hu, G.; Jiang, H.; Chen, K. Structure-based discovery of potassium channel blockers from natural products: virtual screening and electrophysiological assay testing. *Chemistry* **2003**, *10*, 1103–1113.

81. Doman, T. N.; McGovern, S. L.; Witherbee, B. J.; Kasten, T. P.; Kurumbail, R.; Stallings, W. C.; Connolly, D. T.; Shoicht, B. K. Molecular docking and high-throughput screening for novel inhibitors of protein tyrosine phosphatase-1B. *J. Med. Chem.* **2002**, *45*, 2213–2221.

82. Paiva, A. M.; Vanderwall, D. E.; Blanchard, J. S.; Kozarich, J. W.; Williamson, J. M.; Kelly, T. M. Inhibitors of dihydropicolinate reductase, a key enzyme of the diaminopimelate pathway of *Mycobacterium tuberculosis*. *Biochim. Biophys. Acta* **2001**, *1545*, 67–77.

83. Enyedy, I. J.; Ling, Y.; Nacro, K.; Tomita, Y.; Wu, X.; Cao, Y.; Guo, R.; Li, B.; Zhu, X.; Huang, Y.; Long, Y.-Q.; Roller, P. P.; Yang, D.; Wang, S. Discovery of small-molecule inhibitors of Bcl-2 through structure-based computer screening. *J. Med. Chem.* **2001**, *44*, 4313–4234.

84. Iwata, Y.; Arisawa, M.; Hamada, R.; Kita, Y.; Mizutani, M. Y.; Tomioka, N.; Itai, A.; Miyamoto, S. Discovery of novel aldose reductase inhibitors using a protein structure-based approach: 3D-database search followed by design and synthesis. *J. Med. Chem.* **2001**, *44*, 1718–1728.

85. Gradler, U.; Gerber, H.-D.; Goodenough-Lashua, D. A. M.; Garcia, G. A.; Ficner, R.; Reuter, K.; Stubbs, M. T.; Klebe, G. A new target for shigellosis: rational design and crystallographic studies of inhibitors of tRNA-guanine transglycosylase. *J. Mol. Biol.* **2001**, *306*, 455–467.

86. Pang, Y.-P.; Xub, K.; Kollmeyer, T. M.; Perola, E.; McGrathe, W. J.; Greene, D. T.; Mangele, W. F. Discovery of a new inhibitor lead of adenovirus proteinase: steps toward selective, irreversible inhibitors of cysteine proteinases. *FEBS Lett.* **2001**, *502*, 93–97.

87. Hopkins, S. C.; Vale, R. D.; Kuntz, I. D. Inhibitors of kinesin activity from structure-based computer screening. *Biochemistry* **2000**, *39*, 2805–2814.

88. Freymann, D. M.; Wenck, M. A.; Engel, J. C.; Feng, J.; Focia, P. J.; Eakin, A. E.; Craig, S. P., III. Efficient identification of inhibitors targeting the closed active site conformation of the HPRT from *Trypanosoma cruzi*. *Chem. Biol.* **2000**, *7*, 957–968.

89. Wang, J.-L.; Liu, D.; Zhang, Z.-J.; Shan, S.; Han, X.; Srinivasula, S. M.; Croce, C. M.; Alnemri, E. S.; Huang, Z. Structure-based discovery of an organic compound that binds Bcl-2 protein and induces apoptosis of tumor cells. *Proc. Natl. Acad. Sci. USA* **2000**, *97*, 7124–7129.

90. Liu, J.-S.; Cheng, W.-C.; Wang, H.-J.; Chen, Y.-C.; Wang, W.-C. Structure-based inhibitor discovery of *Helicobacter pylori* dehydroquinate synthase. *Biochem. Biophys. Res. Commun.* **2008**, *373*, 1–7.

91. Mukherjee, P.; Desai, P.; Ross, L.; White, E. L.; Avery, M. A. Structure-based virtual screening against SARS-3CLpro to identify novel non-peptidic hits. *Bioorg. Med. Chem.* **2008**, *16*, 4138–4149.

92. Park, H.; Jung, S.-K.; Jeong, D. G.; Ryu, S. E.; Kim, S. J. Discovery of novel PRL-3 inhibitors based on the structure-based virtual screening. *Bioorg. Med. Chem. Lett.* **2008**, *18*, 2250–2255.

93. Ruiz, F. M.; Gil-Redondo, R.; Morreale, A.; Ortiz, A. R.; Fabrega, C.; Bravo, J. Structure-based discovery of novel non-nucleosidic DNA alkyltransferase inhibitors: virtual screening and in vitro and in vivo activities. *J. Chem. Inf. Model.* **2008**, *48*, 844–854.

94. Babaoglu, K.; Simeonov, A.; Irwin, J. J.; Nelson, M. E.; Feng, B.; Thomas, C. J.; Cancian, L.; Costi, M. P.; Maltby, D. A.; Jadhav, A.; Inglese, J.; Austin, C. P.; Shoichet, B. K. Comprehensive mechanistic analysis of hits from high-throughput and docking screens against β-lactamase. *J. Med. Chem.* **2008**, *51*, 2502–2511.

95. Park, H.; Hwang, K. Y.; Oh, K. H.; Kim, Y. H.; Lee, J. Y.; Kim, K. Discovery of novel α-glucosidase inhibitors based on the virtual screening with the homology-modeled protein structure. *Bioorg. Med. Chem.* **2008**, *16*, 284–292.

96. Montes, M.; Braud, E.; Miteva, M. A.; Goddard, M.-L.; Mondesert, O.; Kolb, S.; Brun, M.-P.; Ducommun, B.; Garbay, C.; Villoutreix, B. O. Receptor-based virtual ligand screening for the identification of novel CDC25 phosphatase inhibitors. *J. Chem. Inf. Model.* **2008**, *48*, 157–165.

97. Agarwal, S. M.; Jain, R.; Bhattacharya, A.; Azam, A. Inhibitors of *Escherichia coli* serine acetyltransferase block proliferation of *Entamoeba histolytica* trophozoites. *Int. J. Parasitol.* **2008**, *38*, 137–141.

98. Hellmuth, K.; Grosskopf, S.; Lum, C. T.; Wuertele, M.; Roeder, N.; von Kries, J. P.; Rosario, M.; Rademann, J.; Birchmeier, W. Specific inhibitors of the protein tyrosine phosphatase Shp2 identified by high-throughput docking. *Proc. Natl. Acad. Sci. USA* **2008**, *105*, 7275–7280.

99. Betzi, S.; Restouin, A.; Opi, S.; Arold, S. T.; Parrot, I.; Guerlesquin, F.; Morelli, X.; Collette, Y. Protein-protein interaction inhibition (2P2I) combining high throughput and virtual screening: application to the HIV-1 nef protein. *Proc. Natl. Acad. Sci. USA* **2007**, *104*, 19256–19261.

100. Wang, G.; Huang, N.; Meng, Z.; Liu, Q. Identification of novel inhibitors of the streptogramin group A acetyltransferase via virtual screening. *Yaoxue Xuebao* **2007**, *42*, 47–53.

101. Luzhkov, V. B.; Selisko, B.; Nordqvist, A.; Peyrane, F.; Decroly, E.; Alvarez, K.; Karlen, A.; Canard, B.; Aaqvist, J. Virtual screening and bioassay study of novel inhibitors for dengue virus mRNA cap (nucleoside-2′O)-methyltransferase. *Bioorg. Med. Chem.* **2007**, *15*, 7795–7802.

102. Ragno, R.; Mai, A.; Simeoni, S.; Caroli, A.; Caffarelli, E.; La Neve, P.; Gioia, U.; Bozzoni, I. Structure-based drug discovery of XendoU inhibitors through multi-docking virtual screening. In: *Frontiers in CNS and Oncology Medicinal Chemistry*, Vol. COMC-063. Washington, DC: American Chemical Society; 2007.

103. Park, H.; Kim, Y.-J.; Hahn, J.-S. A novel class of Hsp90 inhibitors isolated by structure-based virtual screening. *Bioorg. Med. Chem. Lett.* **2007**, *17*, 6345–6349.

104. Ostrov, D. A.; Hernandez Prada, J. A.; Corsino, P. E.; Finton, K. A.; Le, N.; Rowe, T. C. Discovery of novel DNA gyrase inhibitors by high-throughput virtual screening. *Antibac. Agents Chemother.* **2007**, *51*, 3688–3698.

105. Szewczuk, L. M.; Saldanha, S. A.; Ganguly, S.; Bowers, E. M.; Javoroncov, M.; Karanam, B.; Culhane, J. C.; Holbert, M. A.; Klein, D. C.; Abagyan, R.; Cole, P. A. De novo discovery of serotonin N-acetyltransferase inhibitors. *J. Med. Chem.* **2007**, *50*, 5330–5338.

106. Liao, C.; Karki, R. G.; Marchand, C.; Pommier, Y.; Nicklaus, M. C. Virtual screening application of a model of full-length HIV-1 integrase complexed with viral DNA. *Bioorg. Med. Chem. Lett.* **2007**, *17*, 5361–5365.

107. Srivastava, S. K.; Dube, D.; Kukshal, V.; Jha, A. K.; Hajela, K.; Ramachandran, R. NAD+-dependent DNA ligase (Rv3014c) from *Mycobacterium tuberculosis*: novel structure-function relationship and identification of a specific inhibitor. *Proteins* **2007**, *69*, 97–111.

108. Brooks, W. H.; McCloskey, D. E.; Daniel, K. G.; Ealick, S. E.; III; Secrist, J. A.; Waud, W. R.; Pegg, A. E.; Guida, W. C. In silico chemical library screening and experimental validation of a novel 9-aminoacridine based lead-inhibitor of human S-adenosylmethionine decarboxylase. *J. Chem. Inf. Model.* **2007**, *47*, 1897–1905.

109. Spannhoff, A.; Machmur, R.; Heinke, R.; Trojer, P.; Bauer, I.; Brosch, G.; Schuele, R.; Hanefeld, W.; Sippl, W.; Jung, M. A novel arginine methyltransferase inhibitor with cellular activity. *Bioorg. Med. Chem. Lett.* **2007**, *17*, 4150–4153.

110. Wang, J.-G.; Xiao, Y.-J.; Li, Y.-H.; Ma, Y.; Li, Z.-M. Identification of some novel AHAS inhibitors via molecular docking and virtual screening approach. *Bioorg. Med. Chem.* **2007**, *15*, 374–380.

111. Hamilton, D.; Wu, J. H.; Batist, G. Structure-based identification of novel human γ-glutamylcysteine synthetase inhibitors. *Mol. Pharm.* **2007**, *71*, 1140–1147.

112. Tsai, K.-C.; Chen, S.-Y.; Liang, P.-H.; Lu, I.-L.; Mahindroo, N.; Hsieh, H.-P.; Chao, Y.-S.; Liu, L.; Liu, D.; Lien, W.; Lin, T.-H.; Wu, S.-Y. Discovery of a novel family of SARS-CoV protease inhibitors by virtual screening and 3D-QSAR studies. *J. Med. Chem.* **2006**, *49*, 3485–3495.

113. Cavasotto, C. N.; Ortiz, M. A.; Abagyan, R. A.; Piedrafita, F. J. In silico identification of novel EGFR inhibitors with antiproliferative activity against cancer cells. *Bioorg. Med. Chem. Lett.* **2006**, *16*, 1969–1974.

114. Dooley, A. J.; Shindo, N.; Taggart, B.; Park, J-.G.; Pang, Y-.P. From genome to drug lead: identification of a small-molecule inhibitor of the SARS virus. *Bioorg. Med. Chem. Lett.* **2006**, *16*, 830–833.

115. Prykhod'ko, A. O.; Yakovenko, O. Y.; Golub, A. G.; Bdzhola, V. G.; Yarmoluk, S. M. Evaluation of 4H-4-chromenone derivatives as inhibitors of protein kinase CCK. *Biopolimeri i Klitina* **2005**, *21*, 287–292.

116. Huang, D.; Lüthi, U.; Kolb, P.; Edler, K.; Cecchini, M.; Audetat, S.; Barberis, A.; Caflisch, A. Discovery of cell-permeable non-peptide inhibitors of β-secretase by high-throughput docking and continuum electrostatics calculations. *J. Med. Chem.* **2005**, *48*, 5108–5111.

117. Liu, Z.; Huang, C.; Fan, K.; Wei, P.; Chen, H.; Liu, S.; Pei, J.; Shi, L.; Li, B.; Yang, K.; Liu, Y.; Lai, L. Virtual screening of novel noncovalent inhibitors for SARS-CoV 3C-like proteinase. *J. Chem. Inf. Model.* **2005**, *45*, 10–17.

118. Soelaiman, S.; Wei, B. Q.; Bergson, P.; Lee, Y.-S.; Shen, Y.; Mrksich, M.; Shoichet, B. K.; Tang, W.-J. Structure-based inhibitor discovery against adenylyl cyclase toxins from pathogenic bacteria that cause anthrax and whooping cough. *J. Biol. Chem.* **2003**, *278*, 25990–25997.

119. McNally, V. A.; Gbaj, A.; Douglas, K. T.; Stratford, I. J.; Jaffar, M.; Freemanan, S.; Bryce, R. A. Identification of a novel class of inhibitor of human and *Escherichia coli* thymidine phosphorylase by in silico screening. *Bioorg. Med. Chem. Lett.* **2003**, *13*, 3705–3709.

120. Peng, H.; Huang, N.; Qi, J.; Xie, P.; Xu, C.; Wang, J.; Yang, C. Identification of novel inhibitors of BCR-Abl tyrosine kinase via virtual screening. *Bioorg. Med. Chem. Lett.* **2003**, *13*, 3693–3699.

121. Pickett, S. D.; Sherborne, B. S.; Wilkinson, T.; Bennett, J.; Borkakoti, N.; Broadhurst, M.; Hurst, D.; Kilford, I.; McKinnell, M.; Jones, P. S. Discovery of novel low molecular weight inhibitors of IMPDH via virtual needle screening. *Bioorg. Med. Chem. Lett.* **2003**, *13*, 1691–1694.

122. Powers, R. A.; Morandi, F.; Shoichet, B. K. Structure-based discovery of a novel, noncovalent inhibitor of AmpC β-lactamase. *Structure* **2002**, *10*, 1013–1023.

123. Kamionka, M.; Rehm, T.; Beisel, H.-G.; Lang, K.; Engh, R. A.; Holak, T. A. In silico and NMR identification of inhibitors of the IGF-I and IGF-Binding Protein-5 interaction. *J. Med. Chem.* **2002**, *45*, 5655–5660.

124. Iino, M.; Furugori, T.; Mori, T.; Moriyama, S.; Fukuzawa, A.; Shibano, T. Rational design and evaluation of new lead compound structures for selective βARK1 inhibitors. *J. Med. Chem.* **2002**, *45*, 2150–2159.

125. Perola, E.; Xu, K.; Kollmeyer, T. M.; Kaufmann, S. H.; Prendergast, F. G.; Pang, Y.-P. Successful virtual screening of a chemical database for farnesyltransferase inhibitor leads. *J. Med. Chem.* **2000**, *43*, 401–408.

126. Sarmiento, M.; Wu, L.; Keng, Y.-F.; Song, L.; Luo, Z.; Huang, Z.; Wu, G.-Z.; Yuan, A. K.; Zhang, Z.-Y. Structure-based discovery of small molecule inhibitors targeted to protein tyrosine phosphatase 1B. *J. Med. Chem.* **2000**, *43*, 146–155.

127. Nordqvist, A.; Nilsson, M. T.; Roettger, S.; Odell, L. R.; Krajewski, W. W.; Andersson, C. E.; Larhed, M.; Mowbray, S. L.; Karlen, A. Evaluation of the amino acid binding site of *Mycobacterium tuberculosis* glutamine synthetase for drug discovery. *Bioorg. Med. Chem.* **2008**, *16*, 5501–5513.

128. Feder, M.; Purta, E.; Koscinski, L.; Cubrilo, S.; Vlahovicek, G. M.; Bujnicki, J. M. Virtual screening and experimental verification to identify potential inhibitors of the ErmC methyltransferase responsible for bacterial resistance against macrolide antibiotics. *ChemMedChem* **2008**, *3*, 316–322.

129. Zeng, Z.; Qian, L.; Cao, L.; Tan, H.; Huang, Y.; Xue, X.; Shen, Y.; Zhou, S. Virtual screening for novel quorum sensing inhibitors to eradicate biofilm formation of *Pseudomonas aeruginosa*. *App. Microbiol. Biotechnol.* **2008**, *79*, 119–126.

130. Kuo, C.-J.; Guo, R.-T.; Lu, I.-L.; Liu, H. G.; Wu, S.-Y.; Ko, T.-P.; Wang, A. H.-J.; Liang, P.-H. Structure-based inhibitors exhibit differential activities against *Helicobacter pylori* and

Escherichia coli undecaprenyl pyrophosphate synthases. *J. Biomed. Biotechnol.* **2008**.

131. Hirayama, K.; Aoki, S.; Nishikawa, K.; Matsumoto, T.; Wada, K. Identification of novel chemical inhibitors for ubiquitin C-terminal hydrolase-L3 by virtual screening. *Bioorg. Med. Chem.* **2007**, *15*, 6810–6818.

132. Song, H.; Wang, R.; Wang, S.; Lin, J. A low-molecular-weight compound discovered through virtual database screening inhibits Stat3 function in breast cancer cells. *Proc. Natl. Acad. Sci. USA* **2005**, *102*, 4700–4705.

133. Westerfors, M.; Tedebark, U.; Andersson, H. O.; Öhrman, S.; Choudhury, D.; Ersoy, O.; Shinohara, Y.; Axén, A.; Carredano, E.; Baumann, H. Structure-based discovery of a new affinity ligand to pancreatic α-amylase. *J. Mol. Recognit.* **2003**, *16*, 396–405.

134. Chowdhury, S. F.; Lucrezia, R. D.; Guerrero, R. H.; Brun, R.; Goodman, J.; Ruiz-Perez, L. M.; Pacanowska, D. G.; Gilbert, I. H. Novel inhibitors of leishmanial dihydrofolate reductase. *Bioorg. Med. Chem. Lett.* **2001**, *11*, 977–980.

135. Malvezzi, A.; de Rezende, L.; Izidoro, M. A.; Cezari, M. H. S.; Juliano, L.; Amaral, A. T. Uncovering false positives on a virtual screening search for cruzain inhibitors. *Bioorg. Med. Chem. Lett.* **2008**, *18*, 350–354.

136. Barreiro, G.; Guimaraes, C. R. W.; Tubert-Brohman, I.; Lyons, T. M.; Tirado-Rives, J.; Jorgensen, W. L. Search for non-nucleoside inhibitors of HIV-1 reverse transcriptase using chemical similarity, molecular docking, and MM-GB/SA scoring. *J. Chem. Inf. Model.* **2007**, *47*, 2416–2428.

137. Brenk, R.; Irwin, J. J.; Shoichet, B. K. Here be dragons: docking and screening in an uncharted region of chemical space. *J. Biomol. Screen.* **2005**, *10*, 667–674.

138. Kanji., G. K. *100 Statistical Tests*, 3rd edition. Thousand Oaks, CA: Sage, **2006**.

139. http://stattrek.com/Tables/ChiSquare.aspx.

140. Snedecor, G. W.; Cochran., W. G. *Statistical Methods, 8th edition.* Ames, IA: Iowa State University Press; **1989**, 135–148.

141. Irwin, J. J. Shoichet, B. K. ZINC – a free database of commercially available compounds for virtual screening. *J. Chem. Inf. Model.* **2005**, *45*, 177–182.

142. Negron-Encarnacion, I.; Arce, R.; Jimenez, M. Characterization of acridine species adsorbed on $(NH_4)2SO_4$, SiO_2, $Al2O_3$, and MgO by steady-state and time-resolved fluorescence and diffuse reflectance techniques. *J. Phys. Chem. A* **2005**, *109*, 787–797.

143. Turek-Etienne, T. C.; Small, E. C.; Soh, S. C.; Xin, T. A.; Gaitonde, P. V.; Barrabee, E. B.; Hart, R. F.; Bryant, R. W. Evalu-

ation of fluorescent compound interference in 4 fluorescence polarization assays: 2 kinases, 1 protease, and 1 phosphatase. *J. Biomol. Screening* **2003**, *8*, 176–184.

144. Feng, B. Y.; Simeonov, A.; Jadhav, A.; Babaoglu, K.; Inglese, J.; Shoichet, B. K.; Austin, C. P. A high-throughput screen for aggregation-based inhibition in a large compound library. *J. Med. Chem.* **2007**, *50*, 2385–2390.

145. Mojumdar, S. C.; Martiska, L.; Valigura, D.; Melnik, M. Thermal and spectral properties of halogenosalicylato-Cu(II) complexes. *J. Therm. Analysis and Calor.* **2003**, *74*, 905–914.

146. Schwarz, K. B.; Arey, B. J.; Tolman, K.; Mahanty, S. Iron chelation as a possible mechanism for aspirin-induced malondialdehyde production by mouse liver microsomes and mitochondria. *J. Clin. Invest.* **1988**, *81*, 165–170.

147. Ha, S.; Andreani, R.; Robbins, A.; Muegge, I. Evaluation of docking/scoring approaches: a comparative study based on MMP3 inhibitors. *J. Comput. Aided Mol. Design* **2000**, *14*, 435–448.

148. http://sampl.eyesopen.com/.

149. Goto, J.; Kataoka, R.; Hirayama, N. Ph4Dock: pharmacophore-based protein-ligand docking. *J. Med. Chem.* **2004**, *47*, 6804–6811.

150. Blow, D. M. A rearrangement of Cruickshanks formulae for the diffraction-component precision index. *Acta Crystallogr., Sect. D* **2002**, *D58*, 792–797.

151. Cruickshank, D. W. J. Remarks about protein structure precision. *Acta Crystallogr., Sect. D* **1999**, *D55*, 583–601.

152. http://www.eyesopen.com/products/applications/omega.html.

153. http://www.eyesopen.com/products/applications/rocs.html.

154. Bohacek, R. S.; McMartin, C. Definition and display of steric, hydrophobic, and hydrogen-bonding properties of ligand binding sites in proteins using Lee and Richards accessible surface: validation of a high-resolution graphical tool for drug design. *J. Med. Chem.* **1992**, *35*, 1671–1684.

155. Wang, Z.; Canagarajah, B. J.; Boehm, J. C.; Kassisà, S.; Cobb, M. H.; Young, P. R.; Abdel-Meguid, S.; Adams, J. L.; Goldsmith, E. J. Structural basis of inhibitor selectivity in MAP kinases. *Structure* **1998**, *6*, 1117–1128.

156. Hare, B. J.; Walters, W. P.; Caron, P. R.; Bemis, G. W. CORES: An automated method for generating three-dimensional models of protein/ligand complexes. *J. Med. Chem.* **2004**, *47*, 4731–4740.

157. http://www.bioinform.com/issues/12˙41/features/150096-1.html.

8

The role of quantum mechanics in structure-based drug design

Kenneth M. Merz, Jr.

INTRODUCTION

The routine use of quantum mechanics (QM) in all phases of in silico drug design is the logical next step in the evolution of this field. The first principles nature of QM allows it to systematically improve the accuracy of the description of the nature of the interactions between molecules. Moreover, the systematic way in which one can approach the use of QM methods to solve chemical and biological problems is quite appealing, but the practical use of many of the appealing features of QM in in silico drug design applications is still to be realized in large part because of computational limitations. In recent years it has become clear that classical potential functions are being pushed to their limits and as many pitfalls of using them are coming to light, one is tempted to explore the use of QM procedures. This is a somewhat naïve view, however, because one of the main observations of a large body of computational work has shown that sampling of relevant conformational states can be as important as providing an accurate representation of an inter-or intramolecular interaction. Hence, even as QM becomes a routine tool used to calculate the energy of individual states of a biological system, one still faces the daunting task of sampling relevant conformational space, which, in our view, will for the near term be largely confined to classical models.

Since the mid-2000s there have been significant advances with respect to use of QM in all aspects of drug design.[1,2] This has in part been fueled by the extraordinary increase in computational power and the plummeting cost of CPU time and storage space, which has in turn sped up development and validation of more sophisticated algorithms for calculating wave functions of macromolecular systems. Moreover, there have been equally impressive improvements in algorithms and software that allow researchers to address large-scale biological questions using QM models. The following sections highlight the evolving role played by QM in all aspects of in silico drug design and describe what, in our view, are significant recent advances. The focus of this review is on the use of QM in drug design, but QM has found broad application, for example, in the study of enzyme catalysis. The latter is not discussed here, but the

interested reader is directed to many of the recent reviews on QM studies of enzyme catalysis.[3,4]

The use of QM in in silico drug design can be divided into two broad categories: receptor- or structure-based and ligand-based methods (see Figure 8.1). Structure-based drug design (SBDD) methods involve the explicit treatment of the receptor as well as its associated ligands and include scoring protein/ligand poses using QM or quantum mechanics/molecular mechanics (QM/MM) methods, homology modeling of the receptor (prior to docking studies, for example), and energy decomposition methods like COMBINE that is based on a quantitative structure/activity relationship (QSAR) of pairwise interaction energies between a receptor and a series of ligand. SBDD requires either an x-ray or nuclear magnetic resonance (NMR) structure of the ligand in complex with the receptor and this information is shown as inputs in Figure 8.1. An important aspect of the structure determination process is the refinement process, which we show below can be impacted by QM-based methods as well. Although ligand-based drug design (LBDD) methods include various QSAR methods, they rely only on the knowledge of the ligand structure. QSAR can be carried out using 2D, 2.5D (structures generated from 2D), or 3D structures and ligand structures can come from NMR or x-ray studies, but they are generally obtained from purely computational means. However, one has to use 3D structures when using QM because of the need to have an all-atom description of the nuclei and associated electrons.

QUANTUM MECHANICS IN X-RAY AND NMR REFINEMENT

X-ray refinement of protein/ligand complexes

Three-dimensional structural information about therapeutic targets and their bound substrates and inhibitors is vitally important to structure-based drug design. To date the majority of this information has been supplied by x-ray crystallography, which captures static snapshots of the protein/inhibitor complexes and can be used to make hypotheses about the interactions that are relevant to the observed binding affinity. Spurred by recent advances in protein

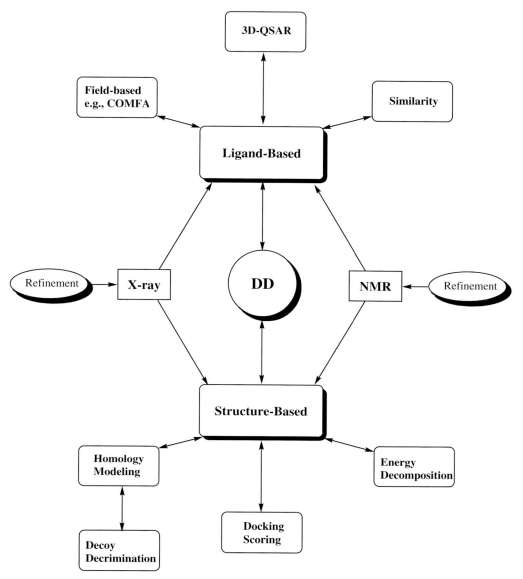

Figure 8.1. Hierarchy of QM methods used in drug design.

production techniques, interest in novel applications of x-ray crystallography in a high-throughput fashion have also been growing. The use of high-throughput crystallography in fragment-based drug discovery, for example, has been explored.[5-7]

For these high-throughput approaches to be practical for drug discovery, structure determination must be rapid enough to provide timely feedback to the design team; meanwhile, the structure of the complex, especially the ligand, must be determined accurately enough to provide adequate reliability on the subsequent hypotheses made about the observed binding interactions. However, it is often overlooked that protein crystallography operates at a resolution that is lower than that observed for small molecules, which gives rise to poor data-to-parameter ratios in protein structure refinements. In particular, the amount of x-ray

diffraction data observed is usually not sufficient to determine the coordinates, occupancies, and temperature factors for all the atoms. It can be shown that at a resolution of 2Å, the data-to-parameter ratio is slightly better than 2, while if the resolution drops to 2.7Å, a resolution that would not be uncommon for high-throughput crystallography, this ratio is less than 1. The issue of poor data-to-parameter ratios is dealt with in the energetically restrained refinement (EREF) formalism by introducing energy restraints to complement the x-ray data:[8]

$$E_{\text{total}} = E_{\text{chem}} + w_{\text{x-ray}} \, E_{\text{x-ray}}, \qquad (8.1)$$

where E_{total} is the function minimized during the refinement, E_{chem} is the energy function conventionally approximated with MM, $E_{\text{x-ray}}$ is the x-ray target function, and $w_{\text{x-ray}}$ is the weight that balances the contributions from

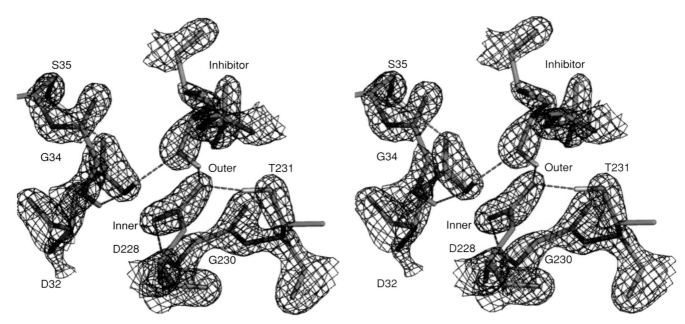

Figure 8.2. Cross-eye stereo view of the key residues of inhibitor-bound β-secretase in a state with Asp32 protonated and Asp228 deprotonated suggested as being most probable by QM/MM x-ray refinement, together with the σ_A-weighted 2Fo-Fc electron density maps contoured at 2.7σ level.

E_{chem} and $E_{x\text{-ray}}$. Although the electron density map computed from the x-ray data can be used to determine the structure on a larger scale, the energy function in Equation (8.1) is necessary to control the stereochemical details of the structure. However, though not yet well recognized, if E_{chem} is accurate enough the EREF formalism allows the use of energetic information to filter out unlikely tautomeric and protonation states, which may not otherwise be clear based solely on the coordinates of nonhydrogen atoms. Conversely, if E_{chem} is represented by approximate or even inaccurate energy functions, the refined structure can be significantly biased.[9,10] Unfortunately even though highly accurate parameters for bond lengths, angles, and torsions are available for amino and nucleic acids,[11–13] those for the small molecules are partially lacking, especially when extremely rare or novel chemical moieties are encountered.[14] QM constitutes an ideal choice for E_{chem} and a major improvement over MM because it does not require a priori knowledge of the potential energy surface of the ligand, which may be actual or virtual, and it is generally more accurate and reliable. Refinement studies on proteins[15,16] and complexes[17–21] have shown that QM-based energy restraints performed comparably with or, in some cases, showed some improvements over the MM-based ones.

Applications involving QM refinements of cocrystal structures have mostly being carried out in the QM/MM manner, which have been focused on two major areas. First, accurate energies calculated with QM and QM/MM have been used to suggest the probable protonation states of the key protein residues[22] and of the metal-bound ligands[17,23] in the context of the crystalline environment. For exam-

ple, QM/MM x-ray structure refinement was employed to construct realistic all-atom models of a complex of human β-secretase bound to a peptidic inhibitor and the relative stability of the resulting structures for different protonation states was evaluated by QM/SCRF calculations, which suggested one of the key aspartates, Asp32, was preferentially protonated in the cocrystal structure.[22] Although the non-hydrogen atom coordinates of the refined structure are not substantially different from those in the crystal structure, QM/MM refinement provided an all-atom model as a reasonable starting point for structure-based virtual screening and de novo design of β-secretase inhibitors. Second, energy restraints derived from high-level QM calculations have been used to refine ligand geometries to enhance the quality of low-resolution structures. Ryde et al. applied this approach to refine a 1.70Å structure of cytochrome c_{553} from *Bacillus pasteurii*. The refined structure was in better agreement with the same structure solved at 0.97Å and also reduced the R value of the lower-resolution structure by 0.018 (Figure 8.2).

A combined molecular dynamics (MD) potential of mean force (PMF) and QM/MM x-ray refinement study[24] has helped further our understanding of the binding preference for 1,6-dihydroxynaphthalene (DHN) to Orf2.[25] From the MD/PMF simulations three minima were located for the binding of DHN to Orf2 [C1 (the x-ray structure) C2 and C3]. C1 leads to the preferential product for the prenylation of DHN, whereas C3 leads to the minor product.[25] Each of these structures were then subjected to QM/MM x-ray refinement using the semiempirical PM3 Hamiltonian. The outcome of the QM/MM refinement versus a standard

Table 8.1. The CNS and QM/MM x-ray refinement of the C1, C2, and C3 conformers of 1,6-dihyroxynaphthalene bound to Orf2

Conformers	Refinement protocol	X-ray weights	R	R_{free}	Distance (Å)	
					D1	D2
C1	QM/MM	0.01	0.2540	0.2674	3.96	7.09
		0.2	0.2419	0.2629	3.97	7.12
		1.0	0.2290	0.2628	4.01	7.21
	CNS	0.01	0.3735	0.4015	5.03	8.17
		0.2	0.2606	0.3004	4.53	7.71
		1.0	0.2307	0.2754	4.10	7.17
C2	QM/MM	0.01	0.2604	0.2894	6.89	9.82
		0.2	0.2432	0.2798	6.78	9.73
		1.0	0.2285	0.2734	6.80	9.79
	CNS	0.01	0.3690	0.4021	8.15	10.48
		0.2	0.2617	0.3015	7.53	10.28
		1.0	0.2320	0.2763	7.10	10.11
C3	QM/MM	0.01	0.2496	0.2795	5.91	4.04
		0.2	0.2414	0.2749	5.81	3.96
		1.0	0.2283	0.2699	5.87	3.97
	CNS	0.01	0.3709	0.4018	7.36	5.27
		0.2	0.2642	0.3057	6.95	4.56
		1.0	0.2315	0.2777	6.42	4.20

CNS refinement (using a classical E_{chem} term) is shown in Table 8.1 and Figure 8.3. In Table 8.1 the weights and the resulting value of R and R_{free} (indicators of the refinement quality where lower is better) for the refinement of the three structures using QM/MM and CNS indicate that the latter refinement is superior to the former for all weights used. The results from this study show the possible improvements in structure quality possible with a QM/MM refinement, but further validation is required on other protein/ligand systems.

The development of high-throughput crystallography has called for improvement of the conventional refinement methods. Recently, Schiffer et al. reviewed the latest advances in simulation techniques that would affect the field of protein crystallography, and the use of QM methods was recognized as one of the three major forefronts.[26] With the capability and efficiency of QM continuing to increase, development and application of QM-based x-ray refinement methodologies will present many new interesting possibilities.

NMR refinement of protein/ligand complexes

Over the past decade, NMR spectroscopy has proven to be a powerful and versatile tool for the study of protein/ligand interactions. The three-dimensional structures of protein/ligand complexes can be determined by combining interproton distance restraints derived from the nuclear Overhauser effect (NOE) with other restraints from J coupling constants, hydrogen bonds, and/or residual dipolar couplings. Up to November 2006, there were over 800 NMR structures of protein/ligand complexes deposited in the Protein Data Bank. However, this determination process is far from automated and high-throughput because it is difficult to obtain accurate NMR restraints. Because Fesik and coworkers introduced SAR (structure/activity relationship) by NMR,[27] many NMR-based screening methods have been developed to identify potential drug molecules in pharmaceutical research (for reviews, see Homans, Lepre et al., and Meyer and Peters).[28–30] A recent interesting application of NMR-based screening methods is to predict protein druggability.[31,32] All these techniques take advantage of the fact that on ligand binding, significant perturbations can be observed in NMR parameters of either the receptor or the ligand. These perturbations can be used qualitatively to detect the complex formation or quantitatively to measure the binding affinity.

Among these NMR parameters, chemical shifts are exquisitely sensitive on the chemical environments of compounds. Therefore, theoretical calculations of chemical shift perturbations (CSP) on ligand binding can provide more insights about protein/ligand interactions at

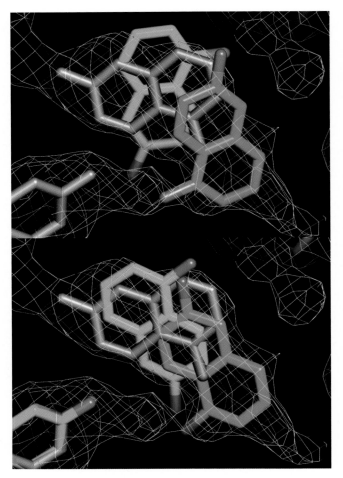

Figure 8.3. The snapshots of the C2 (green) and C3 (cyan) binding states of DHN (top) and the results from the QM/MM x-ray optimization (bottom) superimposed on top of the crystal structure 1ZB6 (gray) and the electron density contour at 0.5σ.

but provide only a limited understanding of the relationship between NMR chemical shifts and molecular structures and conformations. Moreover, it is difficult to extend these approaches to protein/ligand complexes because of the vast diversity of the chemical structures of ligands. Nevertheless, McCoy and Wyss[37] have developed J-surface analysis to map model molecules onto a protein by calculating CSP based on these classical models. Ab initio and DFT methods can be used to accurately predict NMR chemical shifts. However, they are still too computationally expensive to calculate NMR chemical shifts for protein/ligand complexes.

Recently, a relatively fast and accurate approach has been developed[38] to calculate NMR chemical shifts using the divide-and-conquer method at the semiempirical level. This linear-scaling approach allows for the treatment of large biological systems with quantum mechanics. To characterize protein/ligand interactions, this approach was first applied to the FKBP-GPI complex (see Figure 8.4).[39] By comparing calculated proton chemical shifts of the ligand to experimental data, it was possible to determine the binding site structure and identify a key hydrogen bond in this complex. Moreover, the native structure of the complex could be selected from a set of decoy poses (see Figure 8.5). This approach opens a new avenue to score protein/ligand interactions. The typical scoring functions are based on binding energies that are calculated by either knowledge-based or empirical functions derived from classical force fields.[40] One of the limitations in these functions is that they cannot reliably discriminate different poses, especially those that are close to the native structure. By incorporating experimental CSP analysis using QM-derived CSPs, this limitation can be circumvented. To further validate this approach, we have generated several hundred poses of GPI using different docking programs and then scored them by calculating CSPs and then comparing them to experiment.[41] We have found that the deviation of the computed CSPs from experiment can better differentiate decoy poses from native poses than typical scoring functions used in docking studies. This demonstrates that CSP-based approaches can provide an accurate way in which to predict protein/ligand complex structure using in silico NMR approaches.

The J coupling constant is another important NMR parameter that can provide a wealth of information about

the molecular level. There are two categories of computational approaches to calculate NMR chemical shifts: classical models and quantum mechanics.

The classical models[33–36] usually include ring current, magnetic anisotropy, and electrostatic effects on NMR chemical shifts, which are parameterized to experimental data or high-level density functional theory (DFT) results. These approaches are computationally fast so that they can be easily applied to proteins and other biological systems

molecular conformations and dynamics. The Karplus equation, which describes the relationship between J coupling constants and molecular dihedral angles, is widely used in protein structure determination. Recent advances in quantum chemistry make it possible to calculate this NMR observable quite accurately. We have demonstrated that the major conformation of a flexible molecule in solution can be determined by comparing the calculated and experimental J coupling constants.[42] Chou et al.[43] have

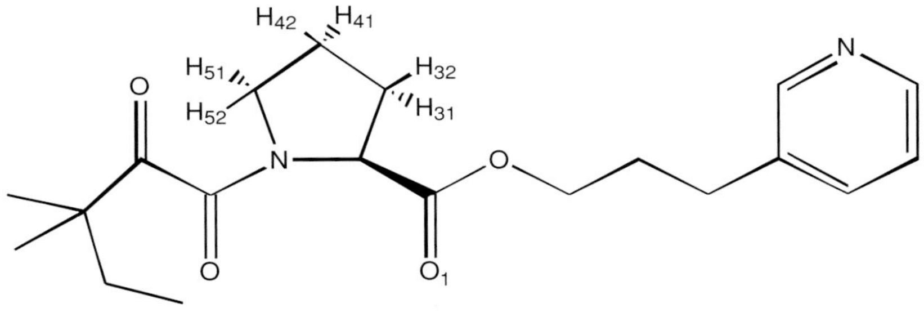

Figure 8.4. Structure of GPI.

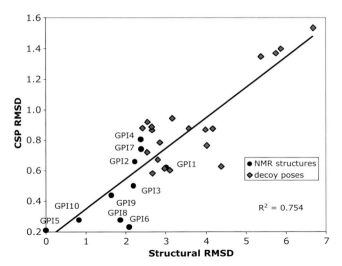

Figure 8.5. Correlation plot of the chemical shift perturbation root-mean-square deviations (rmsds) (in ppm) versus the structural rmsds (in Å) with respect to NMR structure GPI5 for the nine remaining GPI NMR structures and twenty computationally generated structures.

reparameterized the Karplus relationships for Ile, Val, and Thr residues based on DFT calculations to gain improved insights into side-chain dynamics. Trans hydrogen bond scalar J couplings have been detected in nucleic acids and proteins recently. DFT studies of these J coupling constants on peptide models hinted at the cooperative nature of hydrogen bond interactions.[44]

NMR spectroscopy is an important tool to study protein and protein/ligand complexes and novel QM approaches will continue to affect our understanding and interpretation of experimentally observed NMR parameters.

USING QUANTUM MECHANICS TO MODEL PROTEIN STRUCTURE

A major unsolved problem in biology is determining protein structure from sequence (the protein folding problem).[45–47] This includes, in the case of SBDD, predicting the fold from structure or refining homology models. Currently, classical or simplified potentials are used in attempting to solve this problem and significant amounts of very creative effort has been reported, which is beyond the scope of this chapter.[45–47] Instead we focus on the use of QM to discriminate decoy protein structures from native using semiempirical QM methods. Indeed, with the introduction of linear-scaling QM techniques, the modeling of full protein systems is now possible; we briefly review large-scale validations of the method to study protein structure and folding.

Protein geometry validation

To first assess the suitability of semiempirical methods it is important to first demonstrate that the experimental geometries of proteins are reproduced by semiempirical

QM theory. Semiempirical methods were developed to handle a large variety of chemical systems by being parameterized against a wide range of small molecules.[48,49] Proteins are large biopolymers with a small number of unique functional groups, so any error in the semiempirical treatment of those particular groups may potentially be magnified in these systems. Although semiempirical methods are heavily parameterized, they differ from classical approaches such as MM approaches that may employ amino-acid-specific parameters.[13]

A quote from Stewart's development of the semiempirical parameterized model 3 (PM3) method captures the essence of this problem nicely, "The parameter set here has three limitations: in the limit, it is only as good as the reference data used; . . . and it should be used with caution when applied to the prediction of any properties not used either in the parameterization or in subsequent surveys."[49] An analysis of the training compounds used in the parameterization of PM3 highlights the absence of several functional groups present in amino acids. Although the amino acids alanine and glycine were included in the parameterization of PM3, guanidyl-like groups and imidazole-like groups were not included.

Large-scale optimization of protein geometries at the semiempirical level highlights the problems of minimizing in vacuo. Unlike classical methods, QM methods can undergo conformational changes as well as changes in bonding configuration. Bond cleavage and proton transfer involving charged groups were common when optimizing with semiempirical methods in vacuo. These artifacts, not suprisingly, were corrected for when optimizing with an implicit solvent model.

Overall, semiempirical methods match the geometries of proteins surprising well. The largest observed discrepancies were in the torsional angles, in agreement with previous observations.[49,50] Furthermore, optimization with SE methods led to a smaller fraction of side chains in native rotameric states. This is likely to be due to the low energetic differences arising from perturbations in the torsional angles. Also of note, the C–N peptide bonds in proteins are longer by 0.06Å in semiempirical-minimized geometries, and in general C–N bonds were predicted to be longer than those found in crystal structures of proteins. Nonetheless, the optimized structures, although far from perfect, reproduced experimental x-ray geometries satisfactorily.

Approximations to semiempirical geometries

Quantum mechanical calculations are more sensitive to geometries of structures than classical methods. Very large changes in the energy can result from small changes in the structure, particularly with respect to bond lengths and angles. In this regard, it is desirable to first optimize a system before applying QM calculations on the structure. Ideally, it would be preferable to optimize the structure at the QM level so that the resulting structure would be consistent

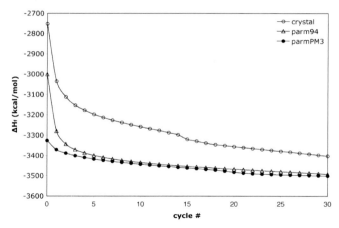

Figure 8.6. Semiempirical minimization profile of N-terminal fragment of NS-1 protein (PDB code 1ail) starting with the crystal structure (circle), the structure preminimized with AMBER (parm94 – triangles), and the structure preminimized with parmPM3 (filled circles).

with the QM treatment employed. However, because of the computational expense associated with minimizing large biomolecules at the QM level, this is often difficult. A more computationally tractable approach that we have developed is to optimize structures using an MM potential that has been parameterized to reproduce geometries that are more consistent with the semiempirical QM treatment.[51]

The AMBER force field has been reparameterized to yield geometries more in register with a semiempirical QM approach, and they are termed parmAM1 and parmPM3 in reference to the semiempirical geometries for which they were parameterized.[51] The advantage of this parameter set is twofold: (1) to reduce the time taken for optimizations by using an MM minimization to arrive at lower energy starting structures and (2) to reduce the overall strain on the system by potentially removing energy and gradient instabilities during subsequent QM minimizations that can lead to bond cleavage or other artifacts.

This approach has been successful in producing initial structures that are generally more stable in subsequent QM optimizations and exhibit much lower energies when scored with QM methods. This is highlighted in Figure 8.6, which compares the semiempirical minimization profile of the N-terminal fragment of the NS-1 protein [Protein Data Bank (PDB) code 1ail] starting with the crystal structure and the structure preminimized with AMBER and preminimized with parmPM3. The structure preminimized with parmPM3 has a lower initial energy and exhibits a smoother minimization profile.

Discrimination of native structures

Another common method used in assessing scoring potentials for proteins is to determine their ability to discriminate native structures from nonnative models.[52] In ab initio folding, large numbers of protein models are generated and a scoring function is used to identify near-native from nonnative structures. The assumption is that the native structure should be at the global minimum of the energy function,[53] so an inability to correctly identify native structures would indicate that there might be deficiencies in the method and, by inference, be less useful in modeling studies of proteins. This is also a particularly challenging problem for QM methods as it entails the scoring of thousands of protein models. This study marked the first large-scale investigation into the utility of semiempirical QM methods for studying protein folding.

Large databases of these computationally generated nonnative protein structures, or decoys, are readily available.[54,55] Many of these decoy sets are generated during ab initio protein structure prediction calculations and contain many of the characteristics of native protein structures, possessing secondary structural elements and favorable packing. During structure prediction simulations, a large set of structures are computationally generated; the aim is to be able to reliably identify those structures that have lower root-mean-square deviations (rmsds) to the native structure. This approach is generally constrained by insufficient sampling and deficiencies in the energy function; a large conformational space must be sampled and the energy function must be robust enough to discriminate nativelike structures from nonnative.

Although classical MM potentials perform very well at identifying the native structure from decoys, they do not identify the native structure in all cases.[56] In our approach, we have used a linear combination of the heat of formation obtained from QM calculations, a classical Lennard-Jones attractive term (LJ6), and a QM-derived Poisson-Boltzmann (PB) solvation term in the scoring function. The attractive term was included to compensate for the poor treatment of dispersive effects by semiempirical methods. Because the individual components of the resulting "DivScore" method were taken from different levels of theory, weighting coefficients were applied to maximize the Z-score of native structures in a test set relative to their decoys and are shown below:

$$E_{tot} = 0.250^*\Delta H_f + 0.225^*\Delta G_{solv} + 0.525^*LJ_6.$$

This approach was used on thirteen large sets of decoys, taken from the four-state reduced set and Rosetta set. Because of the potential for bias when comparing structures generated through different means, an all-atom gradient-based minimization was performed on all decoys and native structures. Both AMBER and parmPM3 were used to clean up the models from any structural anomalies in a consistent fashion. In addition, bond lengths and angles are minimized with a consistent parameterized potential, removing any bias in the force field toward either the native structure or its decoys.

The results of scoring with DivScore show that this scoring function is particularly well suited for identifying the native structure from among all decoys. The native structures can be correctly identified for all thirteen systems,

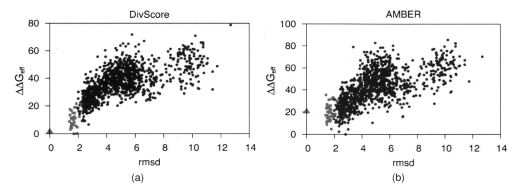

Figure 8.7. Energy versus rmsd plots for the fructose repressor DNA binding domain (PDB id: 1uxd) scored using the DivScore potential (a) and AMBER (b). (▲) NMR minimized mean (taken as the reference for rmsd calculations); (■) individual NMR models; (●) Rosetta decoy. Energies are reported as the difference in energy for a state compared to the lowest energy structure in the decoy set. AMBER scores several decoys better than native models while DivScore correctly identifies several NMR models as native.

although interestingly it is the x-ray structures and not the NMR structures that are generally lowest scoring. The Z-scores for all native structures are large, indicating that the potential function scores the native structure much better than the set of decoys. The energy gaps between the native structure and the best-scoring decoy are large for the four-state-reduced set, although noticeably smaller for the Rosetta decoys. A sample of the resulting plots of Div-Score versus rmsd from native is given in Figure 8.7.

It is interesting that semiempirical methods work so well in identifying native structures from nonnative, considering that proteins contain functional groups that were not explicitly parameterized in the semiempirical Hamiltonians used (AM1[48] and PM3[49]). Furthermore, classical approaches have an advantage in that they have been parameterized for a focused set of functional groups found in biological molecules,[13] whereas SE parameters are implemented at the level of individual elements. In addition, macromolecular effects such as nonlocal van der Waals interactions and multiple charged-charged interactions become significant.

The ability to use semiempirical single-point measurements to discriminate native structures from nonnative indicates that these methods are suitable for applications involving proteins and may be capturing important interactions that lead to protein stability. It is worth considering why semiempirical models score protein decoys as well as we have found in the present study. Semiempirical methods are known not to give phi-psi plots that agree with high-quality ab initio results,[50] while force fields are generally parameterized to reproduce these plots at some level of accuracy. This suggests that other factors play a role like long-range electrostatics or cooperativity effects observed in the folding of secondary structural elements.[57] Possibly these effects are overwhelming the conformational effects when using semiempirical methods in scoring native and decoy protein structures. With this approach in place one can start to consider using semiempirical methods to validate homology models or to use it to study the preferred conformation of loops in proteins.

STRUCTURE-BASED DRUG DESIGN

Qualitative uses of QM in RBDD

The ability to characterize a macromolecule such as a protein using QM opens up a whole new range of descriptors that can aid drug discovery. Many of these descriptors are beyond the reach of classical potentials and by their very nature can be used to gain a qualitative understanding of protein/ligand interactions and then be used in the rational design of drug molecules. Linear-scaling QM methods have made therapeutically important protein targets accessible to qualitative analysis, from a rational drug design perspective. These qualitative insights are often used to predict lig- and binding or metal binding "hot spots" that can be targets for small-molecule inhibitors. Workers have made use of descriptors such as molecular electrostatic potential (ESP) maps, local hardness and softness, Fukui indices, frontier orbital analysis, density of electronic state analysis, and so on, to probe proteins. Below we concentrate on recent studies that have employed QM derived descriptors.

ESP and relative proton potential

ESP maps have been widely used as a tool for characterizing protein or DNA binding sites in RBDD. However, these maps have traditionally been derived from classical point charge models (for example, PARSE) that were used to compute the electrostatic potential on the surface of proteins by solving the linear or nonlinear PB equation. With the advent of linear-scaling QM algorithms, combined with self-consistent reaction field methods to model solvation, ESP maps can now be computed quantum mechanically. Khandogin and York, using linear-scaling QM technology to generate ESP maps, have probed properties of therapeutically important protein targets such as HIV-1 nucleocapsid (NC) protein.[58,59] These authors have clearly demonstrated the advantage of using the PM3/COSMO computed molecular electrostatic potential (MEP) map over the PARSE/PB map, in discerning between the electronegativity of the

C-terminal and N-terminal zinc finger region of NC. These results agree with earlier experimental work that suggests the same.

Another notable aspect of this study is the use of the relative proton potential as a descriptor to predict proton affinity of titratable sites of the ovomucoid third domain (OMTYK3). The agreement between experimental pK_a and relative proton potentials of these residues is very encouraging with a linear correlation coefficient of -0.996. There is a wealth of experimental pK_a data and high-resolution x-ray crystallographic data available for other therapeutically important protein targets. A systematic study of all these targets to confirm the predictive ability of relative proton potential is in order. In related studies, Rajamani and Reynolds have also used linear-scaling QM[60,61] implemented in the computer program DIVCON to model protonation states of catalytic aspartates in β-secretase.[62] These studies suggest that the aspartates prefer the monoprotonated state in the presence of the inhibitor, whereas in its absence they favor the dideprotonated state. Raha and Merz, again using DIVCON, have also formulated a scheme to calculate the proton affinity of the catalytic aspartates of HIV-1 protease in the presence and absence of inhibitors bound to the proteases and discussed the results in light of their binding affinity calculations.[63]

Polarization and charge transfer

Although the role of polarization and charge transfer in macromolecular interaction is well known, only recently has it been quantified in SBDD by the use of QM methods. Hensen and coworkers, using QM/MM methods, have studied the interaction of HIV-1 protease with three high-affinity inhibitors: nelfinavir, mozenavir, and tripnavir.[64] They find that polarization of the ligand by the enzyme environment contributes to up to 39% of the total electrostatic interaction energy. Based on their analysis they propose modifications to one of the inhibitors that can possibly lead to increase in binding affinity. In a similar study, Garcia-Viloca et al. have investigated the role of polarization of the substrate tetrahydrofolate, and the cofactor NADPH, at various stages of dihydrofolate reductase catalyzed hydride transfer reaction.[65] The authors find that polarization contributes to 4% of the total electrostatic interaction and stabilizes the transition state by 9 kcal/mol over the reactants.

Charge transfer in receptor ligand interaction in the context of SBDD has been studied in significant detail by Raha and Merz.[63] In their recent study of 165 noncovalent protein/ligand complexes, they find that in 11% of the complexes more than 0.1 electron units of charge is transferred from the protein to ligand. In the 49 metalloenzyme complexes, there is on average up to 0.6 electron units of charge transferred between the protein and the ligand. The direction of CT depends on the protein/ligand complex. For example, in matrix metalloproteases (MMP), charge is transferred from the protein to the ligand, whereas in human carbonic anhydrase (HCA) and carboxypeptidases (CPA) charge is transferred from the ligand to protein. All

these studies indicate that QM effects are important in protein/ligand interaction and cannot be ignored in SBDD efforts that hope to discover potent inhibitors to protein targets in silico.

Catalysis, QM, and SBDD

The mechanism of recognition of substrates by enzymes, followed by catalysis and product formation, has drawn considerable interest from the drug discovery community as these enzymes are potential targets for therapy. As a result, a thorough understanding of the mechanism with respect to catalysis can lead to effective inhibitor design strategies. QM has come to play a leading role in this area, because the very nature of mechanistic enzymology makes it suitable for sophisticated investigation via use of QM. Recent reviews in this area describe the emerging field of computational enzymology and detail modeling techniques and important advances that involve QM/MM and DFT based approaches.[3,4]

Review of the literature for the past year indicates a host of enzymes that have been the subject of mechanistic investigation using QM-based methods and a thorough review is beyond the scope of the overall topic of this article. However, we touch on two enzymes that have been the subject of detailed investigation and are important SBDD targets. These are β-lactamase and chorismate mutase.[66–70] From the point of view of RBDD, β-lactamases have been particularly well studied to elucidate their mechanism of resistance to β-lactam antibiotics. In one such comprehensive study, Hermann et al. have modeled the acylation mechanism of class A β-lactamase enzyme TEM1 using semiempirical QM/MM and hybrid DFT to correct the semiempirical energies.[71] The insights gleaned from this study will be valuable in the design of β-lactam antibiotics that are not hydrolyzed by β-lactamases. Merz and coworkers have also used QM/MM, DFT, and quantum chemical solvation methods to study the mechanisms and binding preferences of a class of β-lactam antibiotics for these enzymes.[69,72]

Quantitative uses of QM in RBDD

Although QM can provide valuable insights and a different perspective regarding the interaction between receptor and ligand in structure-based drug design, the holy grail of computational drug discovery still remains the ability to accurately calculate the free energy of binding between a protein and its small-molecule inhibitor and thereby discover new inhibitors in silico. Part of this problem involves the prediction of the correct binding mode or "pose" of the inhibitor when bound to a protein target. Several docking programs have been reasonably successful in obtaining the correct binding mode.[73] However, calculating the binding free energy or the correct score has proven to be challenging.[74] This is not surprising, considering that the free energy of binding between two molecular systems depends on a complex interplay of interactions between them and the medium they exist in. Computational methods that strive to calculate the free energy of binding usually use an energy function also known as a "scoring function" that computes a score directly or indirectly, related to the binding free energy. Scoring functions have traditionally been either simplistic empirical or statistical potentials that relate observables to the free energy of binding by using statistical methods, or they are extremely detailed in nature and use physics-based descriptions of the molecular energetics and extensive sampling of receptor-ligand conformations via molecular simulation. Recently we have reviewed all categories of scoring functions and discussed their pros and cons with respect to RBDD.[75]

The use of quantum mechanics in structure-based drug design has until recently been either qualitative as described in the previous section or peripheral. For example, in large-scale virtual screening of databases using docking programs, semiempirical QM methods have been used during the database preparation phase to calculate atomic charges. A database (ZINC) of commercially available drug-like molecules prepared with QM charges and desolvation penalties has been made publicly available.[76] In a recent study Irwin et al., using ZINC, have successfully enriched known ligands that bind to metalloenzymes over non-binders in retrospective docking screens.[77] Although high-quality charges and desolvation penalties are not the only reason for this success, they no doubt play an important role.

Further evidence of the importance of the quality of charges comes from another study by Cho et al., in which ligand charges calculated using QM/MM methods led to significant improvement in the ability of docking programs to obtain the correct binding mode of the inhibitor.[78] The docking method that employed QM charges performed decisively better than force-field-based charges in ranking native binding modes as the best pose. The difference was more pronounced for poses that were predicted within 0.5 to 1.0 Å rmsd of the native pose. Raha and Merz have also designed a classical scoring function – the molecular recognition model – that used CM2 charges calculated using semiempirical QM for modeling electrostatic and solvation effects during binding.[63] It is noteworthy that charges in this case were computed for the entire protein/ligand complex using linear-scaling methods thus accounting for polarization and charge transfer. The molecular recognition model was able to calculate pK_is that agreed with experimental pK_i (correlation coefficient R^2 of 0.78) for thirty-three inhibitors modeled in the active site of HIV-1 protease.

QM/MM and binding affinity calculation
QM/MM methods are widely used to study mechanistic aspects of enzyme catalysis or in peripheral aspects of RBDD such as small-molecule charge calculation in molecular docking as described above. However, few studies have attempted to use QM/MM, either directly or indirectly, for calculating the free energy of binding between a protein and a ligand. In an earlier study, Mlinsek et al. used QM/MM to generate the MEP on the van der Waals surface of thrombin

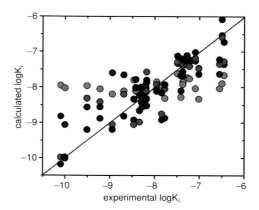

Figure 8.8. Four-tier approach used by Khandelwal et al. Shown is the correlation between the experimental and calculated inhibition constants of a series of hydroxamates against MMP-9 as given by FlexX docking in step 1 (green), QM/MM minimization step 2 (blue), MD simulations with constrained zinc bonds step 3 (red), and by QM/MM energy calculations for the time averaged stuctures from MD simulations step 4 (black).

and then used the MEP as input into an artificial neural network/genetic algorithm engine for data reduction and combination for predicting the pK_i of thrombin inhibitors.[79] Although artificial intelligence methods have shown good success in such studies, often they lack generality. Moreover, the MEPs used in this study were descriptors that ignored other aspects of binding.

In a very recent study, Khandelwal et al. used a four-tier approach that involves docking, QM/MM optimization, MD simulation, and QM/MM interaction energy calculation to predict binding affinity.[80] The authors use a modified version of extended linear response (ELR) theory where the van der Waals and electrostatic terms are replaced by QM/MM interaction energy:

$$\Delta G_{\text{binding}} = \alpha \times \Delta \langle E_{\text{QM/MM}} \rangle + \gamma \times \Delta \langle SASA \rangle + \kappa,$$

where $\langle E_{\text{QM/MM}} \rangle$ is the time average of single-point QM/MM interaction energies obtained from MD simulations. The authors calculated the binding affinity of twenty-eight hydroxamate-based inhibitors of matrix metalloprotease (MMP-9) using this approach with impressive accuracy. The agreement between the calculated and experimental pK_i is excellent ($R^2 = 0.9$ and cross-validated R^2 ranging from 0.77 to 0.88). What is also noteworthy is that the authors clearly demonstrate an improvement in predictive accuracy with every step of their four-tier approach. As shown in Figure 8.8, the agreement with experimental pK_i improves from poor, after the first step of docking ($R^2 = 0.044$; green circles in Figure 8.8) to very good ($R^2 = 0.90$; black circles in Figure 8.2) after the final step of QM/MM single-point interaction energy calculation. This points toward the importance of a quantum mechanical treatment and the sampling of active conformations in accurate binding prediction. Specifically, the QM/MM treatment of the active site is very important (step 3) because it was shown that a proton is transferred from the hydroxamate hydroxyl to the active-site glutamate.

Modeling this phenomenon is more of a challenge when classical potentials are used.

Linear-scaling QM and binding affinity calculation

The QM/MM approaches described above clearly show promise for calculating the binding affinity in protein/ligand interaction. However, it is obvious from the above discussion that, first, these approaches still require extensive sampling of ligand/receptor conformations through molecular simulation and are very time-consuming and, second, in all RBDD QM/MM studies reported to date, only the ligand is treated quantum mechanically, because including even small portions of the protein is computationally too expensive. Third, if bonded regions of the protein/ligand complex are to be divided into QM and MM regions, then there are well-documented pitfalls associated with the boundary region in the QM/MM approach.[81]

These problems have to some extent been surmounted by the development of linear-scaling QM technology in the past decade. Semiempirical Hamiltonians such as AM1 and PM3 can now be employed to calculate the molecular wave function for proteins with thousands of atoms. One of the first applications of linear-scaling methods to RBDD was reported by Raha and Merz, where they calculated the binding affinity of ligands bound to the metalloenzyme human carbonic anhydrase with reasonable accuracy.[82] As described by the authors, the free energy of binding in solution was calculated using the following set of equations:

$$\Delta G_{\text{bind}}^{\text{sol}} = \Delta G_{\text{b}}^{\text{g}} + \Delta G_{\text{solv}}^{\text{PL}} - \Delta G_{\text{solv}}^{\text{P}} - \Delta G_{\text{solv}}^{\text{L}}$$
$$\Delta G_{\text{b}}^{\text{g}} = \Delta H_{\text{b}}^{\text{g}} - T \Delta S_{\text{b}}^{\text{g}}.$$

Here, the free energy of binding in solution was calculated as the sum of the gas phase interaction energy and a solvation correction. The gas phase interaction energy consisted of enthalpic and entropic components. The electrostatic part of the enthalpic component was calculated with the program DivCon, using semiempirical Hamiltonians. The solvation correction was calculated as a difference between the solvation free energies of the protein/ligand complex (PL) with the protein (P) and the ligand (L) free in solution. The solvation free energy was calculated using a Poisson-Boltzmann based self-consistent reaction field (PB/SCRF) method in which the polarization of the solute electron density due to the presence of the solvent reaction field is calculated self-consistently using a QM Hamiltonian.[83] This is a major advantage of using the QM-based solvation method wherein the dielectric relaxation (or the internal dielectric) of the protein in response to a solvent reaction field is not preset.

In subsequent studies, the authors carried out a very large-scale and detailed validation of this quantum-mechanics-based scoring function, named QMScore, for predicting binding affinity. They calculated interaction energies for a diverse range of protein/ligand complexes comprising of 165 noncovalent complexes and 49 metalloenzyme complexes.[63] For the 165 noncovalent complexes the interaction energies, without any fitting, agreed with experimental binding affinity within 2.5 kcal/mol. When different parts of the scoring function were fit to the experimental free energy of binding using regression methods, the agreement was within 2.0 kcal/mol. For metalloenzymes, the agreement with experiments without fitting was within 1.7 kcal/mol and with fitting was within 1.4 kcal/mol. The authors thus demonstrated the inherent predictive ability of this first-generation full QM-based scoring function that takes into account all aspects of binding.

In another study, Nikitina et al., using linear-scaling QM methods, calculated the binding enthalpy of eight ligands bound to protein conformations from the PDB.[84] The authors chose enthalpy to examine the ability of the semiempirical Hamiltonian PM3 to calculate the enthalpy of binding. The choice of the enthalpy of binding instead of the free energy of binding was a prudent choice because the computation of entropy is far more challenging and generally introduces further simplifying approximations. Another important aspect of the study was inclusion of water molecules in the calculation of enthalpy. The structural water molecules were included in the computation of reference state enthalpies of the protein and ligand. They tried two different schemes where water molecules that were hydrogen bonded to both the protein and the ligand in the complex were considered in both reference state calculations of the protein and the ligand. One drawback of the study is the exclusion of solvation effects or the solvation correction to the enthalpy of binding. However, the authors argue that solvation effects are modeled enthalpically by including explicit water molecules. The calculated enthalpies agreed with the experimental enthalpies within 2 kcal/mol.

Other recent examples of using of linear-scaling QM in RBDD include a study by Vasilyev and Bliznyuk where the computer program MOZYME was used to rescore the top 100 predicted ligands from another docking program. The authors evaluated the feasibility of using a linear-scaling QM program for such a task.[85] In another application of MOZYME, Ohno et al. studied the affinity maturation of an antibody by calculating the binding free energy of the hapten bound to a germline antibody and the mature form.[86] The authors emphasize the importance of polarization and charge transfer in the maturation process.

Recent development of linear-scaling technology has focused on higher levels of theory, such as Hatree-Fock or DFT to calculate the wave functions of macromolecules. Gao et al. have described the development and application of a density matrix (DM) scheme based on molecular fractionation with conjugate caps (MFCC).[87] Using this method the density matrix is calculated for capped fragments of a macromolecule at high levels of theory. The total energy is then calculated from the full DM that is assembled from the fragment DMs. In an application of this method, Chen and

Zhang calculated the ligand/DNA/RNA interaction at high levels of theory.[88] Although further validation is needed for evaluating the ability of such a method to calculate binding free energies, it clearly has potential.

Fukuzawa et al. have used another approach – ab intio fragment molecular orbital (FMO) – to calculate the interaction energy of ligands that bind to the human estrogen receptor.[89] Although the agreement between the calculated and observed binding affinity is modest, they have examined the feasibility of modeling the receptor using only a few of the residues surrounding the ligand. They found no significant difference in the computed interaction energy between the complete receptor and the pruned receptor that had residues surrounding only the ligand. This hints toward a strategy to reduce the time taken for such calculations even further. However, a more thorough validation study is still needed.[2]

Interaction energy decomposition with QM and QM/MM

Experimental measures of binding affinity give very little insight into the relationship of the binding pose of an active inhibitor and its interaction with the receptor. Such insights can be very useful for the process of going from a lead to a drug. Computational methods, in general, provide access to the decomposition of the interaction energy between the ligand and the receptor. However, with the application of QM to RBDD, these insights are more grounded theoretically and can often be validated by experiments. These insights can be utilized in design cycles comprising prediction and testing for increasing the potency of submicromolar leads in drug discovery.

Both QM/MM and linear-scaling QM methods have been used to dissect the interaction of a ligand with its receptor. Hensen et al. used MD and QM/MM to dissect the interaction of inhibitors bound to the HIV-1 protease.[64] They demonstrated that a 4-hydroxy-dihydropyrone substructure of the most potent inhibitor, tripnavir, made favorable interactions with the catalytic aspartates and isoluecine residues of the HIV-1 protease. He et al. have used the linear-scaling DM-MFCC approach to dissect the interaction between the HIV-1 reverse transcriptase (RT) and its drug-resistant mutants with the inhibitor nevirapine. The authors calculate a QM interaction spectrum that sheds light on crucial aspects of resistance to RT.[90]

Raha et al., using linear-scaling QM and a pairwise energy decomposition (PWD) scheme, dissected the interaction of a series of fluorine-substituted ligands [N-(4-sulfamylbenzoyl)benzylamine or SBB] with human carbonic anhydrase.[91] They divided the enzyme and inhibitors into subsystems and calculated the exchange energy that consisted of the off-diagonal elements of the density matrix and the one-electron matrix elements between subsystems:

$$E_{AB} = \sum_{\mu}^{A} \sum_{\nu}^{B} P_{\mu\nu}^{AB} \left(2H_{\mu\nu}^{AB} - \frac{1}{2} \sum_{\lambda}^{B} \sum_{\sigma}^{A} P_{\lambda\sigma}^{BA} \left(\mu^{A}\sigma^{A} | \lambda^{B}\nu^{B} \right) \right).$$

Here, A and B are residue subsystems, and P and H are the density matrix and the one-electron matrix, respectively. Using this PWD scheme, the authors investigated the effect of substitution of fluorines on the distal aromatic rings of SBB inhibitors and on its interaction with human carbonic anhydrase. The authors probed at the relationship of various pairwise interactions with the free energy of binding of the inhibitors. It was found that the substitution of fluorine at the distal group did not directly affect the free energy of binding. Rather, it geometrically influenced the strongest interaction between the sulfonamide group of the inhibitor and the Thr199 residue of the protein. This strong interaction, which was chemically identical in each of the inhibitors, was directly correlated with the binding affinity of the ligand. Such insights can be valuable in designing new and potent inhibitors. The PWD scheme was also incorporated into the comparative binding energy analysis (COMBINE)[92] methodology of Ortiz and coworkers to create SE-COMBINE by Peters and Merz.[93] This method elucidated the most important interactions between trypsin and a series of trypsin inhibitors. The multivariate statistical tools, principal component analysis and partial least squares (PLS), were used to mine the interactions between the receptor residues and the ligand fragments to generate QSAR models. The authors introduced so-called IMMs (intermolecular interaction maps), which enable the researcher to graphically view where a candidate drug could be modified or optimized.

LIGAND-BASED DRUG DESIGN

One of the oldest tools used in rational drug design is QSAR. QSAR models are derived for a set of compounds with dependent variables (activity values, e.g., K_i, IC_{50}), and a set of calculated molecular properties or independent variables called descriptors. Each compound in the data set is assumed to be in its active conformation. Models are generated using techniques such as multiple linear regression (MLR), principal component regression (PCR), partial least squares regression (PLSR), and computer neural networks (CNNs) to name a few. Ligand-based methods can be further divided into two categories, 3D-QSAR and field-based methods. Both will be touched on under "3D-QSAR with QM Descriptors."

3D-QSAR WITH QM DESCRIPTORS

The descriptors used in 3D-QSAR are usually divided into three categories: (1) electronic [e.g., highest occupied molecular orbital (HOMO) and lowest unoccupied molecular orbital (LUMO) energies], (2) topological (e.g., connectivity indices), and (3) geometric (e.g., moment of inertia). The models in all cases are often created using multivariate statistical tools due to the large number and high degree of collinearity of descriptors. An excellent review by Karelson, Lobanov, and Katritzky provides details of QM-based descriptors used in QSAR programs such as CODESSA.[94] These include those that can be observed experimentally, such as dipole moments, and those that cannot, such as partial atomic charges. Clark and coworkers have recently used AM1-based descriptors to distinguish between drugs and nondrugs and to understand the relationship between descriptors and their physical properties.[95]

Most descriptors are calculated at the semiempirical level of theory using programs such as AMPAC or MOPAC. However, with computer speed increasing steadily the use of ab initio and DFT methods are becoming increasingly common. These methods allow the descriptors to be calculated from first principals. Yang and coworkers examined various DFT-based descriptors to generate models for a series of protoporphyrinogen oxidase inhibitors. It was shown that the DFT-based model outperformed the PM3-based model.[96]

FIELD-BASED METHODS: CoMFA

Comparative molecular field analysis (CoMFA)[97] and CoMSIA (comparative molecular similarity indices analysis)[98] are field-based or grid-based methods where all the compounds in the data set are aligned on top of one another and steric and electrostatic descriptors are calculated at each grid point using a probe atom. As a result there are many more descriptors than molecules; therefore, a PLS data analysis is used to generate linear equations. A study by Weaver and coworkers compares different field-based methods for QSAR, including CoMFA and CoMSIA, finding that field-based methods provide a robust tool to aid medicinal chemists.[99] Absent from the traditional MFA approaches are quantum mechanically derived descriptors of electronic structure. QMQSAR is a relatively new technique where semiempirical QM methods are used to develop quantum molecular field-based QSAR models.[100] Placing the aligned training set ligands into a finely spaced grid produces quantum molecular fields, where each ligand is characterized by a set of probe interaction energy (PIE) values. A PIE is defined as the "electrostatic potential energy obtained by placing a positively charged carbon 2s electron at a given grid point and summing the attractive and repulsive potentials experienced by that electron as it interacts with the field of the ligand L":

$$PIE = -\langle s_i s_i | V(L) \rangle = \int_{r_1} \chi_{s_i}^*(r_1) \chi_{s_i}(r_2)$$

$$\times \left\{ \sum_{\alpha=1}^{N_{atoms}} \left[\frac{z_\alpha}{|r_1 - r_\alpha|} - \sum_{\mu \in \alpha} \sum_{\mu' \in \alpha} P_{\mu\mu'} \int_{r_2} \frac{\chi_\mu^*(r_2) \chi_{\mu'}(r_1)}{|r_1 - r_2|} dr_2 \right] \right\} dr_1.$$

The nuclear charge z_α is simply the number of valence electrons on atom α and the notation $\mu \in \alpha$ indicates the set of valence atomic orbitals centered on atom α. Density

matrix elements $P_{\mu\mu'}$ are given by the following sum over the occupied MOs:

$$P_{\mu\mu'} = 2 \sum_{k=1}^{N_{occ}} c_{\mu k} c_{\mu' k}.$$

When applied to data sets containing corticosteroids, endothelin antagonists, and serotonin antagonists, linear regression models were produced with similar predictability compared to various CoMFA models.

SPECTROSCOPIC 3-D QSAR

The spectroscopic QSAR methods include EVA (vibrational frequencies),[101] EEVA (MO energies),[102] and CoSA (NMR chemical shifts).[103] It is a requirement of 3D QSAR that all compounds that are being studied contain the same number of descriptors. However, none of the above techniques provides this necessarily. The number of vibrational frequencies is dependent on the number of atoms, N, in a molecule (3N-6 or 3N-5 if linear). The number of NMR chemical shifts depends on N while the number MOs also depends on basis set size. A solution of this problem is to force the information onto a bound scale using a Gaussian smoothing technique, where the upper and lower limits of this scale are consistent for all compounds in the data set. A Gaussian kernel with a standard deviation of σ is placed over each calculated point, EVA, EEVA, or NMR chemical shift. Summing the amplitudes of the overlaid Gaussian functions at intervals x along the defined range results in the descriptors for each molecule, $f(x)$:

$$f(x) = \sum_{i=1}^{3N-6} \frac{1}{\sigma \sqrt{2\pi}} e^{-(x-f_i)^2/2\sigma^2}.$$

These descriptors contain a wealth of structural information when we consider the physical basis of the methods. Infrared spectroscopy provides information concerning the arrangement of molecular functional groups and NMR chemical shifts are highly dependent on substituents effects in a congeneric series of compounds. However, MO energies give the electronic structure of the molecule such as the HOMO/LUMO energies that play an important role in the binding process.

The choice of theory used to calculate these descriptors depends on the number of compounds in the data set and the accuracy that is required; all can be calculated using semiempirical or ab initio methods. The QSAR results also depend on the choice σ and x in the above equation.

These methods have provided predictive models for a number of data sets and have an advantage over the field-based methods because they are "alignment-free"; in other words there is no need to superimpose the structures in the data set. Asikainen and coworkers provided a comparison of these methods in a recent article where they studied estrogenic activity of a series of compounds.[104]

QUANTUM QSAR AND MOLECULAR QUANTUM SIMILARITY

The Carbó group has been involved in the development of the field of quantum QSAR and molecular quantum similarity since the 1980s.[105] The quantum similarity measure (QSM) between any two molecules, A and B, can be calculated using the following:

$$z_{AB} = \langle \rho_A | \Omega | \rho_B \rangle = \iint \rho_A(r_1) \Omega(r_1 r_2) \rho_B(r_2) \, dr_1 \, dr_2,$$

where Ω is some positive definite operator (e.g., kinetic energy or Coulomb) and ρ is the electron density. The QSMs can be transformed into indices ranging between 0 and 1 using

$$r_{AB} = \frac{z_{AB}}{\sqrt{z_{AA} z_{BB}}},$$

yielding the so-called Carbó similarity index (CSI). Calculating an array of QSMs or CSIs between all molecular pairs in some data set provides descriptors for quantum QSAR.[106]

A drawback of the CoMFA-based methods is the need to superimpose the molecules in the training set. This is no easy task due to the many degrees of freedom (both rigid and internal motions). However, the alignment of the molecular structures in a common 3D framework provides a convenient method of determining which regions of the molecules impact activity and which regions can be developed to create new compounds with more favorable properties. QSMs have been developed with a Lamarckian genetic algorithm called the quantum similarity superposition algorithm (QSSA) to superimpose the classic CoMFA data set.[107] The QSSA is performed in such a way as to maximize the molecular similarity and does not rely on atom typing as other empirical based methods do.

Accurate and efficient molecular alignment techniques based on first-principles electronic structure calculations represents a significant challenge due to the associated computational expense. Hence, QSMs tend to use approximate electron densities. Fusti-Molnar and Merz[108] recently described a new scheme that maximizes quantum similarity matrixes in the relative orientation of the molecules using Fourier transform (FT) techniques for two purposes: first, build up the numerical representation of true ab initio electronic densities and their Coulomb potentials and, second, apply the Fourier convolution technique to accelerate optimizations in the translational degrees of freedom. Importantly, to avoid interpolation errors, the necessary analytical formulae were derived for the transformation of the ab initio wave functions in rotational coordinates. The new alignment technique was then shown to be generally applicable for overlap, Coulomb, and kinetic energy quantum similarity measures and can be extended from QSM computation to solving the docking problem with ab initio scoring.

Popelier and coworkers have coupled the atoms-in-molecules (AIM) theory of Bader with quantum molecular similarity to produce quantum topological molecular similarity (QTMS).[109] It uses the so-called Bond critical points of predefined bonds in a series of molecules as descriptors followed by multivariate statistical analysis. The series of compounds must have a common core for this method to remain computationally tractable. QTMS has been used to generate models to estimate the pK_a values for a set of aliphatic carboxylic acids, anilines, and phenols.[110]

OUTLOOK

As with any brief review it is difficult to catalog all the most recent advances. But the use of quantum mechanical approaches in drug design problems using both ligand- and receptor-based drug design applications will certainly experience tremendous growth in the coming years. The ability, in principal, for QM to give extremely accurate interaction energies between a receptor and ligand and its ability to generate novel descriptor classes should attract even more attention to the use of QM in structure-based drug design in the coming years. However, for the use of QM to become standard requires the development of even faster QM methodologies and careful validation studies to demonstrate improved performance over classical methodologies. In the case of RBDD the incorporation of entropy and the role of conformational dynamics still represents a significant hurdle for both classical and QM-based methodologies. Future effort to overcome these problems will certainly be a major focus of researchers involved in SBDD.

ACKNOWLEDGMENTS

The authors acknowledge the generous support of the NIH (GM44974 and GM066859).

REFERENCES

1. Cavalli, A.; Carloni, P.; Recanatini, M. Target-related applications of first principles quantum chemical methods in drug design. *Chem. Rev.* **2006**, *106*, 3497–3519.
2. Fedorov, D. G.; Kitaura, K. Extending the power of quantum chemistry to large systems with the fragment molecular orbital method. *J. Phys. Chem. A* **2007**, *111*, 6904–6914.
3. Mulholland, A. J. Modelling enzyme reaction mechanisms, specifity and catalysis. *Drug. Discov. Today* **2005**, *10*, 1393–1402.
4. Friesner, R. A.; Gullar, V. Ab initio quantum chemical and mixed quantum mechanics/molecular mechanics (QM/MM) methods for studying enzymatic catalysis. *Ann. Rev. Phys. Chem.* **2005**, *56*, 389–427.
5. Blundell, T. L.; Jhoti, H.; Abell, C. High-throughput crystallography for lead discovery in drug design. *Nat. Rev. Drug Discov.* **2002**, *1*(1), 45–54.
6. Hartshorn, M. J.; Murray, C. W.; Cleasby, A.; Frederickson, M.; Tickle, I. J.; Jhoti, H. Fragment-based lead discovery using X-ray crystallography. *J. Med. Chem.* **2005**, *48*(2), 403–413.
7. Nienaber, V. L.; Richardson, P. L.; Klighofer, V.; Bouska, J. J.; Giranda, V. L.; Greer, J. Discovering novel ligands for macromolecules using X-ray crystallographic screening. *Nat. Biotechnol.* **2000**, *18*(10), 1105–1108.

8. Jack, A.; Levitt, M. Refinement of large structures by simultaneous minimization of energy and R factor. *Acta Crystallogr. A* **1978**, *34*, 931–935.

9. Kleywegt, G. J.; Jones, T. A. Where freedom is given, liberties are taken. *Structure* **1995**, *3*(6), 535–540.

10. Kleywegt, G. J.; Jones, T. A. Databases in protein crystallography. *Acta Crystallogr. D Biol. Crystallogr.* **1998**, *54*, 1119–1131.

11. Brooks, B. R.; Bruccoleri, R. E.; Olafson, B. D.; States, D. J.; Swaminathan, S.; Karplus, M. CHARMM: A program for macromolecular energy, minimization, and dynamics calculations. *J. Comput. Chem.* **1983**, *4*, 187–217.

12. Engh, R. A.; Huber, R. Accurate bond and angle parameters for x-ray protein-structure refinement. *Acta Crystallogr. A* **1991**, *47*, 392–400.

13. Cornell, W. D.; Cieplak, P.; Bayly, C. I.; Gould, I. R.; Merz, K. M.; Ferguson, D. M.; Spellmeyer, D. C.; Fox, T.; Caldwell, J. W.; Kollman, P. A. A second generation force field for the simulation of proteins, nucleic acids, and organic molecules. *J. Am. Chem. Soc.* **1995**, *117*(19), 5179–5197.

14. Davis, A. M.; Teague, S. J.; Kleywegt, G. J. Application and limitations of X-ray crystallographic data in structure-based ligand and drug design. *Angew. Chem. Int. Ed. Engl.* **2003**, *42*(24), 2718–2736.

15. Yu, N.; Li, X.; Cui, G.; Hayik, S. A.; Merz, K. M. Critical assessment of quantum mechanics based energy restraints in protein crystal structure refinement. *Protein Sci.* **2006**, in press.

16. Yu, N.; Yennawar, H. P.; Merz, K. M. Refinement of protein crystal structures using energy restraints derived from linear-scaling quantum mechanics. *Acta Crystallogr. D Biol. Crystallogr.* **2005**, *61*, 322–332.

17. Nilsson, K.; Ryde, U. Protonation status of metal-bound ligands can be determined by quantum refinement. *J. Inorg. Biochem.* **2004**, *98*(9), 1539–1546.

18. Ryde, U.; Nilsson, K. Quantum chemistry can locally improve protein crystal structures. *J. Am. Chem. Soc.* **2003**, *125*(47), 14232–14233.

19. Ryde, U.; Nilsson, K. Quantum refinement: a method to determine protonation and oxidation states of metal sites in protein crystal structures. *J. Inorg. Biochem.* **2003**, *96*(1), 39–39.

20. Ryde, U.; Nilsson, K. Quantum refinement: a combination of quantum chemistry and protein crystallography. *J. Mol. Struct.* **2003**, *632*, 259–275.

21. Ryde, U.; Olsen, L.; Nilsson, K. Quantum chemical geometry optimizations in proteins using crystallographic raw data. *J. Comput. Chem.* **2002**, *23*(11), 1058–1070.

22. Yu, N.; Hayik, S. A.; Wang, B.; Liao, N.; Reynolds, C. H.; Merz, K. M. Assigning the protonation states of the key aspartates in beta-secretase using QM/MM x-ray structure refinement. *J. Chem. Theor. Comput.* **2006**, *2*, 1057–1069.

23. Nilsson, K.; Hersleth, H. P.; Rod, T. H.; Andersson, K. K.; Ryde, U. The protonation status of compound II in myoglobin, studied by a combination of experimental data and quantum chemical calculations: quantum refinement. *Biophys. J.* **2004**, *87*(5), 3437–3447.

24. Cui, G.; Xue, L.; Merz, J., K. M. Understanding the substrate selectivity and the product regioselectivity of orf2-catalyzed aromatic prenylations. *Biochemistry* **2006**, submitted.

25. Kuzuyama, T.; Noel, J. P.; Richard, S. B. Structural basis for the promiscuous biosynthetic prenylation of aromatic natural products. *Nature* **2005**, *435*(7044), 983–987.

26. Schiffer, C.; Hermans, J. Promise of advances in simulation methods for protein crystallography: implicit solvent models, time-averaging refinement, and quantum mechanical modeling. *Methods Enzymol.* **2003**, *374*, 412–461.

27. Shuker, S. B.; Hajduk, P. J.; Meadows, R. P.; Fesik, S. W. Discovering high-affinity ligands for proteins: SAR by NMR. *Science* **1996**, *274*(5292), 1531–1534.

28. Homans, S. W. NMR spectroscopy tools for structure-aided drug design. *Angew. Chem. Int. Ed. Engl.* **2004**, *43*(3), 290–300.

29. Lepre, C. A.; Moore, J. M.; Peng, J. W. Theory and applications of NMR-based screening in pharmaceutical research. *Chem. Rev.* **2004**, *104*(8), 3641–3676.

30. Meyer, B., Peters, T. NMR spectroscopy techniques for screening and identifying ligand binding to protein receptors. *Angew. Chem. Int. Ed. Engl.* **2003**, *42*(8), 864–890.

31. Hajduk, P. J.; Huth, J. R.; Fesik, S. W. Druggability indices for protein targets derived from NMR-based screening data. *J. Med. Chem.* **2005**, *48*(7), 2518–2525.

32. Hajduk, P. J.; Huth, J. R.; Tse, C. Predicting protein druggability. *Drug Discov. Today* **2005**, *10*(23–24), 1675–1682.

33. Sitkoff, D.; Case, D. A. Density functional calculations of proton chemical shifts in model peptides. *J. Am. Chem. Soc.* **1997**, *119*(50), 12262–12273.

34. Wishart, D. S.; Watson, M. S.; Boyko, R. F.; Sykes, B. D. Automated 1H and 13C chemical shift prediction using the BioMagResBank. *J. Biomol. NMR* **1997**, *10*(4), 329–336.

35. Iwadate, M.; Asakura, T.; Williamson, M. P. C-alpha and C-beta carbon-13 chemical shifts in proteins from an empirical database. *J. Biomol. NMR* **1999**, *13*(3), 199–211.

36. Xu, X. P.; Case, D. A. Automated prediction of 15N, 13Calpha, 13Cbeta and 13C' chemical shifts in proteins using a density functional database. *J. Biomol. NMR* **2001**, *21*(4), 321–333.

37. McCoy, M. A.; Wyss, D. F., Spatial localization of ligand binding sites from electron current density surfaces calculated from NMR chemical shift perturbations. *J. Am. Chem. Soc.* **2002**, *124*(39), 11758–11763.

38. Wang, B.; Brothers, E. N.; Van Der Vaart, A.; Merz, K. M. Fast semiempirical calculations for nuclear magnetic resonance chemical shifts: a divide-and-conquer approach. *J. Chem. Phys.* **2004**, *120*(24), 11392–11400.

39. Wang, B.; Raha, K.; Merz, K. M., Jr. Pose scoring by NMR. *J. Am. Chem. Soc.* **2004**, *126*(37), 11430–11431.

40. Abagyan, R.; Totrov, M. High-throughput docking for lead generation. *Curr. Opin. Chem. Biol.* **2001**, *5*(4), 375–382.

41. Wang, B.; Westerhoff, L. M.; Merz, K. M., Jr. A critical assessment of the performance of protein−ligand scoring functions based on NMR chemical shift perturbations. *J. Med. Chem.* **2007**, *50*(21), 5128–5134.

42. Cui, G.; Wang, B.; Merz, K. M., Jr. Computational studies of the farnesyltransferase ternary complex part I: substrate binding. *Biochemistry* **2005**, *44*(50), 16513–16523.

43. Chou, J. J.; Case, D. A.; Bax, A. Insights into the mobility of methyl-bearing side chains in proteins from (3)J(CC) and (3)J(CN) couplings. *J. Am. Chem. Soc.* **2003**, *125*(29), 8959–8966.

44. Salvador, P.; Dannenberg, J. J. Dependence upon basis sets of trans hydrogen-bond C-13-N-15 3-bond and other scalar J-couplings in amide dimers used as peptide models: a density functional theory study. *J. Phys. Chem. B* **2004**, *108*(39), 15370–15375.

45. Fersht, A. R.; Daggett, V. Protein folding and unfolding at atomic resolution. *Cell* **2002**, *108*, 1–20.

46. Baldwin, R. L. In search of the energetic role of peptide hydrogen bonds. *J. Biol. Chem.* **2003**, *278*(20), 17581–17588.

47. Dill, K. A.; Ozkan, S. B.; Shell, M. S.; Weikl, T. R. The protein folding problem. *Annu. Rev. Biophys.* **2008**, *37*, 289–316.

48. Dewar, M. J. S.; Zoebisch, E. G.; Healy, E. F.; Stewart, J. J. P. AM1: a new general purpose quantum mechanical molecular model. *J. Am. Chem. Soc.* **1985**, *107*, 3902–3909.

49. Stewart, J. J. P. Optimization of parameters for semiempirical methods I. Method. *J. Comp. Chem.* **1989**, *10*(2), 209–220.

50. Möhle, K.; Hofmann, H. J.; Thiel, W. Description of peptide and protein secondary structures employing semiempirical methods. *J. Comput. Chem.* **2001**, *22*, 509–520.

51. Wollacott, A. M.; Merz, K. M. Development of a parameterized force field to reproduce semiempirical geometries. *J. Chem. Theory Comput.* **2006**, *2*, 1070–1077.

52. Hendlich, M.; Lackner, P.; Weitckus, S.; Floeckner, H.; Froschauer, R.; Gottsbacher, K.; Casari, G.; Sippl, M. J. Identification of native protein folds amongst a large number of incorrect models: the calculation of low energy conformations from potentials of mean force. *J. Mol. Biol.* **1990**, *216*(1), 167–180.

53. Lazaridis, T.; Karplus, M. Effective energy functions for protein structure prediction. *Curr. Opin. Struct. Biol.* **2000**, *10*(2), 139–145.

54. Park, B.; Levitt, M. Energy functions that discriminate X-ray and near native folds from well-constructed decoys. *J. Mol. Biol.* **1996**, *258*(2), 367–392.

55. Simons, K. T.; Kooperberg, C.; Huang, E.; Baker, D. Assembly of protein tertiary structures from fragments with similar local sequences using simulated annealing and Bayesian scoring functions. *J. Mol. Biol.* **1997**, *268*(1), 209–225.

56. Lee, M. R..; Kollman, P. A. Free-energy calculations highlight differences in accuracy between X-ray and NMR structures and add value to protein structure prediction. *Structure* **2001**, *9*(10), 905–916.

57. Morozov, A. V.; Tsemekhman, K.; Baker, D. Electron density redistribution accounts for half the cooperativity of alpha helix formation. *J. Phys. Chem. B* **2006**, *110*(10), 4503–4505.

58. Khandogin, J.; York, D. M. Quantum descriptors for biological macromolecules from linear-scaling electronic structure methods. *Proteins* **2004**, *56*, 724–737.

59. Khandogin, J.; Musier-Forsyth, K.; York, D. M. Insights into the regioselectivity and RNA-binding affinity of HIV-1 nucleocapsid protein from linear-scaling quantum methods. *J. Mol. Biol,* **2003**, *330*, 993–1004.

60. Dixon, S. L.; Merz, K. M. Semiempirical molecular orbital calculations with linear system size scaling. *J. Chem. Phys.* **1996**, *104*(17), 6643–6649.

61. Dixon, S. L.; Merz, K. M. Fast, accurate semiempirical molecular orbital calculations for macromolecules. *J. Chem. Phys.* **1997**, *107*(3), 879–893.

62. Rajamani, R.; Reynolds, C. H. Modeling the protonation states of catalytic aspartates in b-secretase. *J. Med. Chem.* **2004**, *47*, 5159–5166.

63. Raha, K.; Merz, K. M., Jr. Large-scale validation of a quantum mechanics based scoring function: predicting the binding affinity and the binding mode of a diverse set of protein-ligand complexes. *J. Med. Chem.* **2005**, *48*, 4558–4575.

64. Hensen, C.; Hermann, J. C.; Nam, K.; Ma, S.; Gao, J.; Holtje, H. A combined QM/MM approach to protein-ligand interaction: polarization effects of HIV-1 protease on selected high affinity inhibitors. *J. Med. Chem.* **2004**, *47*, 6673–6680.

65. Garcia-Viloca, M.; Truhlar, D. G.; Gao, J. Importance of substrate and cofactor polarization in the active site of dihydrofolate reductase. *J. Mol. Biol.* **2003**, *372*(2), 549–560.

66. Claeyssens, F.; Ranaghan, K. E.; Manby, F. R.; Harvey, J. N.; Mulholland, A. J. Multiple high-level QM/MM reaction paths demonstrate transition-state stabilization in chorismate mutase: correlation of barrier height with transition-state stabilization. *Chem. Commun. (Camb.)* **2005**, *40*, 5068–5070.

67. Xu, D.; Zhou, Y.; Xie, D.; Guo, H. Antibiotic binding to monozinc CphA beta-lactamase from *Aeromonas hydropila*: quantum mechanical/molecular mechanical and density functional theory studies. *J. Med. Chem.* **2005**, *48*(21), 6679–6689.

68. Zhang, X.; Bruice, T. C. A definitive mechanism for chorismate mutase. *Biochemistry* **2005**, *44*(31), 10443–10448.

69. Park, H.; Brothers, E. N.; Merz, K. M. Jr. Hybrid QM/MM and DFT investigations of the catalytic mechanism and inhibition of the dinuclear zinc metallo-beta-lactamase CcrA from Bacteroides fragilis. *J. Am. Chem. Soc.* **2005**, *127*(12), 4232–4241.

70. Szefczyk, B.; Mulholland, A. J.; Ranaghan, K. E.; Sokalski, W. A. Differential transition-state stabilization in enzyme catalysis: quantum chemical analysis of interactions in the chorismate mutase reaction and prediction of the optimal catalytic field. *J. Am. Chem. Soc.* **2004**, *126*(49), 16148–16159.

71. Hermann, J. C.; Hensen, C.; Ridder, L.; Mulholland, A. J.; Holtje, H. D. Mechanisms of antibiotic resistance: QM/MM modeling of the acylation reaction of a class A beta-lactamase with benzylpenicillin. *J. Am. Chem. Soc.* **2005**, *127*(12), 4454–4465.

72. Diaz, N.; Suarez, D.; Merz, K. M., Jr.; Sordo, T. L. Molecular dynamics simulations of the TEM-1 beta-lactamase complexed with cephalothin. *J. Med. Chem.* **2005**, *48*(3), 780–791.

73. Taylor, R.; Jewsbury, P. J.; Essex, J. W. A review of protein-small molecule docking methods. *J. Comput. Aided. Mol. Des.* **2002**, *16*, 151–166.

74. Schneidman-Duhovny, D.; Nussinov, R.; Wolfson, H. J. Predicting molecular interactions in silico. II. Protein-protein and protein-drug docking. *Curr. Med. Chem.* **2004**, *11*, 91–107.

75. Raha, K.; Merz, K. M., Jr. Calculating binding free energy in protein-ligand interaction. *Ann. Rep. Comput. Chem.* **2005**, *1*, 113–130.

76. Irwin, J. J.; Shoichet, B. K. ZINC: a free database of commercially available compounds for virtual screening. *J. Chem. Inf. Model.* **2005**, *45*(1), 177–182.

77. Irwin, J. J.; Raushel, F. M.; Shoichet, B. K. Virtual screening against metalloenzymes for inhibitors and substrates. *Biochemistry* **2005**, *44*(37), 12316–12328.

78. Cho, A. E.; Guallar, V.; Berne, B. J.; Friesner, R. A. Importance of accurate charges in molecular docking: quantum mechanical/molecular mechanical approach. *J. Comp. Chem.* **2005**, *29*, 917–930.

79. Mlinsek, G.; Novic, M.; Hodoscek, M.; Solmajer, T. Prediction of enzyme binding: human thrombin inhibition study by quantum chemical and artificial intelligence methods based on X-ray structures. *J. Chem. Inf. Comput. Sci.* **2001**, *41*(5), 1286–1294.

80. Khandelwal, A.; Lukacova, V.; Comez, D.; Kroll, D. M.; Raha, S.; Balaz, S. A combination of docking, QM/MM methods, and MD simulation for binding affinity estimation of metalloprotein ligands. *J. Med. Chem.* **2005**, *48*(17), 5437–5447.

81. Klahn, M.; Braun-Sand, S.; Rosta, E.; Warshel, A. On possible pitfalls of ab initio quantum mechanics/molecular mechanics minimization approaches for studies of enzymatic reactions. *J. Phys. Chem. B* **2005**, *109*, 15645–15650.

82. Raha, K.; Merz, K. M., Jr. A quantum mechanics based scoring function: study of zinc-ion mediated ligand binding. *J. Am. Chem. Soc.* **2004**, *126*, 1020–1021.

83. Gogonea, V.; Merz, K. M., Jr. Fully quantum mechanical description of proteins in solution. combining linear scaling quantum mechanical methodologies with the Poisson-Boltzmann equation. *J. Phys. Chem. A* **1999**, *103*, 5171–5188.

84. Nikitina, E.; Sulimov, D.; Zayets, V.; Zaitseva, N. Semiempirical calculations of binding enthalpy for protein-ligand complexes. *Int. J. Quantum Chem.* **2004**, *97*(2), 747–763.

85. Vasilyev, V.; Bliznyuk, A. A. Application of semiempirical quantum chemical methods as a scoring function in docking. *Theor. Chem. Acc.* **2004**, *112*, 313–317.

86. Ohno, K.; Mitsuthoshi, W.; Saito, S.; Inoue, Y.; Sakurai, M. Quantum chemical study of the affinity maturation of 48g7 antibody. *Theor. Chem. Acc.* **2005**, *722*, 203–211.

87. Gao, A. M.; Zhang, D. W.; Zhang, J. Z. H.; Zhang, Y. K. An efficient linear scaling method for ab initio calculation of electron density of proteins. *Chem. Phys. Lett.* **2004**, *394*(4–6), 293–297.

88. Chen, X. H.; Zhang, J. Z. H. Theoretical method for full ab initio calculation of DNA/RNA-ligand interaction energy. *J. Chem. Phys.* **2004**, *120*, 11386–11391.

89. Fukuzawa, K.; Kitaura, K.; Uebayasi, M.; Nakata, K.; Kaminuma, T.; Nakano, T. Ab initio quantum mechanical study of the binding energies of human estrogen receptor alpha with its ligands: an application of fragment molecular orbital method. *J. Comput. Chem.* **2005**, *26*(1), 1–10.

90. He, X.; Mei, Y.; Xiang, Y.; Zhang, D. W.; Zhang, J. Z. H. Quantum computational analysis for drug resistance of HIV-1 reverse transcriptase to nevirapine through point mutations. *Proteins* **2005**, *61*(2), 423–432.

91. Raha, K.; Van Der Vaart, A. J.; Riley, K. E.; Peters, M. B.; Westerhoff, L. M.; Kim, H.; Merz, K. M., Jr. Pairwise decomposition of residue interaction energies using semiempirical quantum mechanical methods in studies of protein-ligand interaction. *J. Am. Chem. Soc.* **2005**, *127*(18), 6583–6594.

92. Ortiz, A. R.; Pisabarro, M. T.; Gago, F.; Wade, R. C. Prediction of drug-binding affinities by comparative binding-energy analysis. *J. Med. Chem.* **1995**, *38*(14), 2681–2691.

93. Peters, M. B.; Merz, K. M. Semiempirical comparative binding energy analysis (SE-COMBINE) of a series of trypsin inhibitors. *J. Chem. Theor. Comput.* **2006**, *2*(2), 383–399.

94. Karelson, M.; Lobanov, V. S.; Katritzky, A. R. Quantum-chemical descriptors in QSAR/QSPR studies. *Chem. Rev.* **1996**, *96*(3), 1027–1044.

95. Brüstle, M.; Beck, B.; Schindler, T.; King, W.; Mitchell, T.; Clark, T. Descriptors, physical properties, and drug-likeness. *J. Med. Chem.* **2002**, *45*, 3345–3355.

96. Wan, J.; Zhang, L.; Yang, G.; Zhan, C. Quantitative structure–activity relationship for cyclic imide derivatives of protoporphyrinogen oxidase inhibitors: a study of quantum chemical descriptors from density functional theory. *J. Chem. Inf. Comput. Sci.* **2004**, *44*, 2099–2105.

97. Cramer III, R. D.; Patterson, D. E.; Bunce, J. D. Comparative molecular field analysis (CoMFA). 1. Effect of shape on binding of steroids to carrier proteins. *J. Am. Chem. Soc.* **1988**, *110*, 5959–5967.

98. Klebe, G. Comparative molecular similarity indices: CoMSIA. In: *3D QSAR in Drug Design*, Vol. 3, Kubinyi, H.; Folkers, G.; Martin, Y. C.; Eds. London: Kluwer Academic; **1998**, 87.

99. Sutherland, J. J.; O'Brien, L. A.; Weaver, D. F. A comparison of methods for modeling quantitative structure-activity relationships. *J. Med. Chem.* **2004**, *47*, 5541–5554.

100. Dixon, S.; Merz, K. M., Jr.; Lauri, G.; Ianni, J. C. QMQSAR: utilization of a semiempirical probe potential in a field-based qsar method. *J. Comput. Chem.* **2005**, *26*, 23–34.

101. Turner, D. B.; Willett, P.; Ferguson, A. M.; Heritage, T. Evaluation of a novel infrared range vibration-based descriptor (EVA) for QSAR studies. 1. General application. *J. Comput. Aided Mol. Des.* **1997**, *11*(4), 409–422.

102. Tuppurainen, K. EEVA (electronic eigenvalue): A new QSAR/QSPR descriptor for electronic substituent effects based on molecular orbital energies. Sar and Qsar in *Environ. Res.* **1999**, *10*(1), 39–46.

103. Bursi, R.; Dao, T.; van Wijk, T.; de Gooyer, M.; Kellenbach, E.; Verwer, P. Comparative spectra analysis (CoSA): spectra as three-dimensional molecular descriptors for the prediction of biological activities. *J. Chem. Inf. Comput. Sci.* **1999**, *39*(5), 861–867.

104. Asikainen, A.; Ruuskanen, J.; Tuppurainen, K. Spectroscopic QSAR methods and self-organizing molecular field analysis for relating molecular structure and estrogenic activity. *J. Chem. Inf. Comput. Sci.* **2003**, *43*(6), 1974–1981.

105. Besalu, E.; Girones, X.; Amat, L.; Carbo-Dorca, R. Molecular quantum similarity and the fundamentals of QSAR. *Acc. Chem. Res.* **2002**, *35*, 289–295.

106. Carbó-Dorca, R.; Gironés, X. Foundation of quantum similarity measures and their relationship to QSPR: density function structure, approximations, and application examples. *Int. J. Quantum Chem.* **2005**, *101*, 8–20.

107. Bultinck, P.; Kuppens, T.; Gironés, X.; Carbó-Dorca, R. Quantum similarity superposition algorithm (QSSA): a consistent scheme for molecular alignment and molecular similarity based on quantum chemistry. *J. Chem. Inf. Comput. Sci.* **2003**, *43*, 1143–1150.

108. Fusti-Molnar, L.; Merz, K. M., Jr. An efficient and accurate molecular alignment and docking technique using ab initio quality scoring. *J. Chem. Phys.* **2008**, *129*, 25102–25113.

109. O'Brien, S. E.; Popelier, P. L. A. Quantum molecular similarity. 3. QTMS descriptors. *J. Chem. Inf. Comput. Sci.* **2001**, *41*, 764–775.

110. Chaudry, U. A.; Popelier, P. L. A. Estimation of pK_a using quantum topological molecular similarity descriptors: application to carboxylic acids, anilines and phenols. *J. Org. Chem.* **2004**, *69*, 233–241.

9

Pharmacophore methods

Steven L. Dixon

INTRODUCTION

Paul Ehrlich introduced the pharmacophore concept in the early 1900s while studying the efficacy of dyes and other compounds as potential chemotherapeutic agents. By analogy with chromophores and toxophores, Ehrlich suggested the term *pharmacophore* to refer to the molecular framework that carries (*phoros*) the features that are essential for the biological activity of a drug (*pharmacon*).[1] The modern, widely accepted definition was offered by Peter Gund in 1977: "a set of structural features in a molecule that is recognized at the receptor site and is responsible for that molecule's biological activity."[2] In practice, the modern definition is implicitly restricted to cover only specific, noncovalent interactions between a molecule and receptor. Thus a pharmacophore model is not concerned with binding that occurs solely as a result of short-lived surface-to-surface hydrophobic interactions, nor binding that involves the formation of covalent bonds.

Although a pharmacophore model codifies the key interactions between a ligand and its biological target, neither the structure of the target nor even its identity is required to develop a useful pharmacophore model. For this reason, pharmacophore methods are often considered to be indispensable when the available information is very limited, for example, when one knows nothing more than the structures of a handful of actives.[3] However, pharmacophore approaches can also be vital for accelerating discovery efforts when more extensive data are available by providing a means of superimposing structures for 3D quantitative structure/activity relationship (QSAR) development,[4–7] or by acting as a rapid prefilter[8] on real or virtual libraries that are too large for routine treatment with more expensive structure-based techniques, such as docking.

Pharmacophore methods actually comprise a fairly broad range of computer-aided approaches, including, but not limited to, automated pharmacophore perception,[7,9,10] structure alignment,[11,12] identification and representation of sterically forbidden regions,[13,14] 3D similarity based on pharmacophore fingerprints,[15–18] and 3D database screening.[2,19–21] This chapter will cover the essential elements of these and other concepts that arise in the development and application of pharmacophore-based methodologies. For additional information and numerous examples, readers are referred to other excellent reviews and compendia.[22–27]

HISTORY AND EVOLUTION OF PHARMACOPHORE METHODS

For decades before modern pharmacophore methods emerged as tools in drug discovery, chemists instinctively sought reliable hypotheses to explain the activity of both naturally occurring and human-made ligands of a given biological target. Elucidation of what makes a class of ligands active is of course critical to the discovery of new compounds with affinity for the same target, along with other desirable properties (novel structure, superior absorption, lower toxicity, etc.). Application of these ideas in an automated fashion and on a large scale became possible in the 1970s, when high-level programming languages such as FORTRAN were increasingly in use in academic settings, paving the way for development of numerous computer-assisted techniques in chemistry.

In pioneering work in the early 1970s, Peter Gund introduced concepts to describe the presentation of 3D chemical features in a manner complementary to the receptor and identified the variability of the atoms that can perform the same pharmacophoric function and the variability in the distances among chemical features.[2,28] These concepts provided the foundation of what is now commonly referred to as "3D searching" and were used to develop the first software to search chemical structure files for matches to pharmacophoric patterns.

Although Gund's work answered critical questions about the feasibility of pharmacophore pattern matching, the fundamental problem of deducing plausible pharmacophore models from a set of flexible ligands remained. A number of methods have emerged to address this issue,[7,9–12,21,29–31] but the active analog approach[3] developed in the late 1970s is among the earliest and best known techniques. In practical applications, a set of torsion angles common to all ligands is systematically varied using a grid search, and various constraints are applied to limit the conformational space explored (Figure 9.1). Each combination of torsion angles produces a geometric arrangement of n pharmacophoric features, which is described by the set of

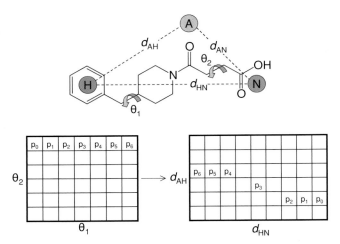

Figure 9.1. Schematic illustration of the active analog approach.[3] A set of torsion angles common to all ligands is systematically varied, and the resulting interfeature distances are tabulated. Common pharmacophores are identified by intersecting the interfeature distance tables from all ligands.

$[n(n-1)]/2$ distances between all pairs of features. Interfeature distances for each ligand are tabulated as a function of its torsion angles, and common pharmacophores are identified by intersecting the interfeature distance tables from all ligands.

In the mid-1980s, Sheridan and coworkers[29] reported an alternate approach, which employed distance geometry techniques[32] to sample the low-energy conformational space of a set of ligands, while constraining interpoint distances among a set of pharmacophore features present in all the ligands. Their "ensemble distance geometry" method was presented in the context of nicotinic receptor agonists and was restricted to consider only three essential interactions with the receptor, although in principle it can be extended to any number of chemical features and distances, provided those features are stipulated at the outset.

The active analog approach and ensemble distance geometry provided solutions to a difficult problem, but neither was easily generalized to arbitrary sets of ligands, and a great deal of input was required from the user for each new data set. This frustration led Yvonne Martin to investigate ways to fully automate the process, which resulted in the development of DISCO (DIStance COmparisons).[9] Starting with a set of precomputed low-energy conformers for each active, DISCO selects as a "reference" the ligand with the fewest conformers and then compares each of its conformers to all conformers of the other actives. A fast clique-detection algorithm[33] is used to identify distance-based arrangements of pharmacophore features in a given reference conformer that also exist, to within some tolerance, in at least one conformer of every other ligand. If no solutions are found, matching tolerances can be increased, or the number of ligands that are required to contain the pharmacophore can be decreased. In principle, then, DISCO identifies common feature pharmacophores for an arbitrary set of

ligands represented by an arbitrary set of conformers, with fairly minimal input from the user. However, one shortcoming in the original implementation is that it did not assign a ranking or score to each solution, which can be somewhat bewildering when a data set yields many common pharmacophore models.

CATALYST/HIPHOP[10] was developed in the mid-1990s with the goal of not only identifying common pharmacophores among flexible ligands but also ascribing to each pharmacophore model an empirically calibrated "rarity" to reflect the likelihood that it will be found in random drug-like molecules. In short, rarity is estimated to be higher for pharmacophores with larger numbers of features, a greater variety of features, particularly those of an ionic nature, and larger interfeature distances. A pharmacophore with high rarity is preferred because it is more likely to be unique to the actives and therefore a more plausible model of selective binding.[21]

HIPHOP carries out a pruned, exhaustive search, which identifies all common two-feature pharmacophores within sets of precomputed ligand conformers, builds on those to produce common three-feature pharmacophores, and so on. HIPHOP allows features to be "missed" by certain ligands, so a given model produced by HIPHOP may not be a true common feature pharmacophore but rather a *union of features* pharmacophore. This relaxation in matching is prized by many users because it increases the chances that *something* will be found, even for a set of fairly diverse ligands. However, care must be exercised to avoid imposing a single pharmacophore model on ligands that are associated with different binding modes, a situation the user is frequently unaware of.

Although CATALYST has enjoyed a great deal of commercial success, HIPHOP is sometimes criticized for failing to yield the most sensible ligand alignments,[34] in part because it incorporates no mechanism for superimposing atoms that are not part of the pharmacophore. GASP (Genetic Algorithm Superposition Program)[11] overcomes this problem by including a volume overlap term in the pharmacophore fitness function, which favors alignments that provide superior superpositions of overall shape. Pharmacophore perception is done in the context of a genetic algorithm,[35] where a chromosome encodes the torsion angles within a set of N ligands, and the mapping of the pharmacophore features in a *base* ligand (the one with the fewest features) to features in the other $N-1$ ligands. Alignments and potential pharmacophores are determined by the common set of mapped features that can be closely aligned, and the overall fitness is a weighted combination of the overlapping volume, a similarity score based on the number and similarity of overlaid features, and the van der Waals energies of the structures. Execution of the GASP algorithm yields a single nondeterministic solution pharmacophore, so the algorithm is typically run many times with different random starting conditions, to produce different pharmacophore models and alignments, all ranked by fitness. The drawback, of course, is that an exhaustive search of pharmacophore space is not done, so any number of valid solutions can be missed.

It is important to recognize that all of the aforementioned methods are designed to operate on relatively small numbers of high-affinity ligands, yet there is sometimes a need to make sense of data arising from hundreds or thousands of heterogeneous compounds of varying activity. In the mid- to late 1990s, recursive partitioning[36] was increasingly recognized for its ability to identify patterns in complex chemical data,[37–41] and pharmacophore-based analysis of large data sets was a natural application for this technique. SCAMPI (Statistical Classification of Activities of Molecules for Pharmacophore Identification)[42] leverages the power of recursive partitioning to construct decision trees that subdivide compounds according to their activities and the pharmacophores they contain. Each node in a tree adds a feature to a pharmacophore from a parent node, and compounds are split into left and right child branches according to whether they contain the proposed pharmacophore. Experimental activities are incorporated into the process to ensure that a given splitting condition yields a statistically significant separation of compounds into less active and more active groups. Addition of features to a particular branch terminates when further separation by activity cannot be achieved. A SCAMPI decision tree produces a number of pharmacophores, usually containing two or three features, which rationalize the observed activities and suggest possible binding modes.

More recently developed pharmacophore perception methods include GALAHAD[12] and PHASE.[7] GALAHAD improves and extends methodologies introduced in GASP by incorporating a multiobjective Pareto scoring function to balance pharmacophore consensus, shape consensus, and conformational energy, while relaxing the requirement that every ligand match all features in the pharmacophore. PHASE provides exhaustive exploration of common pharmacophore space by way of a novel distance-based partitioning algorithm and takes an eclectic approach to scoring with user-adjustable terms to optimize alignment and orientation of features, shape overlap, pharmacophore selectivity, reference ligand conformational energy, and reference ligand activity.

Finally, it should be noted that the past three decades have seen the emergence of numerous other important pharmacophore-based systems, including ALADDIN,[43] DANTE,[21] CAVEAT,[44] APEX-3D,[31] and CHEM-X,[18] to name just a few. Many of the principles on which these systems are based are used routinely in other software packages and will be covered in subsequent sections of this chapter.

PHARMACOPHORE MODEL DEVELOPMENT

Pharmacophore models are created using a variety of methods and workflows, including manual construction, automated perception from ligand structure alone, and receptor-based inference from a crystallographic structure. The particular method or workflow used depends on any

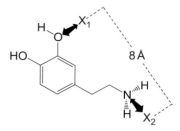

Figure 9.2. Dopamine D_2 agonist pharmacophore model from Seeman et al.[45] Two receptor sites, X_1 and X_2, separated by about 8Å, form hydrogen bonds to an acceptor and a basic center, respectively, on the ligand.

number of factors, including the amount and quality of available experimental data, computational resources, and the ultimate goals and expectations placed on the pharmacophore model itself. The next several sections are concerned with the methodological details and applicability of these different approaches to pharmacophore model development.

MANUAL CONSTRUCTION

The simplest and probably the most widely employed method to create a pharmacophore model is to construct it by hand, using the structure of a known active or based on general characteristics of known actives. Figure 9.2 illustrates the classic Seeman model[45] of dopamine D_2 agonists, which consists of an aromatic ring bearing a hydrogen bond acceptor and a basic nitrogen that form hydrogen bonds with complementary receptor sites X_1 and X_2, respectively, which are separated by about 8Å. In practical applications, such as 3D searching, one would normally designate some variability in the distances between pharmacophore features, or positional tolerances that constrain how far a matching feature may deviate from the corresponding feature in the model after an alignment is performed. Depending on the software used, it may also be possible to define tolerances on the orientation of features, such as a range in the allowed angles between the hydrogen bond acceptor axis and the plane of the ring.

A manually constructed pharmacophore can be quite advantageous, particularly if it's derived from the x-ray structure of a ligand or from a ligand with a rigid backbone. In either case, the locations of pharmacophore features are essentially pinned down, so one of the biggest uncertainties in pharmacophore model development, conformational flexibility, is eliminated. There is still the question of the particular features to incorporate in the model, which is not always easy to infer without additional information, such as the structure of a ligand/receptor complex, activities from a well-designed SAR series, or data from mutagenesis experiments.

AUTOMATED PERCEPTION FROM LIGAND STRUCTURE

A review of the available methods for automated perception of common pharmacophores has already been provided, so the details of each method shall not be repeated here. Rather, the basic tasks that are common to most or all of these methods are presented, with a discussion of various alternatives for achieving a given task and, where applicable, any recognized standard in the field.

PREPARING LIGANDS

Identification of the correct spatial relationships among key ligand/receptor interaction points is ultimately governed by the accuracy of the structures from which pharmacophore models are derived. Thus once an appropriate set of ligands has been identified, realistic models of 3D chemical structure must be developed. Doing so requires not only a procedure for generating a set of low-energy conformers for each ligand but also decisions about ionization and tautomeric states and appropriate treatment of stereochemistry.

Methods for sampling the thermally accessible conformational states of a ligand is a topic that deserves far more attention than can be paid here, but in the context of pharmacophore methods, conformational sampling techniques are usually divided into two classes: those that are appropriate for pharmacophore model development and those that are appropriate for searching large 3D databases. Pharmacophore software frequently provides separate methods to address each of these situations, with thorough sampling and full minimization of structures being done[46,47] for pharmacophore model development and faster, less rigorous approaches[48-50] being used for large databases.

When developing a pharmacophore model from a set of actives, the goal of conformer generation is to produce an ensemble of structures that each ligand can adopt under biological conditions, with a granularity fine enough to ensure that at least one structure is reasonably close to the bioactive conformation. Whether this can be achieved depends on both the initial set of structures generated and the force field (or Hamiltonian) that's employed to minimize them. If the initial sample contains no structure sufficiently close to the bioactive conformation, it is unlikely that subsequent minimization will dramatically improve the situation. Conversely, even if the initial sample contains a reasonable facsimile of the bioactive structure, an inferior force field may drive that structure to a somewhat distant local minimum. As noted previously, pharmacophore packages frequently provide a means for conformer generation, but MacroModel MCMM (Monte Carlo Multiple Minimum)[46] is generally recognized as a standard for thorough exploration and sampling of conformational states along a given potential energy surface, while MMFF (Merck Molecular Force Field)[51] and OPLS (Optimized Potential for Liquid Simulations)[52] are routinely used for energetics and minimization.

A structure's stability and interactions with the receptor are affected by its ionic character, so identification of ionic centers in a ligand is an important consideration. When there is a priori knowledge about the correct ionization state (e.g., a particular secondary amine in the structure is known to be protonated), it is common practice to assign ionization states explicitly based on that knowledge. In other cases, software may be called on to either neutralize all ligands or assign the most probable ionization states based on a set of rules.[53] Whether one starts with neutral or ionized structures is less of an issue when the pharmacophore feature mapping procedure automatically recognizes ionizable centers even if they are expressed in neutral form.

It is worth noting that although docking software routinely generates multiple ionic states for each ligand, doing so within the context of common pharmacophore perception is not a trivial matter. The difficulty stems from the fact that each ligand and its conformers are normally associated with only a single connection table (i.e., the set of atoms and the bonds that connect them), which allows a single set of mappings to be defined between the atoms and the pharmacophore features in a given ligand. When additional ionic states are introduced, each has a different connection table, which requires additional sets of atom→feature mappings, not to mention additional sets of conformers. When perceiving common pharmacophores, then, somewhat arbitrary decisions may be required regarding which ionic form to report for a given parent ligand when a pharmacophore is matched equally well by child structures with different ionization states.

Tautomerization raises many of the same questions as ionization, although less attention is normally paid to this issue, in part because the most commonly recognized tautomeric states are usually just assumed (keto preferred over enol, amide preferred over amidic acid, etc.). There are certainly cases where the location of a proton may be less obvious (e.g., imidazoles, pyrazoles, and triazoles), so if a particular choice is made, the possible consequences should be considered. For example, if a pharmacophore model contains a hydrogen bond donor feature that maps to a proton whose location is in question, one may wish to give equal consideration to the corresponding model that results when the proton is moved to an equally probable location. As in the case of ionization states, a more general treatment of tautomers requires a means for dealing with different connection tables and their associated atom→feature mappings and conformers.

From a mechanical perspective, treating different stereoisomers of a given parent ligand is somewhat less challenging because their structures can share a single connection table. Consequently, their conformers may be readily combined and treated as a single ligand if necessary. Thus if a pair of enantiomers has been resolved and the activities of both isomers are known, they can, and should, be treated as separate ligands. But if the observed activity is based on a racemate, the most sensible approach is to merge the conformers from the two enantiomers. If one enantiomer is far less active than the other, as is often the case, and the data set contains other ligands whose stereochemistry is not in question, the structures of the

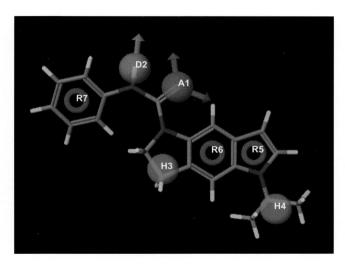

Figure 9.3. Placement of pharmacophoric features on a serotonin antagonist using the default feature mapping rules in Phase 3.0.[7,55]

latter may automatically impose restrictions that eliminate conformers from the less active enantiomer. Nevertheless, indeterminate stereochemistry should always be considered an impediment to pharmacophore perception and should be avoided if possible.

MAPPING PHARMACOPHORE FEATURES

Assigning the locations of potential interaction sites on the ligand is the most fundamental aspect of automated pharmacophore perception. An omission or inconsistency at this stage can prevent the identification of the correct common pharmacophore model and sometimes the identification of common pharmacophores altogether. Therefore, it is critical to recognize all of the ways each ligand may bind to a receptor, which in turn requires a comprehensive set of feature-mapping rules, with some level of customizability to accommodate addition of new rules and modification of existing rules.

The typical types of interaction sites recognized by pharmacophore software include hydrogen bond acceptor (A), hydrogen bond donor (D), hydrophobic (H), negative ionic/ionizable (N), and positive ionic/ionizable (P). The term *ionic/ionizable* refers to centers that are explicitly ionized or are very likely to be ionized under biological conditions, such as carboxylic acids. Some packages provide a separate category for aromatic rings (R) to distinguish them from aliphatic rings, which are typically treated as hydrophobic centers. Figure 9.3 illustrates the placement of various pharmacophoric features on a serotonin receptor antagonist[54] using version 3.0 of PHASE,[7,55] with its default feature-mapping rules.

Many rules can be encoded in the form of a *feature dictionary*, which associates a set of atoms or fragments with a specific type of pharmacophoric feature. For convenience and customizability, feature dictionaries are usually implemented by way of atom typing schemes and/or one-

dimensional chemical structure syntax, such as Sybyl Line Notation[56] or SMARTS.[57] For example, the SMARTS pattern "[#1][O;X2]" matches all hydroxyl groups and thus might be included in a hydrogen bond donor feature dictionary. However, such a general rule requires restrictions to prevent application where improper, such as the hydroxyl group of a carboxylic acid that has been provided in neutral form. Accordingly, a SMARTS pattern of the form "[#1]OC(=O)" could be employed as a rule for excluding carboxylic acids as hydrogen bond donors.

To express directionality in hydrogen bonding features, a vector attribute may be assigned using an explicit mathematical construct, as in Figure 9.4(a), or by including two points in the feature [Figure 9.4(b)]. Directionality may be relaxed altogether by mapping features as pure projected points [Figure 9.4(c)]. The advantage of using pure projected points is that it can model the situation where two ligands form hydrogen bonds to the same receptor site but from different directions.

Ionic features are normally assigned to acidic and basic groups that are likely to be dissociated at biological pH, even if the structures are provided in neutral form. The location of an ionic feature may coincide with a single atom, such as the nitrogen in an ammonium ion, or it may be located at the centroid of atoms that share the ionic charge, such as the oxygens in a carboxylate ion or the nitrogens in an amidinium ion. Because ionic groups frequently form hydrogen bonds with the receptor, some users prefer to model negative and positive groups as hydrogen bond acceptors and donors, respectively. However, in the context of identifying common pharmacophores, one can argue that there is no real advantage to the acceptor/donor treatment, because there is usually not enough information to distinguish, for example, which oxygen in a carboxylate is forming a hydrogen bond. There is also the question of whether neutral and ionic groups are likely to form hydrogen bonds to the same receptor site. For example, should one give credence to a pharmacophore model that overlays a pyridine nitrogen from one ligand with a carboxylate oxygen from another? This is a question the user ultimately must answer, but it is important to recognize that in the absence of receptor information, certain assumptions may offer no actual benefit.

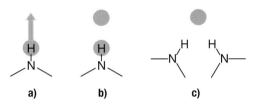

Figure 9.4. Different conventions used to represent hydrogen bonding features. Directionality may be expressed by associating an explicit vector construct with the feature **(a)** or by including two points **(b)**. Use of pure projected points **(c)** models the situation where two ligands form hydrogen bonds to the same receptor site but approach from different directions.

Not all types of pharmacophore features are easily encoded using a fragment dictionary alone. Hydrophobic character, in particular, is not readily identified with any small number of fragments or patterns, and so special techniques are usually called on to assign hydrophobic centers within rings and aliphatic chains of arbitrary length. The method described by Greene et al.[20] has been adopted in HipHop,[10] SCAMPI,[42] and Phase[7] and could therefore be considered a standard in the field. Briefly, rings, isopropyl groups, t-butyl groups, and chains as long as four carbons are treated as a single hydrophobic feature. Chains of five or more carbons are broken into smaller fragments containing between two and four carbons, with each fragment designated as a separate hydrophobic feature. The location r_H of each hydrophobic feature is an average of the positions r_i of the non n-hydrogen atoms in the associated fragment, with each atom weighted by its solvent-accessible surface area s_i and an empirically assigned hydrophobicity factor t_i that ranges between 0 and 1:

$$\mathbf{r}_H = \frac{\sum\limits_i s_i t_i r_i}{\sum\limits_i s_i t_i}.$$

The resulting position is thus skewed in the direction of atoms with greater exposed surface area and away from atoms with greater polarity.

One final note is that the locations of two different types of pharmacophore features may be coincident or nearly coincident. For example, it is common practice to map aromatic rings as both H and R. This allows common pharmacophores to be found if a key interaction incorporates an aliphatic group in some ligands but an aromatic ring in others. Yet it does not eliminate the possibility that an aromatic ring may be required in every ligand to facilitate an interaction that involves pi stacking.

PERCEIVING COMMON PHARMACOPHORES

Although each common pharmacophore identification method discussed previously contains unique characteristics, several of them incorporate an exhaustive or semiexhaustive enumeration of potential common pharmacophores. Doing so almost invariably leads to the use of an interfeature distance representation [Figure 9.5(a)]. By working with interfeature distances, it is possible to compare two pharmacophores without explicitly superimposing them. Superposition normally involves a least squares alignment of points,[58,59] which is far more expensive computationally than simply comparing the distances. Note, however, that close correspondence of interfeature distances is a necessary, but not sufficient, condition for close correspondence of superimposed features. As shown in Figure 9.5(b), pharmacophores that are mirror images exhibit the same interfeature distances, but they may not superimpose well. Consequently, any algorithm that uses interfeature distances to perceive common pharmacophores must

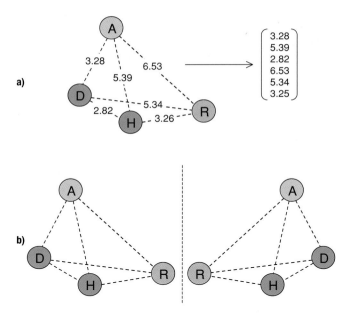

Figure 9.5. (a) Interfeature distance representation of a four-point pharmacophore. **(b)** Mirror image pharmacophores contain the same interfeature distances but may not superimpose well.

be followed by a superposition step to screen out spurious solutions.

To account for ligand flexibility and differences in chemical scaffolds, tolerances must be built into the procedure that matches or associates common pharmacophores. For example, the distance between an acceptor and a hydrophobe may be 5.2Å in one ligand but 5.5Å in another ligand; any sensible algorithm would consider these to be the same. The manner in which tolerances are incorporated depends on how pharmacophore space is explored.

When pharmacophores are enumerated from a single reference ligand, such as in DISCO, a user-defined tolerance may be used to identify arrangements of pharmacophoric features in other ligands that exhibit the same interfeature distances, plus or minus the tolerance. Treating all ligands equivalently, though, requires other means to identify common arrangements. If the number of features in the pharmacophore is relatively small, an analytical approach[21,30] may be practical for determining an exact intersection of interfeature distances from the conformationally accessible space of a set of ligands (Figure 9.6). In other cases,[7,18] interfeature distance space may be formally represented as a set of overlapping bins, into which the pharmacophores from each ligand are mapped. Bins with predefined spacing are readily encoded as a bit string,[18] so common pharmacophores may be identified from bits that are set by all ligands. Alternatively, bins of successively finer granularity may be constructed in a hierarchical manner,[7] with elimination of large regions of interfeature distance space, and many potential mappings, when those regions cannot yield a common pharmacophore (Figure 9.7).

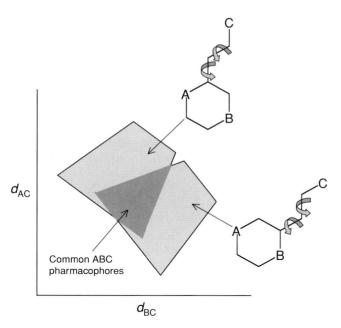

Figure 9.6. Identification of common three-point pharmacophores by intersection of the conformationally accessible spaces of two ligands.[30]

SCORING PHARMACOPHORES

A set of ligands for a given receptor frequently share a single chemical scaffold, which typically affords any number of common pharmacophores that must be screened out because they fail to encode the precise interactions that are essential for activity. Even when the ligands comprise different scaffolds, the enumeration procedure may still find many uninteresting arrangements of features that are unlikely to represent models of specific binding and/or that are ubiquitous in chemical compound space (e.g., three hydrobobes separated by a few angstroms). Yet other arrangements of features may impose an unrealistic superposition of chemical features that are not contained in the pharmacophore, such as a long, hydrophobic tail in one ligand being overlaid with a carboxylate in another. It is desirable, therefore, to be able to assess the quality of each pharmacophore using a scoring method that embodies one or more of these considerations.

The notion of selectivity is central to the scoring functions used in CATALYST/HIPHOP[10] and DANTE,[21] and it is incorporated as a user-weighted term in PHASE.[7] Though the approaches taken are somewhat different, the objective in each is to promote pharmacophores that are more likely to be unique to the ligands being analyzed. A key quantity to minimize, then, is the probability q that a given pharmacophore will be contained in structures of randomly chosen druglike molecules. Although a meaningful estimate of q may be obtained by searching a large medicinal chemistry database for matches to the pharmacophore in question, it is simply not practical to do so when scoring a large number of common pharmacophores. Instead, q is normally approximated using either tabulated data[21] or an empirical probability function that is calibrated using statistics from a large number of pharmacophore searches.[10]

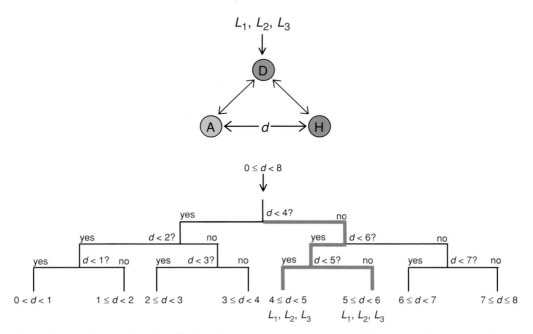

Figure 9.7. Algorithm used by Phase[7] to identify common pharmacophores. In this example, three ligands, L_1, L_2, L_3, are analyzed for instances of three-point pharmacophores containing the features A, D, H. The A–H distance is partitioned through a successively finer tree to identify distance ranges that are observed in at least one conformer from every ligand (green branches). Subtrees that cannot yield a common pharmacophore (black branches) are never traversed.

Closely related to selectivity is the ability of a pharmacophore to distinguish actives from inactives when the two classes of compounds are structurally similar and/or come from the same structure/activity series. A tacit assumption here is that the inactive compounds fail to bind because they lack one or more key features not because of steric clashes with the receptor, poor solubility, or other factors that cannot be explained by the pharmacophore model itself. SCAMPI[42] builds pharmacophore models, feature by feature, incorporating a Student's t-test on the separation of actives and inactives directly into the feature selection process. APEX-3D[31] identifies pharmacophores common to the most active compounds using clique detection and then employs Bayesian statistics to eliminate pharmacophores whose frequencies in the active and inactive populations are not sufficiently different. CATALYST/HYPOGEN[6] constructs a series of HIPHOP pharmacophore models from the most active compounds in a training set, eliminates those that are found in more than half of the inactives, and then refines each model by adding, subtracting, and moving features so the degree to which each compound fits the pharmacophore correlates with experimental activity. Thus all of these methods use activity to drive development of pharmacophore models that can distinguish actives and inactives, while discarding those that do not. PHASE[7] uses a more passive approach, scoring each common pharmacophore model according to how well it matches a set of known inactives but ultimately deferring to the user the decision about which pharmacophores are most relevant.

Reasonable superposition of the ligand features that map to a common pharmacophore model is normally a given, but this does not guarantee that the ligand structures themselves or their overall superpositions will be satisfactory. A number of pharmacophore development approaches[7,11,12,29,60] incorporate a procedure for eliminating or penalizing unrealistic high-energy structures, although methods that accept external conformers[7,9,10,31] will accomplish essentially the same objective if an appropriate energy filter is applied to the conformers before they are supplied. To achieve consensus in the alignment of chemical features that do not contribute to the pharmacophore, the scoring process may favor conformers that match the pharmacophore and yield superior overlap of molecular volumes throughout each ligand structure.[7,11] Volumes may be distinguished by atom type to help ensure that chemically similar fragments in different ligands are superimposed.[7]

RECEPTOR-BASED PHARMACOPHORE MODELS

Previous sections focused on the identification of common feature pharmacophores within flexible ligand structures, which is often a necessary exercise in the absence of crystallographic data. But when explicit knowledge of the receptor binding site is available, it can be a tremendous advantage in pharmacophore model development. Though it is certainly possible to visually inspect a ligand/receptor complex to identify key interactions, and manually construct a pharmacophore model that encodes those interactions, automated procedures to achieve this task are in high demand. A number of important receptor-based pharmacophore techniques have been reported involving ligand docking,[61,62] fragment docking,[63,64] and molecular dynamics simulations,[65,66] but this section is concerned primarily with methodologies that provide an alternative to what are essentially products of structure-based and de novo design.

A fundamental step in developing a receptor-based pharmacophore model is an analysis of the binding site to identify potential interaction points. In structure-based focusing,[67] a sphere with user-adjustable location and radius is used to mark key residues in the binding site, and a LUDI[68] interaction map is generated to describe favorable interactions in which a ligand is expected to engage. The interaction map is translated to an interaction model, which consists of a set of complementary points in the binding pocket, representing possible locations of pharmacophore features on the ligand. A user-defined density controls the number of points created, but it is usually quite large, so hierarchical clustering is performed to select a smaller number of representative points, typically on the order of a dozen. Normally, this is still too many interaction points for a single ligand, so a series of pharmacophore models containing subsets of the representative features is constructed, with restrictions on minimum and maximum separations between points. Excluded volumes (see next section) are added to each model to represent the receptor surface, and a 3D database of known actives is searched to determine which pharmacophore models are most frequently matched.

LIGANDSCOUT[69] takes a somewhat more direct approach, deriving a pharmacophore model from a single ligand/receptor complex. After perceiving hybridization, unsaturated bonds, and aromatic rings, the resulting ligand structure is analyzed for the presence of features encoding hydrogen bonding, hydrophobic character, and charge transfer. Features are mapped in general accordance with CATALYST rules, with customization to allow certain atoms to be associated with more than one type of pharmacophoric feature. Whether a feature is incorporated into the pharmacophore model depends on its location relative to a complementary site on the receptor. For example, a hydrogen bond donor is included if the associated heavy atom X is 2.5–3.8Å from an acceptor atom Y in the receptor and the X−H−Y angle is within 34° of colinearity. Incorporation of hydrophobic and ionic features, which are nondirectional, depends only on a user-defined distance range from a compatible interaction site on the receptor. If the receptor site is hydrophobic, a steric constraint is added to the pharmacophore model by creating a series of excluded volume spheres in the vicinity. A LIGANDSCOUT model normally needs some manual refinement (removal of features, addition of excluded volumes) to improve its hit rate and selectivity toward known actives.[70]

EXCLUDED VOLUMES

An accurate pharmacophore model represents a set of necessary, but not sufficient, conditions for specific, high-affinity binding to a given receptor. Thus a molecule may be capable of presenting a set of features in a manner that is entirely consistent with the pharmacophore yet still fails to bind. One possible reason is that some portion of the molecule would experience a steric clash with the receptor if it were to bind in the mode described by the pharmacophore model. Excluded volumes are designed to emulate this situation by indicating regions of space that a structure may not occupy when it is aligned to the pharmacophore.

A crystallographic receptor structure[13] is by far the most reliable source of excluded volumes, even conceding induced fit effects.[71–73] Receptor-based excluded volumes are most naturally represented as spheres centered on appropriate atoms in and around the binding site, with sizes dictated by the associated atomic van der Waals radii [Figure 9.8(a)]. A hard-sphere approximation is normally made, so a violation occurs whenever a molecule occupies the same volume as any receptor atom. This approximation may be too harsh if the conformational sampling in a 3D database is inadequate to produce a structure that will fit entirely within the binding pocket, so some sort of relaxation is required in such cases to accommodate a degree of penetration into the receptor surface. Relaxation may be accomplished by reducing the size of the excluded volume spheres, by eliminating spheres that are too close to a bound ligand, or by tolerating a certain amount of overlap between the molecule and the excluded volumes.

When the receptor structure is unavailable, as is often the case, assigning meaningful locations of excluded volumes is less straightforward because it's difficult to verify their correctness. One approach is to simply assume that the ligands themselves reflect the overall shape of the binding pocket and can therefore be used to guide the placement of excluded volumes. For example, the "Shrink-Wrap" method[14] analyzes the surfaces of one or more ligands superimposed on a pharmacophore model and constructs a series of solid angles that are pieced together to form a continuous envelope that encloses the ligands. When searching a 3D database, an analogous surface is created for each structure matching the pharmacophore, and the interpenetration of the two surfaces is computed. If the Shrink-Wrap surface of the matching structure lies entirely within the Shrink-Wrap surface of the ligand(s), or if the amount of clashing volume is within a user-defined threshold, then the matching structure is accepted.

A more simplistic approach[7] is to define a grid of points to surround one or more aligned ligands and place an excluded volume sphere at each point sufficiently far from the van der Waals surface of the ligands. Figure 9.8(b)

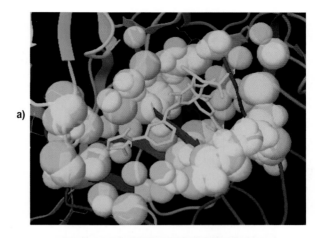

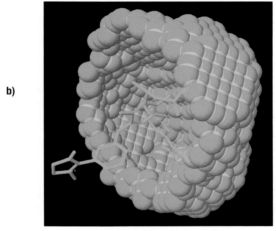

Figure 9.8. (a) Excluded volumes created from protein atoms within 5Å of the bound ligand in the Factor Xa complex 1fjs. **(b)** Cutaway view of an excluded volume shell created using only the structure of the 1fjs ligand.

contains a cutaway view to illustrate the placement of 1Å spheres on a 1Å grid, with a 2Å buffer between the molecular and excluded volume surfaces. The sphere radii and the grid spacing may be reduced to achieve any desired smoothness and precision in the excluded volume shell.

Perhaps the most elusive goal is to infer the locations of excluded volumes from a set of known inactives. The basic assumption normally made is that if one has a sufficiently correct pharmacophore model, and an inactive closely matches that model, there is a good chance that its lack of activity is due to a clash with the receptor. This could be a poor assumption, of course, but continuing with that line of reasoning, regions of space that are occupied only by inactives may therefore be considered as candidate locations for excluded volumes. Many packages allow manual placement of excluded volumes, so a user can visually inspect a set of aligned structures and create spheres at the desired locations. Automated methods are also available to perform this task,[7,74,75] though a healthy level of skepticism should always be exercised, and it is generally not wise to summarily reject a structure simply because it clashes with excluded volumes derived from inactive structures.

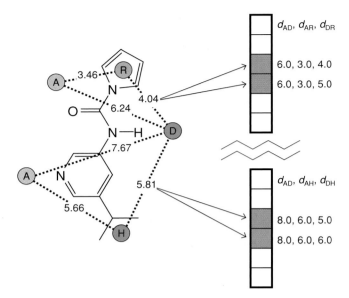

d_{AD}, d_{AR}, d_{DR}

6.0, 3.0, 4.0

6.0, 3.0, 5.0

d_{AD}, d_{AH}, d_{DH}

8.0, 6.0, 5.0

8.0, 6.0, 6.0

Figure 9.9. Encoding of pharmacophore triplets into a bit string with distance bins that are 1Å wide. To prevent loss of information due to the partitioning of distances, each triplet sets not only the bit whose midpoint is closest to the distances in that triplet but also neighboring bits in each distance dimension. For simplicity, neighboring bits are shown for only the last dimension in each triplet.

PHARMACOPHORE FINGERPRINTS

A summary of the pharmacophoric information contained in a structure may be represented in the form of a bit string that encodes the presence, absence, and sometimes the counts of various arrangements of pharmacophore features. These bit strings are referred to by various names, including pharmacophore fingerprints, pharmacophore keys, and pharmacophore tuplets.[15–17] The CHEM-X software system[18] is most closely identified with this concept, though many other packages contain their own implementations.

Pharmacophore fingerprints are usually based on either triplets of features (three-point pharmacophores) or quartets of features (four-point pharmacophores). Each bit in a fingerprint corresponds to a particular set of n pharmacophoric feature types (acceptor, donor, hydrophobe, etc.) separated by a specific set of $[n(n-1)]/2$ interfeature distances. To limit the number of distinct bits, the distance coordinate is divided into bins of predefined width, so a range of distances, and thus a range of pharmacophores, is mapped to a single bit. The bins may be of unequal width to allow greater discrimination in certain regions of the distance coordinate, and the upper limit bin may be defined to include all distances greater than some value, or it may simply ignore distances above that value.[18]

Figure 9.9 illustrates the encoding of pharmacophore triplets into a bit string characterized by distance bins that are 1Å wide. To prevent loss of information due to the partitioning of distances, a given triplet sets not only

the bit whose midpoint is closest to the distances in that triplet but also neighboring bits in each distance dimension. Observe that certain combinations of distances are physically impossible,[2,4,10] so many bits will never be set.

A pharmacophore fingerprint may be created from a conformational ensemble, so it represents the pharmacophore space that is conformationally accessible to a particular molecule. The fingerprint is normally a logical OR (i.e., the union) of the bits set by different conformers, so information to map individual bits back to their source conformers is not retained. Whether a pharmacophore fingerprint comes from a single structure or multiple conformers, it may be used in precisely the same manner as 2D bit string representations[76–79] in applications involving similarity, diversity, clustering, and so on.[80–84]

Pharmacophore fingerprints are perhaps most powerful when used in the context of 3D database screening. When a pharmacophore query is posed, the features and distances in that query can be translated into a fingerprint, with multiple bits being set, as necessary, to account for tolerances on matching the interfeature distances. The pattern of bits set by the query creates a necessary condition for matching the pharmacophore, so if fingerprints have been created for a database of molecules to be searched, very fast logical bit operations may be performed to rapidly eliminate molecules that cannot possibly match the pharmacophore. In general, not every molecule that satisfies the fingerprint query will actually match the pharmacophore, but a majority of false positives can be eliminated, which may result in a drastic reduction in overall searching time.

3D DATABASE SCREENING

By far the most common role a pharmacophore model ultimately plays is that of 3D database query. If the pharmacophore model accurately embodies the key interactions required for binding, molecules in a database that match the query, the so-called *hits*, should have a greater-than-average chance of being active. The degree to which this advantage is actually observed depends on a number of additional factors, including the matching criteria, the presence/absence of steric constraints, and the quality of the database.

Each molecule in a 3D database may be represented by a set of precomputed conformers or by a single, low-energy structure. In the latter case, conformers for a given molecule can be generated during the database screen using systematic or stochastic searching,[7,85,86] or the structure may be flexed in an attempt to fit the query.[87,88] The primary advantage of storing precomputed conformers is searching speed, which may be one to two orders of magnitude faster than when conformers are generated during the search. However, speed comes at the expense of disk space, which grows with the number of conformers stored, although not necessarily in a linear fashion due to compression of redundant data.

At its most basic, a pharmacophore model is just an arrangement of feature points whose relative locations are defined by a set of interpoint distances, internal coordinates, or Cartesian coordinates. A query is created only after conditions on matching the pharmacophore are stipulated. Most pharmacophore packages support user-defined tolerances on matching distances, positions, angles, and so on, but a number of general guidelines have been established that rely on a combination of experimental data and common sense.[20,89] For example, observed variations in hydrogen bond distances X–Y and hydrogen bond angles X–H–Y within crystallographic complexes may be used to conclude that the positional tolerance on matching hydrogen bond acceptors and donors should be about 2Å.[20] It is also possible to use known actives and inactives to derive suitable constraints on matching interfeature distances.[21] Positional tolerances between 1Å and 2Å for various types of features are typical, but much stricter criteria are sometimes used.[86,88]

When automated common pharmacophore perception is employed, it is tempting to argue that matching tolerances should be inferable from positional variations in the superimposed ligand features. However, such variations are really characteristics of the ligands themselves and of the conformational sampling method; they are not indicative of the receptor's flexibility, promiscuity, and so on. For example, consider a common pharmacophore model that is derived from a set of rigid, congeneric ligands. When the ligands are superimposed on the pharmacophore model, there should be essentially no variations in the feature locations from ligand to ligand. If a database query were then posed with matching tolerances consistent with those tiny variations, it is unlikely that any additional actives would be found, unless the database contained molecules with the same rigid framework. This sort of restriction eliminates the possibility of scaffold hopping,[90] an advantage that pharmacophore-based searching is naturally assumed to offer.

As shown in Figure 9.10, a point-based pharmacophore query may be embellished with any number of additional characteristics and constraints, such as a distance between a point and a plane, an angle between planes, or a cone of revolution about a hydrogen bond axis. However, before any of these conditions can be applied, a suitable match to the feature points must be found, which nearly always involves identifying sets of interfeature distances in a database structure that are consistent with the locations of the feature points in the pharmacophore model. Thus, the primary criterion for a match is that a structure must contain all n features in the pharmacophore model and that a particular mapping of those features to the pharmacophore yields an $n \times n$ distance matrix whose elements are sufficiently close to the corresponding elements in the pharmacophore distance matrix. As noted previously, the user normally stipulates how closely the points must match, either by specifying tolerances on the interfeature distances themselves

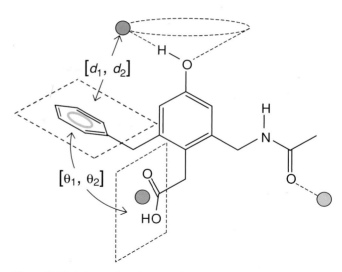

Figure 9.10. A four-point pharmacophore model with additional constraints and features. The angle between two planes and the distance between a hydrogen donor and a plane must lie within specified ranges, while the hydrogen bond donor sweeps out a cone of revolution.

or by specifying positional tolerances on the feature points after least squares alignment.[58,59]

Many pharmacophore packages allow *partial matching*, wherein only m of n points in a query must be matched. There may be user-imposed requirements to match specific points, or matching any subset of m may be sufficient. In either case, the algorithm must be modified to cycle through different subsets of m points in the pharmacophore model and attempt matching on the associated $m \times m$ submatrices. Partial matching is frequently invoked out of necessity when the pharmacophore model contains more points than can reasonably be expected to be matched by any molecule that does not contain the same chemical scaffold as the ligand(s) from which the model was derived. Thus a "kitchen sink" approach may be taken when developing a pharmacophore model, with the database screen being used to determine which parts of the model actually occur in other molecules. This convenience comes with a price, though, because the combinatorics of matching m of n points is governed by the binomial coefficient $n!/[m!(n-m)!]$, so when $m \approx n/2$, a search can be exceedingly slow if n is too large. Furthermore, certain subsets of feature points may correspond to very ordinary pharmacophores, which may cause an inordinate number of database molecules to be matched.

In practice, the matching algorithms just described are normally invoked only after performing one or more rapid prescreens to eliminate molecules that cannot possibly satisfy the query. A prescreen may involve only 2D criteria, such as rejection of molecules that are missing any required feature in the pharmacophore, or it may be 3D in nature. If the database contains precomputed conformers and their associated pharmacophore fingerprints, the strategy described in the previous section may be employed to perform a fast 3D prescreen. The more effective the pre-screen is at eliminating false positives, the faster the overall searching time.

Finally, a database screen may return different levels of information, depending on the capabilities of the software and the user's requirements. When the pharmacophore-based screen is being done as a precursor to docking, the user may need to know only the identities of the molecules that match the query. In other cases, the user may wish to see each matching structure aligned to the pharmacophore model. If multiple conformers are searched, a given molecule may yield more than one match, and the user may wish to examine some or all of them. Sorting of matches according to some fitness measure is also common, which allows the user to focus only on what he considers to be a reasonable number of high-ranking hits.

CONCLUSIONS

The past few decades have seen extensive innovation in pharmacophore modeling and continual expansion in its scope of applicability. Thus while a substantial portion of modeling efforts remain devoted to structure-based design, pharmacophore methods continue to be relied on for analysis of complex SAR data, elucidation of key ligand/receptor interactions when crystallographic data are unavailable, measurement of 3D similarity, rapid screening of large chemical libraries, and as a powerful means of combining structure-based and ligand-based knowledge.

The sheer diversity of available pharmacophore methods is a tremendous asset to modern drug discovery, but recognizing the limitations of a particular technique is absolutely critical to its successful application. Likewise, it is important to have realistic expectations about what can and cannot be achieved. A given pharmacophore method may provide any number of plausible solutions to the structure/activity problem, but it rarely points a user directly to the most correct solution. Nor is there any guarantee that all factors governing activity can be embodied in a pharmacophore model, so the picture one obtains is not always complete. Yet if the advantages are leveraged appropriately in light of the limitations, pharmacophore methods are indispensable tools in the drug discovery paradigm.

REFERENCES

1. Ehrlich, P. Present status of chemotherapy. *Chem. Ber.* **1909**, *42*, 17–47.
2. Gund, P. Three-dimensional pharmacophore pattern searching. In: *Progress in Molecular and Subcellular Biology*, Hahn, F. E.; Ed. Berlin: Springer-Verlag; **1977**, *5*, 117–143.
3. Marshall, G. R.; Barry, C. D.; Bosshard, H. E.; Dammkoehler, R. A.; Dunn, D. A. The conformational parameter in drug design: the active analog approach. In: *Computer-Assisted Drug Design*, Olson, E. C.; Christoffersen, R. E.; Eds. Washington, D.C.: American Chemical Society; **1979**, 205–226.
4. Cramer, R. D.; Patterson, D. E.; Bunce, J. D. Comparative molecular field analysis (CoMFA). 1. Effect of shape on binding of steroids to carrier proteins. *J. Am. Chem. Soc.* **1988**, *110*, 5959–5967.
5. Klebe, G.; Abraham, U.; Mietzner, T. Molecular similarity indices in comparative analysis (CoMSIA) of drug molecules to correlate and predict their biological activity. *J. Med. Chem.* **1994**, *37*, 4130–4146.
6. Li, H.; Sutter, J.; Hoffmann, R. HypoGen: an automated system for generating 3d predictive pharmacophore models. In: *Pharmacophore Perception, Development and Use in Drug Design*, Güner, O. F.; Ed. La Jolla, CA: International University Line; **2000**, 173–189.
7. Dixon, S. L.; Smondyrev, A. M.; Knoll, E. H.; Rao, S. N.; Shaw, D. E.; Friesner, R. A. PHASE: a new engine for pharmacophore perception, 3D QSAR model development, and 3d database screening. 1. Methodology and preliminary results. *J. Comput. Aided Mol. Des.* **2006**, *20*, 647–671.
8. Jacobsson, M.; Gäredal, M.; Schultz, J.; Karlén, A. Identification of plasmodium falciparum spermidine synthase active site binders through structure-based virtual screening. *J. Med. Chem.* **2008**, *51*, 2777–2786.
9. Martin, Y. C. Distance comparisons (DISCO): a new strategy for examining 3d structure-activity relationships. In: *Classical and 3D QSAR in Agrochemistry*, Hansch, C., Fujita, T.; Ed. Washington, D.C.: American Chemical Society; **1995**, 318–329.
10. Barnum, D.; Greene, J.; Smellie, A.; Sprague, P. Identification of common functional configurations among molecules. *J. Chem. Inf. Comput. Sci.* **1996**, *36*, 563–571.
11. Jones, G.; Willett, P.; Glen, R. C. A genetic algorithm for flexible molecular overlay and pharmacophore elucidation. *J. Comput. Aided Mol. Des.* **1995**, *9*, 532–549.
12. Richmond, N. J.; Abrams, C. A.; Wolohan, P. R. N.; Abrahamian, E.; Willet, P.; Clark, R. D. GALAHAD: 1. Pharmacophore identification by hypermolecular alignment of ligands in 3D. *J. Comput. Aided Mol. Des.* **2006**, *20*, 567–587.
13. Greenidge, P. A.; Carlsson, B.; Bladh, L.; Gillner, M. Pharmacophores incorporating numerous excluded volumes defined by x-ray crystallographic structure in three-dimensional database searching: application to the thyroid hormone receptor. *J. Med. Chem.* **1998**, *41*, 2503–2512.
14. Van Drie, J. H. "Shrink-Wrap" surfaces: a new method for incorporating shape into pharmacophoric 3d database searching. *J. Chem. Inf. Comput. Sci.* **1997**, *37*, 38–42.
15. Good, A. C.; Kuntz, I. D. Investigating the extension of pairwise distance pharmacophore measures to triplet-based descriptors. *J. Comput. Aided Mol. Des.* **1995**, *9*, 373–379.
16. Pickett, S. D.; Mason, J. S.; McLay, I. M. Diversity profiling and design using 3d pharmacophores: pharmacophore-derived queries (PDQ). *J. Chem. Inf. Comput. Sci.* **1996**, *36*, 1214–1223.
17. McGregor, M. J.; Muskal, S. M. Pharmacophore fingerprinting. 1. Application to QSAR and focused library design. *J. Chem. Inf. Comput. Sci.* **1999**, *39*, 569–574.
18. Cato, S. J. Exploring pharmacophores with CHEM-X. In: *Pharmacophore Perception, Development, and Use in Drug Design*, Güner, O. F.; Ed. La Jolla, CA: International University Line; **2000**, 110–125.
19. Güner, O. F.; Henry, D. R.; Pearlman, R. S. Use of flexible queries for searching conformationally flexible molecules in databases of three-dimensional structures. *J. Chem. Inf. Comput. Sci.* **1992**, *32*, 101–109.
20. Greene, J.; Kahn, S.; Savoj, H.; Sprague, P.; Teig, S. Chemical function queries for 3d database search. *J. Chem. Inf. Comput. Sci.* **1994**, *34*, 1297–1308.

21. Van Drie, J. H. Strategies for the determination of pharmacophoric 3d database queries. *J. Comput. Aided Mol. Des.* **1997**, *11*, 39–52.

22. Güner, O. F. *Pharmacophore Perception, Development, and Use in Drug Design*. La Jolla, CA: International University Line; **2000**.

23. Mason, J. S.; Good, A. C.; Martin, E. J. 3D pharmacophores in drug discovery. *Curr. Pharm. Des.* **2001**, *7*, 567–597.

24. Güner, O. F. History and evolution of the pharmacophore concept in computer-aided drug design. *Curr. Top. Med. Chem.* **2002**, *2*, 1321–1332.

25. Van Drie, J. H. Pharmacophore discovery: lessons learned. *Curr. Pharm. Des.* **2003**, *9*, 1649–1664.

26. Dror, O.; Shulman-Peleg, A.; Nussov, R.; Wolfson, H. J. Predicting molecular interaction in silico. I. A guide to pharmacophore identification and its applications to drug design. *Curr. Med. Chem.* **2004**, *11*, 71–90.

27. Van Drie, J. Pharmacophore-based virtual screening: A practical perspective. In: *Virtual Screening in Drug Discovery*, Alvarez, J.; Shoichet, B.; Ed. Boca Raton, FL: CRC Press; **2005**.

28. Gund, P.; Wipke, W. T.; Langridge, R. *Computer Searching of a Molecular Structure File for Pharmacophoric Patterns*, Amsterdam: Elsevier; **1974**, *3*, 33–39.

29. Sheridan, R. P.; Nilakantan, R.; Dixon, J. S.; Venkataraghavan, R. The ensemble approach to distance geometry: application to the nicotinic pharmacophore. *J. Med. Chem.* **1986**, *29*, 899–906.

30. Mayer, D.; Naylor, C. B.; Motoc, I.; Marshall, G. R. A unique geometry of the active site of angiotensin-converting enzyme consistent with structure-activity studies. *J. Comput. Aided Mol. Des.* **1987**, *1*, 3–16.

31. Golender, V. E.; Vorpagel, E. R. Computer-assisted pharmacophore identification. In: *3D QSAR in Drug Design: Theory, Methods and Applications*, Kubinyi, H.; Ed. Leiden: ESCOM Science Publishers; **1993**, 137–149.

32. Havel, T. F.; Kuntz, I. D.; Crippen, G. M. The theory and practice of distance geometry. *Bull. Math. Biol.* **1983**, *45*, 665–720.

33. Bron, C.; Kerbosch, J. Algorithm 457: finding all cliques of an undirected graph. *Commun. ACM* **1973**, *16*, 575–577.

34. Patel, Y.; Gillet, V. J.; Bravi, G.; Leach, A. R. A comparison of the pharmacophore identification programs: CATALYST, DISCO and GASP. *J. Comput. Aided Mol. Des.* **2002**, *16*, 653–681.

35. Goldberg, D. E. *Genetic Algorithms in Search, Optimization and Machine Learning*. Reading, MA: Addison-Wesley; **1989**.

36. Breiman, L.; Friedman, J. H.; Olshen, R. A.; Stone, C. J. *Classification and Regression Trees*. Belmont, CA: Wadsworth International Group; **1984**.

37. Young, S. S.; Hawkins, D. M. Analysis of a 29 full factorial chemical library. *J. Med. Chem.* **1995**, *38*, 2784–2788.

38. Hawkins, D. M.; Young, S. S.; Rusinko, A. Analysis of a large structure-activity data set using recursive partitioning. *Quant. Struct.-Act. Relat.* **1997**, *16*, 1–7.

39. Young, S. S.; Hawkins, D. M. Using recursive partitioning to analyze a large sar data set. *SAR QSAR. Eviron. Res.* **1998**, *8*, 183–193.

40. Chen, X.; Rusinko, A., III; Young, S. S. Recursive partitioning analysis of a large structure-activity data set using three-dimensional descriptors. *J. Chem. Inf. Comput. Sci.* **1998**, *38*, 1054–1062.

41. Dixon, S. L.; Villar, H. O. Investigation of classification methods for the prediction of activity in diverse chemical libraries. *J. Comput. Aided Mol. Des.* **1999**, *13*, 533–545.

42. Chen, X.; Rusinki, A., III; Tropsha, A.; Young, S. S. Automated pharmacophore identification for large chemical data sets. *J. Chem. Inf. Comput. Sci.* **1999**, *39*, 887–896.

43. Van Drie, J. H.; Weininger, D.; Martin, Y. C. ALADDIN: an integrated tool for computer-assisted molecular design and pharmacophoric pattern recognition from geometric, steric and substructure searching of three-dimensional molecular structures. *J. Comput. Aided Mol. Des.* **1989**, *3*, 225–251.

44. Lauri, G.; Bartlett, P. A. CAVEAT: a program to facilitate the design of organic molecules. *J. Comput. Aided Mol. Des.* **1994**, *8*, 51–66.

45. Seeman, P.; Watanabe, M.; Grigoriadis, D.; Tedesco, J. L.; George, S. R.; Svensson, U.; Nilsson, J. L. G.; Neumeyer, J. L. Dopamine D-2 receptor binding sites for agonists: a tetrahedral model. *Mol. Pharmacol.* **1985**, *28*, 391–399.

46. Chang, G.; Guida, W.; Still, W. C. An internal coordinate Monte Carlo method for searching conformational space. *J. Am. Chem. Soc.* **1989**, *111*, 4379–4386.

47. Smellie, A.; Teig, S. L.; Towbin, P. Poling: promoting conformational variation. *J. Comput. Chem.* **1995**, *16*, 171–187.

48. Catalyst/ConFirm. San Diego, CA Accelrys.

49. OMEGA. Sante Fe, NM OpenEye Scientific Software. September **2008**.

50. Li, J.; Ehlers, T.; Sutter, J.; Varma-O'Brien, S.; Kirchmair, J. CAESAR: a new conformer generation algorithm based on recursive buildup and local rotational consideration. *J. Chem. Inf. Model.* **2007**, *47*, 1923–1932.

51. Halgren, T. A. Merck molecular force field. I. Basis, form, scope, parameterization and performance of MMFF94. *J. Comput. Chem.* **1996**, *17*, 520–552.

52. Jorgensen, W. L.; Maxwell, D. S.; Tirado-Rives, J. Development and testing of the opls all-atom force field on conformational energetics and properties of organic liquids. *J. Am. Chem. Soc.* **1996**, *118*, 11225–11236.

53. Shelley, J.; Cholleti, A.; Frye, L. L.; Greenwood, J. R.; Timlin, M. R.; Uchimaya, M. EPIK: a software program for pKa prediction and protonation state generation for drug-like molecules. *J. Comput. Aided Mol. Des.* **2007**, *21*, 681–691.

54. Forbes, I. T.; Dabbs, S.; Duckworth, M. D.; Ham, P.; Jones, G. E.; King, F. D.; Saunders, D. V.; Blaney, F. E.; Naylor, C. B.; Baxter, G. S.; Blankburn, T. P.; Kennett, G. A.; Wood, M. D. Synthesis, biological activity, and molecular modeling studies of selective 5-HT2C/2B receptor antagonists. *J. Med. Chem.* **1996**, *39*, 4966–4977.

55. Phase 3.0. New York: Schrödinger, LLC; **2008**.

56. Ash, S.; Cline, M. A.; Homer, R. W.; Hurst, T.; Smith, G. B. SYBYL line notation (SLN): a versatile language for chemical structure representation. *J. Chem. Inf. Comput. Sci.* **1997**, *37*, 71–79.

57. SMARTS: Smiles ARbitrary Target Specification. Aliso Viejo, CA: Daylight Chemical Information Systems.

58. Schonemann, P. A generalized solution of the orthogonal procrustes problem. *Psychometrika* **1966**, *31*, 1–10.

59. Ferro, D.; Hermans, J. A. A different best rigid-body molecular fit routine. *Acta Crystallogr.* **1977**, *A33*, 345–347.

60. Beusen, D. D.; Marshall, G. R. Pharmacophore definition using the active analog approach. In: *Pharmacophore Perception, Development, and Use in Drug Design*, Güner, O. F.; Ed. La Jolla, CA: International University Line; **2000**, 23–45.

61. Griffith, R.; Bremner, J. B.; Coban, B. Docking-derived pharmacophores from models of receptor-ligand complexes. In: *Pharmacophore Perception, Development, and Use in Drug Design*, Güner, O. F.; Ed. La Jolla, CA: International University Line; **2000**, 387–408.

62. Claussen, H.; Gastreich, M.; Apelt, V.; Greene, J.; Hindle, S. A.; Lemmen, C. The FlexX database docking environment: rational extraction of receptor based pharmacophores. *Curr. Drug Discov. Technol.* **2004**, *1*, 49–60.

63. Tschinke, V.; Cohen, N. C. The NEWLEAD program: a new method for the design of candidate structures from pharmacophoric hypotheses. *J. Med. Chem.* **1993**, *36*, 3863–3870.

64. Gastreich, M.; Lilienthal, M.; Briem, H.; Claussen, H. Ultrafast de novo docking combining pharmacophores and combinatorics. *J. Comput. Aided Mol. Des.* **2006**, *20*, 717–734.

65. Carlson, H. A.; Masukawa, K. M.; Rubins, K.; D., B. F.; Jorgensen, W. L.; Lins, R. D.; Briggs, J. M.; McCammon, J. A. Developing a dynamic pharmacophore model for HIV-1 integrase. *J. Med. Chem.* **2000**, *43*, 2100–2114.

66. Deng, J.; Lee, K. W.; Sanchez, T.; Cui, M.; Neamati, N.; Briggs, J. M. Dynamic receptor-based pharmacophore model development and its application in designing novel HIV-1 integrase inhibitors. *J. Med. Chem.* **2005**, *48*, 1496–1505.

67. Kirchhoff, P. D.; Brown, R.; Kahn, S.; Waldman, M. Application of structure-based focusing to the estrogen receptor. *J. Comput. Chem.* **2001**, *22*, 993–1003.

68. Böhm, H.-J. LUDI: rule-based automatic design of new substituents for enzyme inhibitor leads. *J. Comput. Aided Mol. Des.* **1992**, *6*, 593–606.

69. Wlber, G.; Langer, T. LigandScout: 3-D pharmacophores derived from protein-bound ligands and their use as virtual screening filters. *J. Chem. Inf. Model.* **2005**, *45*, 160–169.

70. Markt, P.; Schuster, D.; Kirchmair, J.; Laggner, C.; Langer, T. Pharmacophore modeling and parallel screening for PPAR ligands. *J. Comput. Aided Mol. Des.* **2007**, *21*, 575–590.

71. Murray, C. W.; Baxter, C. A.; Frenkel, A. D. The sensitivity of the results of molecular docking to induced fit effects: application to thrombin, thermolysin and neuraminidase. *J. Comput. Aided Mol. Des.* **1999**, *13*, 547–562.

72. Carlson, H. A.; McCammon, J. A. Accommodating protein flexibility in computational drug design. *Mol. Pharmacol.* **2000**, *57*, 213–218.

73. Sherman, W.; Day, T.; Jacobson, M. P.; Friesner, R. A.; Farid, R. Novel procedure for modeling ligand/receptor induced fit effects. *J. Med. Chem.* **2006**, *49*, 534–553.

74. Catalyst/HypoRefine. San Diego, CA: Accelrys.

75. Schuster, D.; Laggner, C.; Steindl, T. M.; Palusczak, A.; Hartmann, R.; Langer, T. Pharmacophore modeling and in silico screening for new P450 19 (aromatase) inhibitors. *J. Chem. Inf. Model.* **2006**, *46*, 1301–1311.

76. Brown, R. D.; Martin, Y. C. Use of structure-activity data to compare structure-based clustering methods and descriptors for use in compound selection. *J. Chem. Inf. Comput. Sci.* **1996**, *36*, 572–584.

77. Brown, R. D.; Martin, Y. C. The information content of 2D and 3D structural descriptors relevant to ligand-receptor binding. *J. Chem. Inf. Comput. Sci.* **1997**, *37*, 1–9.

78. Flower, D. R. On the properties of bit string-based measures of chemical similarities. *J. Chem. Inf. Comput. Sci.* **1998**, *38*, 379–386.

79. Dixon, S. L.; Koehler, R. T. The hidden component of size in two-dimensional fragment descriptors: side effects on sampling in bioactive libraries. *J. Med. Chem.* **1999**, *42*, 2287–2900.

80. Patterson, D. E.; Cramer, R. D.; Ferguson, A. M.; Clark, R. D.; Weinberger, L. E. Neighborhood behavior: a useful concept for validation of "molecular diversity" descriptors. *J. Med. Chem.* **1996**, 3049–3059.

81. Matter, H. Selecting optimally diverse compounds from structure databases: a validation study of two-dimensional and three-dimensional molecular descriptors. *J. Med. Chem.* **1997**, *40*, 1219–1229.

82. Lajiness, M. S. Dissimilarity-based compound selection techniques. *Perspect. Drug Discov. Des.* **1997**, *7/8*, 65–84.

83. Pötter, T.; Matter, H. Random or rational design? Evaluation of diverse compound subsets from chemical structure databases. *J. Med. Chem.* **1998**, *41*, 478–488.

84. Ajay, A.; Walters, W. P.; Murcko, M. A. Can we learn to distinguish between "drug-like" and "nondrug-like" molecules? *J. Med. Chem.* **1998**, *41*, 3314–3324.

85. Murrall, N. W.; Davies, E. K. Conformational freedom in 3-D databases. 1. Techniques. *J. Chem. Inf. Comput. Sci.* **1990**, *30*, 312–316.

86. Clark, D. E.; Jones, G.; Willett, P. Pharmacophoric pattern matching in files of three-dimensional chemical structures: comparison of conformational searching algorithms for flexible searching. *J. Chem. Inf. Comput. Sci.* **1994**, *34*, 197–206.

87. Moock, T. E.; Henry, D. R.; Ozkabak, A. G.; Alamgir, M. Conformational searching in ISIS/3D databases. *J. Chem. Inf. Comput. Sci.* **1994**, *34*, 184–189.

88. Hurst, T. Flexible 3D searching: the directed tweak technique. *J. Chem. Inf. Comput. Sci.* **1994**, *34*, 190–196.

89. Martin, Y.; Bures, M.; Danaher, E.; DeLazzer, J. New strategies that improve the efficiency of the 3D design of bioactive molecules. In: *Trends in QSAR and Molecular Modelling 92*, Wermuth, C.; Ed. Leiden: ESCOM; **1993**, 20–26.

90. Schneider, G.; Neidhart, W.; Giller, T.; Schmid, G. "Scaffold-hopping" by topological pharmacophore search: a contribution to virtual screening. *Angew. Chem. Int. Ed. Engl.* **1999**, *38*, 2894–2896.

10

QSAR in drug discovery

Alexander Tropsha

INTRODUCTION

With nearly fifty years of rich history of methodology developments and applications (the Hansch article of 1963[1] is often considered first in the field), quantitative structure/activity relationship (QSAR) modeling is a well-established area of research. As is true perhaps for any computational field, QSAR modeling has been both blessed and sometimes cursed in the literature. In the first volume of the famous book series titled *Reviews in Computational Chemistry*, Boyd summarized several documented cases when QSAR modeling was instrumental in discovering new drugs of drug candidates in advanced phases of clinical trials.[2] The methodologies used by that time were relatively simple, employing a small number of physical chemical descriptors and statistical methods such as multiple linear regression. QSAR modeling was viewed solely as a tool for lead optimization; that is, it was employed to elucidate the relationship between structure and activity in relatively small congeneric compound series and predict relatively small structural modifications leading to enhanced activity.

Since the late 1980s the field has changed dramatically, fueled by changes in the size, complexity, and availability of experimental data sets of biologically active compounds. These changes have been coincidental with the advances in chemometrics, resulting in a significant increase in the number of chemical descriptors as well as growing implementation of machine learning and advanced statistical modeling techniques available for QSAR studies. The dramatic shift in the content and complexity of QSAR modeling away from original simple and easily interpretable linear models built with a small number of descriptors toward complex multiparametric and mostly nonlinear approaches was not recognized and acknowledged by many users of the technique. Indeed, many modern QSAR modeling approaches are much closer to such subdisciplines of computational science as data mining and knowledge discovery in databases than to physical organic chemistry where the field actually originated. Ignorance of this paradigm shift led to many studies that confused model fitness with its predictive power, lacked model validation, and misinterpreted correlation as causation as discussed in a recent critical

review[3]; the author even posed the question whether QSAR is dead or alive.

Not surprisingly, the field was indeed criticized harshly in several recent publications. Our group was one of the first emphasizing the importance of statistical validation of QSAR models.[4] Another important article examined reasons behind the failure of in silico absorption/distribution/metabolism/excretion (ADME)/Tox models.[5] The unfortunate abundance of poorly executed QSAR studies led to a recent editorial published by the leading cheminformatics periodical, *Journal of Chemical Information and Modeling* (also reproduced by the *Journal of Medicinal Chemistry*) that introduced severe limitations on the quality of QSAR articles to be considered acceptable.[6] Another editorial opinion outlined limitations and some reasons for failures of QSAR modeling that relate to the so-called activity cliffs. In most cases the authors looked deeply into possible sources of errors or offered approaches to improve the robustness of models.[7] However, in a negative opinion letter published in early 2008 the author made an unfortunate attempt to equate the fraction of articles that did not pay enough attention to the statistical quality of models with the entire field.[8]

The limited if not falsified representation of modern QSAR modeling in the latter publication only emphasizes the need to present deeper analysis of the nature and role that modern QSAR continues plays in drug discovery, which is the focus of this chapter. Indeed, the attention to failures of QSAR modeling expressed in aforementioned publications naturally begs an important and perhaps critical question as to whether there is any room for further advancement of the field via innovative methodologies and important applications. A large body of previous and ongoing research in the area of QSAR suggests that the answer is a resounding yes. We believe strongly that many examples of low-impact QSAR research have been due to frequent exploration of data sets of limited size with little attention paid to model validation. This limitation leads to models having questionable "mechanistic" explanatory power but perhaps little if any forecasting ability outside of the training sets used for model development. We believe that the latter ability along with the capabilities of QSAR models to explore chemically diverse data sets with complex biological properties should become the chief focus of QSAR studies. This focus requires the reevaluation of the success criteria for the modeling as well as the development of novel chemical data mining algorithms and model validation approaches. In fact, we think that the most interesting era in QSAR modeling is just beginning with the rapid growth of the experimental publicly available SAR data space due to such projects as PubChem.[9]

This chapter examines the strategy and the output of the modern QSAR modeling approaches especially as applied to increasingly more complex biomolecular data sets. We discuss a data-analytical modeling workflow developed in our laboratory that incorporates modules for combinatorial QSAR model development (i.e., using all possible binary combinations of available descriptor sets and statistical data-modeling techniques), rigorous model validation, and virtual screening of available chemical databases to identify novel biologically active compounds. Our approach places particular emphasis on model validation as well as on the need to define model applicability domains in the chemistry space. We present examples of studies where the application of rigorously validated QSAR models for virtual screening identified computational hits that were confirmed by subsequent experimental investigations. The emerging focus of QSAR modeling on target property forecasting brings it forward as a predictive, as opposed to evaluative, modeling approach that is suitable not only for traditional lead optimization but also for lead discovery.

The subsequent sections of this chapter present a brief overview of the modern QSAR modeling field without going into specific details of any particular technique, introduce the predictive QSAR modeling workflow developed in our group, present examples of successful applications of the workflow to several data sets resulting in experimentally confirmed computational predictions of biologically active compounds by the means of virtual screening, address the issue of fruitful collaborations between QSAR modelers in developing and supporting "best practices" in QSAR modeling, and summarize most important challenges that the field of QSAR modeling is facing today.

THE COMPLEXITY OF MODERN DATA SETS

In the early days of QSAR modeling the experimental data sets were relatively small and chemically congeneric and the techniques employed were relatively unsophisticated. Since then, the size and complexity of experimental data sets has increased dramatically as have the complexity and challenges of data-analytical approaches. Traditionally, QSAR approaches have been applied to modeling data sets tested against a single target (e.g., in specific enzymatic or receptor-binding assays). Recent experimental advances in high-throughput screening and multitarget testing of compound libraries have led to the establishment of data sets of biologically active compounds (often publicly

available) that we define as complex. A complex data set could include a library of compounds tested against multiple targets, have the target property measured in the form of gene or protein expression profiles across many genes (chemical genomics), or be formed by diverse compounds tested against a complex assay where multiple mechanisms leading to the measured response could be involved (e.g., carcinogenicity or mutagenicity). The examples of complex data sets include Pubchem,[9] PDSP,[10] NCI,[11] U.S. FDA,[12] NIEHS,[13] and EPA DSS-Tox [14] (see more examples in a recent review[15]). In most cases the biological end point (e.g., any toxicity) is very complex with many possible underlying biological mechanisms. Naturally, the complex data sets call for the development of more sophisticated computational tools and corresponding models that place particular emphasis on statistical model validation and external predictive power rather than mechanistic interpretation.

BRIEF NOTES ON QSAR METHODOLOGY

Modern QSAR modeling is a very complex and complicated field requiring deep understanding and thorough practice to develop robust models. Multiple types of chemical descriptors and numerous statistical model development approaches can be found in specialized literature and so need not be discussed in this chapter. Instead, we present several unifying concepts that underlie practically any QSAR methodology.

Any QSAR method can be generally defined as an application of mathematical and statistical methods to the problem of finding empirical relationships (QSAR models) of the form $P_i = \hat{k}(D_1, D_2, \ldots, D_n)$, where P_i are biological activities (or other properties of interest) of molecules, $D_1, D_2, \ldots, D_n$ are calculated (or, sometimes, experimentally measured) structural properties (molecular descriptors) of compounds, and $\hat{k}$ is some empirically established mathematical transformation that should be applied to descriptors to calculate the property values for all molecules. The relationship between values of descriptors D and target properties P can be linear or nonlinear. The example of the former relationship is given by multiple linear regression (MLR) common to the Hansch QSAR approach,[16] where target property can be predicted directly from the descriptor values. On the contrary, nearest-neighbor QSAR methods serve as examples of nonlinear techniques where descriptor values are used in characterizing chemical similarities between molecules, which are then used to infer compound activity.[17] The goal of QSAR modeling is to establish a trend in the descriptor values, which parallels the trend in biological activity. In essence, all QSAR approaches imply, directly or indirectly, a simple similarity principle, which for a long time has provided a foundation for experimental medicinal chemistry: compounds with similar structures are expected to have similar biological activities.

Modern QSAR approaches are characterized by the use of multiple descriptors of chemical structure combined with the application of both linear and nonlinear optimization approaches and a strong emphasis on rigorous model validation to afford robust and predictive models. As mentioned above, the most important recent developments in the field concur with a substantial increase in the size of experimental data sets available for the analysis and an increased application of QSAR models as virtual screening tools to discover biologically active molecules in chemical databases and/or virtual chemical libraries.[18] The latter focus differs substantially from the traditional emphasis on developing so-called explanatory QSAR models characterized by high statistical significance but only as applied to training sets of molecules with known chemical structure and biological activity.

The differences in various QSAR methodologies can be understood in terms of the types of *target property* values, *descriptors*, and *optimization* algorithms used to relate descriptors to the target properties and generate statistically significant models. Target properties (regarded as dependent variables in a statistical data modeling sense) can be generally of three types: *continuous* (i.e., real values covering certain range, e.g., IC_{50} values or binding constants), *categorical related* or *rank based* (e.g., classes of rank-ordered target properties covering certain range of values, e.g., classes of metabolic stability such as unstable, moderately stable, stable), or *categorical unrelated* (i.e., classes of target properties that do not relate to each other in any continuum, e.g., compounds that belong to different pharmacological classes). As simple as it appears, understanding this classification is actually very important because the choice of descriptor types and modeling techniques as well as model accuracy metrics is often dictated by the type of the target properties. Thus, in general the latter two types require classification modeling approaches, whereas the former type of the target properties allows the use of (multi-)linear regression type modeling. The corresponding methods of data analysis are referred to as either classification or continuous property QSAR.

Many QSAR approaches have been developed during the past few decades.[4,19] The major differences between various approaches are due to structural parameters (descriptors) used to characterize molecules and the mathematical approaches used to establish a correlation between descriptor values and biological activity. Most of the modeling techniques assume a linear relationship between molecular descriptors and a target property, which may be an adequate methodology for many data sets. However, the advances in combinatorial chemistry and high-throughput screening technologies have resulted in the explosive growth of the amount of structural and biological data, making the problem of developing robust QSAR models more challenging. This progress has provided an impetus for the development of fast, nonlinear QSAR methods that can capture structure/activity relationships for large and complex data. New nonlinear methods of multivariate analysis such as different types of artificial neural networks,[20–23] generalized linear models,[21,24–26] classification and regression trees,[24,27–30] random forests,[31–33] multivariate adaptive regression splines (MARS),[33,34] support vector machines,[35–38] and some other methods have become routine tools in QSAR studies. Interesting examples of applications have been reported for all types of the above methods. In some cases the comparisons between different techniques as applied to the same data set have been made but in general there appears to be no universal QSAR approach that produces the best QSAR models for any data sets.

CRITICAL IMPORTANCE OF MODEL VALIDATION

It should sound almost axiomatic that validation should be a natural part of any model development process. Indeed, what is the (ultimate) purpose of any modeling approach such as QSAR if not to develop models with a significant external predictive power? Unfortunately, as we and others have indicated in many publications,[39–41] the field of QSAR modeling has been plagued with insufficient attention paid to the subject of external validation. Indeed, most practitioners have merely presumed that internally cross-validated models built from available training set data should be externally predictive. As mentioned in the Introduction, the large number of QSAR publications exploring small- to medium-size data sets to produce models with little statistical significance led to the editorial published by the *Journal of Chemical Information and Modeling* two years ago that explicitly discouraged researchers from submitting the "introspective" QSAR/QSPR publications and requested that "evidence that any reported QSAR/QSPR model has been properly validated using data not in the training set must be provided."[6] We and others have demonstrated (as we detail below) that the training set statistics using most common internal validation techniques such as leave-one-out or even leave-many-out cross-validation approaches is insufficient and the statistical figures of merit of such models serve as misleading indicators of the external predictive power of QSAR models.[40]

In our highly cited publication "Beware of q^2!" we demonstrated the insufficiency of the training set statistics for developing externally predictive QSAR models and formulated the main principles of model validation.[39] At the time of that publication in 2002, the majority of articles on QSAR analysis ignored any model validation except for the cross-validation, performed during model development. Despite earlier observations of several authors warning that a high cross-validated correlation coefficient R^2 (q^2) is the necessary, but not sufficient, condition for the model to have high predictive power,[42–44] many authors continued to consider q^2 as the only parameter characterizing the predictive power of QSAR models. In Golbraikh and Tropsha (2002a) we have shown that the predictive power of QSAR models can be claimed only if the model was successfully applied for prediction of the external test set compounds, which were not used in the model development.[39] We have demonstrated that the majority of the models with high q^2 values have poor predictive power when applied for prediction of compounds in the external test set. In another publication the importance of rigorous validation was again emphasized as a crucial, integral component of model development.[4] Several examples of published QSPR models with high fitted accuracy for the training sets, which failed rigorous validation tests, have been considered. We presented a set of simple guidelines for developing validated and predictive QSPR models and discussed several validation strategies such as the randomization of the response variable (Y-randomization) external validation using rational division of a data set into training and test sets. We highlighted the need to establish the domain of model applicability in the chemical space to flag molecules for which predictions may be unreliable and discussed some algorithms that can be used for this purpose. We advocated the broad use of these guidelines in the development of predictive QSPR models.[4,45,46]

At the 37th Joint Meeting of Chemicals Committee and Working Party on Chemicals, Pesticides & Biotechnology, held in Paris November 17–19, 2004, the Organization for Economic Co-operation and Development (OECD) member countries adopted the following five principles that valid (Q)SAR models should follow to allow their use in regulatory assessment of chemical safety: (1) a defined end point; (2) an unambiguous algorithm; (3) a defined domain of applicability; (4) appropriate measures of goodness-of-fit, robustness, and predictivity; and (5) a mechanistic interpretation, if possible. Since then, most of the European authors publishing in QSAR include a statement that their models fully comply with OECD principles.[47–50] For instance, two aspects of QSAR modeling outlined in the OECD principles are considered by Estrada and Patlewicz.[51] The first aspect concerns the theoretical approaches used in chemistry in general and in QSAR in particular, specifically, which method should be selected for theoretical studies: more sophisticated and complex or more simple. The authors criticized the common belief that applying more sophisticated methods should always lead to significantly better results. They considered an example of polycyclic aromatic hydrocarbons (PAHs), the toxicity of which is believed to depend on the energy gap between HOMO and LUMO values. The authors showed that a simple Hückel molecular orbital theory gives practically the same values of HOMO and LUMO as the sophisticated ab initio methods yet the calculations are 10^{-4} to 10^{-7} times faster. They reach the conclusion that if a more simple method is capable of giving results better or similar to those of more sophisticated method, one should naturally use a more simple method!

We shall also comment on the issue of so-called mechanistic QSAR. Some authors prefer descriptors that are mechanistically interpretable.[52] However, Estrada and Patlewicz argued that in many cases a biological response is a result of a multitude of different processes, some of which cannot even be known, and its a posteriori mechanistic interpretation is difficult if not impossible.[51] The authors suggested an alternative approach where a biological system is considered as a black box and no specific underlying mechanism is implied. At the same time, some variables included in the model can describe several different mechanisms of biological action simultaneously (e.g., $\log P$), so in many cases it makes no sense to suggest that the use of this descriptor in QSAR models affords any mechanistic interpretation.[53] We would add that descriptors that give better models in terms of their predictive power are actually preferable. We consider building predictive models as the main goal of QSAR analysis. Of course, the interpretation of the model is also important, and, if possible, it should be done. However, in many cases it is impossible, even when models with high predictive power have been obtained (e.g., the best models were found to be those built using the molecular connectivity indices but these models were disregarded by the authors for the lack of mechanistic interpretability.[52]) We believe that mechanistic interpretation of the *externally validated* QSAR model is an important a posteriori exercise that should be done after the model has been internally and externally validated, and descriptors that afford models with the highest predictive power should be always used preferentially.

Validation of QSAR models remains one of the most critical problems of QSAR. Recently, we have extended our requirements for the validation of multiple QSAR models selected by acceptable statistics criteria of prediction of the test set.[54] Additional studies in this critical component of QSAR modeling should establish reliable and commonly accepted "good practices" for model development.

APPLICABILITY DOMAINS OF QSAR MODELS

One of the most important problems in QSAR analysis is establishing the models' domain of applicability in the chemistry space. In the absence of the applicability domain, each model can formally predict the activity of any compound, even with a completely different structure from those included in the training set. Thus, the absence of the model applicability domain as a mandatory component of any QSAR model would lead to the unjustified extrapolation of the model in the chemistry space and, as a result, a high likelihood of inaccurate predictions. In our research we have always paid particular attention to this issue.[40,55–61] The need for establishing the applicability domain for every model adds another critical degree of complexity to the model-building process.

The applicability domain problem has been addressed by many researchers. Mandel introduced the so-called effective prediction domain that was based on the ranges of descriptors included in the regression equation.[62] Afantitis et al. built a multiple linear regression model for a data set of apoptotic agents.[63] They defined the applicability domain for each compound as a leverage defined as a corresponding diagonal element of the hat matrix. In fact, it is a method for detecting possible leverage outliers. If for some compound leverage is higher than $3K/N$, where K is the number of descriptors and N is the number of compounds, the compound is an outlier. To use this approach, for each external compound it would be necessary to recalculate the leverage. Netzeva et al. and Saliner et al. defined the applicability domain by ranges of descriptors (i.e., in fact, as a subspace occupied by representative points in the descriptor space).[49,64] This definition of the applicability domain has a significant drawback, because the representative points could be found only in a small part of the hyperparallelepiped corresponding to descriptor ranges rather than distributed uniformly. A similar definition of the applicability domain was proposed by Tong et al.[65] The authors built QSAR models for two data sets of estrogen receptor ligands using the decision forest method and studied the dependence of the model predictive power versus the applicability domain threshold. The prediction accuracy within the domain is defined as a ratio of the number of correct predictions to the total number of compounds in the domain. The accuracy was changing from about 90% for the initial applicability domain to about 50% when the applicability domain increased by 30%. Interestingly, for one of the data sets the prediction accuracy was increasing until the domain was extended by about 20%. Another important aspect of this study was that the authors defined the confidence level of prediction. The probability that a compound belongs to a certain class was defined as the percentage of active compounds in the leaf node that the compound belongs to. The authors found (as expected) that the confidence level correlated with the prediction accuracy.

Helma used a lazy learning k-nearest-neighbor- (kNN) like method for the prediction of rodent carcinogenicity and *Salmonella* mutagenicity.[66] The applicability domain was defined by a so-called confidence index. A compound was assigned to one of the two classes by a weighted majority vote of its nearest neighbors. The confidence index is the weighted majority vote divided by the number of nearest neighbors. If the absolute value of the confidence index is low (<0.05) a compound is said to be out of the applicability domain. This definition of the applicability domain captures the areas in the descriptor space where compounds of both classes are close to each other and possibly mixed. In this area the precise and accurate prediction of a compound's class is impossible. A Tanimoto-like coefficient is used as a similarity measure. Nearest neighbors are defined by the value of this coefficient higher than 0.3, which limits the possibility of overextrapolation.

In most of our QSAR studies we have defined the applicability domain as the distance cutoff value $D_{cutoff} = <D> + Zs$, where Z is a similarity threshold parameter defined by a user and $<D>$ and s are the average and standard deviation of all Euclidian distances in the multidimensional

descriptor space between each compound and its nearest neighbors for all compounds in the training set.[46] This definition of the applicability domain has several major drawbacks that we continue to address in our ongoing studies: (1) Currently, the applicability domain is direction independent in the descriptor space. We shall consider the directions in the descriptor space in which the distribution of representative points has smaller spread as less important than those that have higher spread. Thus, the applicability domain will be represented as a multidimensional ellipsoid in the principal component space. (2) Too strict definition of the applicability domain: if a compound is outside of the model applicability domain, we currently do not predict its activity. Naturally, we shall establish the lower and upper bounds for the applicability domain. (3) Finally, it seems reasonable to introduce a confidence level of prediction, which will depend on the distance of the compound under prediction from its nearest neighbor of the training set. These considerations provide just a few examples that illustrate the importance of ongoing research in this area of QSAR modeling. Not surprisingly, the model applicability domain was the subject of a special symposium organized at a recent 235th meeting of the American Chemical Society in New Orleans, Louisiana.

COMBINATORIAL QSAR AND MODEL ACCEPTABILITY CRITERIA

The chief hypothesis of the combi-QSAR approach that we introduced in recent publications[67–70] is that, if an implicit structure/activity relationship exists for a given data set, it can be formally manifested via a variety of QSAR models obtained with different descriptors and optimization protocols. Our experience indicates that there is no universal QSAR method that is guaranteed to give the best results for any data set. Thus we believe that multiple alternative QSAR models should be developed (as opposed to a single model using some favorite QSAR method) for each data set to identify the most successful technique in the context of the given data set. Because QSAR modeling is relatively fast, these alternative models could be explored simultaneously when making predictions for external data sets. The consensus predictions of biological activity for novel test set compounds on the basis of several QSAR models, especially when they converge, are more reliable and provide better justification for the experimental exploration of hits.

Our current approach to combi-QSAR modeling is summarized on the workflow diagram (Figure 10.1). Our experience suggests that QSAR is a highly experimental area of statistical data modeling where it is impossible to decide a priori which particular QSAR modeling method will prove most successful. To achieve QSAR models of the highest internal and, most importantly, *external* accuracy, the combi-QSAR approach explores all possible binary combinations of various descriptor types and optimization methods along with external model validation. Each

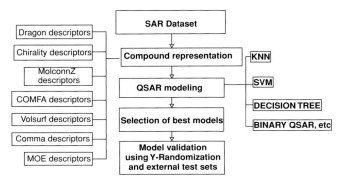

Figure 10.1. Flowchart of the combinatorial QSAR methodology. All descriptor sets and methods currently implemented in our laboratory are listed.

combination of descriptor sets and optimization techniques is likely to capture certain unique aspects of the structure/activity relationship. Because our ultimate goal is to use the resulting models as reliable activity (property) predictors, application of different combinations of modeling techniques and descriptor sets will increase our chances for success.

In our critical publications we have recommended a set of statistical criteria that must be satisfied by a predictive model.[4,39] For continuous QSAR, parameters that we use in developing activity/property predictors are as follows: (1) correlation coefficient R between the predicted and observed activities, (2) coefficients of determination[71] (predicted versus observed activities R_0^2, and observed versus predicted activities $R_0'^2$ for regressions through the origin), and (3) slopes k and k' of regression lines through the origin. We consider a QSAR model *predictive* if the following conditions are satisfied: (i) $q^2 > 0.5$; (ii) $R^2 > 0.6$; (iii) $-\frac{(R^2 - R_0^2)}{R^2} < 0.1$ and $0.85 \leq K \leq 1.15$ or $\frac{(R^2 - R_0^2)}{R^2} < 0.1$ and $0.85 \leq K' \leq 1.15$; and (iv) $|R_0^2 - R_0'^2| < 0.3$, where q^2 is the cross-validated correlation coefficient calculated for the training set, but all other criteria are calculated for the test set.

AN EXAMPLE OF "GOOD PRACTICES" IN QSAR MODEL DEVELOPMENT AND THE IMPORTANCE OF CONSENSUS PREDICTION

We discuss below the results of a recent important study of aquatic toxicity.[72] In our opinion this particular study may serve as a useful example to illustrate the complexity and power of modern QSAR modeling approaches and highlight the importance of collaborative and consensual model development.

The combinatorial QSAR modeling approach was applied to a diverse series of organic compounds tested for aquatic toxicity in *Tetrahymena pyriformis* in the same laboratory over nearly a decade.[73–80] The unique aspect of this research was that it was conducted in collaboration

between six academic groups specializing in cheminformatics and computational toxicology. The common goals for our virtual collaboratory were to explore the relative strengths of various QSAR approaches in their ability to develop robust and externally predictive models of this particular toxicity end point. We have endeavored to develop the most statistically robust, validated, and *externally* predictive QSAR models of aquatic toxicity. The members of our collaboratory included scientists from the University of North Carolina at Chapel Hill in the United States, the University of Louis Pasteur in France, the University of Insubria in Italy, the University of Kalmar in Sweden, the Virtual Computational Chemistry Laboratory in Germany, and the University of British Columbia in Canada. Each group relied on its own QSAR modeling approaches to develop toxicity models using the same modeling set, and we agreed to evaluate the realistic model performance using the same external validation set(s) (cf. Table 10.1 for the summary of approaches).

The *T. pyriformis* toxicity data set used in this study was compiled from several publications of the Schultz group as well as from data available at the Tetratox database Web site (http://www.vet.utk.edu/TETRATOX/). After deleting duplicates as well as several compounds with conflicting test results and correcting several chemical structures in the original data sources, our final data set included 983 unique compounds. The data set was randomly divided into two parts: (1) the modeling set of 644 compounds and (2) the validation set including 339 compounds. The former set was used for model development by each participating group and the latter set was used to estimate the external prediction power of each model as a universal metric of model performance. In addition, when this project was already well under way, a new data set had become available from the most recent publication by the Schultz group.[81] It provided us with an additional *external* set to evaluate the predictive power and reliability of all QSAR models. Among compounds reported, 110 were unique (i.e., not present among the original set of 983 compounds); thus, these 110 compounds formed the second independent validation set for our study.[81]

Universal statistical figures of merit for all models

Different groups have employed different techniques and (sometimes) different statistical parameters to evaluate the performance of models developed independently for the modeling set (described below). To harmonize the results of this study the same standard parameters were chosen to describe each model's performance as applied to the modeling and external test set predictions. Thus, we have employed q_{abs}^2 (squared leave-one-out cross-validation correlation coefficient) for the modeling set, R_{abs}^2 (frequently described as the coefficient of determination) for the external validations sets, and MAE (mean absolute error) for the

Table 10.1. Overview of QSAR modeling approaches employed by six cheminformatic groups in the study of aquatic toxicity

Group ID[a]	Modeling techniques	Descriptor type	Applicability domain definition
UNC	kNN, SVM	MolconnZ, Dragon	Euclidean distance threshold between a test compound and compounds in the modeling set
ULP	MLR, SVM, kNN	Fragments (ISIDA), Molecular (CODESSA-Pro)	Euclidean distance threshold between a compound and compounds in the modeling set; bounding box
UI	MLR/OLS	Dragon	Leverage approach
UK	PLS	Dragon	Residual standard deviation and leverage within the PLSR model
VCCLAB	ASNN	E-state indices	Maximal correlation coefficient of the test molecule to the training set molecules in the space of models
UBC	MLR, ANN, SVM, PLS	IND_I	Undefined

[a] *Abbreviations:* UNC = University of North Carolina at Chapel Hill; ULP = University of Louis Pasteur; UI = University of Insubria; UK = University of Kalmar; VCCLAB = Virtual Computational Chemistry Laboratory; UBC = University of British Columbia.

linear correlation between predicted (Y_{pred}) and experimental (Y_{exp}) data (here, $Y = pIGC_{50}$); these parameters are defined as follows:

$$Q_{abc}^2 = 1 - \sum_Y (Y_{exp} - Y_{100})^2 \, Q_{abc}^2 / \sum_Y (Y\exp - <y>_{exp})^2 \tag{10.1}$$

$$R_{abc}^2 = 1 - \sum_Y (Y_{exp} - Y_{pred})^2 / \sum_R (Y_{exp} - <Y>_{exp})^2 \tag{10.2}$$

$$MAE = \sum_Y |Y - Y_{pred}| / n. \tag{10.3}$$

Many other statistical characteristics can be used to evaluate model performance; however, we restricted ourselves to these three parameters that provide minimal but sufficient information concerning any model's ability to reproduce both the trends in experimental data for the test sets as well as mean accuracy of predicting all experimental values. The models were considered acceptable if R_{abs}^2 exceeded 0.5.

Consensus QSAR models of aquatic toxicity; comparison between methods and models

The objective of this study from a methodological perspective was to explore the suitability of different QSAR modeling tools for the analysis of a data set with an important toxicological end point. Typically, such data sets are analyzed with one (or several) modeling techniques, with a great emphasis on the (high value of) statistical parameters of the training set models. In this study, we went well beyond the modeling studies reported in the original publications in several respects. First, we have compiled all reported data on chemical toxicity against *T. pyriformis* in a single large data set and attempted to develop global QSAR models for the entire set. Second, we have employed multi-

ple QSAR modeling techniques thanks to the engagement of six collaborating groups. Third, we have focused on defining model performance criteria not only using training set data but most importantly using external validation sets that were not used in model development in *any* way (unlike any common *cross*-validation procedure).[82] This focus afforded us the opportunity to evaluate and compare all models using simple and objective universal criteria of *external* predictive accuracy, which in our opinion is the most important single figure of merit for a QSAR model that is of practical significance for experimental toxicologists. Fourth, we have explored the significance of applicability domains and the power of consensus modeling in maximizing the accuracy of external predictivity of our models.

We believe that results of our analysis lend strong support for our strategy. Indeed, all models performed quite well for the training set (Table 10.2) with even the lowest q_{abs}^2 among them as high as 0.72. However, there was much greater variation between these models when looking at their (universal and objective) performance criteria as applied to the validation sets I and II (Table 10.2).

Of fifteen QSAR approaches used in this study, nine implemented method-specific applicability domains. Models that did not define the AD showed a reduced predictive accuracy for the validation set II even though they yielded reasonable results for the validation set I. Only CODESSA-MLR (which did not employ any AD) approached in accuracy the lower bound of the models using the AD as measured by $R_{abs}^2 = 0.58$ but still had one of the highest MAE of 0.47 (Table 10.2). However, among models employing the AD only kNN-MOLCONNZ had a relatively low accuracy of prediction for the validation set II, with R_{abs}^2 below 0.5. For all other models the R_{abs}^2 ranged between 0.55 and 0.83. On average, the use of applicability domains improved the performance of individual models although the improvement came at the expense of the lower chemistry space coverage (cf. Table 10.2).

Table 10.2. Statistical results obtained with all toxicity QSAR models for the modeling and external validation sets

Model	Group ID	Modeling Set ($n = 644$)			Validation Set I ($n = 339$)			Validation Set II ($n = 110$)		
		Q^2_{abs}	MAE	(Coverage %)	R^2_{abs}	MAE	(Coverage %)	R^2_{abs}	MAE	(Coverage %)
kNN-Dragon	UNC	0.92	0.22	100	0.85	0.27	80.2	0.72	0.33	52.7
kNN-MolconnZ	UNC	0.91	0.23	99.8	0.84	0.30	84.3	0.44	0.39	53.6
SVM-Dragon	UNC	0.93	0.21	100	0.81	0.31	80.2	0.83	0.27	52.7
SVM-MolconnZ	UNC	0.89	0.25	100	0.83	0.30	84.3	0.55	0.37	53.6
ISIDA-kNN	ULP	0.77	0.37	100	0.73	0.36	78.5	0.63	0.37	42.7
ISIDA-SVM	ULP	0.95	0.15	100	0.76	0.32	100	0.38	0.50	100
ISIDA-MLR	ULP	0.94	0.20	100	0.81	0.31	95.9	0.65	0.41	51.8
CODESSA-MLR	ULP	0.72	0.42	100	0.71	0.44	100	0.58	0.47	100
OLS	UI	0.86	0.30	92.1	0.77	0.35	97.0	0.59	0.43	98.2
PLS	UK	0.88	0.28	97.7	0.81	0.34	96.1	0.59	0.40	95.5
ASNN	VCCLAB	0.83	0.31	83.9	0.87	0.28	87.4	0.75	0.32	71.8
PLS-IND_I	UBC	0.76	0.39	100	0.74	0.39	99.7	0.45	0.54	100
MLR-IND_I	UBC	0.77	0.39	100	0.75	0.40	99.7	0.46	0.53	100
ANN-IND_I	UBC	0.77	0.39	100	0.76	0.39	99.7	0.46	0.53	100
SVM-IND_I	UBC	0.79	0.31	100	0.79	0.35	99.7	0.53	0.46	100
Consensus model[a]	–	0.92	0.22	100	0.87	0.27	100	0.70	0.34	100

[a] Consensus model: average of the nine models (kNN-Dragon, kNN-MolconnZ, SVM-Dragon, SVM-MolconnZ, ISIDA-kNN, ISIDA-MLR, OLS, PLS, and ASNN) using their individual applicability domains.

For the most part all models succeeded in achieving reasonable accuracy of external prediction especially when using the AD. It then appeared natural to bring all models together to explore the power of *consensus prediction*. Thus, the *consensus model* was constructed by averaging all available predicted values taking into account the applicability domain of each individual model. In this case we could use only nine of fifteen models that had the AD defined. Because each model had its unique way of defining the AD, each external compound could be found within the AD of anywhere between one and nine models so for averaging we only used models covering the compound. The advantage of this data treatment is that the overall coverage of the prediction is still high because it was rare to have an external compound outside of the ADs of all available models. The results (Table 10.2) showed that the prediction accuracy for both the modeling set (MAE = 0.22) and the validation sets I and II (0.27 and 0.34, respectively) was the best compared to any individual model. The same observation could be made for the correlation coefficient R^2_{abs}. The coverage of this consensus model II was 100% for all three data sets. This observation suggests that consensus models afford both high space coverage and high accuracy of prediction.

In summary, this study presented an example of a fruitful international collaboration between researchers that use different techniques and approaches but share general principles of QSAR model development and validation. Significantly, we made no assumptions about the purported mechanisms of aquatic toxicity yet were able to develop statistically significant models for all experimentally tested compounds. In this regard it is relevant to cite an opinion expressed in an earlier publication by T. Schultz that "models that accurately predict acute toxicity without first identifying toxic mechanisms are highly desirable."[80] However, the most significant single result of our studies is the demonstrated superior performance of the *consensus modeling* approach when all models are used concurrently and predictions from individual models are averaged. We have shown that both the predictive accuracy and coverage of the final consensus QSAR models were superior as compared to these parameters for individual models. The consensus models appeared robust in terms of being insensitive to both incorporating individual models with low prediction accuracy and the inclusion or exclusion of the AD. Another important result of this study is the power of addressing complex problems in QSAR modeling by forming a virtual collaboratory of independent research groups leading to the formulation and empirical testing of *best modeling practices*. This latter endeavor is especially critical in light of the growing interest of regulatory agencies to developing the most reliable and predictive models for environmental risk assessment[83] and placing such models in the public domain.

PREDICTIVE QSAR MODELING WORKFLOW AND ITS APPLICATION TO VIRTUAL SCREENING

Our experience in QSAR model development and validation has led us to establishing a complex strategy that is summarized in Figure 10.2. It describes the predictive QSAR modeling workflow focused on delivering validated models and, ultimately, computational hits confirmed for the experimental validation. We start by randomly selecting a fraction of compounds (typically, 10–15%) as an external validation set. The remaining compounds are then divided rationally (using the sphere exclusion protocol implemented in our laboratory[46]) into multiple training and test sets that are used for model development and validation, respectively, using criteria discussed in more detail below. We employ multiple QSAR techniques based on the combinatorial exploration of all possible pairs of descriptor sets coupled with various statistical data-mining techniques (combi-QSAR) and select models characterized by high accuracy in predicting both training and test sets data. Validated models are finally tested using the evaluation set. The critical step of the external validation is the use of applicability domains. If external validation demonstrates the significant predictive power of the models we use all such models for virtual screening of available chemical databases (e.g., ZINC[84]) to identify putative active compounds and work with collaborators who could validate such hits experimentally. The entire approach is described in detail in several recent articles and reviews.[18,19,40]

In our recent studies we were fortunate to recruit experimental collaborators who have validated computational hits identified through our modeling of anticonvulsants,[59] HIV-1 reverse transcriptase inhibitors,[85] D1 antagonists,[37] antitumor compounds,[86] and β-lactamase inhibitors.[88] Thus, models resulting from this workflow could be used to prioritize the selection of chemicals for the experimental validation. However, because we cannot generally guarantee that every prediction resulting from our modeling effort will be validated experimentally we cannot include the experimental validation step as a mandatory part of the workflow in Figure 10.2, which is why we used the dotted line for this component. We note that our approach shifts the emphasis on ensuring good (best) statistics for the model that fits known experimental data toward generating testable hypo-

thesis about purported bioactive compounds. Thus, the output of the modeling has exactly the same format as the input [i.e., chemical structures and (predicted) activities making model interpretation and utilization completely seamless for medicinal chemists].

The development of truly validated and predictive QSAR models affords their growing application in chemical data mining and combinatorial library design.[88,89] For example, 3D stereoelectronic pharmacophore based on QSAR modeling was used recently to search the National Cancer Institute Repository of Small Molecules[11] to find new leads for inhibiting HIV type 1 reverse transcriptase at the nonnucleoside binding site.[90]

Our studies have shown that QSAR models could be used successfully as virtual screening tools to discover compounds with the desired biological activity in chemical databases or virtual libraries.[18,37,59,86,87,91] The discovery of novel bioactive chemical entities is the primary goal of computational drug discovery, and the development of validated and predictive QSAR models is critical to achieve this goal. We present several examples of these studies below to illustrate the use of QSAR models as virtual screening tools for lead identification.

EXAMPLES OF APPLICATIONS OF THE PREDICTIVE QSAR MODELING WORKFLOW FOR LEAD OPTIMIZATION

To illustrate the power of validated QSAR models as virtual screening tools we shall discuss the examples of studies that resulted in experimentally confirmed hits. We note that such studies could only be done if there is sufficient data available for a series of tested compounds such that robust validated models could be developing using the workflow described in Figure 10.2.

The first example is *anticonvulsant compounds*. In the first phase of modeling, we have applied kNN[17] and simulated annealing-partial least squares (SA-PLS)[89]

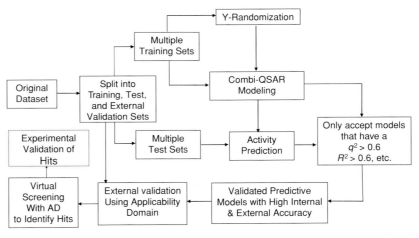

Figure 10.2. Flowchart of predictive QSAR modeling framework based on the validated combi-QSAR models.

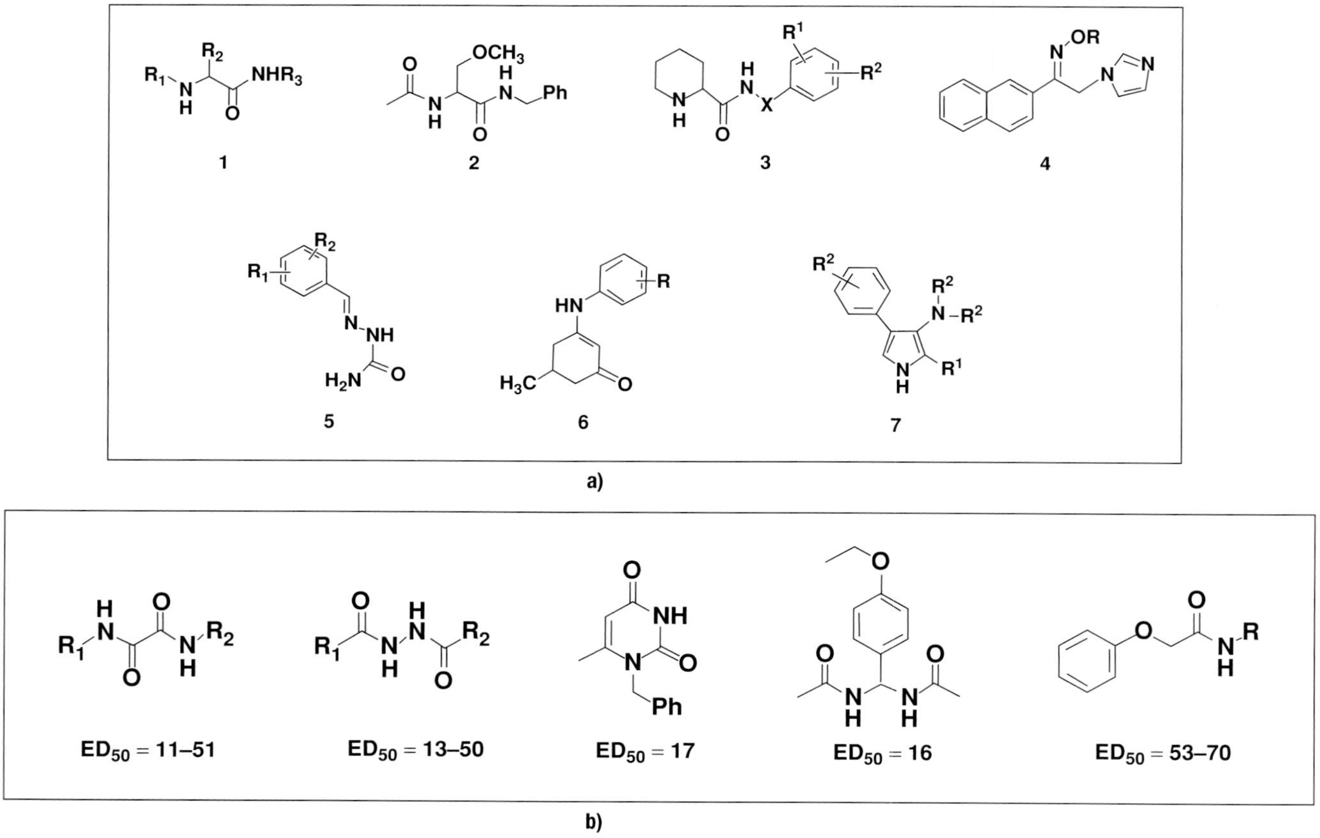

Figure 10.3. Uniqueness of scaffolds for QSAR-based experimentally confirmed virtual screening hits (b) as compared to training set compounds (a).

QSARapproaches to a data set of forty-eight chemically diverse functionalized amino acids (FAA) with anticonvulsant activity that were synthesized previously, and successful QSARmodels of FAA anticonvulsants have been developed[58] (see Fig. 10.3a for chemical structures). Both methods used multiple descriptors such as molecular connectivity indices or atom pair descriptors, which are derived from two-dimensional molecular topology. QSAR models with high internal accuracy were generated, with leave-one-out cross-validated R^2 (q^2) values ranging between 0.6 and 0.8. The q^2 values for the actual data set were significantly higher than those obtained for the same data set with randomly shuffled activity values, indicating that models were statistically significant. The original data set was further divided into several training and test sets, and highly predictive models providing q^2 values for the training sets greater than 0.5 and R^2 values for the test sets greater than 0.6.

In the second phase of modeling, we have applied the validated QSAR models to mining available chemical databases for new lead FAA anticonvulsant agents. Two databases have been explored: the National Cancer Institute[11] and Maybridge[92] databases, including (at the time of that study) 237,771 and 55,273 chemical structures, respectively. Database mining was performed independently using ten individual QSAR models that have been extensively validated using several criteria of robustness and accuracy. Each individual model selected some number of hits as a result of independent database mining, and the consensus hits (i.e., those selected by all models) were further explored experimentally for their anticonvulsant activity. As a result of computational screening of the NCI database, twenty-seven compounds were selected as potential anticonvulsant agents and submitted to our experimental collaborators. Of these twenty-seven compounds, our collaborators chose two for synthesis and evaluation; their choice was based on the ease of synthesis and the fact that these two compounds had structural features that would not be expected to be found in active compounds based on prior experience. Several additional compounds, which were close analogs of these two, were either taken from the literature or designed in our collaborator's laboratory. In total, seven compounds were resynthesized and sent to National Institutes of Health (NIH) for the maximum electroshock test (a standard test for anticonvulsant activity, which was used for the training set compounds as well). The biological results indicated that on initial and secondary screening, *five of seven compounds tested showed anticonvulsant activity* with ED_{50} less than 100 mg/kg (Fig. 10.3b), which is considered promising by NIH standards. Interestingly, all seven compounds were also found to be very active in the same tests performed on rats (a complete set of experimental data on rats for the training set were not available, and therefore no QSAR models for rats were built).

Mining of the Maybridge database yielded two additional promising compounds that were synthesized and sent to NIH for the MES anticonvulsant test. One of the compounds showed moderate anticonvulsant activity of ED_{50} between 30 and 100 mg/kg (in mice), while the other was found to be a *very* potent anticonvulsant agent with ED_{50} of 18 mg/kg in mice (intraperitoneal). In summary, both compounds were found to be very active in both mice and rats. Figure 10.3 summarizes the results of using validated QSAR models for virtual screening as applied to the anticonvulsant data set. It presents a practical example of using the predictive QSAR modeling workflow (cf. Fig. 10.2) that can be generalized for any data set where sufficient data to develop reliable QSAR models is available. It is important to note that *none* of the compounds identified in external databases as potent anticonvulsants and validated experimentally belong to the same class of FAA molecules as the training set. This observation was very stimulating because it underscored the power of our methodology to identify potent anticonvulsants of novel chemical classes as compared to the training set compounds, which is one of the most important goals of virtual screening.

Anticancer agents

A combined approach of validated QSAR modeling and virtual screening was successfully applied to the discovery of novel tylophorine derivatives as anticancer agents.[86] QSAR models have been initially developed for fifty-two chemically diverse phenanthrine-based tylophorine derivatives (PBTs) with known experimental EC_{50} using chemical topological descriptors (calculated with the MOLCONNZ program) and variable selection *k*NN method. Several validation protocols have been applied to achieve robust QSAR models. The original data set was divided into multiple training and test sets, and the models were considered acceptable only if the leave-one-out cross-validated R^2 (q^2) values were greater than 0.5 for the training sets and the correlation coefficient R^2 values were greater than 0.6 for the test sets. Furthermore, the q^2 values for the actual data set were shown to be significantly higher than those obtained for the same data set with randomized target properties (Y-randomization test), indicating that models were statistically significant. Ten best models were then employed to mine a commercially available ChemDiv Database (ca. 500,000 compounds) resulting in thirty-four consensus hits with moderate to high predicted activities. Ten structurally diverse hits were experimentally tested and eight were confirmed active with the highest experimental EC_{50} of 1.8 μM implying an exceptionally high hit rate (80%). The same ten models were further applied to predict EC_{50} for four new PBTs, and the correlation coefficient (R^2) between the experimental and predicted EC_{50} for these compounds

plus eight active consensus hits was shown to be as high as 0.57.

AmpC β-lactamase inhibitors

This example provides an interesting comparison between QSAR-based and structure-based virtual screening.[87] The use of inaccurate scoring functions in docking algorithms may result in the selection of compounds with high predicted binding affinity that nevertheless are known experimentally not to bind to the target receptor. Such falsely predicted binders have been termed "binding decoys." We posed a question as to whether true binders and decoys could be distinguished based only on their structural chemical descriptors using approaches commonly used in ligand-based drug design. We applied the *k*NN classification QSAR approach to a data set of compounds characterized as binders or binding decoys of AmpC β-lactamase. Models were subjected to rigorous internal and external validation as part of our standard workflow (Figure 10.2) and a special QSAR modeling scheme was employed that took into account the imbalanced ratio of inhibitors to nonbinders (1:4) in this data set. Three hundred forty-two predictive models were obtained with correct classification rate (CCR) for both training and test sets as high as 0.90 or higher. The prediction accuracy was as high as 100% (CCR = 1.00) for the external validation set composed of ten compounds (ten true binders and ten decoys) selected randomly from the original data set. For an additional external set of fifty known nonbinders, we have achieved a CCR of 0.87 using very conservative model applicability domain threshold. The validated binary *k*NN QSAR models were further employed for mining the NCGC AmpC screening data set (69,653 compounds). The consensus prediction of sixty-four compounds identified as screening hits in the AmpC PubChem assay disagreed with their annotation in PubChem but was in agreement with the results of secondary assays.[93] At the same time, fifteen compounds were identified as potential binders contrary to their annotation in PubChem. Five of them were tested experimentally and showed inhibitory activities in millimolar range with the highest binding constant K_i of 135 μM. Our studies suggest that validated QSAR models could complement structure-based docking and scoring approaches in identifying promising hits by virtual screening of molecular libraries. This study also illustrates that robust QSAR models could be used to recover false negatives resulting from the high-throughput screening.

CONCLUSIONS: EMERGING QSAR RESEARCH STRATEGIES AND FOCUS ON LEAD DISCOVERY

In the past fifteen years, innovative technologies that enable rapid synthesis and high-throughput screening of large libraries of compounds have been adopted in almost all major pharmaceutical and biotech companies. As a result, there has been a huge increase in the number of compounds available on a routine basis to quickly screen for novel drug candidates against new targets or pathways. In contrast, such technologies have rarely become available to the academic research community, thus limiting its ability to conduct large-scale chemical genetics or chemical genomics research. The NIH Molecular Libraries Roadmap Initiative has changed this situation by forming the national Molecular Library Screening Centers Network (MLSCN)[94] with the results of screening assays made publicly available via PubChem.[9] These efforts have already led to the unprecedented growth of *available* databases of biologically tested compounds (cf. our recent review where we list about twenty available databases of compounds with known bioactivity).[15]

This growth creates new challenges for QSAR modeling such as developing novel approaches for the analysis and visualization of large databases of screening data, novel biologically relevant chemical diversity or similarity measures, and novel tools for virtual screening of compound libraries to ensure high expected hit rates. Application studies discussed in this chapter have established that QSAR models could be used successfully as virtual screening tools to discover compounds with the desired biological activity in chemical databases or virtual libraries.[18,37,59,86,87,91] The discovery of novel bioactive chemical entities is the primary goal of computational drug discovery, and the development of validated and predictive QSAR models is critical to achieve this goal. Due to the significant recent increase in publicly available data sets of biologically active compounds and the critical need to improve the hit rate of experimental compound screening *there is a strong need in developing widely accessible and reliable computational QSAR modeling techniques and specific end-point predictors.*

ACKNOWLEDGMENTS

The studies described in this review were supported in parts by the National Institutes of Health's Cheminformatics Center planning grant P20-RR20751 and the research grants R01GM066940 and R21GM076059.

REFERENCES

1. Hansch, C.; Streich, M.; Geiger, F.; Muir, R. M.; Maloney, P. P.; Fujita, T. Correlation of biological activity of plant growth regulators and chloromycetin derivatives with Hammett constants and partition coefficients. *J. Am. Chem. Soc.* **1963**, *85*, 2817–2824.
2. Boyd D. Successes of computer-assisted molecular design. In: *Reviews in Computational Chemistry*, Boyd, D.; Lipkowitz, K. B.; Eds. New York, NY: VCH; **1990**, 355–371.
3. Doweyko, A. M. QSAR: dead or alive? *J. Comput. Aided. Mol. Des.* **2008**, *22*, 81–89.
4. Tropsha A. Recent trends in quantitative structure-activity relationships. In: *Burger's Medicinal Chemistry and Drug Discovery*, Abraham, D.; Ed. New York, NY: John Wiley & Sons, **2003**; 49–77.
5. Stouch, T. R.; Kenyon, J. R.; Johnson, S. R.; Chen, X. Q.; Doweyko, A.; Li, Y. In silico ADME/Tox: why models fail. *J. Comput. Aided Mol. Des.* **2003**, *17*, 83–92.
6. Jorgensen, W. L.; Tirado-Rives, J. QSAR/QSPR and proprietary data. *J. Chem. Inf. Model.* **2006**, *46*, 937.
7. Maggiora, G. M. On outliers and activity cliffs: why QSAR often disappoints. *J. Chem. Inf. Model.* **2006**, *46*, 1535.
8. Johnson, S. R. The trouble with QSAR (or how I learned to stop worrying and embrace fallacy). *J. Chem. Inf. Model.* **2008**, *48*, 25–26.
9. PubChem. http://pubchem.ncbi.nlm.nih.gov/. **2008.**
10. Roth, B. L.; Kroeze W. K. Screening the receptorome yields validated molecular targets for drug discovery. *Curr. Pharm. Des.* **2006**, *12*, 1785–1795.
11. NCI. http://dtp nci nih gov/docs/3d_database/structural_information/smiles_strings html **2007.**
12. FDA. http://www.fda.gov/cder/Offices/OPS_IO/. **2005.**
13. NTP. http://ntp.niehs.nih.gov/ntpweb/. **2005.**
14. DSSTox. http://www.epa.gov/nheerl/dsstox/About.html. **2005.**
15. Oprea, T.; Tropsha, A. Target, chemical and bioactivity databases: integration is key. *Drug Discov. Today* **2006**, *3*, 357–365.
16. Hansch, C.; Fujita, T. r-s-p analysis: a method for the correlation of biological activity and chemical structure. *J. Am. Chem. Soc.* **1964**, *86*, 1616–1626.
17. Zheng, W.; Tropsha, A. Novel variable selection quantitative structure–property relationship approach based on the k-nearest-neighbor principle. *J. Chem. Inf. Comput. Sci.* **2000**, *40*, 185–194.
18. Tropsha, A. Application of predictive QSAR models to database mining. In: *Cheminformatics in Drug Discovery*, Oprea, T.; Ed. Weinheim: Wiley-VCH; **2005**, 437–455.
19. Tropsha, A. Predictive QSAR (quantitative structure activity relationships) modeling. In: *Comprehensive Medicinal Chemistry II*, Martin, Y. C.; Ed. Amsterdam: Elsevier, **2006**; 113–126.
20. Papa, E.; Villa, F.; Gramatica, P. Statistically validated QSARs, based on theoretical descriptors, for modeling aquatic toxicity of organic chemicals in *Pimephales promelas* (fathead minnow). *J. Chem. Inf. Model.* **2005**, *45*, 1256–1266.
21. Tetko, I. V. Neural network studies. 4. Introduction to associative neural networks. *J. Chem. Inf. Comput. Sci.* **2002**, *42*, 717–728.
22. Zupan, J.; Novic, M.; Gasteiger, J. Neural networks with counter-propagation learning-strategy used for modeling. *Chemometrics Intelligent Lab. Syst.* **1995**, *27*(2), 175–187.
23. Devillers, J. Strengths and weaknesses of the back propagation neural network in QSAR and QSPR studies. In: *Genetic Algorithms in Molecular Modeling*, Devillers, J.; Ed. San Diego, CA: Academic Press; **1996**; 1–24.
24. Engels, M. F. M.; Wouters, L.; Verbeeck, R.; Vanhoof, G. Outlier mining in high throughput screening experiments. *J. Biomol. Screen.* **2002**; (7): 341–351.
25. Schuurmann, G.; Aptula, A. O.; Kuhne, R.; Ebert, R. U. Stepwise discrimination between four modes of toxic action of phenols in the *Tetrahymena pyriformis* assay. *Chem. Res. Toxicol.* **2003**, *16*, 974–987.
26. Xue, Y.; Li, H.; Ung, C. Y.; Yap, C. W.; Chen, Y. Z. Classification of a diverse set of *Tetrahymena pyriformis* toxicity chemical compounds from molecular descriptors by statistical learning methods. *Chem. Res. Toxicol.* **2006**, *19*, 1030–1039.

27. Breiman, L.; Friedman, J. H.; Olshen, R. A.; Stone, C. J. *Classification and Regression Trees*. Florence, KY: Wadsworth; **1984**.

28. Deconinck, E.; Hancock, T.; Coomans, D.; Massart, D. L.; Vander Heyden, Y. Classification of drugs in absorption classes using the classification and regression trees (CART) methodology. *J. Pharm. Biomed. Anal.* **2005**, *39*, 91–103.

29. MOE. http://www.chemcomp.com/fdept/prodinfo.htm# Cheminformatics. **2005**.

30. Put, R.; Perrin, C.; Questier, F.; Coomans, D.; Massart, D. L.; Vander Heyden, Y. V. Classification and regression tree analysis for molecular descriptor selection and retention prediction in chromatographic quantitative structure-retention relationship studies. *J. Chromatogr. A* **2003**, *988*, 261–276.

31. Breiman L. Random forests. *J. Mach. Learn. Res.* **2001**, *45*, 5–32.

32. Svetnik, V.; Liaw, A.; Tong, C.; Culberson, J. C.; Sheridan, R. P.; Feuston, B. P. Random forest: a classification and regression tool for compound classification and QSAR modeling. *J. Chem. Inf. Comput. Sci.* **2003**, *43*, 1947–1958.

33. Put, R.; Xu, Q. S.; Massart, D. L.; Heyden. Y. V. Multivariate adaptive regression splines (MARS) in chromatographic quantitative structure-retention relationship studies. *J. Chromatogr. A* **2004**, *1055*, 11–19.

34. Friedman, J. H. Multivariate adaptive regression splines. *Ann. Stat.* **1991**, *19*, 1–67.

35. Vapnik, V. N. *The Nature of Statistical Learning Theory*. New York, NY: Springer-Verlag; **1995.**

36. Aires-de-Sousa, J.; Gasteiger, J. Prediction of enantiomeric excess in a combinatorial library of catalytic enantioselective reactions. *J. Comb. Chem.* **2005**, *7*, 298–301.

37. Oloff, S.; Mailman, R. B.; Tropsha, A. Application of validated QSAR models of D1 dopaminergic antagonists for database mining. *J. Med. Chem.* **2005**, *48*, 7322–7332.

38. Chohan, K. K.; Paine, S. W.; Waters, N. J. Quantitative structure activity relationships in drug metabolism. *Curr. Top. Med. Chem.* **2006**, *6*, 1569–1578.

39. Golbraikh, A.; Tropsha, A. Beware of q2! *J. Mol. Graph. Model.* **2002a**, *20*, 269–276.

40. Tropsha, A.; Gramatica, P.; Gombar, V. K. The importance of being earnest: validation is the absolute essential for successful application and interpretation of QSPR models. *QSAR Comb. Sci.* **2003** *22*, 69–77.

41. Kubinyi, H.; Hamprecht, F. A.; Mietzner, T. Three-dimensional quantitative similarity-activity relationships (3D QSiAR) from SEAL similarity matrices. *J. Med. Chem.* **1998**, *41*, 2553–2564.

42. Novellino, E.; Fattorusso, C.; Greco, G. Use of comparative molecular field analysis and cluster analysis in series design. *Pharm. Acta Helv.* **1995**, *70*, 149–154.

43. Norinder, U. Single and domain made variable selection in 3D QSAR applications. *J. Chemomet.* **1996**, *10*, 95–105.

44. Tropsha, A.; Cho, S. J. Cross-validated R2-guided region selection for CoMFA studies. In: *3D QSAR in Drug Design*, Vol. III, Kubinyi, H.; Folkers, G.; Martin, Y. C.; Eds. Dordrecht: Kluwer Academic; **1998**, 57–69.

45. Golbraikh, A.; Tropsha, A. Predictive QSAR modeling based on diversity sampling of experimental datasets for the training and test set selection. *J. Comput. Aided Mol. Des.* **2002b**, *16*, 357–369.

46. Golbraikh, A.; Shen, M.; Xiao, Z.; Xiao, Y. D.; Lee, K. H.; Tropsha, A. Rational selection of training and test sets for the development of validated QSAR models. *J. Comput. Aided. Mol. Des.* **2003b**, *17*, 241–253.

47. Pavan, M.; Netzeva, T. I.; Worth, A. P. Validation of a QSAR model for acute toxicity. *SAR QSAR Environ. Res.* **2006**, *17*, 147–171.

48. Vracko, M.; Bandelj, V.; Barbieri, P.; Benfenati, E.; Chaudhry, Q.; Cronin, M.; Devillers, J.; Gallegos, A.; Gini, G.; Gramatica, P.; Helma, C.; Mazzatorta, P.; Neagu, D.; Netzeva, T.; Pavan, M.; Patlewicz, G.; Randic, M.; Tsakovska, I.; Worth, A. Validation of counter propagation neural network models for predictive toxicology according to the OECD principles: a case study. *SAR QSAR Environ. Res.* **2006**, *17*, 265–284.

49. Saliner, A. G.; Netzeva, T. I.; Worth A. P. Prediction of estrogenicity: validation of a classification model. *SAR QSAR Environ. Res.* **2006**, *17*, 195–223.

50. Roberts, D. W.; Aptula, A. O.; Patlewicz, G. Mechanistic applicability domains for non-animal based prediction of toxicological endpoints: QSAR analysis of the schiff base applicability domain for skin sensitization. *Chem. Res. Toxicol.* **2006**, *19*, 1228–1233.

51. Estrada, E.; Patlewicz, G. On the usefulness of graph-theoretic descriptors in predicting theoretical parameters: phototoxicity of polycyclic aromatic hydrocarbons (PAHs). *Acta Clin. Croat.* **2004**, *77*, 203–211.

52. Moss, G. P.; Cronin, M. T. D. Quantitative structure-permeability relationships for percutaneous absorption: re-analysis of steroid data. *Int. J. Pharm.* **2002**, *238*, 105–109.

53. Leo, A. J.; Hansch, C. Role of hydrophobic effects in mechanistic QSAR. *Perspectives in Drug Discov. Des.* **1999**, *17*, 1–25.

54. Zhang, S.; Golbraikh, A.; Tropsha, A. Development of quantitative structure-binding affinity relationship models based on novel geometrical chemical descriptors of the protein-ligand interfaces. *J. Med. Chem.* **2006b**, *49*, 2713–2724.

55. Golbraikh, A.; Bonchev, D.; Tropsha, A. Novel chirality descriptors derived from molecular topology. *J. Chem. Inf. Comput. Sci.* **2001**, *41*, 147–158.

56. Kovatcheva, A.; Buchbauer, G.; Golbraikh, A.; Wolschann, P. QSAR modeling of alpha-campholenic derivatives with sandalwood odor. *J. Chem. Inf. Comput. Sci.* **2003**, *43*, 259–266.

57. Shen, M.; Xiao, Y.; Golbraikh, A.; Gombar, V. K.; Tropsha, A. Development and validation of k-nearest-neighbor QSPR models of metabolic stability of drug candidates. *J. Med. Chem.* **2003**, *46*, 3013–3020.

58. Shen, M.; LeTiran, A.; Xiao, Y.; Golbraikh, A.; Kohn, H.; Tropsha, A. Quantitative structure-activity relationship analysis of functionalized amino acid anticonvulsant agents using k nearest neighbor and simulated annealing PLS methods. *J. Med. Chem.* **2002**, *45*, 2811–2823.

59. Shen, M.; Beguin, C.; Golbraikh, A.; Stables, J. P.; Kohn, H.; Tropsha, A. Application of predictive QSAR models to database mining: identification and experimental validation of novel anticonvulsant compounds. *J. Med. Chem.* **2004**, *47*, 2356–2364.

60. Zhang, S.; Golbraikh, A.; Oloff, S.; Kohn, H.; Tropsha, A. A novel automated lazy learning QSAR (ALL-QSAR) approach: method development, applications, and virtual screening of chemical databases using validated ALL-QSAR models. *J. Chem. Inf. Model.* **2006a**, *46*, 1984–1995.

61. Golbraikh, A.; Shen, M.; Xiao, Z.; Xiao, Y. D.; Lee, K. H.; Tropsha, A. Rational selection of training and test sets for the development of validated QSAR models. *J. Comput. Aided. Mol. Des.* **2003a**, *17*, 241–253.

62. Mandel, J. Use of the singular value decomposition in regression-analysis. *Am. Stat.* **1982**, *36*, 15–24.

63. Afantitis, A.; Melagraki, G.; Sarimveis, H.; Koutentis, P. A.; Markopoulos, J.; Igglessi-Markopoulou, O. A novel QSAR model for predicting induction of apoptosis by 4-aryl-4H-chromenes. *Bioorg. Med. Chem.* **2006**, *14*, 6686–6694.

64. Netzeva, T. I.; Gallegos, S. A.; Worth, A. P. Comparison of the applicability domain of a quantitative structure-activity relationship for estrogenicity with a large chemical inventory. *Environ. Toxicol. Chem.* **2006**, *25*, 1223–1230.

65. Tong, W.; Xie, Q.; Hong, H.; Shi, L.; Fang, H.; Perkins, R. Assessment of prediction confidence and domain extrapolation of two structure-activity relationship models for predicting estrogen receptor binding activity. *Environ. Health Perspect.* **2004**, *112*, 1249–1254.

66. Helma, C. Lazy structure-activity relationships (lazar) for the prediction of rodent carcinogenicity and *Salmonella* mutagenicity. *Mol. Divers.* **2006**, *10*, 147–158.

67. Zhu, H.; Tropsha, A.; Fourches, D.; Varnek, A.; Papa, E.; Gramatica, P.; Oberg, T.; Dao, P.; Cherkasov, A.; Tetko, I. V. Combinatorial QSAR modeling of chemical toxicants tested against *Tetrahymena pyriformis*. *J. Chem. Inf. Model.* **2008**, *48*, 766–784.

68. Wang, X. S.; Tang, H.; Golbraikh, A.; Tropsha, A. Combinatorial QSAR modeling of specificity and subtype selectivity of ligands binding to serotonin receptors 5HT1E and 5HT1F. *J. Chem. Inf. Model.* **2008**, *48*, 997–1013.

69. de Cerqueira, L. P.; Golbraikh, A.; Oloff, S.; Xiao, Y.; Tropsha, A. Combinatorial QSAR modeling of P-glycoprotein substrates. *J. Chem. Inf. Model.* **2006**, *46*, 1245–1254.

70. Kovatcheva, A.; Golbraikh, A.; Oloff, S.; Xiao, Y. D.; Zheng, W.; Wolschann, P.; Buchbauer, G.; Tropsha, A. Combinatorial QSAR of ambergris fragrance compounds. *J. Chem. Inf. Comput. Sci.* **2004**, *44*, 582–595.

71. Sachs, L. *Handbook of Statistics*. New York, NY: Springer-Verlag; **1984.**

72. Zhu, H.; Tropsha, A.; Fourches, D.; Varnek, A.; Papa, E.; Gramatica, P.; Oberg, T.; Dao, P.; Cherkasov, A.; Tetko, I. V. Combinatorial QSAR modeling of chemical toxicants tested against *Tetrahymena pyriformis*. *J. Chem. Inf. Model.* **2008**, *48*(4), 766–784.

73. Aptula, A. O.; Roberts, D. W.; Cronin, M. T. D.; Schultz, T. W. Chemistry-toxicity relationships for the effects of di- and trihydroxybenzenes to *Tetrahymena pyriformis*. *Chem. Res. Toxicol.* **2005**, *18*, 844–854.

74. Netzeva, T. I.; Schultz, T. W. QSARs for the aquatic toxicity of aromatic aldehydes from *Tetrahymena* data. *Chemosphere* **2005**, *61*, 1632–1643.

75. Schultz, T. W.; Sinks, G. D.; Miller, L. A. Population growth impairment of sulfur-containing compounds to *Tetrahymena pyriformis*. *Environ. Toxicol.* **2001**, *16*, 543–549.

76. Schultz, T. W.; Cronin, M. T.; Netzeva, T. I.; Aptula, A. O. Structure-toxicity relationships for aliphatic chemicals evaluated with *Tetrahymena pyriformis*. *Chem. Res. Toxicol.* **2002**, *15*, 1602–1609.

77. Schultz, T. W.; Netzeva, T. I. Development and evaluation of QSARs for ecotoxic endpoints: the benzene response-surface model for *Tetrahymena* toxicity. In: *Modeling Environmental Fate and Toxicity*, Cronin, M. T. D.; Livingstone, D. J.; Eds. Boca Raton, FL: CRC Press; **2004**, 265–284.

78. Schultz, T. W.; Netzeva, T. I.; Roberts, D. W.; Cronin, M. T. Structure-toxicity relationships for the effects to *Tetrahymena pyriformis* of aliphatic, carbonyl-containing, alpha,beta-unsaturated chemicals. *Chem. Res. Toxicol.* **2005**, *18*, 330–341.

79. Schultz, T. W.; Yarbrough, J. W.; Woldemeskel, M. Toxicity to *Tetrahymena* and abiotic thiol reactivity of aromatic isothiocyanates. *Cell Biol. Toxicol.* **2005**, *21*, 181–189.

80. Schultz, T. W. Structure-toxicity relationships for benzenes evaluated with Tetrahymena pyriformis. *Chem. Res. Toxicol.* **1999**, *12*, 1262–1267.

81. Schultz, T. W.; Hewitt, M.; Netzeva, T. I.; Cronin. M. T. D. Assessing applicability domains of toxicological QSARs: definition, confidence in predicted values, and the role of mechanisms of action. *QSAR Comb. Sci.* **2007**, *26*, 238–254.

82. Gramatica P. Principles of QSAR models validation: internal and external. *QSAR Comb. Sci.* **2007**, *26*, 694–701.

83. Yang, C.; Richard, A. M.; Cross, K. P. The art of data mining the minefields of toxicity databases to link chemistry to biology. *Curr. Comput. Aided Drug Des.* **2006**, *2*, 135–150.

84. Irwin, J. J.; Shoichet, B. K. ZINC – a free database of commercially available compounds for virtual screening. *J. Chem. Inf. Model.* **2005**, *45*, 177–182.

85. Medina-Franco, J. L.; Golbraikh, A.; Oloff, S.; Castillo, R.; Tropsha, A. Quantitative structure-activity relationship analysis of pyridinone HIV-1 reverse transcriptase inhibitors using the k nearest neighbor method and QSAR-based database mining. *J. Comput. Aided Mol. Des.* **2005**, *19*, 229–242.

86. Zhang, S.; Wei, L.; Bastow, K.; Zheng, W.; Brossi, A.; Lee, K. H.; Tropsha, A. Antitumor Agents 252. Application of validated QSAR models to database mining: discovery of novel tylophorine derivatives as potential anticancer agents. *J. Comput. Aided Mol. Des.* **2007**, *21*, 97–112.

87. Hsieh, J. H.; Wang, X. S.; Teotico, D.; Golbraikh, A.; Tropsha, A. Differentiation of AmpC beta-lactamase binders vs. decoys using classification kNN QSAR modeling and application of the QSAR classifier to virtual screening. *J. Comput. Aided Mol. Des.* **2008**, *22*(9), 593–609.

88. Tropsha, A.; Cho, S. J.; Zheng, W. "New tricks for an old dog": development and application of novel QSAR methods for rational design of combinatorial chemical libraries and database mining. In: *Rational Drug Design: Novel Methodology and Practical Applications*, Parrill, A. L.; Reddy, M. R.; Eds. Washington, DC: American Chemical Society; **1999**, 198–211.

89. Cho, S. J.; Zheng, W.; Tropsha, A. Rational combinatorial library design. 2. Rational design of targeted combinatorial peptide libraries using chemical similarity probe and the inverse QSAR approaches. *J. Chem. Inf. Comput. Sci.* **1998**, *38*, 259–268.

90. Gussio, R.; Pattabiraman, N.; Kellogg, G. E.; Zaharevitz, D. W. Use of 3D QSAR methodology for data mining the National Cancer Institute Repository of Small Molecules: application to HIV-1 reverse transcriptase inhibition. *Methods* **1998**, *14*, 255–263.

91. Tropsha, A.; Zheng, W. Identification of the descriptor pharmacophores using variable selection QSAR: applications to database mining. *Curr. Pharm. Des.* **2001**, *7*, 599–612.

92. Maybridge. http://www.daylight.com/products/databases/Maybridge.html **2005.**

93. Babaoglu, K.; Simeonov, A.; Irwin, J. J.; Nelson, M. E.; Feng, B.; Thomas, C. J.; Cancian, L.; Costi, M. P.; Maltby, D. A.; Jadhav, A.; Inglese, J.; Austin, C. P.; Shoichet, B. K. Comprehensive mechanism analysis of hits from high-throughput and docking screens against beta-lactamase. *J. Med. Chem.* **2008**, *51*, 2502–2511.

94. Austin, C. P.; Brady, L. S.; Insel, T. R.; Collins, F. S. NIH Molecular Libraries Initiative. *Science* **2004**, *306*, 1138–1139.

11

Predicting ADME properties in drug discovery

William J. Egan

INTRODUCTION

Drug discovery is an extremely risky business. Practically every molecule ever made in a drug discovery research project will be a failure. It is estimated that for every ten research projects producing molecules of high-enough quality to begin clinical testing in man, 10,000 to 20,000 molecules will need to be synthesized. Of those ten clinical candidates, nine will fail, leaving just one new drug in the end. In short, the pharmaceutical industry has a failure rate on the order of 99.99%.[1,2] These many failures do not come cheaply. The cost of developing a new drug is estimated to be between $500 million and $2 billion, depending on the indication and company.[3]

As Dr. Arthur Patchett of Merck said, "Current, major stumbling blocks in drug development are often the clumsy, empirical, and time-consuming efforts required to go from an exquisitely potent in vitro inhibitor to one with good bioavailability and an adequate duration of action. This is the unglamorous part of drug development but often separates highly successful ventures from those which lag behind them."[4] Medicinal chemists commonly synthesize potent molecules only to find out later they have poor exposure in vivo and thus poor efficacy.

The broad term *exposure* can be broken down into its component factors: absorption, distribution, metabolism, and excretion, which are commonly known as ADME. Solubility is also very important and tends to be implicitly included in discussions of ADME.

Poor ADME properties contribute significantly to the high failure rate. Kola and Landis[2] reported that at ten large pharmaceutical companies, ADME/formulation problems were responsible for ~40% of clinical failures in the year 1991 but only ~12% of clinical failures in the year 2000. Clinical safety and toxicity were responsible for ~22% of clinical failures in 1991 and ~33% of clinical failures in 2000. Clinical failures due to poor efficacy/pharmacodynamics were just under 30% at both time points.

Computational modeling to predict ADME properties of molecules began in earnest in the late 1990s. This work was spurred by a number of factors. First, there was an increasing awareness of the importance of poor ADME properties as a cause of failures in drug discovery. Second, higher throughput in vitro assays for ADME properties became available (e.g., the Caco-2 cell permeability assay designed to estimate the intestinal absorption potential of drug candidates). Third, databases, computer processing power, and algorithms all matured and enabled these modeling efforts.

As Dr. Richard Hamming said, "The purpose of computing is insight, not numbers."[5] By analogy, we should conduct our ADME modeling work to help answer the two questions we always ask in drug discovery research: "Is this molecule any good?" and "How can we make it better?" We need insight and guidance, not yet another column of numbers to go into a spreadsheet.

ADME models can help drug discovery efforts by (1) aiding chemists in triaging large numbers of molecules to select interesting examples for testing, (2) providing alerts of ADME risks so that those risks can be investigated earlier in the drug discovery process, (3) helping chemists interpret experimental ADME data, and (4) guiding decision-making and prioritizing syntheses.

The physiological and physicochemical mechanisms of ADME and solubility are amazingly complex and not fully understood even today. This is a fertile area for industrial and academic research due to its importance in drug discovery. This review will discuss recent research (through mid-2008) with a focus on practical findings and insights.

DRUG-LIKENESS MEASURES

One of the simplest and most common ways to evaluate a molecule for ADME properties is a qualitative examination of its basic descriptor values such as molecular weight (MW), lipophilicity (log$P$), polar surface area (PSA), counts of hydrogen bond donors and acceptors (HBD, HBA), and count of rotatable bonds (RB). This type of approach was popularized by Lipinski's famous Rule of 5.[6] Lipinski's cutoffs were MW > 500, computed log$P$ > 5, HBA > 10, and HBD > 5. The Rule of 5 considers a violation of any two of these cutoffs to be an alert for poor absorption or permeability. These cutoffs were based on the 90th percentile of distributions of molecules in the World Drug Index having USAN or INN names.

More recent studies have expanded on this type of analysis by subcategorizing descriptor distributions by oral versus nonoral marketed drugs, temporal patterns of development candidates versus marketed drugs, target family differences, and targeted simple analyses. Wenlock et al.[7] compared the mean and standard deviations of MW, logP, logD$_{7.4}$, HBD, HBA, and RB for orally administered clinical candidates from Phase I clinical trials to preregistration, as well as a set of 594 marketed oral drugs. The results showed that the mean molecular weight declined consistently as drug candidates advanced through the clinical trial process, going from 423 at Phase I to 337 in marketed oral drugs. Mean lipophilicity, as measured by ACD logP, was roughly constant (2.6 at to 2.5) but the discontinued development candidates at each phase had higher mean logP values (3.5 at Phase I, 3.5 at Phase II, 3.2 at Phase III). These differences were statistically significant and indicate there is an increased chance of clinical failure for high MW and/or logP compounds. Vieth et al.[8] examined the distributions of computed descriptors for 1,729 marketed drugs, including 1,193 orally administered drugs. They tabulated means, min/max, and different percentiles for 12 descriptors by six categories. One interesting and statistically significant difference was that injectable drugs have higher MW, greater polarity, lower lipophilicity, and are more flexible than oral drugs.

Two studies examined the changes in computed descriptors over time. For oral drugs launched prior to 1983, mean MW, HBA, RB, and number of rings are lower than for drugs launched during 1983–2002, whereas mean %PSA, ClogP, and HBD do not change significantly.[9] Similarly, Proudfoot[10] found that mean MW increased steadily from below 300 in 1950 to often above 400 in 1997 and that only seven drugs were marketed between 1937 and 1951 with MW > 500 but that 32 drugs exceeding MW 500 were marketed 1983–1997. Lipophilicity did not increase. Increasing MW and steady lipophilicity causes an increase in polarity that would lower the probability of absorption. Also, Proudfoot notes that less than 5% of oral drugs have HBD > 4, which may be related to their propensity for Phase II metabolism.

Studies of proteomic or target families show large differences in the distribution of computed descriptors between classes. Vieth and Sutherland[11] were able to assign a specific proteomic family to 642 of 1,210 marketed oral drugs. Mean descriptor values were not statistically different from overall oral drugs for drugs in the cytochrome P450, phosphodiesterase, kinase, and transporter families. Drugs targeting G-protein-coupled receptors (GPCRs) and proteases had significantly greater means for one or more of MW, ClogP, HBD, or HBA. Drugs targeting ion channels were significantly smaller than the overall distribution. Morphy[12] analyzed the computed property distributions of a literature and internal compound database at Organon containing data on 1,860 optimization projects. All target families showed increases in MW during optimization. Differences between families were due to differences in the properties of the leads. High property values were consis-

tently observed for drugs targeting peptide GPCRs, integrin receptors, proteases, and transferases, whereas drugs targeting monoamine GPCRs, ion channels, oxidases, and transporters had lower property values. Antibacterial compounds have descriptor averages that are different from the average descriptor values reported for oral drug. Gram-positive antibacterials have average MW = 813, clogD$_{7.4}$ = −0.2, and PSA = 243. Gram-negative antibacterials have average MW = 414, clogD$_{7.4}$ = −2.8, and PSA = 165.[13]

Gleeson at GlaxoSmithKline has analyzed internal ADMET data on thousands of drug discovery compounds using only three simple descriptors: MW, logP, and ionization state. The analyses show general trends in line with common beliefs, but are imprecise.[14] Correcting computed logP for ionization by using computed logD$_{7.4}$ < 5 as a cutoff was shown to pass approximately 50% of molecules with computed logP > 5 in a Lipinski-type analysis.[15]

Overall, several useful concepts emerge from these analyses. Different targets and routes of administration may require biased property distributions and screening libraries for successful lead optimization. This could influence the eventual chances of project success and should be taken into account early by project leaders. Once more, optimization focused on potency has been shown again to lead to larger molecules which increases the potential for poor ADME properties. The extent of any ADME issues would of course depend on the structure of lead molecules. Larger, more lipophilic molecules historically have an increased rate of failure in the clinic. Finally, more rules using simple descriptors have been identified for culling molecules with poor ADME properties.

SOLUBILITY

Solubility is a property that depends on many complex factors. It is important to know the exact solid form of the molecule that was tested, the solvent used, and the performance characteristics of the experimental method. Molecules are commonly amorphous in form early in the research process, less pure, and are dissolved in dimethyl sulfoxide (DMSO) to create stock solutions for archival storage and high-throughput screening. These DMSO stocks are then diluted with buffer for activity and ADME in vitro screening assays. In later stage research, larger quantities of promising molecules are synthesized with the aim of producing a crystalline solid suitable for formulation and dosing in animal studies for pharmacology, pharmacokinetics, and toxicity. Salt forms, pH-dependent ionization, the existence of polymorphs with their varying solubilities, melting point of the crystal lattice, and the many available formulation solvents (water, polyethylene glycol, methylcellulose, organics, etc.) all influence measured solubility. Solubility can be measured with varying degrees of accuracy ranging from cheaper and faster, but less accurate and more variable, kinetic approaches using nephelometry or flow cytometry detection to "gold standard" thermodynamic solubility using shake-flask with high-pressure liquid chromatography with UV detector (HPLC-UV) or liquid chromatograph/mass spectrometry detection. These factors can cause a single molecule to have widely differing solubility values that are not comparable.

From a modeling standpoint, the prediction of a molecule's solubility is a very difficult task because of the issues listed above.[16–18] The problem of predicting solubility has been attacked with some success with complex neural network models. Although not interpretable, neural networks can function as a black-box in silico assay. Other techniques that are more interpretable have also been applied to the problem.

An interesting approach for estimating the effects of small modifications on molecular properties such as solubility was published by Leach et al.[19] The technique is called "matched molecular pairs analysis." First, a set of specific structural transformations are used to search a set of molecules having some type of property data. Subsets of almost identical molecules having each transformation are identified (e.g., all molecules differing by *p*-fluorine on a phenyl ring). The percentage of molecules with a positive property value change is computed, and the binomial distribution is used as a statistical test to ascertain if the change is significant. For example, the authors reported that when an amide is methylated, 112 of 142 pairs had increased solubility by an average of +0.64 log units. The percentage of pairs with increased solubility was 79% with a 95% confidence interval of 71–85%, indicating the effect is statistically significant. This technique is not limited to solubility but can be applied to any property of a molecule, ADME or otherwise. The authors also show examples of insights gained from matched molecular pairs analysis of data on protein binding and oral exposure in rats. Matched molecular pairs analysis is clearly interpretable and as the authors state, "can be used as a tool to test many of the 'rules of thumb' that abound within medicinal chemistry."

Another simple approach to classifying molecules as soluble or insoluble was published by Lamanna et al.[20] They used recursive partitioning to classify 3,563 molecules as soluble/insoluble using a small set of descriptors. Multiple models were found which were predictive. The best model used only two simple descriptors: MW and the descriptor "aromatic proportion" and had an accuracy of 81% for a test set of 1,200 molecules using a cutoff of 30 μM.

Huuskonen[21] assembled aqueous solubility data for 1,297 organic molecules and modeled it using neural network and linear regression models trained on 55 connectivity, shape, and electrotopological state descriptors. Test set results were $r^2 = 0.92$ and standard deviation (s) = 0.60 for the neural network and $r^2 = 0.88$ and $s = 0.71$ for the linear regression model. Yan et al.[22] were able to build neural network and linear regression models of comparable quality for the Huuskonen data set using only 18 topological descriptors. Test set results were $r^2 = 0.94$ and $s = 0.52$ for the neural network model and $r^2 = 0.89$ and $s = 0.68$ for the

linear regression model. Further work by Yan et al.[23] modeled the aqueous solubility of a set of 2,743 drug discovery molecules from Merck KGaA, resulting in a neural network model using 18 2D topological descriptors with $r = 0.92$ and $s = 0.62$. The authors note that the Huuskonen set is limited in diversity in comparison to the Merck KGaA data set.

One problem highlighted by several reviewers[17,24] is that data sets like the Huuskonen set cover unnecessarily large ranges of solubility. The Huuskonen set covers the range log$S$ (log of solubility in mol/l) from -11.62 to $+1.58$, which converts approximately to 9.6×10^{-7} to 1.5×10^{7} μg/ml for a MW of 400 Da. Johnson and Zheng[17] recommend a pharmaceutically relevant range of 0.1 to 250 μg/ml as more appropriate.

However, the issue is more complex than a simple range. Lipinski[25] provides better guidance for minimum acceptable solubility based on maximal absorbable dose calculations. These take into account dose amount and permeability both of which have significant effects on required solubility. For example, the minimum acceptable solubility for a 0.1 mg/kg human dose (a 7 mg pill) of a high-permeability molecule is 1 μg/ml, whereas the minimum acceptable solubility for a 10 mg/kg human dose (a 700 mg pill) of a low permeability molecule is 2,100 μg/ml. This range is somewhat similar to the range recommended by Johnson and Zheng, but it is important for both medicinal chemists and modelers to be aware of the factors modifying the minimum acceptable solubility values within the solubility range relevant for drug discovery.

Goeller et al.[26] at Bayer modeled buffer solubility at pH 6.5 using a data set containing 5,000 molecules whose solubility was measured in a consistent fashion. The Bayer assay was a high-throughput assay starting from DMSO stock diluted to 1% DMSO in phosphate-buffered saline at pH 6.5 and using HPLC detection. The log$S$ range is approximately -6 to -3. The model used 65 VAMP/PROPGEN descriptors computed from 3D structures plus eight common 2D descriptors. These descriptors were used to train various neural networks. The best neural network had a root-mean-squared error (rmse) of 0.73 and 83% of predictions had <1.0 log unit error on a test data set of 7,222 molecules.

Recently, Gaussian process nonlinear regression was used to model a set of combined literature aqueous solubility data and shake flask buffer solubility data for 632 molecules at pH 7.0–7.4 from Schering AG.[27] This machine learning algorithm is just beginning to be used in drug discovery modeling. Gaussian process models can provide error estimates for predictions and can automatically select features. Other studies on modeling solubility using Gaussian processes have also been published. The error bars shown in these articles are wide enough to be alarming.[28,29]

As mentioned, solubility in DMSO is important for compound storage and high-throughput screening efforts. Computational models for the prediction of DMSO solubility have been reported by Balakin et al. and Lu and

Bakken.[30,31] Balakin et al. modeled a large set of 65,500 molecules with measured DMSO solubility. Molecules were classified as insoluble if they were not soluble at 0.01 mol/l. A Kohonen neural network was able to correctly classify 93% of compounds using only eight descriptors. Such models work by mapping the input data into a smaller dimensional space based on the nodes and making predictions based on node membership. In essence, a molecule is predicted as soluble or insoluble in DMSO based on the neighboring molecules in its assigned node. Surprisingly, a standard neural network performed worse on the same data, having approximately 75% accuracy. At Pfizer, 33,329 compounds dissolved in 30 mM DMSO stock solutions were visually inspected for precipitates. They computed 200 2D descriptors (78 E-state keys and a set of 122 from the MOE software package) to build five models to classify compounds that showed precipitation versus those that showed no precipitation. Test set accuracy was reasonably good across all five models: recursive partitioning 81%, random forest 81%, binary quantitative structure/activity relationship (QSAR) 74%, self-organizing map 69%, and linear discriminant analysis 76%.

Little work has been performed to model solubility while taking into account crystal packing. Johnson et al.[32] published an initial attempt using calculated intrinsic solubility corrected for effects of ionization, and crystal-packing forces derived from an escalating temperature molecular dynamics simulation. Although the model requires crystal structure information, it can be applied to analogs that do not have crystal structures simply by overlaying those analogs onto the known crystal form to begin the simulation. Results suggest this type of model could be useful to understand the solubility of late-stage optimization and early development candidates, although it is highly dependent on pK_a estimates.

INTESTINAL ABSORPTION

Theory and computational aspects of intestinal permeability have been reviewed in detail by Egan and Lauri.[33] A drug must be somewhat permeable through the membrane of the intestinal tract if it is to be administered orally and achieve systemic exposure. The rate of membrane permeability is strongly related to the lipophilicity and hydrophilicity of the molecule.

Egan et al.[33,34] demonstrated that a statistically based classification model built using only PSA and Alog$P$98 could predict the region of chemical space occupied by well-absorbed (>90% absorbed) molecules and exclude poorly absorbed molecules (<30% absorbed). Molecules with absorption in the range 30–90% were not used because of large data variability. Actively transported molecules were excluded. These results were validated on Caco-2 permeability assay data from drug discovery projects at Pharmacopeia. The Caco-2 permeabilities were shown to have a hill-shape in PSA-Alog$P$98 space. The sides of the hill

declined rapidly at the edge of the well-absorbed region and less than 10% of highly permeable molecules were outside the well-absorbed region, while only 21% of poorly permeable molecules were inside the well-absorbed region.

In an excellent article, Zhao et al.[35] assembled a carefully reviewed literature set of human absorption data on 241 drugs. They showed that a linear regression model built with five Abraham descriptors could fit percent human absorption data reasonably well ($r^2 = 0.83$, rmse = 14%). The descriptors are excess molar refraction (E), polarizability (S), hydrogen bond acidity (A), hydrogen bond basicity (B), and McGowan volume (V), all related to lipophilicity, hydrophilicity, and size. In a follow-up article, data on rat absorption for 151 drugs was collected from the literature and modeled using the Abraham descriptors.[36] A model with only descriptors A and B had $r^2 = 0.66$, rmse = 15%.

All in vivo data, including the human and rat absorption data used by both Egan and Zhao et al., have considerable variability. Zhao et al. comment that measurements of percent absorbed for the same molecule may vary by 30% and that the 95% confidence interval for a prediction is approximately 30% given a model rmse of 15%. This is approximately the same as the normal experimental error for absorption values. This means that models predicting percent absorbed have to be carefully interpreted (i.e., a prediction of 30% absorbed really means the molecule is predicted to have absorption from 15–45%). For this problem, regression models are really no better than classification models because of the variability in absorption data.

A classification regression tree model using 28 descriptors to predict the fraction absorbed for a large set of 1,260 drugs and drug candidates has been published.[37] The training set was 899 molecules and fraction absorbed was split into six classes (0–0.19, 0.2–0.31, 0.32–0.43, 0.44–0.59, 0.6–0.75, 0.76–1). Predicted values were reported as the median of each class. Average absolute error (AAE) for the test set of 362 molecules was 0.169 and 80.4% of molecules were predicted within one class of their actual class. For 37 proprietary molecules having human data, AAE = 0.14 and 86.4% of molecules were predicted correctly within one class.

Descriptors such as PSA, Clog$P$, and the Abraham descriptors can be interpreted in terms of chemical structure without much difficulty. Jones et al.[38] showed that quantum mechanical descriptors can be used to successfully predict intestinal absorption and at the same time provide an interpretable model. They used the data set of Zhao et al.[35] and computed molecular surface charges using density functional theory. The model quality was almost identical to the Abraham descriptor model reported by Zhao et al. (rmse = 15% for the same test set). The surface charges were mapped to the 3D structure of drugs creating an easily interpretable image.

Intramolecular hydrogen bonds can have an effect on membrane permeability. If a polar molecule can adopt a conformation that forms intramolecular hydrogen bonds, it will be able to present a more lipophilic surface to the membrane and solvent and thus have greater permeability than standard measures of polarity would suggest. Rezai et al.[39,40] conducted two experiments testing this effect. The first experiment synthesized nine cyclic hexapeptide diastereomers and measured their parallel artificial membrane permeability assay (PAMPA) permeabilities. The least and most permeable cyclic hexapeptides had permeabilities differing by two orders of magnitude. NMR and molecular modeling studies suggested that the most permeable cyclic peptide exposed only one amide to solvent, whereas the least permeable cyclic peptide exposed three to five amides to solvent.

In the second experiment, virtual libraries of 128 hexapeptides and 320 heptapeptides were analyzed computationally using extensive conformational sampling in low (membrane) and high (water) dielectric environments. They hypothesized that the partition coefficient between two different environments (the free energy of insertion) of the lowest energy conformer in the low dielectric environment would be proportional to the PAMPA permeability. Eleven peptides with varied predicted properties were synthesized and their PAMPA permeabilities did have a high correlation ($r^2 = 0.96$) with the computed free energy of insertion. These approaches could give insights into the mechanisms of permeability of drug candidates with larger molecular weight and greater flexibility that are capable of forming multiple intermolecular hydrogen bonds.

Computational models are increasingly being added to drug discovery workflows. At Pfizer, computational models for passive permeability and active efflux were developed using internal Caco-2 data on 3,018 molecules.[41] Two models were built because the apical to basolateral measurements of permeability normally used to estimate passive permeability will be affected if a compound is an efflux substrate. Logistic regression was used to fit molecular operating environment (MOE) 2D graph fingerprints. Model predictions and results for similar compounds are reported to chemists. Receiver operating characteristic curve analysis was used to evaluate model quality: AUC = 0.9 for the efflux model and AUC = 0.83 for the passive permeability model (a perfect classifier has an AUC score of 1.0). Guidance is provided to project teams based on the predictions (e.g., molecules predicted to have low passive permeability without active efflux should be submitted to the cheaper PAMPA assay and not to cellular assays during lead optimization efforts).

BLOOD-BRAIN-BARRIER PENETRATION

Computational models for blood-brain-barrier penetration have been well reviewed in detail by Clark.[42] Penetration of the blood-brain-barrier (BBB) *via* passive diffusion is dependent on the hydrophilicity and lipophilicity of a molecule. However, the BBB is a thicker, more lipophilic membrane than the intestinal membrane. Kelder et al.[43] showed that very few of 776 orally administered central

nervous system (CNS) drugs had PSA > 90, while a substantial fraction of 1,590 orally administered non-CNS had PSA > 90. These results demonstrate hydrophilic molecules have poor BBB penetration.

A simple two-variable linear regression model using PSA and ClogP was used to successfully predict logBB with $r = 0.887$, $s = 0.354$ (logBB = $\log_{10}$ [brain]/[blood]).[44] Lobell et al.[45] compared a set of 14 models designed to predict logBB and concluded two of the 14 models had advantages. Lobell used a stepwise linear regression on 34 2D and 3D variables to produce a model with five terms plus intercept with $r^2 = 0.837$ and MAE = 0.26. This model was judged best for low-medium-throughput applications. The 2D Cerius^2 ADME model for predicting logBB was judged the best compromise between speed and accuracy for ultra-high-throughput processing of large data sets. The 2D Cerius^2 ADME model fit AlogP98 and 2D PSA to predict logBB with a robust regression and uses an exclusionary region to prevent extrapolation.

The calculated cross-sectional area of a molecule (A_{Dcalc}) based on the internal amphiphilic gradient of a molecule has been used as the basis for a novel BBB model.[46] For each molecule, a conformational ensemble was generated and the smallest A_{Dcalc} was chosen. A simple biplot of $\log D_{7.4}$ vs. A_{Dcalc} was sufficient to correctly predict the BBB penetration of 85.2% of 122 drugs.

Abraham et al.[47] modeled literature data of rat in vivo BBB penetration measured in blood, plasma, or serum. They concluded that the three types could be combined because the systematic differences were so small. A linear regression model built using the Abraham descriptors for 116 molecules had $r^2 = 0.73$ and $s = 0.34$ and performed well on a test set with AAE = 0.25 and $s = 0.31$. They note the experimental error(s) for logBB should be approximately 0.3 log units, which is the error of the fitted model. Work by Zhao et al.[48] further demonstrates the ability of models built using one to five descriptors (Abraham, PSA, HBA, HBD, RB, etc.) to provide useful predictions of BBB penetration. Models were built using a 1,093-compound training set and tested on a 500-compound set. Models built using one to five simple descriptors had test set accuracies for +/− classifications in the range 96.5–99.8% for BBB+ molecules and 65.3–79.6% for BBB− molecules.

A concern about the use of logBB values as the index of brain permeability/penetration has been raised by Pardridge.[49] He argues that logBB is a simplistic and incorrect distributional measure that does not take into account actual permeabilities. Pardridge advocates using the BBB PS product that is a measure of unidirectional clearance from blood across the BBB to the brain and predicts the level of free drug in the brain. Modeling results for two small data sets of BBB PS data suggest that models similar to those discussed above can readily predict BBB PS. Liu et al.[50] measured the BBB PS and fit a linear regression model to predict logPS of 23 molecules with only three terms (logD, PSA, and van der Waals surface area of basic atoms) and $r^2 = 0.74$

and $s = 0.50$. Abraham[51] achieved similar results modeling literature data on logPS for 30 molecules using a linear regression model fit to five Abraham descriptors, with $r^2 = 0.87$ and $s = 0.52$.

P-GLYCOPROTEIN EFFLUX

P-glycoprotein is an ABC cassette transporter encoded by the *MDR1* gene in humans that is responsible for the efflux of drugs from cells. It plays a significant role in limiting brain penetration and to a lesser extent limits intestinal absorption of drugs. For oral drugs dosed in quantities greater than 50 mg with reasonable dissolution rates, P-glycoprotein transport will be saturated and thus unable to limit absorption. It should be noted that drugs with poor solubility effectively have a "low dose" and may have limited absorption due to P-glycoprotein efflux (e.g., paclitaxel). Unfortunately, the blood concentrations of drugs at the BBB do not achieve the levels found for most drugs in the intestines. Thus, P-glycoprotein transporters at the BBB cannot be saturated and will decrease the brain penetration of substrates.[52,53]

In a study of P-glycoprotein substrates versus nonsubstrates, Varma et al.[54] concluded that substrate molecules with high passive permeability overwhelmed the transporter while substrate molecules with moderate passive permeability were more affected by P-glycoprotein. Approximately half of 63 P-glycoprotein substrates studied had MW > 400 and PSA > 75, indicating that larger, more polar molecules are more likely to be P-glycoprotein substrates.

Several QSAR models have been used to predict whether a molecule is a P-glycoprotein substrate. Gombar et al.[55] modeled a set of 95 P-glycoprotein substrates and nonsubstrates using stepwise linear discriminant analysis. Class assignment was based on efflux ratios measured by an in vitro Madin–Darby canine kidney cell assay run at GlaxoSmithKline. The initial 254 descriptors were trimmed down to a set of 27 descriptors with an accuracy of 98.9%. Performance on a test set was also good, with 50/58 (86.2%) correctly predicted. A single E-state descriptor, MolES, representing molecular bulk, was particularly good at discriminating substrates. For MolES > 110, eighteen of nineteen molecules were substrates, and for MolES < 49, eleven of thirteen molecules were nonsubstrates.

Cabrera et al.[56] modeled a set of 163 drugs using topological substructural molecular design (TOPS-MODE) descriptors with a linear discriminant model to predict P-glycoprotein efflux. Model accuracy was 81% for the training set and 77.5% for a validation set of 40 molecules. A "combinatorial QSAR" approach was used by de Lima et al.[57] to test multiple model types (kNN, decision tree, binary QSAR, SVM) with multiple descriptor sets from various software packages (MolconnZ, Atom Pair, VoSurf, MOE) for the prediction of P-glycoprotein substrates for a data set of 192 molecules. Best overall performance on a test set of

51 molecules was achieved with an SVM and AP or VolSurf descriptors (81% accuracy each).

Analyses of molecules that are P-glycoprotein substrates have suggested a number of possible pharmacophores. For example, based on an analysis of 100 molecules, Seelig[58] proposed that molecules containing at least one Type I or Type II unit would be P-glycoprotein substrates, and their binding increases with the strength and number of these groups. Type I units contain two electron donor groups 2.5 ± 0.3Å apart, and Type II units contain two or three electron donor groups whose maximum distance apart is 4.6 ± 0.6Å. Pajeva and Wiese[59] proposed a pharmacophore containing two hydrophobic groups, three HBA groups, and one HBD group. They conclude that binding depends on the number of these pharmacophore points present and that different drugs interact with varied groups with multiple possible binding modes. This pharmacophore hypothesis was shown to agree with a homology model of P-glycoprotein created using *Escherichia coli MsbA* as the template.[60]

Two 3D QSAR models were built using GRIND descriptors for P-glycoprotein substrate recognition. Cianchetta et al.[61] selected 100 proprietary molecules and 29 publicly available molecules having Caco-2 A-B/B-A ratios > 1 and screened them for inhibition of P-glycoprotein activity in a calcein-AM assay. The inhibition values were modeled using GRIND and VolSurf descriptors. The 3D alignment independent GRIND descriptors fit the data well, with $r^2 = 0.83$. VolSurf descriptors produced a model that was slightly better than random. The pharmacophoric GRIND features suggested the following features were important for P-glycoprotein substrate recognition: two hydrophobic groups 16.5Å apart, two HBA groups 11.5Å apart, plus the size of the molecule (21.5Å distance required between edges of the molecule). Crivori et al.[62] similarly compared VolSurf and GRIND descriptors for the prediction of P-glycoprotein substrates. Fifty-three drugs were classified as substrates or nonsubstrates by a cutoff of two for their Caco-2 efflux ratio and modeled using VolSurf descriptors; the model was 89% accurate. When tested on a proprietary data set of 272 molecules, the VolSurf model correctly classified 72% of the data set. Thirty of the 53 drugs were assayed in a calcein-AM assay and the data were used to select nine substrates and fourteen nonsubstrates for modeling with GRIND descriptors. The model was tested on a set of 125 drugs from the literature and accurately predicted 82% of them. Two GRIND features were important in the model: two hydrophobic regions 11.5Å apart and two HBA groups 8Å apart.

The effect of P-glycoprotein efflux limiting brain penetration has been examined by two analyses. A bagged recursive-partitioning model was built using the R software on 190 compounds with literature logBB data and three sets of descriptors.[63] The literature-based model was tested on 250 Pfizer compounds, of which approximately 60% showed significant P-glycoprotein mediated efflux based on brain penetration experiments in knockout versus wild-type *mdr1a* mice. Results were much worse for the Pfizer compounds than for the training set ($Q^2 \sim 0.5$ vs. ~ 0.2), indicating the effect of P-glycoprotein efflux. Garg and Varma[64] used a prediction of P-glycoprotein efflux probability as an input into a neural network model with good results ($r = 0.89$, $s = 0.32$ for test set of 50 molecules).

Raub[53] has published an excellent review with examples discussing the SAR of P-glycoprotein substrate recognition. He notes that "the SAR for P-gp is obviously complicated and poorly understood" and "no single functional group alone is recognized, but one group can accentuate the recognition points existing within a scaffold. It is likened to a rheostat, rather than an on/off switch, where addition or removal of a key group can increase or decrease the pumping efficiency." Raub concludes that the best approach to reduce P-glycoprotein efflux effects is to increase passive diffusion to overwhelm the P-glycoprotein transporter.

Raub's point is well made. P-glycoprotein transports many of the same substrates that the liver enzyme CYP3A4 metabolizes. CYP3A4 is responsible for half the metabolic clearance marketed drugs. For the P-glycoprotein transporter to recognize so many different types of substrates, it requires multiple binding modes and/or multiple sites with wide tolerances. However, the 2D and 3D models reviewed above demonstrate that useful insights can be attained from computational models. For specific chemical series, local models could be tried to better predict P-glycoprotein efflux.

PLASMA PROTEIN BINDING

The binding of drugs to plasma proteins has a significant effect on pharmacokinetics and pharmacodynamics. The biological effect of a drug is due to the free fraction. The most abundant plasma proteins to which drugs can bind are human serum albumin (HSA) and α_1-acid glycoprotein. The fraction of unbound drug, also called the free fraction, directly affects V_d and thus half-life. The volume of distribution at a steady state (V_{ss}) is related to the volume of plasma, tissue, and fraction of the drug unbound in plasma and tissue. The half-life ($t_{1/2}$) of a drug is related to the volume of distribution (V_d) and clearance (CL) by the equation $t_{1/2} = 0.693 \times V_d/CL$.

The lipophilicity of molecules can strongly affect their plasma protein binding. Van de Waterbeemd et al.[65] showed that percent plasma protein binding had similar, but offset, sigmoidal relationships to log$D$ at pH 7.4 for acids, bases, and neutral compounds. Molecules with log$D > 3$ were greater than 90% bound. Yamazaki and Kanaoka[66] performed a more complete analysis of the relationship between lipophilicity and protein binding for 302 drugs. They successfully used a simple nonlinear equation to predict the percent protein bound for neutral/basic/zwitterions using only log$D$ at pH 7.4 ($r^2 = 0.80$, MAE =

10.4%). A similar attempt for acidic drugs gave a poorly fitting model. When a simple pharmacophore was used to classify acidic drugs, the protein binding of the acidic drugs matching the pharmacophore could be fit using a simple nonlinear model. Kratochwil et al.[67] have reviewed the effects of lipophilicity on protein binding and conclude that for smaller data sets the correlation may depend on the nature of the data sets.

The log of the primary binding affinities for HSA for a set of 138 molecules was used to build a QSAR model for protein binding.[68] Topological pharmacophore descriptors were subjected to dimensionality reduction and fit using partial least squares. The model fit parameters were $r^2 = 0.72$, $s = 0.62$ and the experimental variability of the binding constants was estimated to be 0.54 log units. Validation results gave error estimates on the order of $s = 0.7$–0.9. Interestingly, for a subset of 76 molecules, measured log$D$ values had moderate to poor correlation with binding constants.

Leeson[69] analyzed several large sets of protein binding data on GlaxoSmithKline internal compounds using partial least squares and 30 descriptors related to ionization, size, lipophilicity, and polarity. The percent protein bound values were converted to a pseudo-log equilibrium constant. For 1,081 compounds measured in rat, the model performance was reasonable ($r^2 = 0.44$, rmse = 0.62) with similar performance on test 347 test compounds. A model based on human protein binding data for 686 compounds had somewhat better results, $r^2 = 0.56$, rmse = 0.55. For these large data sets, protein binding increased with increasing lipophilicity and acidity, while addition of a basic group decreased binding, as did increasing a basic pK_a. Leeson comments that models with this level of predictive error can be used to rank compounds, because the 95% confidence limits for predictions of protein binding less than 95% rule out the possibility of protein binding of greater than 99%, which is usually the level of protein binding causing the greatest concern. A variety of other QSAR type models for the prediction of plasma protein binding have also been published recently, including neural networks/support vector machines,[70] 4D fingerprints,[71] and TOPS-MODE descriptors.[72]

A crystallographic study of drug binding to HSA provides a valuable resource for structure-based design efforts to modify protein binding affinity of drug candidates. Ghuman et al.[73] published 17 co-complexes of drugs and small toxins with HSA. Both binding sites of HSA were occupied by various compounds revealing specific binding interactions. The binding pockets were determined to be flexible, with distinct subspaces, and overlapped with binding sites for fatty acids, the endogenous ligand.

Rodgers et al. proposed and tested the concept of correction libraries for QSAR models of plasma protein binding.[74] The correction library is simply a list of prediction errors for compounds previously modeled but that have not been used to retrain the model. If the new compound is similar enough to training data as measured by Mahalanobis distance, three nearest neighbors are used to correct the prediction. Improvements were statistically significant and greater than achieved by simply retraining.

TISSUE DISTRIBUTION

Three recent articles have presented computational models for the prediction of tissue distribution of drugs. Zhang and Zhang[75] modeled the distribution into brain, kidney, muscle, lung, liver, heart, and fat of eighty diverse molecules. A complex, nonlinear regression model was fit to a set of physicochemical descriptors generated by the HYPERCHEM software package. The model also incorporated known weight fractions of lipid, protein, and water for each tissue type. The model performance on the training set of sixty-seven molecules for the prediction of the log partition coefficient was $r = 0.877$ and $s = 0.352$, and on a test set of thirteen molecules the model gave similar results, with $r = 0.844$ and $s = 0.342$.

Gleeson et al.[76] reported the first purely computational models for large data sets of volume of distribution at steady state in rat and human. The rat data set contained 2,086 in-house measurements for AstraZeneca compounds and the human data set contained data from 199 marketed drugs. Individual models for each species were built using Bayesian neural networks, classification and regression trees, and partial least squares algorithms with physicochemical descriptors. Best performance on the test sets was given by a combined three-way model for rat, rmse = 0.374 log units, and for human, rmse = 0.479 log units. Lombardo et al.[77] also developed a model of human volume of distribution. Their model fit intravenous clinical data reported for 384 drugs using a mixture linear discriminant analysis/random forest model using thirty-one descriptors. For the training data, the geometric-mean-fold error was ~2, and for a test set of twenty-three proprietary compounds, the geometric-mean-fold-error was 1.78.

CLEARANCE

Hirom[78,79] demonstrated more than three decades ago that the route of excretion of xenobiotics is dependent on MW by testing up to seventy-five compounds in rats, guinea pigs, and rabbits. Lower MW compounds (<350) were mainly eliminated in the urine (>90%). As MW increased from 350 to 450, a sharp increase in the fraction of compound eliminated in the bile occurred, and for MW > 450, compounds were eliminated 50–100% in the bile in all three species. Smith[80] correlated the log of free metabolic and renal clearance (ml/min/kg) with $\log D$ and found a similar relationship. Metabolic clearance increases with increasing $\log D$, while renal clearance decreases with increasing $\log D$.

Percent renal clearance was modeled for a set of 130 compounds from the literature using partial least squares applied to 3D VolSurf or 2D Molconn-Z descriptors.[81] The model based on VolSurf descriptors gave the best prediction quality: model $r^2 = 0.844$, training set $s = 11\%$, test set $s = 13.4\%$. Yap et al.[82] tested a variety of algorithms and descriptors to develop a model for total clearance using a large set of literature data on 503 drugs administered intravenously to males. General regression neural network and support vector regression algorithms performed best, particularly when using the full set of 645 descriptors. Average fold error was on the order of $1.6\times$ for the best models.

METABOLISM

Oxidative drug metabolism is extremely complex and possibly the most poorly understood ADME property. Rapid metabolism is unacceptable for drug candidates, except for drugs whose metabolite is the active moiety, because it causes duration of action to be too short. Considerable work has focused on the liver enzyme CYP3A4, which is responsible for half the metabolic clearance of marketed drugs. Recent approaches used to model and understand drug metabolism include database matching, quantum mechanics, QSAR, and structure-based analyses.

For a commercial database of known metabolic transformations, Borodina et al.[83] extracted all known sites of aromatic hydroxylations. These observed transformations were used to generate all possible transformations for each molecule, giving an estimate of the probability that each transformation would actually occur. The method was 85% accurate in predicting site of aromatic hydroxylation when tested against a second metabolism database containing 1,552 molecules. Boyer et al.[84] took a similar approach using reaction center fingerprints to estimate the occurrence ratio of a particular metabolic transformation. The method successfully predicted the three most probable sites of metabolism in 87% of compounds tested.

Quantum mechanical approaches have been successfully used to predict hydrogen abstraction potentials and likely sites of metabolism of drug molecules.[85–88] AM1, Fukui functions, and density functional theory calculations could identify potential sites of metabolism. Activation energies for hydrogen abstraction were calculated by Olsen et al.[88] to be below 80 kJ/mol, suggesting most CH groups can be metabolized; which particular one depends on steric accessibility and intrinsic reactivities.

Shen et al.[89] reported the use of a k-nearest-neighbor QSAR model trained to predict the metabolic stability of 631 molecules in human hepatic S9 homogenate. The model was accurate for ~85% of molecules in both training and test data sets. A GRIND QSAR model was shown to be able to predict the stability of molecules incubated with human CYP3A4 with 75–85% accuracy on test data sets.[90] A Bayesian regularized neural network using electrotopological descriptors was used to predict the K_m values of CYP3A4 substrates.[91] Lee et al. report a random forest model of human liver microsomal stability ($CL_{int,app}$) using 2D MOE and E-state descriptors trained on a large data set that had 75% accuracy on a test set of 2,911 compounds.[92] At Bayer, a Gaussian process model has been trained to predict the probability of stability of molecules in human, mouse, and rat microsomes from internal Bayer data.[93]

Until recently, structure-based analyses of CYP450 metabolizing enzymes were limited to homology model studies due to the lack of crystal structures of human CYP450s.[94–97] In the last few years, multiple crystal structures of human CYP4503A4 have been solved.[98–100] Ekroos and Sjoegren published several extremely interesting crystal structures.[100] They found that CYP3A4 is much more flexible than previously reported and that the active site can enlarge by greater than 80% on binding to ketoconazole, a potent CYP450 inhibitor. In fact, the crystal structure showed two molecules of ketoconazole were bound within the active site. A CYP3A4-erythromycin complex suggested multiple binding modes. These results suggest further experimental studies will be needed to improve modeling results for CYP3A4.

Cruciani et al.[101] have developed the program MetaSite for the prediction of the site of oxidative metabolism by CYP450 enzymes. MetaSite uses GRID molecular interaction fields to fingerprint both structures of CYP450s (from homology models or crystal structures) and test substrates. The fingerprints are generated from hydrophobic, hydrogen bond donor/acceptor, and charge GRID probes. The accessibility of each reactive group to the heme is determined using the field measures from the probes, and quantum and fragment recognition calculations are used to estimate the reactivity of each atom. A final probability for each site of metabolism is computed using both accessibility and reactivity.

Zhou et al.[102] showed that MetaSite was able to correctly predict the site(s) of metabolism 78% of the time for 227 CYP3A4 substrates with 325 metabolic pathways. For molecules with multiple sites of metabolism, the MetaSite model quality was evaluated using the three sites wit the greatest probability of metabolism. In comparison, the GLUE docking method in combination with a homology model of CYP3A4 was 69% accurate. Kjellander et al. also studied the GLUE docking method in comparison to MetaSite.[103] Caron et al.[104] used MetaSite to analyze the oxidative metabolism of seven statins and found Meta-Site was 77% accurate. However, the 77% accuracy value involved considering the top five sites of metabolism, not the top three. The CYP2C9 metabolism of celecoxib and analogs have been studied using MetaSite and docking methods.[105,106] The molecular alignment program ROCS was used to align seventy CYP2C9 substrates with the known CYP2C9 substrate flurbiprofen with good results: thirty-nine of the first forty-four best scoring molecules had alignments that agreed with the known experimental site of metabolism.[107]

Sheridan et al. developed QSAR models to predict regioselectivity for CYP3A4, CYP2D6, and CYP2C9.[108] Results were comparable or superior to MetaSite but did depend on the data set size. They noted that overall, the QSAR models and MetaSite are correct 70% of the time and more work is needed. Docking plus an activation energy calculation compared favorably for CYP3A4 regioselectivity versus MetaSite and Sheridan's QSAR.[109] Terfloth et al. conducted a large comparison of multiple QSAR modeling algorithms applied to a set of 379 drugs to predict which CYP450 isoform metabolized the drugs.[110] All algorithms performed at least reasonably well, with support vector machines giving the best results. The significant differences in model performance were caused by variable selection and how the data set was partitioned into training and test sets. The final model was 83% accurate on a test set of 233 compounds.

CONCLUSION

Many advances have been made in computational ADME modeling. For many ADME properties, models now exist that provide reasonably good predictive quality and can be deployed to aid medicinal chemists in drug discovery projects.

The usefulness of computational ADME models depends on many factors, including the quality and breadth of data used to build them, how well the model approximates the physiological or physicochemical mechanism of interest, how the model is made available to chemists, and how well the chemist understands and uses the model. Ideally, ADME models are made available on the desktop, are easy to use, and are fast enough to help a chemist to better evaluate and prioritize a variety of molecular designs or even libraries each day. ADME models can also play a crucial role in helping the interpretation of experimental data by directly highlighting structural features the model associates with a particular ADME property, or at least allowing a chemist to quickly sketch different analogs and remove portions of a molecule to observe how the model's predictions change. A number of companies are reporting ADME/cheminformatics systems designed to aid in these efforts.[111–114]

Two major issues for ADME modeling are data availability and optimization. The lack of larger data sets has hampered development of ADME models and reduced their potential quality; however, articles reviewed here show that this situation is improving. More human and animal ADME data would provide significant benefits. The fact that many ADME properties interact means that we must optimize a molecule's ADME properties simultaneously or much work will be wasted traversing chemical space fixing one poor property but inadvertently causing a second to worsen.[115,117] This requires more work to develop systems with scoring functions for molecule quality based on models for multiple ADME properties (e.g., Segall et al.)[114]

REFERENCES

1. Mervis, J. Productivity counts – but the definition is key. *Science* **2005**, *309*, 726.

2. Kola, I.; Landis, J. Opinion: Can the pharmaceutical industry reduce attrition rates? *Nature Rev. Drug Disc.* **2004**, *3*, 711.

3. Adams, C.; Brantner, V. Estimating the cost of new drug development: is it really 802 million dollars? *Health Affairs* **2006**, *25*, 420.

4. Patchett, A. Excursions in drug discovery. *J. Med. Chem.* **1993**, *36*, 2051.

5. Hamming, R. *Numerical Methods for Scientists and Engineers.* New York: McGraw-Hill; **1962**.

6. Lipinski, C. A.; Lombardo, F.; Dominy, B. W.; Feeney, P. J. Experimental and computational approaches to estimate solubility and permeability in drug discovery and development settings. *Adv. Drug Deliv. Rev.* **1997**, *23*, 3.

7. Wenlock, M. C.; Austin, R. P.; Barton, P.; Davis, A. M.; Leeson, P. D. A comparison of physiochemical property profiles of development and marketed oral drugs. *J. Med. Chem.* **2003**, *46*, 1250.

8. Vieth, M.; Siegel, M. G.; Higgs, R. E.; Watson, I. A.; Robertson, D. H.; Savin, K. A.; Durst, G. L.; Hipskind, P. A. Characteristic physical properties and structural fragments of marketed oral drugs. *J. Med. Chem.* **2004**, *47*, 224.

9. Leeson, P. D.; Davis, A. M. Time-related differences in the physical property profiles of oral drugs. *J. Med. Chem.* **2004**, *47*, 6338.

10. Proudfoot, J. R. The evolution of synthetic oral drug properties. *Bioorg. Med. Chem. Lett.* **2005**, *15*, 1087.

11. Vieth, M.; Sutherland, J. Dependence of molecular properties on proteomic family for marketed oral drugs. *J. Med. Chem.* **2006**, *49*, 3451.

12. Morphy, R. The influence of target family and functional activity on the physicochemical properties of pre-clinical compounds. *J. Med. Chem.* **2006**, *49*, 2969.

13. O'Shea, R.; Moser, H. E. Physicochemical properties of antibacterial compounds: implications for drug discovery. *J. Med. Chem.* **2008**, *51*, 2871.

14. Gleeson, M. P. Generation of a set of simple, interpretable ADMET rules of thumb. *J. Med. Chem.* **2008**, *51*, 817.

15. Bhal, S. K.; Kassam, K.; Peirson, I. G.; Pearl, G. M. The Rule of Five revisited: applying log D in place of log P in drug-likeness filters. *Mol. Pharm.* **2007**, *4*, 556.

16. Faller, B.; Wang, J.; Zimmerlin, A.; Bell, L.; Hamon, J.; Whitebread, S.; Azzaoui, K.; Bojanic, D.; Urban, L. High-throughput in vitro profiling assays: lessons learnt from experiences at Novartis. *Expert Opin. Drug Metab. Tox.* **2006**, *2*, 823.

17. Johnson, S. R.; Zheng, W. Recent progress in the computational prediction of aqueous solubility and absorption. *AAPS J.* **2006**, *8*, E27.

18. Balakin, K. V.; Savchuk, N. P.; Tetko, I. V. In silico approaches to prediction of aqueous and DMSO solubility of drug-like compounds: trends, problems and solutions. *Curr. Med. Chem.* **2006**, *13*, 223.

19. Leach, A. G.; Jones, H. D.; Cosgrove, D. A.; Kenny, P. W.; Ruston, L.; MacFaul, P.; Wood, J. M.; Colclough, N.; Law, B. Matched molecular pairs as a guide in the optimization of pharmaceutical properties; a study of aqueous solubility, plasma protein binding and oral exposure. *J. Med. Chem.* **2006**, *49*, 6672.

20. Lamanna, C.; Bellini, M.; Padova, A.; Westerberg, G.; Maccari, L. Straightforward recursive partitioning model for discarding insoluble compounds in the drug discovery process. *J. Med. Chem.* **2008**, *51*, 2891.

21. Huuskonen, J. Estimation of aqueous solubility for a diverse set of organic compounds based on molecular topology. *J. Chem. Inf. Comp. Sci.* **2000**, *40*, 773.

22. Yan, A.; Gasteiger, J. Prediction of aqueous solubility of organic compounds by topological descriptors. *QSAR Combin. Sci.* **2003**, *22*, 821.

23. Yan, A.; Gasteiger, J.; Krug, M.; Anzali, S. Linear and nonlinear functions on modeling of aqueous solubility of organic compounds by two structure representation methods. *J. Comput. Aided Mol. Des.* **2004**, *18*, 75.

24. Delaney, J. S. Predicting aqueous solubility from structure. *Drug Discov. Today* **2005**, *10*, 289.

25. Lipinski, C. A. Drug-like properties and the causes of poor solubility and poor permeability. *J. Pharmacol. Toxicol. Meth.* **2000**, *44*, 235.

26. Goeller, A. H.; Hennemann, M.; Keldenich, J.; Clark, T. In silico prediction of buffer solubility based on quantum-mechanical and HQSAR- and topology-based descriptors. *J. Chem. Inf. Model.* **2006**, *46*, 648.

27. Schwaighofer, A.; Schroeter, T.; Mika, S.; Laub, J.; Ter Laak, A.; Suelzle, D.; Ganzer, U.; Heinrich, N.; Mueller, K.-R. Accurate solubility prediction with error bars for electrolytes: a machine learning approach. *J. Chem. Inf. Model.* **2007**, *47*, 407.

28. Obrezanova, O.; Csanyi, G.; Gola, J. M. R.; Segall, M. D. Gaussian processes: a method for automatic QSAR modeling of ADME properties. *J. Chem. Inf. Model.* **2007**, *47*, 1847.

29. Obrezanova, O.; Gola, J. M. R.; Champness, E. J.; Segall, M. D. Automatic QSAR modeling of ADME properties: blood-brain barrier penetration and aqueous solubility. *J. Comput. Aided Mol. Des.* **2008**, *22*, 431.

30. Balakin, K. V.; Ivanenkov, Y. A.; Skorenko, A. V.; Nikolsky, Y. V.; Savchuk, N. P.; Ivashchenko, A. A. In silico estimation of DMSO solubility of organic compounds for bioscreening. *J. Biomolec. Screen.* **2004**, *9*, 22.

31. Lu, J.; Bakken, G. A. Building classification models for DMSO solubility: comparison of five methods. 228th ACS National Meeting, Philadelphia, PA, United States, August 22–26, **2004**, CINF-045.

32. Johnson, S. R.; Chen, X. Q.; Murphy, D.; Gudmundsson, O. A. Computational model for the prediction of aqueous solubility that includes crystal packing, intrinsic solubility, and ionization effects. *Mol. Pharm.* **2007**, *4*, 513.

33. Egan, W. J.; Lauri, G. Prediction of intestinal permeability. *Adv. Drug Deliv. Rev.* **2002**, *54*, 273.

34. Egan, W. J.; Merz, K. M.; Baldwin, J. J. Prediction of drug absorption using multivariate statistics. *J. Med. Chem.* **2000**, *43*, 3867.

35. Zhao, Y. H.; Le, J.; Abraham, M. H.; Hersey, A.; Eddershaw, P. J.; Luscombe, C. N.; Boutina, D.; Beck, G.; Sherborne, B.; Cooper, I.; Platts, J. A. Evaluation of human intestinal absorption data and subsequent derivation of a quantitative structure-activity relationship (QSAR) with the Abraham descriptors. *J. Pharm. Sci.* **2001**, *90*, 749.

36. Zhao, Y. H.; Abraham, M. H.; Hersey, A.; Luscombe, C. N. Quantitative relationship between rat intestinal absorption and Abraham descriptors. *Eur. J. Med. Chem.* **2003**, *38*, 939.

37. Bai, J. P. F.; Utis, A.; Crippen, G.; He, H. D.; Fischer, V.; Tullman, R.; Yin, H. Q.; Hsu, C. P.; Jing, Hwang, K. K. Use of classification regression tree in predicting oral absorption in humans. *J. Chem. Inf. Comp. Sci.* **2004**, *44*, 2061.

38. Jones, R.; Connolly, P. C.; Klamt, A.; Diedenhofen, M. Use of surface charges from DFT calculations to predict intestinal absorption. *J. Chem. Inf. Model.* **2005**, *45*, 1337.

39. Rezai, T.; Bock, J. E.; Zhou, M. V.; Kalyanaraman, C.; Lokey, R. S.; Jacobson, M. P. Conformational flexibility, internal hydrogen bonding, and passive membrane permeability: successful in silico prediction of the relative permeabilities of cyclic peptides. *J. Am. Chem. Soc.* **2006**, *128*, 14073.

40. Rezai, T.; Yu, B.; Millhauser, G. L.; Jacobson, M. P.; Lokey, R. S. Testing the conformational hypothesis of passive membrane permeability using synthetic cyclic peptide diastereomers. *J. Am. Chem. Soc.* **2006**, *128*, 2510.

41. Stoner, C. L.; Troutman, M.; Gao, H.; Johnson, K.; Stankovic, C.; Brodfuehrer, J.; Gifford, E.; Chang, M. Moving in silico screening into practice: a minimalist approach to guide permeability screening!! *Lett. Drug Design Discov.* **2006**, *3*, 575.

42. Clark, D. E. Computational prediction of blood-brain barrier permeation. *Ann. Rep. Med. Chem.* **2005**, *40*, 403.

43. Kelder, J.; Grootenhuis, P. D.; J. Bayada, D. M.; Delbressine, L. P. C.; Ploemen, J. P. Polar molecular surface as a dominating determinant for oral absorption and brain penetration of drugs. *Pharm. Res.* **1999**, *16*, 1514.

44. Clark, D. E. Rapid calculation of polar molecular surface area and its application to the prediction of transport phenomena. 2. Prediction of blood-brain barrier penetration. *J. Pharm. Sci.* **1999**, *88*, 815.

45. Lobell, M.; Molnar, L.; Keseru, G. M. Recent advances in the prediction of blood-brain partitioning from molecular structure. *J. Pharm. Sci.* **2003**, *92*, 360.

46. Gerebtzoff, G.; Seelig, A. In silico prediction of blood-brain barrier permeation using the calculated molecular cross-sectional area as main parameter. *J. Chem. Inf. Model.* **2006**, *46*, 2638.

47. Abraham, M. H.; Ibrahim, A.; Zhao, Y.; Acree, W. E. A data base for partition of volatile organic compounds and drugs from blood/plasma/serum to brain, and an LFER analysis of the data. *J. Pharm. Sci.* **2006**, *95*, 2091.

48. Zhao, Y. H.; Abraham, M. H.; Ibrahim, A.; Fish, P. V.; Cole, S.; Lewis, M. L.; de Groot, M. J.; Reynolds, D. P. Predicting penetration across the blood-brain barrier from simple descriptors and fragmentation schemes. *J. Chem. Inf. Model.* **2007**, *47*, 170.

49. Pardridge, W. M. Log(BB), PS products and in silico models of drug brain penetration. *Drug Disc. Today* **2004**, *9*, 392.

50. Liu, X.; Tu, M.; Kelly, R. S.; Chen, C.; Smith, B. J. Development of a computational approach to predict blood-brain barrier permeability. *Drug Metab. Dispos.* **2004**, *32*, 132.

51. Abraham, M. H. The factors that influence permeation across the blood-brain barrier. *Eur. J. Med. Chem.* **2004**, *39*, 235.

52. Lin, J. H.; Yamazaki, M. Role of P-glycoprotein in pharmacokinetics: clinical implications. *Clin. Pharmacokinet.* **2003**, *42*, 59.

53. Raub, T. J. P-glycoprotein recognition of substrates and circumvention through rational drug design. *Mol. Pharm.* **2006**, *3*, 3.

54. Varma, M. V. S.; Sateesh, K.; Panchagnula, R. Functional role of P-glycoprotein in limiting intestinal absorption of drugs: contribution of passive permeability to P-glycoprotein mediated efflux transport. *Mol. Pharm.* **2005**, *2*, 12.

55. Gombar, V. K.; Polli, J. W.; Humphreys, J. E.; Wring, S. A.; Serabjit-Singh, C. S. Predicting P-glycoprotein substrates by a quantitative structure-activity relationship model. *J. Pharm. Sci.* **2004**, *93*, 957.

56. Cabrera, M. A.; Gonzalez, I.; Fernandez, C.; Navarro, C.; Bermejo, M. A topological substructural approach for the prediction of P-glycoprotein substrates. *J. Pharm. Sci.* **2006**, *95*, 589.

57. de Lima, P.; Golbraikh, A.; Oloff, S.; Xiao, Y.; Tropsha, A. Combinatorial QSAR modeling of P-glycoprotein substrates. *J. Chem. Inf. Model.* **2006**, *46*, 1245.

58. Seelig, A. A general pattern for substrate recognition by P-glycoprotein. *Eur. J. Biochem.* **1998**, *251*, 252.

59. Pajeva, I. K.; Wiese, M. Pharmacophore model of drugs involved in P-glycoprotein multidrug resistance: explanation of structural variety (hypothesis). *J. Med. Chem.* **2002**, *45*, 5671.

60. Vandevuer, S.; Van Bambeke, F.; Tulkens, P. M.; Prevost, M. Predicting the three-dimensional structure of human P-glycoprotein in absence of ATP by computational techniques embodying crosslinking data: insight into the mechanism of ligand migration and binding sites. *Proteins* **2006**, *63*, 466.

61. Cianchetta, G.; Singleton, R. W.; Zhang, M.; Wildgoose, M.; Giesing, D.; Fravolini, A.; Cruciani, G.; Vaz, R. A pharmacophore hypothesis for P-glycoprotein substrate recognition using GRIND-based 3D-QSAR. *J. Med. Chem.* **2005**, *48*, 2927.

62. Crivori, P.; Reinach, B.; Pezzetta, D.; Poggesi, I. Computational models for identifying potential P-glycoprotein substrates and inhibitors. *Mol. Pharm.* **2006**, *3*, 33.

63. Mente, S. R.; Lombardo, F. A recursive-partitioning model for blood-brain barrier permeation. *J. Comput. Aided Mol. Design* **2005**, *19*, 465.

64. Garg, P.; Verma, J. In silico prediction of blood brain barrier permeability: an artificial neural network model. *J. Chem. Inf. Model.* **2006**, *46*, 289.

65. Van de Waterbeemd, H.; Smith, D. A.; Jones, B. C. Lipophilicity in PK design: methyl, ethyl, futile. *J. Comput. Aided Mol. Des.* **2001**, *15*, 273.

66. Yamazaki, K., Kanaoka, M. Computational prediction of the plasma protein-binding percent of diverse pharmaceutical compounds. *J. Pharm. Sci.* **2004**, *93*, 1480.

67. Kratochwil, N. A.; Huber, W.; Mueller, F.; Kansy, M.; Gerber, P. R. Predicting plasma protein binding of drugs – revisited. *Curr. Opin. Drug Disc. Devel.* **2004**, *7*, 507.

68. Kratochwil, N. A.; Huber, W.; Muller, F.; Kansy, M.; Gerber, P. R. Predicting plasma protein binding of drugs: a new approach. *Biochem. Pharmacol.* **2002**, *64*, 1355.

69. Gleeson, M. P. Plasma protein binding affinity and its relationship to molecular structure: an in-silico analysis. *J. Med. Chem.* **2007**, *50*, 101.

70. Votano, J. R.; Parham, M.; Hall, L. M.; Hall, L. H.; Kier, L. B.; Oloff, S.; Tropsha, A. QSAR modeling of human serum protein binding with several modeling techniques utilizing structure-information representation. *J. Med. Chem.* **2006**, *49*, 7169.

71. Liu, J.; Yang, L.; Li, Y.; Pan, D.; Hopfinger, A. J. Constructing plasma protein binding model based on a combination of cluster analysis and 4D-fingerprint molecular similarity analyses. *Bioorg. Med. Chem.* **2006**, *14*, 611.

72. Estrada, E.; Uriarte, E.; Molina, E.; Simon-Manso, Y.; Milne, G. W. A. An integrated in silico analysis of drug-binding to human serum albumin. *J. Chem. Inf. Model.* **2006**, *46*, 2709.

73. Ghuman, J.; Zunszain, P. A.; Petitpas, I.; Bhattacharya, A. A.; Otagiri, M.; Curry, S. Structural basis of the drug-binding specificity of human serum albumin. *J. Mol. Biol.* **2005**, *353*, 38.

74. Rodgers, S. L.; Davis, A. M.; Tomkinson, N. P.; Van de Waterbeemd, H. QSAR modeling using automatically updating correction libraries: application to a human plasma protein binding model. *J. Chem. Inf. Model.* **2007**, *47*, 2401.

75. Zhang, H.; Zhang, Y. Convenient nonlinear model for predicting the tissue/blood partition coefficients of seven human tissues of neutral, acidic, and basic structurally diverse compounds. *J. Med. Chem.* **2006**, *49*, 5815.

76. Gleeson, M. P.; Waters, N. J.; Paine, S. W.; Davis, A. M. In silico human and rat Vss quantitative structure-activity relationship models. *J. Med. Chem.* **2006**, *49*, 1953.

77. Lombardo, F.; Obach, R. S.; DiCapua, F.; Bakken, G. A.; Lu, J.; Potter, D. M.; Gao, F.; Miller, M. D.; Zhang, Y. A hybrid mixture discriminant analysis-random forest computational model for the prediction of volume of distribution of drugs in human. *J. Med. Chem.* **2006**, *49*, 2262.

78. Hirom, P. C.; Millburn, P.; Smith, R. L.; Williams, R. T. Species variations in the threshold molecular-weight factor for the biliary excretion of organic anions. *Biochem. J.* **1972**, *129*, 1071.

79. Hirom, P. C.; Millburn, P.; Smith, R. L. Bile and urine as complementary pathways for the excretion of foreign organic compounds. *Xenobiotica* **1976**, *6*, 55.

80. Smith, D. A. Physicochemical properties in drug metabolism and pharmacokinetics. In: *Computer-Assisted Lead Finding and Optimization: Current Tools for Medicinal Chemistry*, van de Waterbeemd, H.; Testa, B.; Folkers, G.; Eds. Weinheim: Wiley-VCH; **1997**, 267.

81. Doddareddy, M. R.; Cho, Y. S.; Koh, H. Y.; Kim, D. H.; Pae, A. N. In silico renal clearance model using classical Volsurf approach. *J. Chem. Inf. Model.* **2006**, *46*, 1312.

82. Yap, C. W.; Li, Z. R.; Chen, Y. Z. Quantitative structure-pharmacokinetic relationships for drug clearance by using statistical learning methods. *J. Mol. Graph. Model.* **2006**, *24*, 383.

83. Borodina, Y.; Rudik, A.; Filimonov, D.; Kharchevnikova, N.; Dmitriev, A.; Blinova, V.; Poroikov, V. A new statistical approach to predicting aromatic hydroxylation sites. Comparison with model-based approaches. *J. Chem. Inf. Comp. Sci.* **2004**, *44*, 1998.

84. Boyer, S.; Arnby, C.; Hasselgren, C.; Carlsson, L.; Smith, J.; Stein, V.; Glen, R. C. Reaction site mapping of xenobiotic biotransformations. *J. Chem. Inf. Model.* **2007**, *47*, 583.

85. Singh, S. B.; Shen, L. Q.; Walker, M. J.; Sheridan, R. P. A model for predicting likely sites of CYP3A4-mediated metabolism on drug-like molecules. *J. Med. Chem.* **2003**, *46*, 1330.

86. Lewin, J. L.; Cramer, C. J. Rapid quantum mechanical models for the computational estimation of C-H bond dissociation energies as a measure of metabolic stability. *Mol. Pharm.* **2004**, *1*, 128.

87. Beck, M. E. Do Fukui function maxima relate to sites of metabolism? A critical case study. *J. Chem. Inf. Model.* **2005**, *45*, 273.

88. Olsen, L.; Rydberg, P.; Rod, T. H.; Ryde, U. Prediction of activation energies for hydrogen abstraction by Cytochrome P450. *J. Med. Chem.* **2006**, *49*, 6489.

89. Shen, M.; Xiao, Y.; Golbraikh, A.; Gombar, V. K.; Tropsha, A. Development and validation of k-nearest-neighbor QSPR models of metabolic stability of drug candidates. *J. Med. Chem.* **2003**, *46*, 3013.

90. Crivori, P.; Zamora, I.; Speed, B.; Orrenius, C.; Poggesi, I. Model based on GRID-derived descriptors for estimating CYP3A4 enzyme stability of potential drug candidates. *J. Comput. Aided Mol. Des.* **2004**, *18*, 155.

91. Wang, Y. H.; Li, Y.; Li, Y. H.; Yang, S. L.; Yang, L. Modeling Km values using electrotopological state: substrates for cytochrome P450 3A4-mediated metabolism. *Bioorg. Med. Chem. Lett.* **2005**, *15*, 4076.

92. Lee, P. H.; Cucurull-Sanchez, L.; Lu, J.; Du, Y. J. Development of in silico models for human liver microsomal stability. *J. Comput. Aided Mol. Des.* **2007**, *21*, 665.

93. Schwaighofer, A.; Schroeter, T.; Mika, S.; Hansen, K.; ter Laak, A.; Lienau, P.; Reichel, A.; Heinrich, N.; Mueller, K. R. A probabilistic approach to classifying metabolic stability. *J. Chem. Inf. Model.* **2008**, *48*, 785.

94. Lewis, D. F. V.; Ito, Y.; Goldfarb, P. S. Structural modeling of the human drug-metabolizing cytochromes P 450. *Curr. Med. Chem.* **2006**, *13*, 2645.

95. Lewis, D. F. V.; Lake, B. G.; Dickins, M.; Goldfarb, P. S. Homology modelling of CYP3A4 from the CYP2C5 crystallographic template: analysis of typical CYP3A4 substrate interactions. *Xenobiotica* **2004**, *34*, 549.

96. Tanaka, T.; Okuda, T.; Yamamoto, Y. Characterization of the CYP3A4 active site by homology modeling. *Chem. Pharm. Bull.* **2004**, *52*, 830.

97. Park, H.; Lee, S.; Suh, J. Structural and dynamical basis of broad substrate specificity, catalytic mechanism, and inhibition of cytochrome P 450 3A4. *J. Am. Chem. Soc.* **2005**, *127*, 13634.

98. Yano, J. K.; Wester, M. R.; Schoch, G. A.; Griffin, K. J.; Stout, C. D.; Johnson, E. F. The structure of human microsomal Cytochrome P450 3A4 determined by x-ray crystallography to 2.05-.ANG. resolution. *J. Biol. Chem.* **2004**, *279*, 38091.

99. Williams, P. A; Cosme, J.; Vinkovic, D. M.; Ward, A.; Angove, H. C.; Day, P. J.; Vonrhein, C.; Tickle, I. J.; Jhoti, H. Crystal structures of human cytochrome P450 3A4 bound to metyrapone and progesterone. *Science* **2004**, *305*, 683.

100. Ekroos, M.; Sjoegren, T. Structural basis for ligand promiscuity in cytochrome P 450 3A4. *Proc. National Acad. Sci. U.S.A.* **2006**, *103*, 13682.

101. Cruciani, G.; Carosati, E.; De Boeck, B.; Ethirajulu, K.; Mackie, C.; Howe, T.; Vianello, R. MetaSite: understanding metabolism in human cytochromes from the perspective of the chemist. *J. Med. Chem.* **2005**, *48*, 6970.

102. Zhou, D.; Afzelius, L.; Grimm, S. W.; Andersson, T. B.; Zauhar, R. J.; Zamora, I. Comparison of methods for the prediction of the metabolic sites for CYP3A4-mediated metabolic reactions. *Drug Metab. Dispos.* **2006**, *34*, 976.

103. Kjellander, B.; Masimirembwa, C. M.; Zamora, I. Exploration of enzyme-ligand interactions in CYP2D6 & 3A4 homology models and crystal structures using a novel computational approach. *J. Chem. Inf. Model.* **2007**, *47*, 1234.

104. Caron, G.; Ermondi, G.; Testa, B. Predicting the oxidative metabolism of statins: an application of the MetaSite algorithm. *Pharm. Res.* **2007**, *24*, 480.

105. Ahlstroem, M. A.; Ridderstrom, M.; Zamora, I.; Luthman, K. CYP2C9 structure-metabolism relationships: optimizing the metabolic stability of COX-2 inhibitors. *J. Med. Chem.* **2007**, *50*, 4444.

106. Ahlstroem, M. A.; Ridderstrom, M.; Zamora, I. CYP2C9 structure-metabolism relationships: substrates, inhibitors, and metabolites. *J. Med. Chem.* **2007**, *50*, 5382.

107. Sykes, M. J.; McKinnon, R. A.; Miners, J. O. Prediction of metabolism by cytochrome P450 2C9: alignment and docking studies of a validated database of substrates. *J. Med. Chem.* **2008**, *51*, 780.

108. Sheridan, R. P.; Korzekwa, K. R.; Torres, R. A.; Walker, M. J. Empirical regioselectivity models for human cytochromes P450 3A4, 2D6, and 2C9. *J. Med. Chem.* **2007**, *50*, 3173.

109. Oh, W. S.; Kim, D. N.; Jung, J.; Cho, K. H.; No, K. T. New combined model for the prediction of regioselectivity in cytochrome P450/3A4 mediated metabolism. *J. Chem. Inf. Model.* **2008**, *48*, 591.

110. Terfloth, L.; Bienfait, B.; Gasteiger, J. Ligand-based models for the isoform specificity of cytochrome P450 3A4, 2D6, and 2C9 substrates. *J. Chem. Inf. Model.* **2007**, *47*, 1688.

111. Delisle, R. K.; Lowrie, J. F.; Hobbs, D. W.; Diller, D. J. Computational ADME/Tox modeling: aiding understanding and enhancing decision making in drug design. *Curr. Comput. Aided Drug Des.* **2005**, *1*, 325.

112. Stoner, C. L.; Gifford, E.; Stankovic, C.; Lepsy, C. S.; Brodfuehrer, J.; Prasad, J.; Surendran, N. Implementation of an ADME enabling selection and visualization tool for drug discovery. *J. Pharm. Sci.* **2004**, *93*, 1131.

113. Lobell, M.; Hendrix, M.; Hinzen, B.; Keldenich, J.; Meier, H.; Schmeck, C.; Schohe-Loop, R.; Wunberg, T.; Hillisch, A. In silico ADMET traffic lights as a tool for the prioritization of HTS hits. *ChemMedChem* **2006**, *1*, 1229.

114. Segall, M. D.; Beresford, A. P.; Gola, J. M. R.; Hawksley, D.; Tarbit, M. H. Focus on success: using a probabilistic approach to achieve an optimal balance of compound properties in drug discovery. *Expert Opin. Drug Metab. Toxicol.* **2006**, *2*, 325.

115. Appell, K.; Baldwin, J. J.; Egan, W. J. Combinatorial chemistry and high-throughput screening in drug discovery and development. In: *Handbook of Modern Pharmaceutical Analysis*, Ahuja, S; Scypinski, S.; Eds. San Diego, Academic Press; **2001**, 23.

116. Biller, S. A.; Custer, L.; Dickinson, K. E.; Durham, S. K.; Gavai, A. V.; Hamann, L. G.; Josephs, J. L.; Moulin, F.; Pearl, G. M.; Flint, O. P.; Sanders, M.; Tymiak, A. A.; Vaz, R. The challenge of quality in candidate optimization. In: *Biotechnology: Pharmaceutical Aspects, 1(Pharmaceutical Profiling in Drug Discovery for Lead Selection)*, Arlington, AAPS Press, **2004**, 413.

117. Egan, W. J.; Walters, W. P.; Murcko, M. A. Guiding molecules towards drug-likeness. *Curr. Opin. Drug Discov. Devel.* **2002**, *5*, 540.

PART III

Applications to drug discovery

Computer-aided drug design: a practical guide to protein-structure-based modeling

Charles H. Reynolds

INTRODUCTION

The role of computation in drug discovery has grown steadily since the late 1960s.[1–3] In the early days emphasis was on statistical and extrathermodynamic approaches aimed at quantifying the relationship of chemical structure to biological properties.[4–6] From these early efforts the field has grown enormously as evidenced by the chapters in this book. In addition, recent computational approaches place a greater focus on the three-dimensional structure of the ligand and/or protein. Modeling has become a critical tool in the drug discovery process.

The growth in protein-structure-based approaches has mirrored the exponential growth in available protein structures, as evidenced by the number of structures deposited in the Research Collaboratory for Structural Bioinformatics (RCSB).[7] Whereas in the late 1980s only a few protein structures were available, we now have tens of thousands across many classes of therapeutically relevant proteins. This trend shows no sign of abating. To the contrary, new target classes that have been resistant to structure determination are beginning to become available, including G-protein-coupled receptors (GPCRs) and ion channels.[8–13] This wealth of structures provides a good starting point for modeling protein/ligand interactions, and the application of computer models to identify improved ligands for these targets (Figure 12.1).

CHALLENGES

There are many obstacles that stand in the way of successful modeling of protein/ligand interactions. First is the high degree of computational accuracy required to predict significant changes in binding affinity. Ligand binding is an equilibrium property that is related to free energy by the relationship

$$\Delta G = -RT \ln K,$$

where K is a binding measurement such as K_d or K_i. The logarithmic relationship means that very small changes in free energy lead to large changes in affinity. For example, a tenfold change in binding affinity results from only a 1.4 kcal/mol difference in the binding free energy. As a consequence meaningful affinity predictions require computed free energies, or at least relative free energies, within less than a kcal/mol. This is a daunting task, particularly when one considers that the absolute energies that go into calculating these differences are relatively huge. For example, the total molecular mechanics energy for a medium-sized protein ligand complex can be several thousand kcal/mol. This would mean that a tenfold change in potency represents a change of only 0.04% of the total energy. This is analogous to weighing the ship's captain by measuring the difference in the ship's weight when he is aboard and then on the dock.[14]

Clearly one of the first challenges for calculating reliable protein-ligand binding affinities is a high-quality molecular model. In most cases this means a classical force field such as AMBER,[15,16] CHARMM,[17,18] or OPLS.[19] In principle this model could also be a quantum method and, as described in Chapter 8, progress is being made in this direction. This level of accuracy is a great challenge, and is routinely accomplished only with very high-level quantum calculations for relatively small molecules.[20,21] In the case of proteins this problem is made even more difficult by the complexity of the surrounding medium. Most biological systems operate in an aqueous environment and the proteins themselves are essentially polyelectrolytes with many ionizable groups. The treatment of electrostatics in terms of simple atomic point charges is one of the most significant limitations of force field methods and is one of the reasons quantum-based methods may hold so much promise for the future.

A second overarching challenge for modeling protein-ligand complexes is the issue of sampling. The number of degrees of freedom in a large drug molecule can by itself be great enough to provide a significant hurdle for sampling all of the possible energetically accessible conformations. Even a modest-sized protein has many times more rotatable bonds. Because the number of conformations increases by the relationship in Equation (12.1), the number of conformations available for sampling undergoes a combinatorial explosion:

Total confs.

$$= (\text{Confs. per rotatable bond})^{(\text{number of rotatable bonds})} \quad (12.1)$$

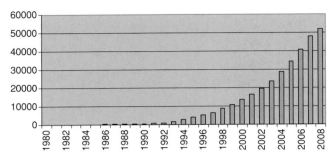

Figure 12.1. Growth of total crystal structures in the RCSB PDB database as of July 22, 2008 (www.rcsb.org).

Table 12.1. Resolution of protein crystal structures

Resolution (Å)	Structural features observable for a good data set[a]
5.5	Overall shape of the protein. Helices as rods.
3.5	Protein main chain (often some ambiguity).
3.0	Protein side chains partly resolved.
2.5	Side chains well resolved.
1.5	Heavy atoms well resolved.

[a] Data taken from *Enzyme Structure and Mechanism*, 2nd edition.[27]

Assuming only three conformations per rotatable bond, even a ligand with only five rotatable bonds would have 243 possible conformations. This is a manageable number, but the numbers increase rapidly going to 59,049 for ten bonds and 3.5×10^9 for twenty rotatable bonds. Because even a small protein would have hundreds of rotatable bonds the magnitude of the problem is apparent.

The most common computational approaches for addressing this sampling problem are molecular dynamics[22] and Monte Carlo[23,24] simulations. But the cost of these methods in terms of computer resources is very high. It should also be pointed out that the benefit of either approach may be suspect unless the simulations are run long enough to assure convergence, another factor that drives up the computational cost. It is possible that inadequate sampling may in some cases be worse than no sampling at all. All of this means that it is important to carefully consider strategies for dealing with conformational flexibility when undertaking any modeling project.

ACCEPTING THE CHALLENGE

One could be forgiven for looking at the challenges outlined above and simply deciding that any efforts to model protein-ligand binding interactions are doomed to failure. Fortunately, this is not the case. Indeed the literature is full of examples where modeling has been successfully applied to the design of ligands and, ultimately, drugs. But it is important to carefully design model systems to take as much advantage as possible of cancellation in the errors that exist. It is also true that the errors in computed geometries are typically much less pronounced than energies. This has been observed for many years with small-molecule quantum calculations[25,26] where the calculated geometries of organic compounds tend to be very good even at relatively low levels of theory. So one can be relatively more confident in predicted structures and these structures are of great practical value in drug discovery.

PROTEIN STRUCTURE

All protein crystal structures have errors of varying severity due to the inherent resolution of the structure (i.e., error

in the diffraction data) and errors associated with fitting a protein structure to that data. The latter model-building step is subject to considerable trial and error and also relies, in most cases, on relatively crude force fields. Thus it is important to carefully prepare protein structures before using them for any significant modeling. General guidelines for preparing protein structures are outlined below. It is also worth reminding medicinal chemists, who sometimes do not know any better, that (1) crystal structures are not handed down on stone tablets (they are models), (2) proteins are flexible beasts while crystal structures are only a single snapshot of the structure under some pretty extreme conditions, and (3) the structures provide little information with regard to many important protein properties that are thermodynamic in nature. Simply having a picture of how a ligand interacts with a protein says nothing about the energetics of that interaction. A general guide to crystal structure resolution is provided in Table 12.1.[27] Davis et al. have published two excellent reviews[28,29] that describe the issues and limitations inherent in x-ray protein structures. These reviews are highly recommended to any modeler or medicinal chemist who is involved in structure-based drug design.

For the modeler, there are a number of practical concerns when working with a crystal structure, either from the RCSB Protein Data Bank (PDB) or internal sources. First, there may be missing residues or side chains. This is a common situation due to areas of the protein that are disordered or poorly resolved for whatever reason. If these are remote from the active site they may not be a problem. If near the site of interest then one may need to attempt to fill in the gaps.

Of course, the first step before any calculations can be carried out is to correctly set the bond orders, charges, and add hydrogens. Commercial modeling packages automate most of this, although there may be a few decisions to make, especially regarding the protonation states of titratable residues. These decisions can have a significant effect on the final results because charges fall off slowly with respect to distance, at least if a constant dielectric is employed. In some cases the protonation state of a given residue is a significant scientific question in its own right such as the catalytic aspartates in aspartyl proteases [e.g., renin, HIV-protease, and beta-site APP cleaving enzyme (BACE)].[30,31]

A great deal of experimental and computational effort has been expended to try to determine the correct protonation state for these residues.[32-38]

My experience suggests that many structures also contain bad contacts and/or structural elements that are highly strained. Structural problems are often most prevalent in the bound ligand.[39,40] Unfortunately this is precisely the region of the protein that is of the greatest interest from a modeling point of view. Many modeling studies have probably been done with the coordinates as they come from the crystal structure, but it is generally a good idea to do at least a small amount of geometry optimization to remediate the most serious structural problems. In most cases limited minimization will result in a protein structure that is little changed in terms of the overall geometry, and even fit to the x-ray data, but the overall strain and the most severe geometric problems can be greatly reduced.

One of the final decisions is the following: water or no water? For docking and many modeling tasks it is common to remove the water molecules from the protein. This makes sense from the point of view of having an unbiased structure for docking, for example. It is also simple – just remove them all. However, there are circumstances where waters do make critical contacts not only with the protein, but in some cases also with the ligand. In such cases removing these critical waters is suspect. Leaving them all in can also pose problems. For example, most docking programs will not displace waters automatically, so any waters in the protein are essentially treated as an unchangeable part of the protein. Selective removal of waters is an intermediate course. This makes sense when a few waters are seen consistently across a number of crystal structures and/or where the water is involved in a key mediating interaction between protein and ligand. Of course this approach is not without hazard because the choice of waters for inclusion can have a big effect on the protein-binding site.

I have personally been bitten by this particular bug in a study of the protonation state of BACE. In our first publication[31] we elected to include a key water in the active site. Although this had no effect on our prediction that the preferred overall protonation state of the two catalytic asps in BACE was the −1 state (i.e., monoprotonated), it did lead to a surprising difference in energy between two specific states involving protonation of Asp32 or Asp228. In retrospect, this significant asymmetry in the active site appears to be due to this water that cooperates with Ser35 in stabilizing Asp32 when it is deprotonated. A later quantum mechanics/molecular mechanics (QM/MM) structure refinement study[30] showed that the energy for protonation of these aspartates were very nearly equivalent. It seems likely that one of the primary reasons for this discrepancy was the treatment of waters that were all included or all replaced by a continuum model in the later QM/MM refinement. This serves as a cautionary tale with respect to selective inclusion of waters in the active site. The protonation state question also highlights one of the other potential pitfalls in crystallography, namely that the crystallization conditions and environment where the enzyme is actually active may be quite different. In the case of BACE, many, if not most, of the crystals have been grown[34,41,42] at a pH near 7 while the enzyme itself is most active under more acidic conditions. This pH difference may be inconsequential, but that cannot be known for certain, particularly for a property as sensitive to medium effects as the protonation state.

In summary, it is important to carefully consider how the protein structure has been prepared. Protein preparation can have a meaningful impact on the quality of any subsequent modeling using that structure. This probably becomes more critical as one asks more from the results, such as computing relative binding affinities, or, as in the case mentioned above, energetically sensitive properties such as protonation states.

DOCKING AND SCORING

Docking and scoring is described in great detail in Chapter 7, but it is worth reiterating some of the practical conclusions of the many validation studies that have been done.[43-47] First, in most drug discovery efforts docking is used for one of two purposes. It may be used to determine the most probable docking pose for a ligand in a protein-binding site where a crystal structure is unavailable. Here the goal is just to find the correct orientation and conformation of the ligand in the protein. The second use for docking is in a virtual screening mode. In this mode the specific docking pose is not as important as ranking a set, usually a very large set, of chemical structures in terms of their propensity to bind to the target of interest. In the first mode the correct structure is the key result. In the second mode, enrichment of a screening set, in terms of potent ligands, is the desired result.

The literature suggests that it is possible in many cases to predict the best binding pose. At least the best binding pose is often near the top of possibilities unless there is a significant change in the protein structure, such as an allosteric modification or significant induced fit on the part of the ligand. Apparently available scoring algorithms are able to differentiate between good and bad binding poses for any one specific ligand. It is also true that decent enrichment factors often result from docking-based virtual screening, albeit perhaps not as significant as we might hope in most cases. It is very clear that scoring functions used in evaluating docking poses are exceedingly poor when asked to rank compounds in terms of their affinities. Most evaluations show essentially no correlation between docking score and affinity. Our experience at J&J has been consistent with this result. Therefore, it is important to consider docking-based virtual screening more as a filter than any kind of ordered list. Docking does filter out compounds that fit the active site poorly, but it does not differentiate well between weak and potent binders. This fact is important to keep in mind when analyzing docking results, and when presenting them to medicinal chemists.

One can speculate as to why scoring functions are better in terms of predicting the ligand pose. One possibility is that this is partly due to cancellation of errors because the ligand structure is a constant and the scoring function merely compares different poses. In addition, although the classical electrostatics are probably a good guide to the orientation of a ligand in the active site, determining their energetic contribution is a much more complex problem.

LIGAND BINDING AFFINITY

The Holy Grail, at least for protein-structure-based modeling, is the accurate calculation of relative binding free energies. This is at the heart of virtually all mechanistic approaches to drug discovery, at least as it pertains to potency. Unfortunately, the free energy of binding of a ligand to a protein is a very complex calculation,[48] as mentioned already. Nevertheless there are a number of approaches that have been employed with some success.

The most theoretically rigorous, at least from a sampling point of view, are the free-energy perturbation methods that were described in Chapter 5. These methods have two significant drawbacks that limit their impact in typical drug discovery efforts. They are extremely expensive in terms of computer resources. This becomes less of an issue with each passing year as computers continue to become faster and faster, but it still stretches the computer resources of most companies. The other issue is that these calculations work best for small perturbations and so are limited to very conservative changes in the ligands of interest. In recent work Jorgensen[49] has proposed a paradigm for using small structural changes and free-energy perturbation (FEP) to guide the development of structure/activity relationships (SAR).

There have been many approaches developed that, unlike FEP, rely only on calculations for the "end points" of ligand, protein, and complex. These methods might all be described as linear interaction energy (LIE) models[50–55] because they all rely on some fitted model based on computed interaction energies,[56] but people differ in their precise terminology. Some of the most well-known approaches are the linear response method[50,51] or the molecular mechanics-Poisson-Boltzman [(MM-PB) or molecular mechanics/generalized Born model/solvent accessibility (MM-GB/SA)] methods.[57,58] Approaches that use interaction energies for the reactants and products of ligand binding are much more commonly pursued in drug discovery because of their more tenable computational cost. They have also in many cases proven themselves to be quite effective.

We have used simple linear interaction energy (LIE) calculations as a tool for comparing the relative affinities of prospective ligands. For example, we made great use of this approach in our BACE program at J&J.[56,59,60] BACE

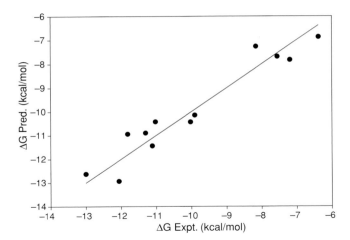

Figure 12.2. LIE model for BACE [Equation (12.2)].

is an aspartyl protease that plays a critical role in processing the amyloid precursor protein (APP) that has been implicated as a causative factor in Alzheimer's disease. We, and other groups, have shown that it is possible to construct reasonable models for BACE using some variation of the LIE approach. Our initial models were derived using a series of peptidic inhibitors reported by Ghosh and his collaborators.[41] These structures and their corresponding affinities are given in Table 12.2. Our procedure was to optimize the ligand in the protein-binding site using OPLS and GB/SA water. Either the protein can be held frozen or a subset of residues near the active site can be allowed to relax. The optimized ligand is then extracted from the protein and allowed to minimize in GB/SA[61] water. The van der Waals and electrostatic interaction energies are then computed and used to fit the LIE model.

We used OPLS and GB/SA calculations for the protein, ligands, and protein-ligand complexes to fit the model for BACE binding given in Equation (12.2):

$$\Delta G_{\text{Bind}} = 0.2228^* \Delta U_{\text{vdw}} + 0.0577^* \Delta U_{\text{ele}} + 12.7464. \quad (12.2)$$

This model provides a root-mean-squared deviation (rmsd) of 0.58 kcal/mol and an r^2 of 0.92 (Figure 12.2), and it has shown itself to be reasonably predictive with respect to compounds outside the training set.[56,59,60]

A similar model was derived for our internal series of BACE inhibitors[63] in spite of the fact that the structures are very different. The initial low micromolar lead for our BACE program (**11**) was identified in a high-throughput screen. Unlike most of the previously reported ligands, it was a nonpeptidic inhibitor:

11

Table 12.2. Experimental binding energies[62]

R_1	R_2	R_3	K_i (nM)	ΔG^{Expt} (kcal/mol)
1	Me	Me	22423.0	−6.38
2	Me	CHMe$_2$	3134.0	−7.55
3	Me	CHMe$_2$	1129.0	−8.16
4	Me	Me	61.4	−9.90
5	Me	CHMe$_2$	5.9	−11.30
6	Me	CHMe$_2$	50.1	−10.02
7	Me	CHMe$_2$	9.4	−11.02
8	Me	CHMe$_2$	5808.0	−7.19
9	Me	CHMe$_2$	2.5	−11.81
10	Me	CHMe$_2$	8.0	−11.11
OM99-2			1.6	−12.06
OM00-3			0.32	−13.05

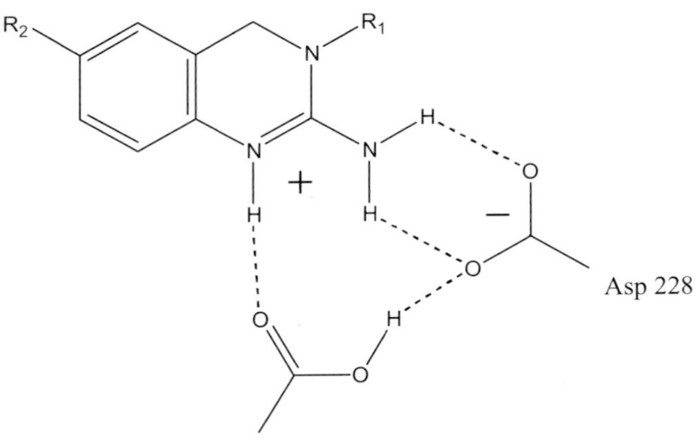

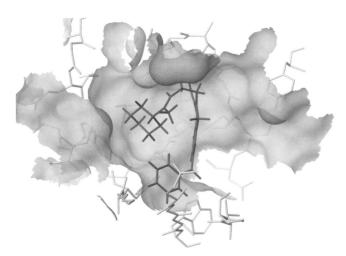

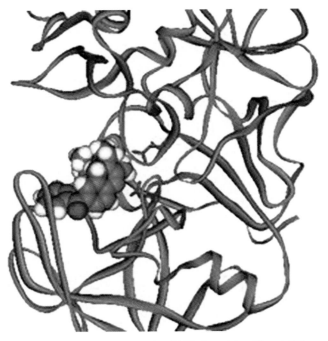

Figure 12.3. Hydrogen bond network between heterocycle in **11** and catalytic aspartates in BACE.

Compound **11** is a particularly interesting inhibitor of BACE in that it forms a strong hydrogen-bond network with the two catalytic aspartates via a unique protonated heterocycle (Figure 12.3).

Compound **11** is also unusual with respect to its binding mode. This ligand binds to BACE in a folded conformation where the terminal cyclohexyl bends completely around to bind in the S_1 pocket (Figures 12.4 and Figure 12.5).

BACE presents a few particular problems with respect to modeling. One is the previously mentioned issue of the protonation state for the catalytic aspartates. Asp32 and Asp228 can adopt seven potential protonation states

Figure 12.4. Compound **11** bound to BACE. Aspartates 32 and 228 are shown in red. The benzoyl substitutent binds under the flap that is displaced relative to previous peptidic inhibitors.

Figure 12.5. Compound **11** in the BACE active site. Structure is rotated 90° relative to Figure 12.4 and the flap has been removed for clarity. Notice the severe bend in the ligand.

(Figure 12.6). Modeling suggests that the most favorable states are the monoprotonated (charge $= -1$) states, **c-f**,[30,31,64] at least when the ligand contains a hydroxyl transition state mimic. The precise state might, of course, vary depending on the structure of the ligand.

Another problem is that two of the ligands in the study above are themselves potentially charged. Modeling systems where the formal charges differ is quite difficult. It is one of the reasons that it is important to carefully select charges for the protein. This can be illustrated very simply using OM00–3 from Table 12.2. There are two ionizable fuctional groups in OM00–3 that have the potential to form salt bridges with complementary residues in BACE. Table 12.3 gives the Δ_{vdw} and $\Delta_{coulombic}$ interaction terms[56] for OM00–3 with BACE for a variety of protonation states, using OPLS and GB/SA water. This comparison highlights the huge influence of these charged groups on the computed interaction energies.

The electrostatic term becomes extremely negative for the -2 state, even in the presence of the GB/SA solvation model. The electrostatics also exert a significant influence on the Δ_{vdw} term as van der Waals clashes are tolerated to make the coulombic term even more negative. This effect can be modulated by including a counterion for the unbound ligand. Indeed, inclusion of the counterion makes the change in electrostatics positive. None of these states are really satisfactory, but they illustrate how dominating

Table 12.3. Comparison of Δ_{vdw} and Δ_{coul} terms (kcal/mol) for different charged treatments of OM00–3

Compound	Charge	Counter ion	Δ_{vdw}	Δ_{coul}
OM00-3	Neutral	None	−95.48	−58.23
OM00-3	−2	None	−83.02	−333.61
OM00-3	−2	2 Na$^+$	−94.23	20.58

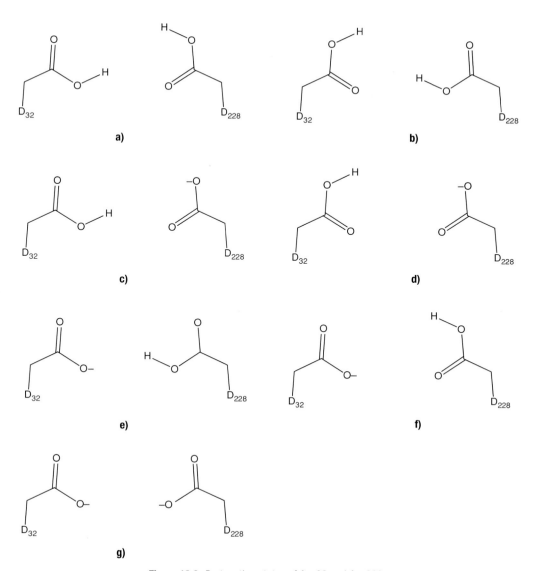

Figure 12.6. Protonation states of Asp32 and Asp228.

the electrostatics can be and why it is better to avoid modeling systems where the overall charge varies.

One is on more solid ground when modeling structural changes that are primarily mediated by changes in van der Waals interactions or where the predicted structure itself is more significant. An example of this is the modification of our internal J&J lead compound for BACE to incorporate a macrocycle.

BACE OPTIMIZATION

The HTS hit, **11**,[63] was modeled in the BACE active site to identify potential modifications to improve potency. A number of modifications were proposed based on this modeling work, but only two are discussed here. First, the hit structure binds exclusively on the N-terminal P (S) side of the enzyme, including the binding pocket that is created

by the flap transition (Figure 12.5). The protein binding sites (S_n) and corresponding binding residues (P_n) are defined with respect to the scissile bond as suggested by Schecter and Berger.[27,65] Sites on the N-terminal side of the scissile bond are denoted S_1, S_2, S_n as one moves away from the catalytic site. Similarly the sites on the C-terminal side are denoted as S_1', S_2', S_n':

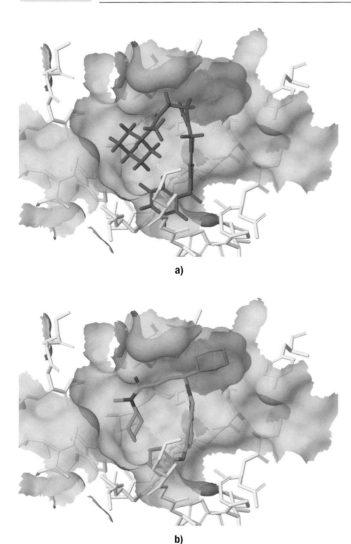

a)

b)

Figure 12.7. S$_1'$ pocket is highlighted in blue **(a)**. Structure **12** presents a cyclohexyl in the hydrophobic S$_1'$ pocket **(b)**.

Model structures showed that it was possible to substitute **11** in such a way as to occupy the S$_1'$ pocket, an interaction that was calculated to be energetically favorable (Figure 12.7). This led to the synthesis of analogs such as **12**. These analogs also have the potential to improve binding by reducing the rotational barrier for adopting the bound conformation.

Compound **12** is itself an interesting modeling problem. Substitution adjacent to the heterocylic core introduces a stereocenter. One of the first questions with regard to this compound was which isomer should be most favorable. Both enantiomers of **12** were manually docked into the BACE active site and subjected to simple minimization using the OPLS force field and GB/SA solvation. This was done with the protein structure frozen and by allowing the residues within 4Å of the ligand to relax. The results were qualitatively the same. Both calculations

predicted that the S-enantiomer should be most energetically favorable by approximately 1.5 kcal/mol, a result that was later confirmed experimentally. As was discussed previously, these simple interaction energy comparisons are most likely to be successful for a homologous series where one can expect a significant amount of cancellation of errors. This represents the ideal case because the stereoisomers are identical except for the configuration of the stereocenter. Substitution with a cyclohexyl (**12**) produces a very sizeable improvement in potency, with **12** being two orders of magnitude more potent than **11** at ~10 nM. This is consistent with the modeling results (Figure 12.7) and represented a very large step in optimizing the affinity of this series.

12

The structure of **11** (Figure 12.5) also suggested another avenue for optimization. This structure binds to the BACE active site in a bent conformation. Another strategy for improving affinity was to enforce this bend by introducing rigid structural elements that enforce this conformation for the ligand. One approach was just to incorporate the structural elements of **12** into a macrocycle by connecting the phenoxy moiety back to the amide. The chemists could have begun making macrocycles of varying sizes in an attempt to find the optimal macrocycle, but instead we built and modeled a variety of macrocycles in order to propose an optimal size before undertaking

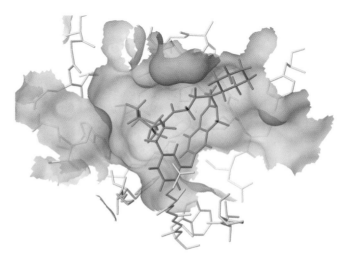

Figure 12.8. Computed structure for a macrocycle bound to BACE.

a large synthetic effort. Several combinations of spacer methylenes on either side of the amide were identified that fit the active site and appeared to be reasonably unstrained. One of these (**13**) with two methylenes connecting the amide to the phenoxy is shown in Figure 12.8 and was found to be quite potent at ~5 nM. This is an example where the structure is probably more important than the computed ΔE values. Just the ability to compute reasonably accurate structures for the prototype macrocycles is enough to be very useful in expediting the design of these compounds.

13

LIGAND BINDING RULES OF THUMB

The binding free energy is usually dominated by hydrophobic effects. This is not well understood by most medicinal chemists, who often focus much more attention on polar interactions, such as hydrogen bonds and salt bridges. Although hydrogen bonds are important, the fact is that in an aqueous environment they can be rather weak.[66] This may not be well appreciated by chemists who spent most of their formative years working in organic solvents where hydrogen bonds rein supreme. The issue is twofold: First the strength of a hydrogen bond is greatly influenced by the surrounding medium. In the gas phase (or a very non-polar solvent) a typical hydrogen bond would be worth on the order of 7 kcal/mol.[67] This is huge in terms of binding affinity. But in aqueous solution the same hydrogen bond may be worth only a fraction of a kcal/mol. Second, while hydrogen bonds in polar groups are typically very well satisfied in water, they are sometimes only poorly satisfied in the protein. This can mean that there is a significant free-energy cost for removing the polar group from solution and placing it in the protein active site.[68] The practical consequence of this is that one should be careful in drug design about putting too much weight on hydrogen bonds between the ligand and protein. In some cases they provide little in terms of potency. However, it is generally always the case that putting a polar functional group on a ligand in a part of the protein that cannot satisfy the polar group is very bad.

It is possible to make some general comments with regard to the introduction of polar substituents into a ligand structure. Hydrogen bonds or salt bridges that are near the solvent interface are much less favorable than the same interactions in deep protein pockets. When the ligand can satisfy the hydrogen bonding requirements of the protein in a sterically constrained pocket, the interaction is favorable because the polar partner in the protein is poorly solvated and because there is an entropy gain from liberating one or more tightly bound waters from the protein. As mentioned above, any substitution of the ligand that forces a polar group into a hydrophobic pocket in the protein is very detrimental to binding. Thus, the polar groups sometimes have more influence on selectivity (i.e., only certain enzymes or receptors have complementary polar regions) than overall potency. This is also why the most certain way to increase affinity is usually to add grease – a well-worn medicinal chemistry strategy and the primary reason for guidelines such as Lipinski's rules. Finally, in my view, finding the proper balance between polar groups in the protein versus water is part of the reason computing binding affinities is so difficult in the first place. It may be a particular problem for most scoring functions used in docking since polar interactions between the protein and ligand probably play a very major role in assessing potential docked poses but are less informative with regard to affinity. All of this is sometimes summarized in the rule: hydrophobic interactions provide potency; polar interactions provide specificity.

BEYOND POTENCY

Computational modeling is not confined to improving potency. It has become clear in recent years that most drug discovery organizations have become very adept at optimizing ligand potency. But that is not enough for a drug candidate. To have a chance at making its way to the market a drug candidate must also have good bioavailability, favorable pharmacokinetic properties, and, of course, very low toxicity or off-target activity. Structure-based drug design can play a significant role in these areas as well. Access to a crystal structure and computational modeling can allow us to design ligands with improved physical properties that do not destroy binding. For example, one might add a metabolic handle to a molecule in a region where it might actually contribute favorably to binding or add a solubilizing group where it either interacts with solvent or satisfies a key polar interaction in the protein. An example of this at J&J involves our efforts to improve the solubility of a BACE lead series (e.g., **12**). In this case we observed a Lys

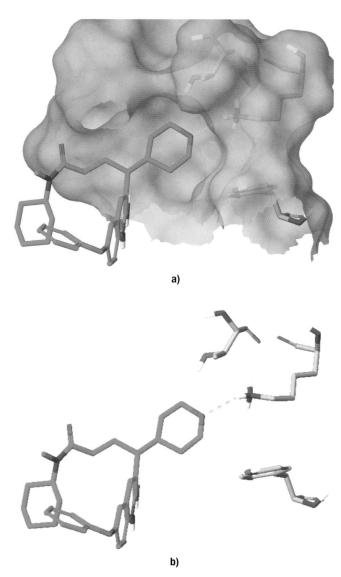

a)

b)

Figure 12.9. S1 region showing interaction between the tetrahydrofuran ether oxygen and Lys224 with **(a)** and without **(b)** the molecular surface displayed.

in the otherwise mostly hydrophobic S'_1 pocket that might interact with the 4-position in a series of potent cyclohexyl-susbstituted analogs. Modification of this ring to include 4-hydroxyl or replacing it by the tetrahydropyranyl (**14**) analog led to structures that were significantly more soluble and maintained potency because of the favorable interaction between the ether oxygen and positively charged Lys (Figure 12.9). Again the goal of identifying favorable interactions such as these is not always so much to improve potency but to improve physical properties such as solubility without *reducing* potency. As discussed earlier it is often difficult to assess how introduction of a favorable electrostatic interaction between the ligand and protein will affect potency due to all the confounding factors (desolvation penalty, etc.). But if we do introduce polar groups into a ligand structure for other reasons we must be sure they are

accommodated in the protein-ligand complex or there will almost surely be a severe loss of activity.

14

In this case the tetrahydropyran oxygen is well accommodated and preserves potency ($K_i = 6$ nM). Ethers can be particularly useful in this context because they can form a favorable polar or hydrogen bonding interaction with the protein[69,70] and are not as difficult to desolvate as other polar groups such as acids or alcohols. This simple substitution has a remarkable impact on solubility with the resulting compound (**14**) being orders of magnitude more soluble (Table 12.4).

hERG modeling

It is also possible to employ structural models to understand and mitigate toxicity. An example of this at J&J is the hERG channel. The human ether-à-go-go related gene (hERG) controls repolarization of the cardiac action potential and therefore proper cardiac function. Impairment of this repolarization process is a cause of long QT syndrome and in some cases severe cardiac arrhythmia. Many drugs are known to have affinity for this potassium channel, a situation that has serious implications for cardiac safety.[71,72]

We developed a multicomponent homology model[73] for the hERG channel that allows us to evaluate ligands with respect to their propensity to bind and, even more importantly, predict a possible binding mode. This predicted binding mode can be used to suggest structural changes that might reduce hERG binding.

It is difficult to determine the structure of the hERG channel experimentally because it is a membrane-bound protein. Membrane-bound proteins are difficult targets for crystallography because they are typically difficult to express in large quantity and do not readily crystallize outside the membrane. There have been a few successes in this area. The first, and perhaps best known, is the bovine rhodopsin GPCR structure.[11] More recently a β-adrenergic GPCR structure has also been solved.[8,12] Perhaps more relevant to hERG, a series of bacterial ion channel structures have also been solved through heroic means.[9,10,13] These ion channel structures provide a possible template for construction of a homology model for hERG. The first effort to build a homology model was reported by Culberson and Sanguinetti.[74] Since that time most modeling efforts relative to hERG have focused on development of either quantitative structure/activity relationship (QSAR) models

Table 12.4. Measured solubility of BACE ligands. Potencies for **12** and **14** are essentially equivalent at 10 and 6 nM, respectively

Compound	Structure	Solubility mg/ml	
		pH = 2	pH = 7.4
12	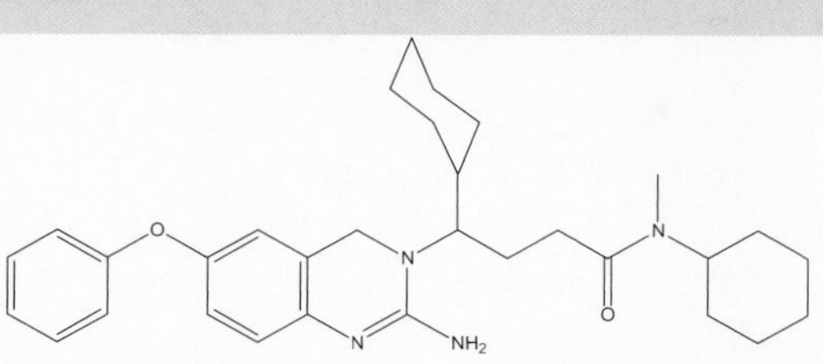	0.008	0.01
14	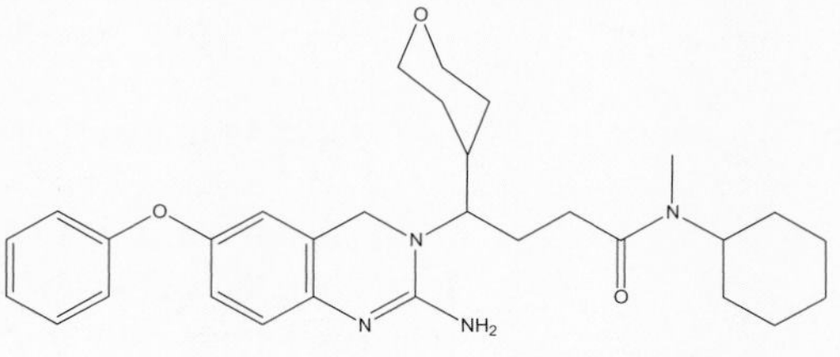	0.91	0.44
		114×	44×

or pharmacophore models for the ion channel. Although these may have some utility in drug discovery they are both relatively weak approaches for understanding how hERG activity might be mitigated in a particular series of interest. We reexamined the issue of a homology model but with one difference: Given the known flexibility of the channel, both open and closed structures of the bacterial ion channels have been observed experimentally, and we decided to include this flexibility explicitly in our model. We did this through the simple expedient of constructing multiple models where the channel is in different states with respect to channel opening. It has been thought that part of the reason hERG is so promiscuous is the fact that it can accommodate ligands of different shapes and sizes as the channel opens and closes. The first step is to align the hERG sequence with one or more of the available bacterial ion channel sequences (Figure 12.10). The homology in the filter region is very high and provides considerable insight into the alignment. There are also a few key residues in the S6 domain that are conserved. One residue of note is the conserved Gly in the S6 domain. Examination of homology models constructed from the closed KcsA[13] and open MthK[9,10] structures shows that the channel can be converted from open to closed by rotation of this hinge Gly.

To obtain potential intermediate states for the hERG channel, the conformation of the hinge Gly was rotated to mimic the open MthK channel. This structure was then

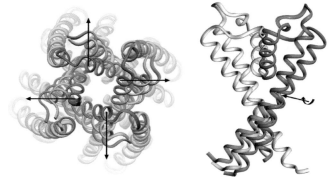

Figure 12.11. Rotation of S6 about the glycine hinge. The closed KcsA structure is shown in red, the partially open structure (10°) in yellow, and the open structure (19°) in green.

rotated in small increments to close the channel until a structure more similar to KcsA (closed) was obtained (Figure 12.11). At each 1° increment molecular dynamics simulations were used to relax the side chains. The protocol at each increment was 0.4 ps of heating followed by 5 ps of equilibration using the CHARMM force field.[17,18] Two states were selected for study: the 10° partially open structure and the 19° fully open structure.

These two states were then evaluated using a series of compounds with known hERG affinities from the literature.[75] In each case the ligand was docked to both states using GLIDE and then submitted for an LIE calculation of the ΔE_{vdw} and ΔE_{elec} values using OPLS and GB/SA water. Our first effort was to see if either state would provide a reasonable model for hERG activity. The compounds evaluated are listed in Table 12.5.

```
< Filter ><            S6 helix              >
hERG:  ...YFTFSSLTSVGFGNVSPNTNSEKIFSICVMLIGSLMYASIFGNVSAII...
KcsA:  ...WWSVETATTVGYGDLYPVTLWGRCVAVVVMVAGITSFGLVTAALATWF...
```

Figure 12.10. Sequence alignment.

Table 12.5. Compounds and their computed and observed pIC$_{50}$ for hERG binding

Compound	pIC$_{50}$ observed	pIC$_{50}$ computed	Δ pIC$_{50}$
		Open state	
Amitriptyline	5.00	4.59	0.41
Astemizole	9.04	8.10	0.94
Azimilde	6.25	6.06	0.19
Bepridil	6.26	5.99	0.27
Diltiazem	4.76	5.80	−1.04
Dolasetron	5.22	4.80	0.42
Domperidone	6.79	7.06	−0.27
Droperidol	7.49	6.67	0.82
Fexofenadine	4.67	5.58	−0.91
Gatifloxacin	3.89	4.21	−0.32
Grepafloxacin	4.11	4.29	−0.18
Halofantrine	6.70	6.89	−0.19
Haloperidol	7.55	5.05	2.50[a]
Mibefradil	5.84	6.68	−0.84
Moxifloxacin	3.93	5.04	−1.11
Norastemizole	7.55	4.65	2.90[a]
Pimozide	7.74	6.29	1.45[a]
Risperidone	6.79	6.77	0.02
Sertindole	7.85	5.15	2.70[a]
Sparfloxacin	4.58	4.82	−0.24
Verapamil	6.84	6.64	0.20
		Partially open state	
Chlorpromazine	5.83	5.75	0.08
Cisapride	8.19	7.36	0.83
Clozapine	6.72	5.47	1.25[a]
Cocaine	5.24	5.14	0.10
Granisetron	5.42	6.03	−0.61
Imipramine	5.47	5.06	0.41
Mizolastine	6.45	6.90	−0.45
Perhexiline	5.11	5.33	−0.22
Terfenadine	6.89	7.06	−0.17
Thioridazine	7.45	7.10	0.35
Ziprasidone	6.82	5.98	0.84

[a] Omitted from final model.

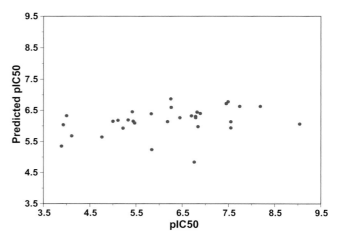

Figure 12.12. Plot of LIE model against experimental pIC$_{50}$.

Initial results were not very promising. The best LIE model for the partially open state is given in Figure 12.12. The correlation is poor with an r^2 of 0.24, as was the model for the open state.

As a next step, the compounds were partitioned between the two homology models. Each compound was docked in each state and the interaction energy was computed as above. But the compounds were then partitioned into two sets: set 1 that gave the most negative interaction energy with the open model and set 2 that gave the most negative interaction energy with the partially open model. We then constructed two separate models for these two sets of compounds. These models were much improved, as can be seen in Figures 12.13 and 12.14.

Interestingly, the two models also had essentially the same coefficients for the van der Waals and electrostatics terms. This allowed us to fit a single LIE equation using the interaction energy terms for each compound that arise from the hERG state with the most negative interaction energy. This model is given in Equation (12.3) and plotted in Figure 12.15:

$$\text{pIC}_{50(\text{Combined})} = -0.163(\Delta E_{\text{vdw}}) + 0.0009(\Delta E_{\text{ele}}). \quad (12.3)$$

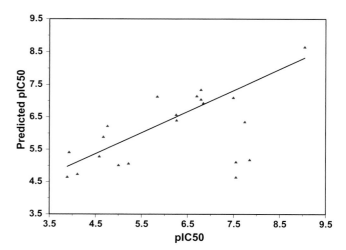

Figure 12.13. Open structure.

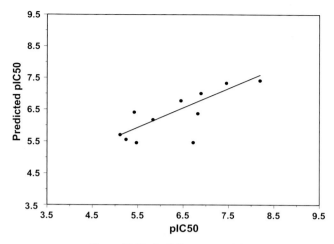

Figure 12.14. Partially open model.

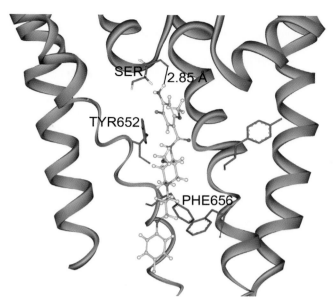

Figure 12.16. Cisapride docked into the partially open state (10°).

There are five structures that give a very poor fit between computed and experimental IC$_{50}$ values. It is not surprising that some structures would not fit the model. This could be due to many factors given the complexity of the system and the computational procedure. A problem with docking or the LIE calculations could lead to large errors. It is also possible that these structures bind in an alternative location or perhaps yet another intermediate state of the pore.

The real strength of this approach over previous QSAR and pharmacophore approaches is not the accuracy of the predicted affinities but the fact that we also get hypothetical binding modes. This is very useful if the goal is to mitigate hERG binding in a series of interest. This approach has been used with some success within J&J, particularly for an opioid target that was plagued with significant hERG liability. Structural changes suggested by the models were critical to efforts that eventually led to a clinical candidate. An example of the kind of docked structure that results from this model is cisapride in the partially open state (Figure 12.16).

CONCLUSION

There have been significant advances in recent years in the application of modeling techniques to the discovery of new drug candidates. In particular, our ability to model protein-ligand interactions has improved greatly with access to more structures, improvements in computational methods, and access to ever faster computers. Moreover, modeling is not just a matter of optimizing potency, it is being used increasingly to answer other questions, such as how to improve physical properties and reduce the potential for toxicity. Molecular modeling has become an indispensable tool for drug discovery.

ACKNOWLEDGMENTS

The work described in this chapter was done with the assistance of several extremely talented collaborators. I acknowledge the contributions of Ramkumar Rajamani (Bristol-Myers Squibb), Jian Li (WuXi AppTec), and Brett Tounge (J&J). I also acknowledge professor Kennie Merz at the University of Florida and his group who collaborated with us on the QM/MM structure refinement and DivCon work.

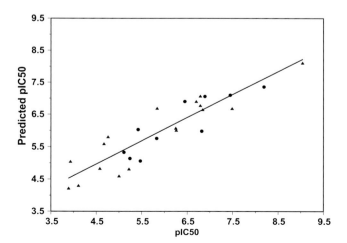

Figure 12.15. Plot of combined model. Triangles and circles represent open and partially open states, respectively.

REFERENCES

1. Clark, D. E. What has computer-aided molecular design ever done for drug discovery? *Exp. Opin. Drug Discov.* **2006**, *1*(2), 103–110.
2. Jorgensen, W. L. The many roles of computation in drug discovery. *Science* **2004**, *303*(5665), 1813–1818.
3. Richon, A. B. An early history of the molecular modeling industry. *Drug Discov. Today* **2008**, *13*, 659–664.
4. Hansch, C.; Leo, A. *Exploring QSAR: Fundamentals and Applications in Chemistry and Biology*, American Chemical Society, Washington, D.C., **1995**.
5. Hansch, C.; Fukunaga, J. Designing biologically active materials. *ChemTech* **1977**, *7*(2), 120–8.

6. Hansch, C. Quantitative approach to biochemical structure-activity relationships. *Acc. Chem. Res.* **1969**, *2*(8), 232–239.

7. www.rcsb.org.

8. Cherezov, V.; Rosenbaum, D. M.; Hanson, M. A.; Rasmussen, S. G. F.; Thian, F. S.; Kobilka, T. S.; Choi, H.-J.; Kuhn, P.; Weis, W. I.; Kobilka, B. K.; Stevens, R. C.; Takeda, S.; Kadowaki, S.; Haga, T.; Takaesu, H.; Mitaku, S.; Fredriksson, R.; Lagerstrom, M. C.; Lundin, L. G.; Schioth, H. B.; Pierce, K. L.; Premont, R. T.; Lefkowitz, R. J.; Lefkowitz, R. J.; Shenoy, S. K.; Rosenbaum, D. M. High-resolution crystal structure of an engineered human β2-adrenergic G protein-coupled receptor. *Science* **2007**, *318*, (5854), 1258–1265.

9. Jiang, Y.; Lee, A.; Chen, J.; Cadene, M.; Chait, B. T.; MacKinnon, R. The open pore conformation of potassium channels. *Nature* **2002**, *417*(6888), 523–526.

10. Jiang, Y.; Lee, A.; Chen, J.; Ruta, V.; Cadene, M.; Chait, B. T.; MacKinnon, R. X-ray structure of a voltage-dependent K+ channel. *Nature* **2003**, *423*(6935), 33–41.

11. Palczewski, K.; Kumasaka, T.; Hori, T.; Behnke, C. A.; Motoshima, H.; Fox, B. A.; Le Trong, I.; Teller, D. C.; Okada, T.; Stenkamp, R. E.; Yamamoto, M.; Miyano, M. Crystal structure of rhodopsin: a G protein-coupled receptor. *Science* **2000**, *289*(5480), 739–745.

12. Rasmussen, S. G. F.; Choi, H.-J.; Rosenbaum, D. M.; Kobilka, T. S.; Thian, F. S.; Edwards, P. C.; Burghammer, M.; Ratnala, V. R. P.; Sanishvili, R.; Fischetti, R. F.; Schertler, G. F. X.; Weis, W. I.; Kobilka, B. K. Crystal structure of the human β2 adrenergic G-protein-coupled receptor. *Nature* **2007**, *450*(7168), 383–387.

13. Zhou, Y., Morals-Cabral, J. H.; Kaufman, A.; MacKinnon, R. Chemistry of ion coordination and hydration revealed by a K+ channel-Fab complex at 2.0.ANG. resolution. *Nature* **2001**, *414*(6859), 43–48.

14. Coulson, C. A. Coulson is credited with using this analogy to describe the accuracy required to compute the energy of interaction between two molecules.

15. Cornell, W. D.; Cieplak, P.; Bayly, C. I.; Gould, I. R.; Merz, K. M., Jr.; Ferguson, D. M.; Spellmeyer, D. C.; Fox, T.; Caldwell, J. W.; Kollman, P. A. A second generation force field for the simulation of proteins, nucleic acids, and organic molecules. *J. Am. Chem. Soc.* **1995**, *117*(19), 5179–5197.

16. Weiner, P. K.; Kollman, P. A. AMBER: assisted model building with energy refinement: a general program for modeling molecules and their interactions. *J. Comput. Chem.* **1981**, *2*(3), 287–303.

17. MacKerell, A. D., Jr.; Bashford, D.; Bellott, M.; Dunbrack, R. L.; Evanseck, J. D.; Field, M. J.; Fischer, S.; Gao, J.; Guo, H.; Ha, S.; Joseph-McCarthy, D.; Kuchnir, L.; Kuczera, K.; Lau, F. T. K.; Mattos, C.; Michnick, S.; Ngo, T.; Nguyen, D. T.; Prodhom, B.; Reiher, W. E., III; Roux, B.; Schlenkrich, M.; Smith, J. C.; Stote, R.; Straub, J.; Watanabe, M.; Wiorkiewicz-Kuczera, J.; Yin, D.; Karplus, M. All-atom empirical potential for molecular modeling and dynamics studies of proteins. *J. Phys. Chem. B* **1998**, *102*(18), 3586–3616.

18. Brooks, B. R.; Bruccoleri, R. E.; Olafson, B. D.; States, D. J.; Swaminathan, S.; Karplus, M. CHARMM: a program for macromolecular energy, minimization, and dynamics calculations. *J. Comput. Chem.* **1983**, *4*(2), 187–217.

19. Jorgensen, W. L.; Tirado-Rives, J. The OPLS (optimized potentials for liquid simulations) potential functions for proteins, energy minimizations for crystals of cyclic peptides and crambin. *J. Am. Chem. Soc.* **1988**, *110*(6), 1657–66.

20. Curtiss, L. A.; Redfern, P. C.; Raghavachari, K.; Pople, J. A. Gaussian-3X (G3X) theory: use of improved geometries, zero-point energies, and Hartree-Fock basis sets. *J. Chem. Phys.* **2001**, *114*(1), 108–117.

21. Curtiss, L. A.; Raghavachari, K.; Redfern, P. C.; Rassolov, V.; Pople, J. A. Gaussian-3 (G3) theory for molecules containing first and second-row atoms. *J. Chem. Phys.* **1998**, *109*(18), 7764–7776.

22. Karplus, M. Molecular dynamics of biological macromolecules: a brief history and perspective. *Biopolymers* **2003**, *68*(3), 350–358.

23. Guimaraes, C. R. W.; Boger, D. L.; Jorgensen, W. L. Elucidation of fatty acid amide hydrolase inhibition by potent a-ketoheterocycle derivatives from monte carlo simulations. *J. Am. Chem. Soc.* **2005**, *127*(49), 17377–17384.

24. Ulmschneider, J. P.; Jorgensen, W. L. Monte Carlo backbone sampling for polypeptides with variable bond angles and dihedral angles using concerted rotations and a Gaussian bias. *J. Chem. Phys.* **2003**, *118*(9), 4261–4271.

25. Dewar, M. J. S.; Zoebisch, E. G.; Healy, E. F.; Stewart, J. J. P. Development and use of quantum mechanical molecular models. 76. AM1: a new general purpose quantum mechanical molecular model. *J. Am. Chem. Soc.* **1985**, *107*(13), 3902–3909.

26. Dewar, M. J. S.; Thiel, W. Ground states of molecules. 39. MNDO results for molecules containing hydrogen, carbon, nitrogen, and oxygen. *J. Am. Chem. Soc.* **1977**, *99*(15), 4907–4917.

27. Fersht, A. *Enzyme Structure and Mechanism*, 2nd ed. New York: Freeman & Co.; **1985**.

28. Davis, A. M.; Teague, S. J.; Kleywegt, G. J. Application and limitations of X-ray crystallographic data in structure-based ligand and drug design. *Angew. Chem. Int. Ed. Engl.* **2003**, *42*(24), 2718–2736.

29. Davis, A. M.; St. Gallay, S. A.; Gerard, J. K. Limitations and lessons in the use of X-ray structural information in drug design. *Drug Discov. Today* **2008**, *13*, 831–841.

30. Yu, N.; Hayik, S. A.; Wang, B.; Liao, N.; Reynolds, C. H.; Merz, K. M., Jr. Assigning the protonation states of the key aspartates in β-secretase using QM/MM x-ray structure refinement. *J. Chem. Theor. Comput.* **2006**, *2*(4), 1057–1069.

31. Rajamani, R.; Reynolds, C. H. Modeling the protonation states of the catalytic aspartates in b-secretase. *J. Med. Chem.* **2004**, *47*(21), 5159–5166.

32. Piana, S.; Sebastiani, D.; Carloni, P.; Parrinello, M. Ab initio molecular dynamics-based assignment of the protonation state of pepstatin A/HIV-1 protease clevage site. *J. Am. Chem. Soc.* **2001**, *123*, 8730–8737.

33. Smith, R.; Brereton, I. M.; Chai, R. Y.; Kent, S. B. H. Ionization states of the catalytic residues in HIV-1 protease. *Nature Struct. Biol.* **1996**, *3*, 946–950.

34. Hong, L.; Koelsch, G.; Lin, X.; Wu, S.; Terzyan, S.; Ghosh, A. K.; Zhang, X. C.; Tang, J. Structure of the protease domain of memapsin 2 (β-secretase) complexed with inhibitor. *Science* **2000**, *290*, 150–153.

35. Harte, W. E., Jr.; Beveridge, D. L. Prediction of the protonation state of the active site aspartyl residues in HIV-1 protease-inhibitor complexed via molecular dynamics simulation. *J. Am. Chem. Soc.* **1993**, *115*, 3883–3886.

36. Piana, S.; Carloni, P. Conformational flexibility of the catalytic asp dyad in HIV-1 protease: an ab initio study on the free enzyme. *Proteins* **2000**, *39*, 26–36.

37. Wang, Y.; Freedberg, D. I.; Yamazaki, T.; Wingfield, P. T.; Stahl, S. J.; Kaufman, J. D.; Kiso, Y.; Torchia, D. A. Solution NMR

evidence that the HIV-1 protease catalytic aspartyl groups have different ionization states in the complex formed with the assymetric drug KNI-272. *Biochemistry* **1996**, *35*, 9945–9950.

38. Yamazaki, T.; Nicholson, L. K.; Torchia, D. A.; Wingfield, P.; Stahl, S. J.; Kaufman, J. D.; Eyermann, C. J.; Hedge, C. N.; Lam, P. Y. S.; R u, Y.; Jadhav, P. K.; Chang, C.; Webers, P. C. NMR and x-ray evidence that the HIV protease catalytic aspartyl groups are protonated in the complex formed by the protease and a non-peptide cyclic urea-based inhibitor. *J. Am. Chem. Soc.* **1994**, *116*, 10791–10792.

39. Kleywegt, G. J. Crystallographic refinement of ligand complexes. *Acta Crystallogr. D Biol. Crystallogr.* **2007**, *D63*(1), 94–100.

40. Kleywegt, G. J.; Henrick, K.; Dodson, E. J.; Van Aalten, D. M. F. Pound-wise but penny-foolish: how well do micromolecules fare in macromolecular refinement? *Structure* **2003**, *11*(9), 1051–1059.

41. Hong, L.; Turner, R. T.; Koelsch, G.; Shin, D.; Ghosh, A. K.; Tang, J. Crystal structure of memapsin 2 (β-secretase) in complex with an inhibitor OM00-3. *Biochemistry* **2002**, *41*, 10963–10967.

42. Patel, S.; Vuillard, L.; Cleasby, A.; Murray, C. W.; Yon, J. Apo and inhibitor complex structures of BACE (β-secretase). *J. Mol. Biol.* **2004**, *343*(2), 407–416.

43. Cummings, M. D.; DesJarlais, R. L.; Gibbs, A. C.; Mohan, V.; Jaeger, E. P. Comparison of automated docking programs as virtual screening tools. *J. Med. Chem.* **2005**, *48*(4), 962–976.

44. Perola, E.; Walters, W. P.; Charifson, P. S. A detailed comparison of current docking and scoring methods on systems of pharmaceutical relevance. *Proteins* **2004**, *56*(2), 235–249.

45. McGaughey, G. B.; Sheridan, R. P.; Bayly, C. I.; Culberson, J. C.; Kreatsoulas, C.; Lindsley, S.; Maiorov, V.; Truchon, J.-F.; Cornell, W. D. Comparison of topological, shape, and docking methods in virtual screening. *J. Chem. Inf. Model.* **2007**, *47*(4), 1504–1519.

46. Warren, G. L.; Andrews, C. W.; Capelli, A.-M.; Clarke, B.; LaLonde, J.; Lambert, M. H.; Lindvall, M.; Nevins, N.; Semus, S. F.; Senger, S.; Tedesco, G.; Wall, I. D.; Woolven, J. M.; Peishoff, C. E.; Head, M. S. A critical assessment of docking programs and scoring functions. *J. Med. Chem.* **2006**, *49*(20), 5912–5931.

47. DesJarlais, R. L.; Cummings, M. D.; Gibbs, A. C. Virtual docking: how are we doing and how can we improve? *Front. Drug Des. Discov.* **2007**, *3*, 81–103.

48. Gilson, M. K.; Zhou, H.-X. Calculation of protein-ligand binding affinities. *Annu. Rev. Biophys. Biomol. Struct.* **2007**, *36*, 21–42.

49. Zeevaart, J. G.; Wang, L.; Thakur, V. V.; Leung, C. S.; Tirado-Rives, J.; Bailey, C. M.; Domaoal, R. A.; Anderson, K. S.; Jorgensen, W. L. Optimization of azoles as anti-human immunodeficiency virus agents guided by free-energy calculations. *J. Am. Chem. Soc.* **2008**, *130*(29), 9492–9499.

50. Aqvist, J.; Marelius, J. The linear interaction energy method for predicting ligand binding free energies. *Comb. Chem. High Throughput Screen.* **2001**, *4*(8), 613–626.

51. Hansson, T.; Marelius, J.; Aqvist, J. Ligand binding affinity prediction by linear interaction energy methods. *J. Comput. Aided Mol. Des.* **1998**, *12*(1), 27–35.

52. Wesolowski, S. S.; Jorgensen, W. L. Estimation of binding affinities for celecoxib analogues with COX-2 via Monte Carlo-extended linear response. *Bioorg. Med. Chem. Lett.* **2002**, *12*(3), 267–270.

53. Lamb, M. L.; Tirado-Rives, J.; Jorgensen, W. L. Estimation of the binding affinities of FKBP12 inhibitors using a linear response method. *Bioorg. Med. Chem.* **1999**, *7*(5), 851–860.

54. Smith, R. H., Jr.; Jorgensen, W. L.; Tirado-Rives, J.; Lamb, M. L.; Janssen, P. A. J.; Michejda, C. J., Smith, M. B. K. Prediction of binding affinities for TIBO inhibitors of HIV-1 reverse transcriptase using Monte Carlo simulations in a linear response method. *J. Med. Chem.* **1998**, *41*(26), 5272–5286.

55. Holloway, M. K. A priori prediction of ligand affinity by energy minimization. *Perspectives in Drug Discovery and Design.* 3D QSAR in Drug Design: Ligand/Protein Interactions and Molecular Similarity. New York: Springer-Verlag; **1998**, 63–84.

56. Tounge, B. A.; Rajamani, R.; Baxter, E. W.; Reitz, A. B.; Reynolds, C. H. Linear interaction energy models for β-secretase (BACE) inhibitors: role of van der Waals, electrostatic, and continuum-solvation terms. *J. Mol. Graph. Model.* **2006**, *24*(6), 475–484.

57. Kuhn, B.; Donini, O.; Huo, S.; Wang, J.; Kollman, P. A. MM-PBSA applied to computer-assisted ligand design. In: *Free Energy Calculations in Rational Drug Design*, Rami Reddy, R.; Erion, M. D.; Eds. New York: Kluwer Academic/Plenum; **2001**, 243–251.

58. Wang, J.; Morin, P.; Wang, W.; Kollman, P. A. Use of MM-PBSA in reproducing the binding free energies to HIV-1 RT of TIBO derivatives and predicting the binding mode to HIV-1 RT of efavirenz by docking and MM-PBSA. *J. Am. Chem. Soc.* **2001**, *123*(22), 5221–5230.

59. Tounge, B. A.; Reynolds, C. H. Calculation of the binding affinity of β-secretase inhibitors using the linear interaction energy method. *J. Med. Chem.* **2003**, *46*, 2074–2082.

60. Rajamani, R.; Reynolds, C. H. Modeling the binding affinities of β-secretase inhibitors: application to subsite specificity. *Bioorg. Med. Chem. Lett.* **2004**, *14*(19), 4843–4846.

61. Qiu, D.; Shenkin, P. S.; Hollinger, F. P.; Still, W. C. The GB/SA continuum model for solvation: a fast analytical method for the calculation of approximate born radii. *J. Phys. Chem. A* **1997**, *101*(16), 3005–3014.

62. Ghosh, A. K.; Bilcer, G.; Harwood, C.; Kawahama, R.; Shin, D.; Hussain, K. A.; Hong, L.; Loy, J. A.; Nguyen, C.; Koelsch, G.; Ermolieff, J.; Tang, J. Structure-based design: potent inhibitors of human brain memapsin 2 (β-secretase). *J. Med. Chem.* **2001**, *44*(18), 2865–2868.

63. Baxter, E. W.; Conway, K. A.; Kennis, L.; Bischoff, F.; Mercken, M. H.; De Winter, H. L.; Reynolds, C. H.; Tounge, B. A.; Luo, C.; Scott, M. K.; Huang, Y.; Braeken, M.; Pieters, S. M. A.; Berthelot, D. J. C.; Masure, S.; Bruinzeel, W. D.; Jordan, A. D.; Parker, M. H.; Boyd, R. E.; Qu, J.; Alexander, R. S.; Brenneman, D. E.; Reitz, A. B. 2-amino-3,4-dihydroquinazolines as inhibitors of BACE-1 (β-site APP cleaving enzyme): use of structure based design to convert a micromolar hit into a nanomolar lead. *J. Med. Chem.* **2007**, *50*(18), 4261–4264.

64. Park, H.; Lee, S. Determination of the active site protonation state of b-secretase from molecular dynamics simulation and docking experiment: implications for structure-based inhibitor design. *J. Am. Chem. Soc.* **2003**, *125*, 16416–16422.

65. Schechter, I.; Berger, A. On the size of the active site in proteases. I. Papain. *Biochem. Biophys. Res. Commun.* **1967**, *27*, 157–162.

66. Tobias, D. J.; Sneddon, S. F.; Brooks, C. L., III. Stability of a model β-sheet in water. *J. Mol. Biol.* **1992**, *227*(4), 1244–1252.

67. Frey, J. A.; Leutwyler, S. An ab initio benchmark study of hydrogen bonded formamide dimers. *J. Phys. Chem. A* **2006**, *110*(45), 12512–12518.

68. Kangas, E.; Tidor, B. Optimizing electrostatic affinity in ligand-receptor binding: theory, computation, and ligand properties. *J. Chem. Phys.* **1998**, *109*(17), 7522–7545.

69. Ghosh, A. K.; Krishnan, K.; Walters, D. E.; Cho, W.; Cho, H.; Koo, Y.; Trevino, J.; Holland, L.; Buthod, J. Structure based design: novel spirocyclic ethers as nonpeptidal P2-ligands for HIV protease inhibitors. *Bioorg. Med. Chem. Lett.* **1998**, *8*(8), 979–982.

70. Graham, S. L.; Ghosh, A. K.; Huff, J. R.; Scholz, T. H. HIV protease inhibitors with n-terminal polyether substituents. *Eur. Pat. Appl.* **1993**.

71. Pearlstein, R.; Vaz, R.; Rampe, D. Understanding the structure-activity relationship of the human ether-a-go-go-related gene cardiac K+ channel: a model for bad behavior. *J. Med. Chem.* **2003**, *46*(11), 2017–2022.

72. Vandenberg, J. I.; Walker, B. D.; Campbell, T. J. HERG K+ channels: friend and foe. *Trends Pharmacol. Sci.* **2001**, *22*(5), 240–246.

73. Rajamani, R.; Tounge, B. A.; Li, J.; Reynolds, C. H. A two-state homology model of the hERG K+ channel: application to ligand binding. *Bioorg. Med. Chem. Lett.* **2005**, *15*(6), 1737–1741.

74. Sanchez-Chapula, J. A.; Navarro-Polanco, R. A.; Culberson, C.; Chen, J.; Sanguinetti, M. C. Molecular determinants of voltage-dependent human ether-a-go-go related gene (HERG) K+ channel block. *J. Biol. Chem.* **2002**, *277*(26), 23587–23595.

75. Cavalli, A.; Poluzzi, E.; De Ponti, F.; Recanatini, M. Toward a pharmacophore for drugs inducing the long QT syndrome: insights from a CoMFA study of HERG K+ channel blockers. *J. Med. Chem.* **2002**, *45*(18), 3844–3853.

Structure-based drug design case study: p38

Arthur M. Doweyko

INTRODUCTION

The overproduction of cytokines has been implicated in a wide variety of inflammatory diseases such as rheumatoid arthritis, inflammatory bowel disease, psoriasis, multiple sclerosis, osteoporosis, Alzheimer's disease, and congestive heart failure. The ability of p38 mitogen-activated protein kinase (p38 MAPK) to regulate the release and activity of multiple pro-inflammatory cytokines has attracted the interest of numerous pharmaceutical companies and independent researchers during the past decade or so. Since its initial discovery in 1994 as a potential molecular target for a novel class of cytokine suppressive inhibitors (SB-203580),[1] more than 150 patent applications from at least thirty pharmaceutical companies have been published, all claiming novel p38 inhibitors. Four distinct isoforms of p38 MAPK are known: p38α and p38β are widely expressed in eukaryotic cells, including endothelial and inflammatory cells; p38γ is found in skeletal muscle; and p38δ is predominantly found in the small intestine, kidneys, and lung tissue.[2,3] Of these four isoforms, p38α has been the most studied and is believed to be the most physiologically relevant. Numerous reviews have been published that focus on both the biology[4–7] and chemistry of p38 inhibitors.[8–17] The focus of this chapter is an illustration of p38 inhibitor design guided by structural information obtained both from modeling and actual x-ray crystallographic data. Structure references with a ".pdb" suffix refer to those obtained from the Research Collaboratory for Structural Bioinformatics.[18]

TRIAZINES AND PYRIMIDINES

We begin with a collaborative venture by Bristol-Myers Squibb and Pharmacopeia aimed at the development of a novel series of trisubstituted triazines. High-throughput screening applied to a collection of 2.1 million compounds derived from a combinatorial library based on the template shown in Scheme 13.1 yielded the 1,3,5-triaminotriazine aniline amide PS200981, having a p38α IC$_{50}$ of 1 μM.[19] Further analyses identified PS166276 with a p38α IC$_{50}$ of 28 nM having 10× less cytotoxicity and superior inhibition of lipopolysaccharide-(LPS) induced TNFα production in THP-1 monocytes (170 nM). These inhibitors were found to compete for the ATP binding site in p38α. Additionally, statistical analysis of the combinatorial data indicated a significant contribution to activity in this series correlated to the presence of the 4-methyl-3-benzamido aniline moiety. When the x-ray crystal structure of the protein-inhibitor complex for a member of this triaminotriazine aniline amide series was determined, the structure/activity relationship (SAR) for the series was quickly rationalized. Specifically, N-methoxy-4-methyl-3-(4-(methyl(neopentyl)amino)-6-(4-methyl-1,4-diazepan-1-yl)-1,3,5-triazin-2-ylamino)benzamide (**1**) was cocrystallized with unactivated p38α protein (Figure 13.1), confirming that the series binds to the ATP pocket.[20] In a manner similar to ATP, **1** binds to the hinge region of p38α (characterized by residues 106–110), forming an anchoring H-bond interaction with Met109. Unlike ATP, **1** makes use of an intervening water molecule to form the interaction between Met109 backbone NH and the triazine N3. Also characteristic of other kinases is the presence of a deep hydrophobic pocket near the so-called gatekeeper residue (Thr106, not shown) which provides for one of the more interesting features of kinase inhibitor design in that it represents a space not occupied by ATP and, thus, of potential value in the search for inhibitor selectivity against off-target kinases. In the present case, the 4-methyl-3-benzamido aniline moiety occupies that space. Further interactions in the binding site include H-bonds among Lys53, Glu71, and amido NH, between Asp168 backbone NH and amido C=O, and between the protonated diazepan nitrogen and Asp168 carboxylate. Interestingly, the distance between triazine N1 and Lys53 is suggestive of an intervening water molecule; however, none was evident from the crystallography. The potential for H-bonding between Lys53 and an acceptor atom in other ligands was eventually realized with subsequent inhibitors. Synthetic efforts targeted variation at all three positions (2,4,6) of the triazine core, and the emergent SAR dovetailed nicely with the crystallographically determined binding mode. For example, the methylhydroxamate ester was found to have superior binding affinity compared to amides in general, a consequence of both its small size (complementing the relatively narrow pocket at that position) and its electron-deficient NH proton H-bond donor. The use of branched alkyl amines at the

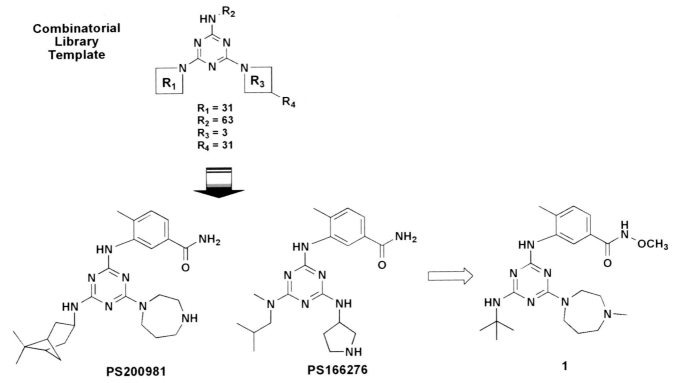

Scheme 13.1. Progression of synthetic efforts that culminated in the design and synthesis of trisubstituted triazines with significant p38α inhibition. Combinatorial libraries of the type shown led to the identification of triazines PS200981 and PS166276 (Pharmacopeia) having the unique 4-methyl-3-benzamido aniline head group. Subsequent SAR work (BMS) led to triazines exemplified by **1**, with superior p38α inhibition and in vitro activity.

4-position of the triazine was found to yield a number of active congeners, locating an angular lipophilic element of the inhibitor along a secondary hydrophobic pocket in p38α. This pocket is created by the lower rim of the P-loop

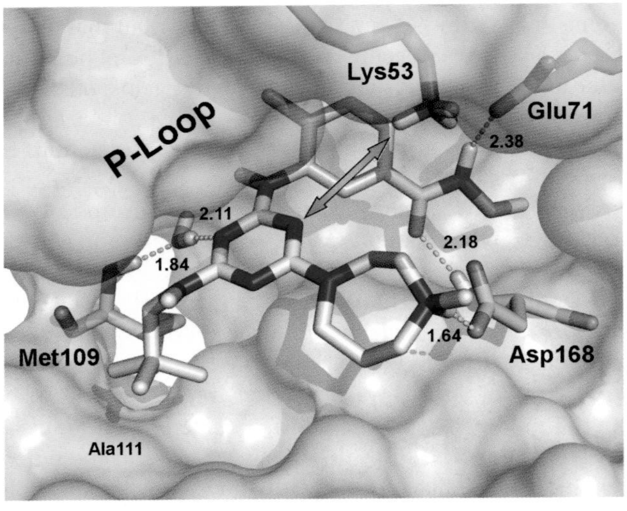

Figure 13.1. Major interactions observed in the complex between p38α and triazine **1**. H-bonds include Met109 backbone NH/H2O/triazine N3, Glu71/hydroxamate NH, Asp168/protonated diazapan, and backbone Asp168 NH/Glu71/hydroxamate O. Hydrophobic interactions include deep pocket/4-methyl-3-benzamido aniline and neopentylmethylamino/hinge hydrophobic pocket. Arrow indicates a potential through water H-bonding motif between triazine N3 and Lys53 not observed.

closing down on the binding site near Ala111. For the sake of consistency and facile orientation, the coloring scheme (yellow P-loop and Ala111) is maintained in subsequent figures.

The through-water H-bond to Met109 observed for **1** represented an intriguing observation that led to a consideration for its replacement by an H-bond acceptor built onto an inhibitor core. Such replacements have been reported as successful in using a cyano moiety to provide the H-bonding acceptor and span the necessary distance with inhibitors of scytalone dehydratase[21] and epidermal growth factor receptor kinase.[22] In the present case, a pyrimidine core was substituted for the triazine of **1** and a cyano group installed at the 5-position leading to the p38α active pyrimidine series illustrated in Scheme 13.2.[23] The 5-position was suggested by modeling to have an optimal trajectory, which was confirmed by the x-ray crystal structure of the p38α complex with **2** (Figure 13.2). The position of the cyano N was found almost precisely where the displaced water O had resided in the **1** complex. The two hydrophobic pockets (deep and hinge) are occupied in a similar manner, with the additional benefit of a likely H-bond between aniline NH and Thr106. In addition to the H-bonding array between ligand amide and Lys53, Glu71, and Asp168, a water molecule is clearly visible between pyrimidine N1, Lys53 and Asp168. The strong p38α binding affinity (IC_{50} 0.41 nM) and hPBMC TNFα inhibition

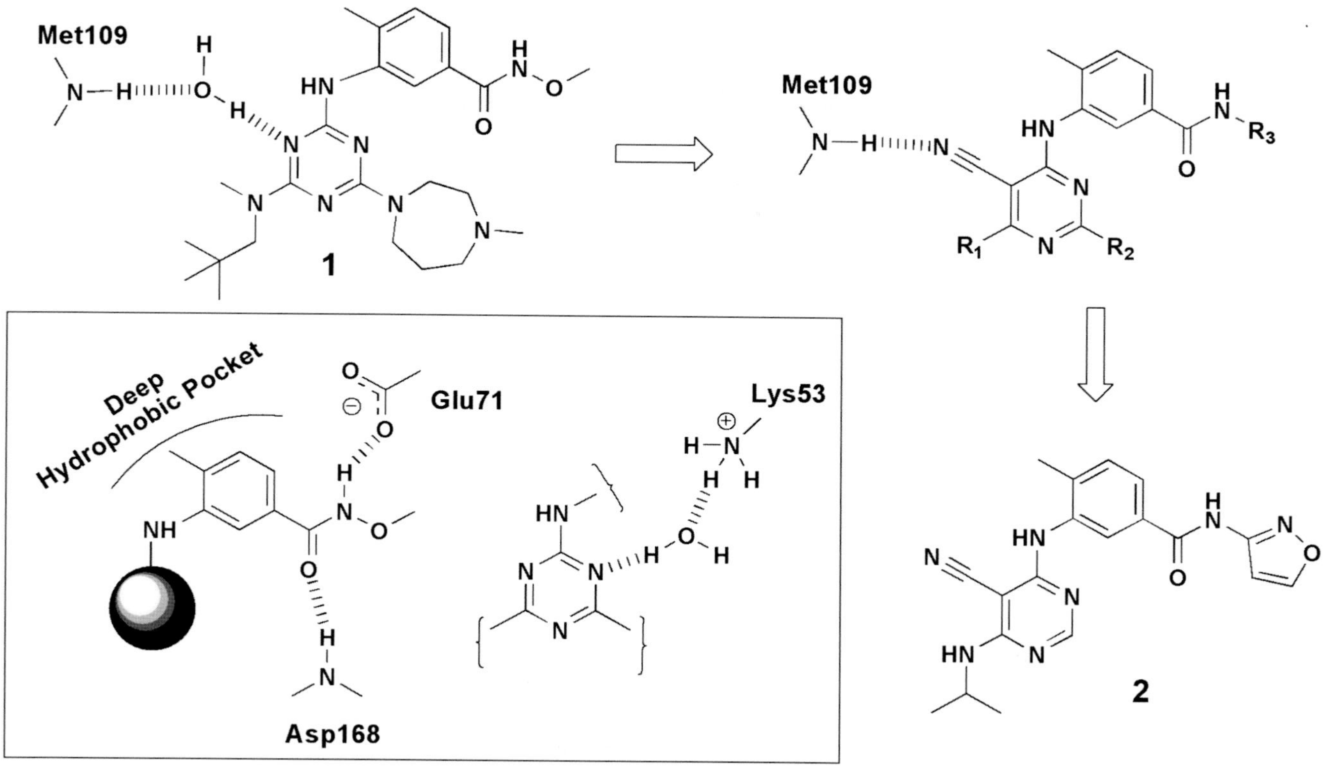

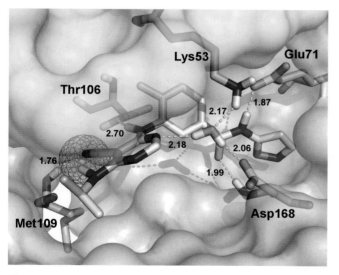

Scheme 13.2. The x-ray crystal structure of **1** revealed the presence of a key water molecule providing an H-bonding interaction between backbone NH at Met109 and triazine N3. The pryimidine scaffold (upper right) provided a means to replace that water molecule with a 5-cyano. Further synthesis identified **2** as a potent p38α inhibitor. The inset illustrates the major hydrophobic and H-bonding interactions observed at the 4-methyl-3-benzamido aniline head group and points to a possible water-mediated H-bonding interaction between triazine N1 and Lys53 (not observed).

Figure 13.2. The complex between **2** and p38α confirms that the 5-cyano group that makes a key H-bonding interaction between inhibitor and p38α is located in the same position as the water molecule in **1**. A water molecule was observed in an H-bonding position among pyridyl N1, Asp168, and Lys53, while backbone NH at Asp168 and Glu71 anchor the pendant amide.

(IC$_{50}$ 8.7 nM) is consistent with the number of strong interactions observed in the p38α ATP binding site, despite the absence of a substituent at the 2-position (6-position in the triazine). As the overall binding affinity for either the triazines or the pyrimidines is significantly affected by the combination and type of substituents it is difficult to directly assess the binding contribution due to a specific substituent. However, in this series, the best combinations included an amine at the 2-position and a branched alkylamine at the 4-position. The ultimate choice of best amine relies not only on observed p38α binding affinity but on cytotoxicity screens and cellular activity.

FUSED HETEROCYLICS

A novel structural class of p38α MAP kinase inhibitors was developed as a result of the high-throughput screening (HTS) hit, pyrrolo[2,1-*f*][1,2,4]triazine oxindoles, shown in Scheme 13.3, which exhibited p38α IC$_{50}$ values in the 60- to 80-nM range.[24] Substituted phenylaminopyrrolo[2, 1-*f*][1,2,4]triazines had been used previously as a template for kinase inhibitor design,[25] and it was envisioned that the incorporation of a 4-methyl-3-benzamido aniline (as

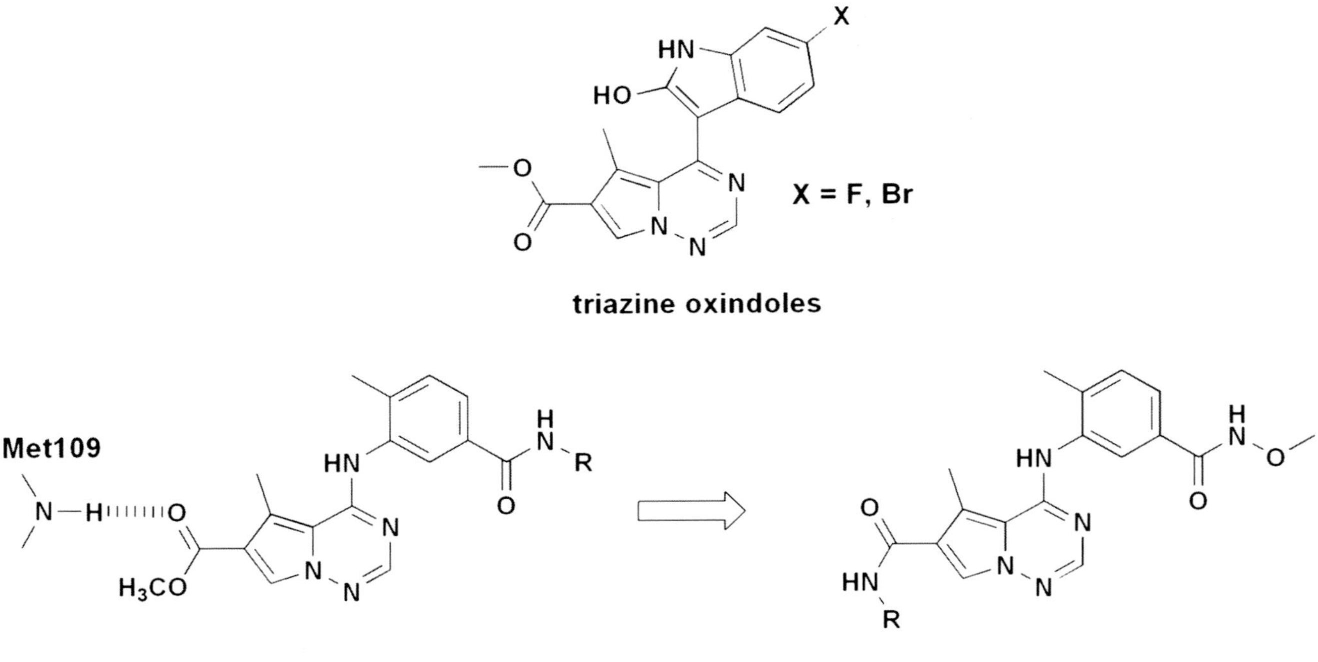

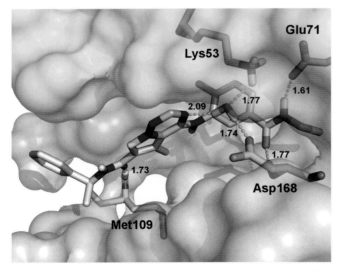

triazine oxindoles

X = F, Br

3   R = Ethyl
4   R = (S)-α-MeBenzyl

Scheme 13.3. High-throughput screening efforts led to the identification of compounds containing the triazine oxindole core pictured above. Incorporation of the 4-methyl-3-benzamido aniline head group led to a series of analogs with variations at both ends of this chemotype, namely the use of amides, reverse amides, carbamates, and hydroxamate esters. Two examples for which x-ray structures with p38α were obtained were **3** and **4**.

Figure 13.3. The x-ray crystal structure of the p38α complex with **4** reveals Met109 NH H-bonding to the carboxamide O and the presence of a water molecule engaged in H-bonding between pyrrolotriazine N3, Asp168, and Lys53. The deep pocket is occupied by the 4-methyl-3-benzamido aniline head group while the (S)-α-methylbenzyl group is located in a hydrophobic channel between P-loop and Ala111 (2RG6.pdb). [*Source:* H.M. Berman, J. Westbrook, Z. Feng, G. Gilliland, T.N. Bhat, H. Weissig, I.N. Shindyalov, P.E. Bourne. The Protein Data Bank Nucleic Acids Research, 28, pp. 235–242 (2000); see also www.pdb. org]

employed in **1** and **2**) together with this novel core would provide an alternative class of p38α inhibitors. A number of analogs were generated with variation at the ester to increase metabolic stability. These analogs included the use of amides, reverse amides, and carbamates at the ester position as well as variations at the 4-methyl-3-benzamido aniline (amides, reverse amides, carbamates, and hydroxamate esters). The series exhibited potent p38α inhibition (IC$_{50}$ 1–680 nM) and submicromolar cell activity (LPS/TNFα). The question of binding mode arose early in the synthetic effort and was answered with x-ray crystal structures of the p38α complexes of **3** and **4**, having p38α IC$_{50}$ values of 3.1 and 2.2 nM, respectively. The crystal structure of **4** is shown in Figure 13.3. Despite the distinct possibility that Met109 NH could H-bond with N1 of the pyrrolotriazine core, the x-ray data confirmed that this key H-bonding interaction was occurring with the pendant amide carbonyl O. This observation was consistent with the emerging SAR as broader types of substitutions were tolerated at the C6 position, presumably reflecting their trajectories along the hinge region and out into solvent. Once again, as found for **2**, a water molecule was found in an H-bonding complex between the N3 of the pyrrolotriazine core, Lys53, and Asp168. The hydroxamate methyl ester was locked in by H-bonding interactions with backbone Asp168 NH and Glu71. The deep hydrophobic pocket was occupied by the

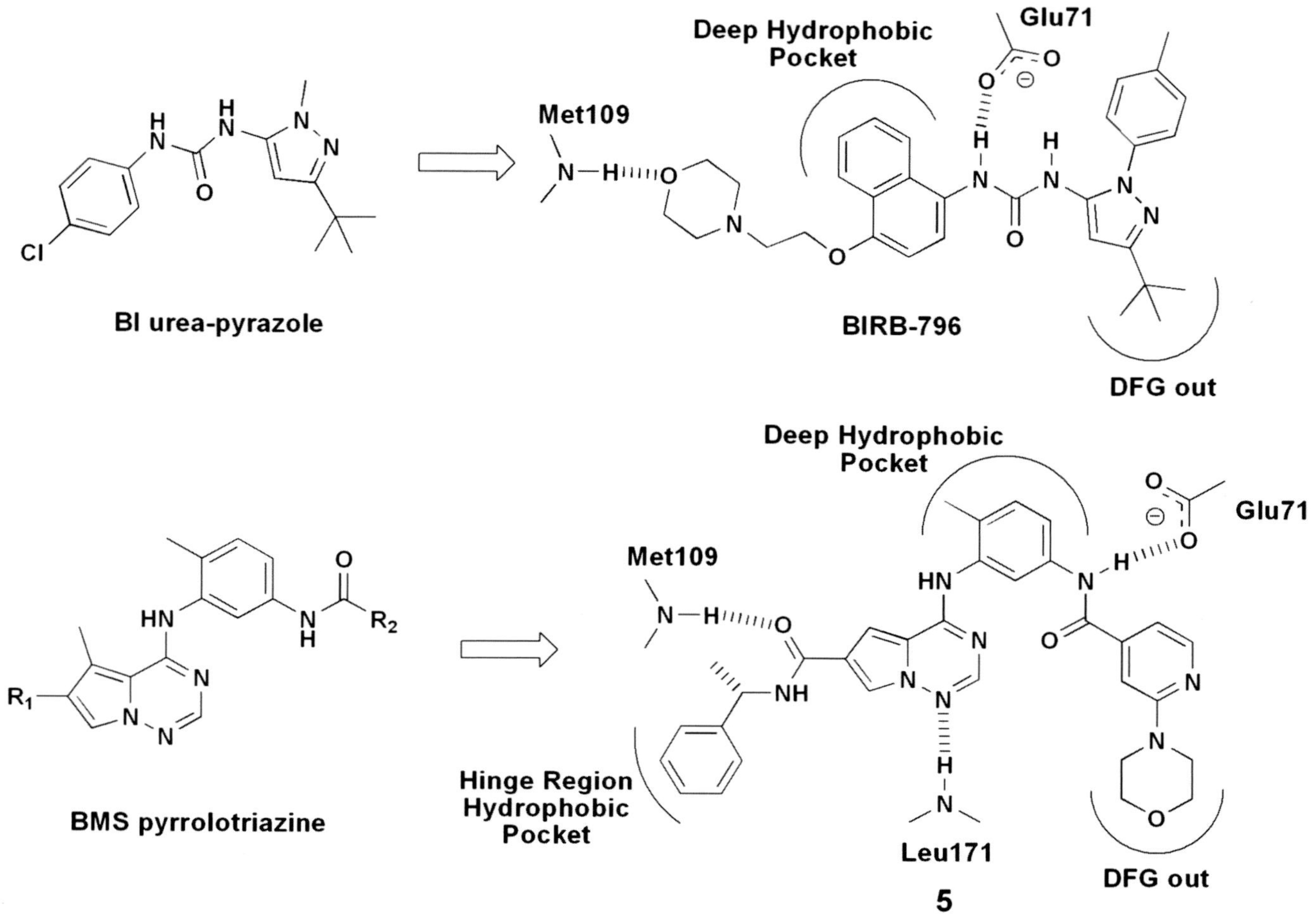

Scheme 13.4. The structures of the Boehringer Ingelheim "allosteric" inhibitors (BI urea-pyrazole and BIRB-796) are shown at top along with an indication of BIRB-796 interactions with p38α. The DFG-out conformation of p38α refers to the displacement of several residues along the activation loop (Asp168-Phe169-Gly170) providing for a hydrophobic pocket as an extension of the ATP binding site. The BMS pyrrolotriazines were further developed to include a structure (3-morpholinobenzamide, **5**) that was found to occupy the same DFG-out pocket.

4-methyl-3-benzamido aniline while the ethyl of **3** (not shown) and the (S)-α-methylbenzyl of **4** rested in the outer hinge pocket.

ACCESSING THE DFG-OUT BINDING POCKET

In 2002 researchers at Boehringer Ingelheim reported a limited set of inhibitors that used a novel p38 MAP kinase allosteric binding site.[26] The urea-pyrazole and the more elaborate BIRB-796 are illustrated in Scheme 13.4. The x-ray crystal structure for BIRB-796 (1KV2.pdb) is shown in Figure 13.4. Although part of the inhibitor is located in the ATP-binding site and H-bonds with Met109, the opposite end locates itself in a pocket created by the displacement of part of the activation loop, namely Asp168-Phe169-Gly170 (or DFG). This relocation of the DFG loop (sometimes referred to as DFG-out) vacates a hydrophobic pocket formerly occupied by Phe169. The DFG-out configuration of p38 results in an extended ATP-binding site. Its

reference as an allosteric site may be somewhat misleading, as the inhibitory effect of binding a small molecule to Phe169 site is not allosteric in the classical sense. When a molecule binds to this newly formed site located adjacent to the ATP binding pocket, it directly interferes with ATP binding by providing a steric block. Normally, allosteric interactions are relegated to those requiring indirect communication between isolated sites. The remaining interactions observed in the x-ray structure for BIRB-796 entail those that have been seen before, namely hinge region Met109 H-bonding to pendant morpholino O and an H-bonding matrix among urea, Glu71, and Asp168 backbone NH.

Accessing the DFG-out conformation of p38 was accomplished through an extension of the pyrrolotriazines exemplified by **3** and **4**. It was found that the installation of larger amide groups off the 4-methyl-3-benzamido aniline head group led to congeners with potent p38α inhibition (Scheme 13.4). For example, the use of a

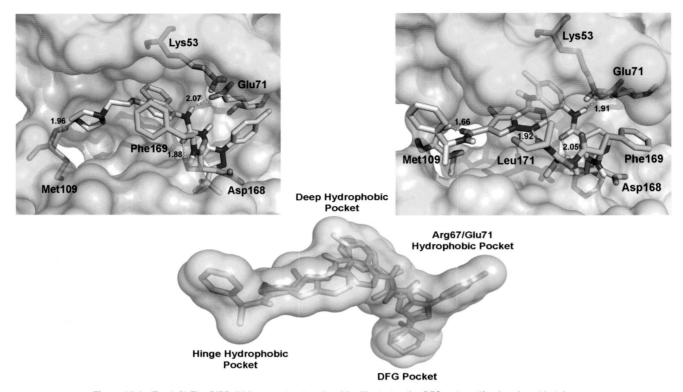

Figure 13.4. (Top left) The BIRB-796 x-ray structure in p38α illustrates the DFG-out motif, wherein a *t*-butyl group occupies the Phe169 pocket while the pendant morpholino O H-bonds to backbone NH at Met109 (1KV2.pdb). (Top right) Pyrrolotriazine **5** occupies the same Phe169 pocket while the displaced activation loop adopts a different pose with Leu171 backbone NH engaged in an H-bond to pyrrolotriazine N1 (3BV2.pdb). (Center) A comparison of overall shape between BIRB-796 and **5** illustrating similar occupation of the deep hydrophobic and DFG-out pockets.

3-morpholinobenzamide in combination with a C6-(S)-α-methylbenzylamide (**5**) exhibited a p38α K_i of 0.44 nM and a LPS/TNFα IC$_{50}$ of 18 nM.[27] The x-ray crystal structure of the p38α complex of **5** confirmed the DFG-out configuration (Figure 13.4). The binding mode of **5** is similar to that of **4** in that the H-bonding patterns to Met109, Glu71, and backbone NH at Asp168 are conserved. The notable distinction here is that the pendant morpholinobenzamide group is found deep within the hydrophobic Phe169 pocket. In addition, part of the activation loop has relocated itself along the outer rim of the ATP-binding site so as to form a seal, as evidenced by the H-bond between pyrrolotriazine N1 and backbone NH at Leu171. This feature is distinct from that reported for BIRB-796. A further comparison between BIRB-796 and **5** is shown in Figure 13.4, wherein the molecular volume overlap between the two inhibitors is highlighted. Although BIRB-796 does not make use of the hinge hydrophobic pocket, both inhibitors occupy the deep hydrophobic pocket and the Phe169 pocket in similar ways. It is clear that relatively large inhibitors can be accommodated by the DFG-out version of p38α.

PYRAZOLOPYRIMIDINES

A further elaboration of the pyrimidine chemotype exemplified by **2** led to the discovery of the pyrazolopyrimidine core (Scheme 13.5). The presumption was that presentation of an H-bond acceptor at roughly the same location and trajectory as the cyano group in **2** could lead to a novel series of inhibitors that retain the Met109 NH interaction thought to be a key H-bonding interaction for nearly all kinase inhibitors. This was achieved by conceptually cyclizing the 5-cyano to the 6-aminoalkyl function, yielding a pyrazolopyrimidine core, which was further elaborated both at the N1 and the 4-methyl-3-benzamido aniline head group to more fully develop an SAR.[28] The x-ray crystal structure of the unphosphorylated p38α complex of **6**, shown in Figure 13.5, confirms that the N2 acceptor in the pyrazolopyrimidine core forms an H-bond with Met109 and the pendant methyl amide forms the usual H-bonding complex with Glu71 and Asp168. Additionally, the N1-phenyl is located along the hinge region hydrophobic pocket. Although **6** exhibited a good inhibition profile (p38α IC$_{50}$ 14 nM, LPS/TNFα IC$_{50}$ 513 nM), further SAR exploration identified the 1,2-oxazolamide (same as in **2**) as superior (p38α IC$_{50}$ 5 nM, LPS/TNFα IC$_{50}$ 6 nM).

THIAZOLES

The discovery of an active thiazole central core represents an unobvious elaboration of the pyrrolotriazine motif. Focused deck screening identified a C2-alkylaminothiazole

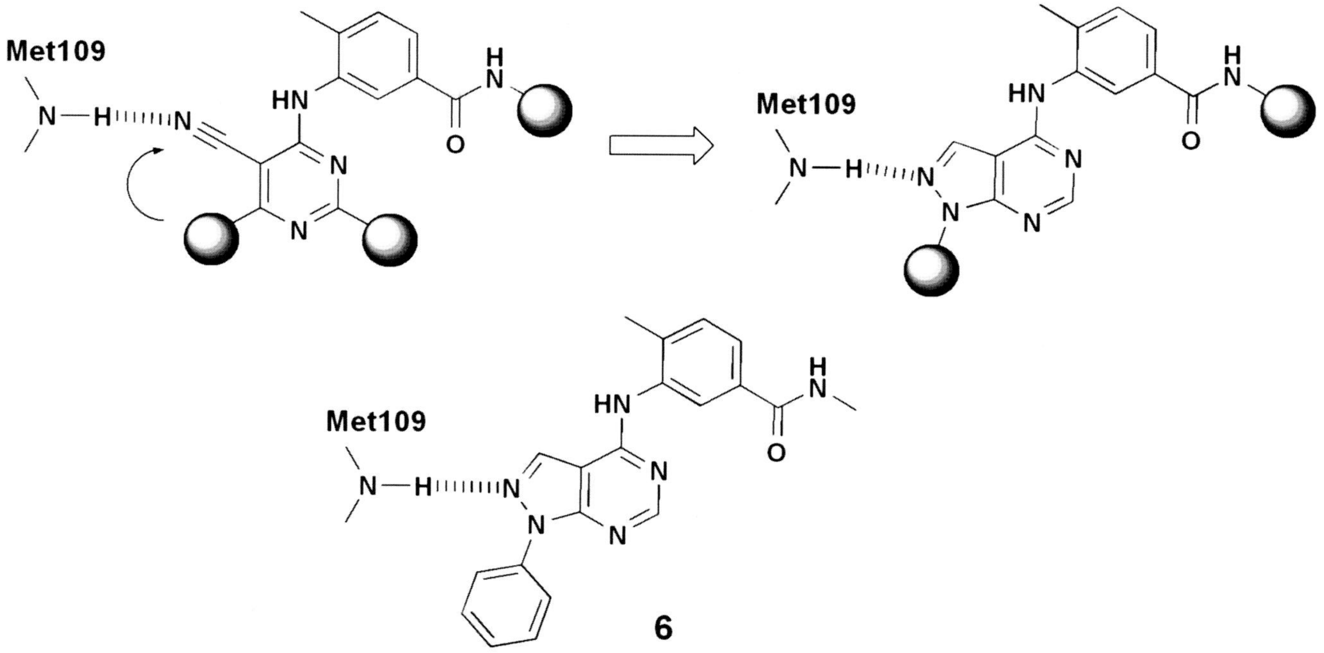

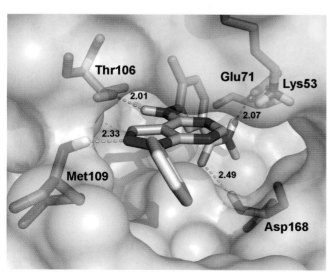

Scheme 13.5. The conceptual "cyclization" of the 5-cyanopyrimidine core led to the synthesis of the pyrazolopyrimidine scaffold, capable of a similar H-bonding trajectory to backbone NH at Met109. An x-ray structure of the p38α complex of **6** confirmed the presence of this key H-bonding interaction.

with moderate p38 activity. This observation suggested that replacement of the triazinyl-aniline link with a carboxanilide may be a way to retain possible "backside" H-bonding through water or directly to Lys53, substituting the carboxanilide O for the triazinyl N3. In addition, the fused 5-membered pyrrolo ring could be replaced with a thiazole containing a potential H-bond acceptor N. These two concepts were embodied in the conceptual transformation

illustrated in Scheme 13.6. Synthetic efforts led to the discovery of **7** which was found to be a potent inhibitor (p38α IC$_{50}$ 3.5 nM, LPS/TNFα IC$_{50}$ 2.9 nM).[29] The x-ray crystal structure of its p38α complex is illustrated in Figure 13.6. Although **7** is slightly shorter than **3**, the added flexibility of the carboxanilide linker allows the molecule to adapt itself

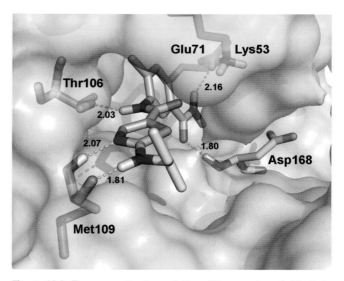

Figure 13.6. The x-ray structure of the p38α complex of C2-alkyl-aminothiazole, **7**, illustrates the characteristic deep hydrophobic pocket occupancy by the 4-methyl-3-benzamido aniline head group and H-bonding interactions between inhibitor and Met109, Thr106, Glu71, and Asp168. Interestingly, both backbone carbonyl O and NH at Met109 are involved in a tandem set of H-bonds. (3BX5.pdb)

Figure 13.5. The x-ray structure of the p38α complex of pyrazolopyrimidine, **6**, illustrates the successful replacement of the 5-cyano group in **2** with the pyrazolyl N2. (3CG2.pdb)

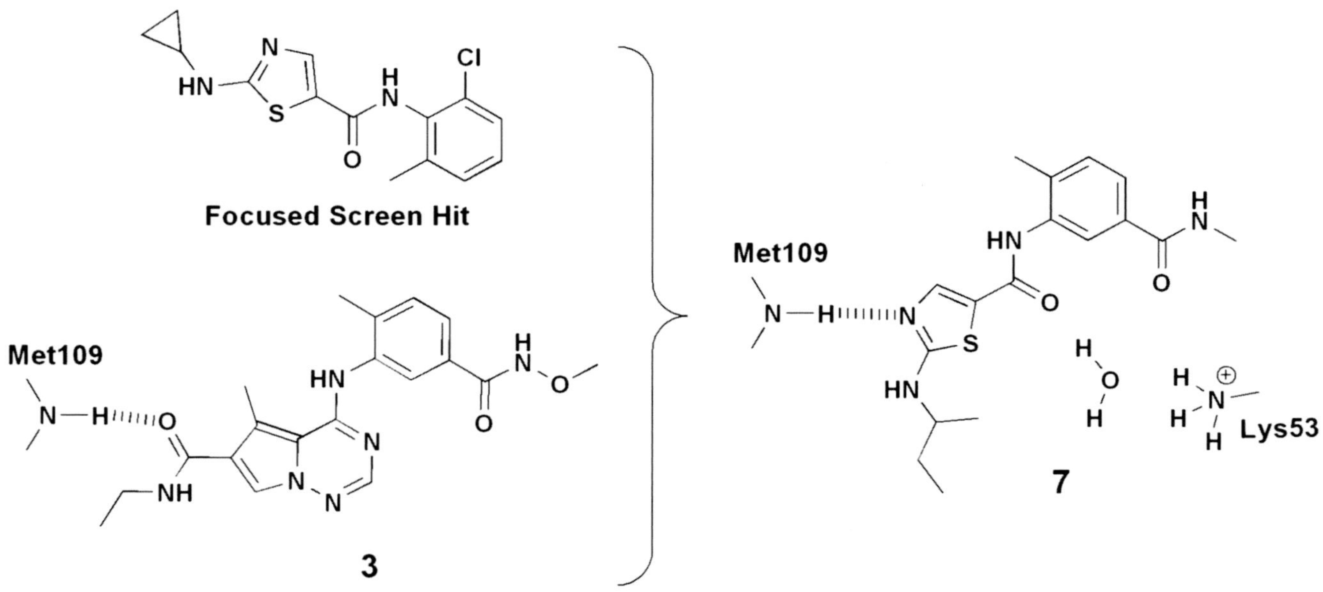

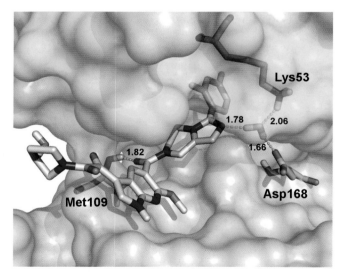

Focused Screen Hit

Scheme 13.6. The thiazole pictured at top was identified through focused deck screening with modest p38α activity. Coupling this observation with the structure of the pyrrolotriazine, **3**, led to the synthesis of **7**. Conceptually, the strategy was to replace the pendant amido carbonyl O–Met109 interaction with the thiazolyl N and incorporate a possible H-bond acceptor replacement (potential for H-bonding to Lys53/water) for the triazinyl N1 with the central carboxamido O.

sufficiently to the binding site to engage in productive H-bonding not only to Met109, Glu71, and Asp168 but also to Thr106 and backbone C=O at Met109 as well. This observation also reflects previous analyses highlighting the flexibility of p38α, specifically regarding the variation in the width of the ATP pocket as determined by a comparison of available x-ray structures.[11]

INDOLES

Scios recently reported the synthesis and SAR of indole-based heterocyclic inhibitors of p38α shown in Scheme 13.7.[30] The authors found that rigidifying the piperidine linker in **Scios 1** led to a significant increase in binding affinity (~fourteenfold, **Scios 2**). Further modifications eventually led to Scios's first p38 clinical compound, **Scios-469** (p38α IC$_{50}$ 9 nM). These observations suggested that a similar conformational restraint might be achieved through the incorporation of a fused ring system, specifically, a connection between the benzyl methylene position and a proximal piperazine or piperidine ring (as illustrated in Scheme 13.7). A number of such analogs were synthesized and found to exhibit double-digit nanomolar p38α inhibition.[31] The binding mode of **8** (p38α IC$_{50}$ 13 nM) was determined by x-ray crystallography (Figure 13.7). Several key H-bonding interactions are evident and consistent with previous observations: through-water Lys53/Asp168 H-bond to the exposed imidazo N and Met109 backbone NH H-bonding to the central carboxamide O. The major hydrophobic interaction occurs through the pendant difluorophenyl occupancy of the deep pocket created by Thr106

(not shown) and the aliphatic chain of Lys53. Curiously, the oxalamide portion extends upward and out along the hinge region, making no direct interactions with protein. It would appear that the occupancy of the deep hydrophobic pocket is critical in this series and that the Scios design, incorporating a conformationally constrained linker, directs the pendant benzyl group into that pocket.

Figure 13.7. The x-ray structure of the complex between p38α and an analog of Scios-469 using a conformational constraint in the form of a fused ring system (imidazopyrazine, **8**) illustrates several key interactions: central amido carbonyl O H-bonding to Met109 and water molecule H-bonding among imidazo N, Asp168, and Lys53. The deep hydrophobic pocket created between Thr106 (not shown) and Lys53 is occupied by the pendant difluorophenyl. (2QD9.pdb)

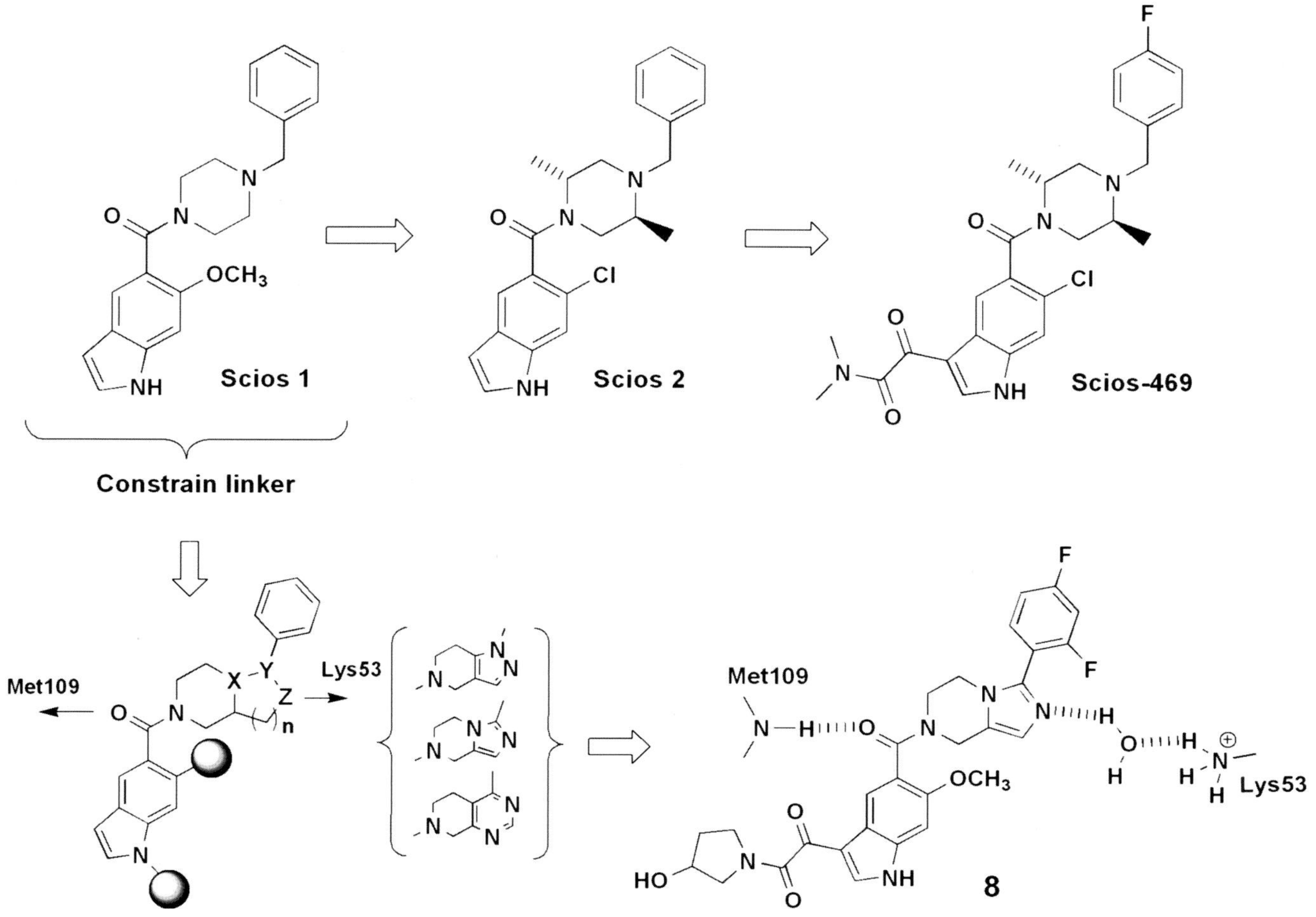

Scheme 13.7. Scios reported enhanced p38α inhibition through the incorporation of conformational constraints in their series (**Scios 1**, **Scios 2**, and **Scios-469**). The installation of a fused ring system (such as shown in parentheses) was considered as an alternate approach to conformational constraint, culminating in the potent p38α inhibitor, **8**.

THE 5-MEMBERED HETEROCYCLIC CORE

A very popular p38α inhibitor design is based on the early work of SmithKline Beecham (SKB) that described the trisubstituted imidazole, SB-203580 (Scheme 13.8).[1,32] Much effort has been expended on the successful replacement of the central imidazole core with other five-membered ring systems. Recent efforts have expanded the approach by focusing on fused ring systems as central cores. Examples in this regard include the Roche pyrrolopyridine.[33] Replacement of the Met109-targeting moiety has also been pursued, exemplified by the two Pfizer structures shown in Scheme 13.8.[34,35] Parallel efforts at Bristol-Myers Squibb (BMS) yielded the benzothiazole series that included the use of oxazoles and imidazoles as central cores.[36] An example oxazole, **9** (p38α IC$_{50}$ 6.4 nM, LPS/TNFα IC$_{50}$ 40 nM), was successfully crystallized with p38α (Figure 13.8). As expected, the fluorophenyl moiety is located in the deep hydrophobic pocket. Interestingly, the hinge region Met109 is engaged in two H-bonds to the ligand 2-aminothiazole system. Lys53 is found close enough

to the oxazole N to consider a possible additional H-bond at that location. Unexpectedly, the P-loop of p38α is collapsed on the inhibitor in such a way that Tyr35 makes a tight van der Waals contact with the thiazole sulfur. This may represent a unique hydrophobic interaction scheme not typically used by p38 inhibitors. Finally, there is the subtle, yet important, hydrophobic interaction engaged by the 2-isopropylamine at the hinge entry. Small alkyl substituents at this position were observed to modulate the binding affinity (ethyl-butyl, 1.6–16 nM).

In summary, a number of structure-based design strategies were highlighted that focused on the use of novel lig- and head groups to access the deep hydrophobic pocket (most notably, the 3-methyl-5-benzamide system), the incorporation of H-bond acceptor atoms in the core that target both the hinge region Met109 interaction as well as Lys53/Glu71/Asp168 deeper in the binding site, the exploitation of the Tyr169 pocket available in the DFG-out configuration, the subtle effect of alkyl/aryl group occupancy of the hinge region hydrophobic channel, and unique interactions such as the Tyr35 van der Waals interaction

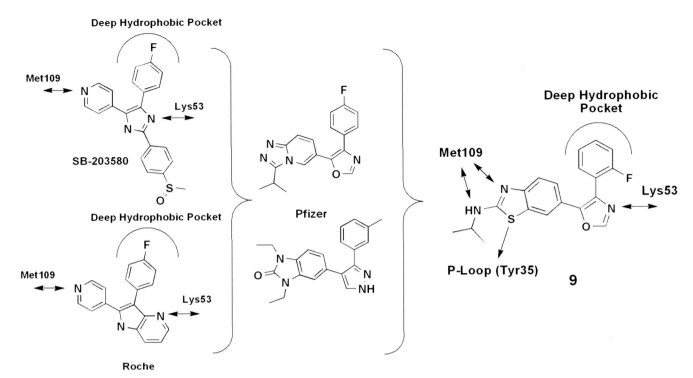

Scheme 13.8. The early work of SKB led to the synthesis of SB-203580 whose p38α x-ray structure revealed key interactions with Met109, Lys53, and the deep hydrophobic pocket. Subsequent efforts by Roche and Pfizer represent just a few of the variations around the SKB theme that led to potent inhibitors. The use of a fused heterocycle to access the backbone Met109 NH H-bond was successfully realized with **9**. In addition to the usual interactions, **9** exhibited a unique P-loop collapse that included a tight van der Waals contact between thiazolyl S and the ring face of Tyr35.

with thiazole sulfur. All of these approaches have led to the development of leads currently being investigated as potential drug candidates, testifying to the value and impact of a structure-based design approach in modern drug discovery.

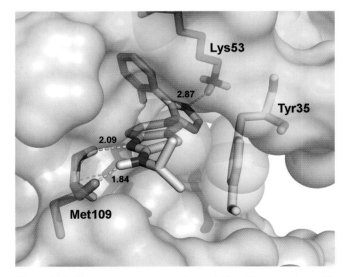

Figure 13.8. The x-ray crystal structure of the p38α complex with benzothiazole-oxazole, **9**, illustrates the expected H-bonding interactions at Met109 and Lys53. In addition, the collapse of the P-loop unto the inhibitor is evident, along with a tight van der Waals contact between thiazolyl S and Tyr35. (3C5U.pdb)

REFERENCES

1. Lee, J. C.; Laydon, J. T.; McDonnell, P. C.; Gallagher, T. F.; Kumar, S.; Green, D.; McNulty, D.; Blumenthal, M. J.; Heyes, J. R.; Landvatter, S. W.; Strickler, J. E.; McLaughlin, M. M.; Siemens, I. R.; Fisher, S. M.; Livi, G. P.; White, J. R.; Adams, J. L.; Young, P. R. A protein kinase involved in the regulation of inflammatory cytokine biosynthesis. *Nature* **1994**, *372*, 739–746

2. Hale, K. K.; Trollinger, D.; Rihanek, M.; Manthey, C. L. Differential expression and activation of p38 mitogen-activated protein kinase α, β, γ and δ in inflammatory cell lineages *J. Immunol.* **1999**, *162*, 4246–4252.

3. Lee, J. C.; Kassis, S.; Kumar, S.; Badger, A.; Adams, J. L. p38 mitogen-activated protein kinase inhibitors – mechanisms and therapeutic potentials. *Pharmacol. Ther.* **1999**, *82*, 389–397.

4. Chen, Z.; Gibson, T. B.; Robinson, F.; Silvestro, L.; Pearson, G.; Xu, B.-E.; Wright, A.; Vanderbilt, C.; Cobb, M. H. MAP kinases. *Chem. Rev.* **2001**, *101*, 2449–2476.

5. Dambach, D. M. Potential adverse effects associated with inhibition of p38. α/β MAP kinases *Curr. Top. Med. Chem.* **2005**, *5*, 929–939.

6. Pearson, G.; Robinson, F.; Gibson, T. B.; Xu, B.-E.; Karandikar, M.; Berman, K.; Cobb, M. H. Mitogen-activated protein (MAP) kinase pathways: Regulation and physiological functions. *Endocr. Rev.* **2001**, *22*, 153–183.

7. Schieven, G. L. The biology of p38 kinase: a central role in inflammation. *Curr. Top. Med. Chem.* **2005**, *5*, 921–928.

8. Boehm, J. C.; Adams, J. L. New inhibitors of p38 kinase. *Expert Opin. Ther. Pat.* **2000**, *10*, 25–37.

9. Chakravarty, S.; Dugar, S. Inhibitors of p38a MAP kinase. *Ann. Rep. Med. Chem.* **2002**, *37*, 177–186.

10. Cirillo, P. F.; Pargellis, C.; Regan, J. The non-diaryl heterocycle class of p38 MAP kinase inhibitors. *Curr. Top. Med. Chem.* **2002**, *2*, 1021–1035.

11. Doweyko, A. M.; Wrobleski, S. T. A comparison of p38 inhibitor-protein structures. *Am. Drug Discov.* **2006**, *1*, 47–52.

12. Dumas, J.; Sibley, R.; Riedl, B.; Monahan, M. K.; Lee, W.; Lowinger, T. B.; Redman, A. M.; Johnson, J. S.; Kingery-Wood, J.; Scott, W. J.; Smith, R. A.; Bobko, M.; Schoenleber, R.; Ranges, G. E.; Housley, T. J.; Bhargava, A.; Wilhelm, S. M.; Shrikhande, A. Discovery of a new class of p38 kinase inhibitors. *Bioorg. Med. Chem. Lett.* **2000**, *10*, 2047–2050.

13. Dumas, J.; Smith, R. A.; Lowinger, T. B. Recent developments in the discovery of protein kinase inhibitors from the urea class. *Curr. Opin. Drug Discov. Dev.* **2004**, *7*, 600–616.

14. Hanson, G. Inhibitors of p38 kinase. *Expert Opin. Ther.* **1997**, *7*, 729–733.

15. Jackson, P. F.; Bullington, J. L. Pyridinylimidazole based p38 MAP kinase inhibitors. *Curr. Top. Med. Chem.* **2002**, *2*, 1011–1020.

16. Salituro, F. G.; Germann, U. A.; Wilson, K. P.; Benis, G. W.; Fox, T.; Su, M. S.-S. Inhibitors of p38 MAP kinase: therapeutic intervention in cytokine-mediated diseases. *Curr. Med. Chem.* **1999**, *6*, 807–823.

17. Wrobleski, S. T.; Doweyko, A. M. Structural comparison of p38 inhibitor-protein complexes: a review of recent p38 inhibitors having unique binding interactions. *Curr. Top. Med. Chem.* **2005**, *5*, 1005–1016.

18. Berman, H. M.; Westbrook, J.; Feng, Z.; Gilliland, G.; Bhat, T. N.; Weissig, H.; Shindyalov, I. N.; Bourne, P. E. The Protein Data Bank. *Nucleic Acids Res.* **2000**, *28*, 235–242.

19. Lin, T. H.; Metzger, A.; Diller, D. J.; Desai, M.; Henderson, I.; Ahmed, G.; Kimble, E. F.; Quadros, E.; Webb, M. L. Discovery and characterization of triaminotriazine aniline amides as highly selective p38 kinase inhibitors. *J. Pharmacol. Exp. Ther.* **2006**, *318*, 495–502.

20. Leftheris, K.; Ahmed, G.; Chan, R.; Dyckman, A. J.; Hussain, Z.; Ho, K.; Hynes, J., Jr.; Letourneau, J.; Li, W.; Lin, S.; Metzger, A.; Moriarty, K. J.; Riviello, C.; Shimshock, Y.; Wen, J.; Wityak, J.; Wrobleski, S. T.; Wu, H.; Wu, J.; Desai, M.; Gilllooly, K. M.; Lin, T. H.; Loo, D.; McIntyre, K. W.; Pitt, S.; Shen, D. R.; Shuster, D. J.; Zhang, R.; Diller, D.; Doweyko, A.; Sack, J.; Baldwin, J.; Barrish, J.; Dodd, J.; Henderson, I.; Kanner, S.; Schieven, G. L.; Webb, M. The discovery of orally active triaminotriazine aniline amides as inhibitors of p38 MAP kinase *J. Med. Chem.* **2004**, *47*, 6283–6291.

21. Chen, J. C.; Xu, S. L.; Wawrzak, Z.; Basarab, G. S.; Jordan, D. B. Structure-based design of potent inhibitors of scytalone dehydratase: displacement of a water molecule from the active site. *Biochemistry* **1998**, *37*, 17735–17744.

22. Wissner, A.; Berger, D. M.; Boschelli, D. H.; Floyd, B.; Greenberger, L. M.; Gruber, B. C.; Johnson, B. D.; Mamuya, N.; Nilakantan, R.; Reich, M. F.; Shen, R.; Tsou, H.-R.; Upeslacis, E.; Wang, Y. F.; Wu, B.; Ye, F.; Zhang, N. 4-Anilino-6,7-dialkoxyquinoline-3-carbonitrile inhibitors of epidermal growth factor receptor kinase and their bioisosteric relationship to the 4-anilino-6,7-dialkoxyquinazoline inhibitors. *J. Med. Chem.* **2000**, *43*, 3244–3256.

23. Liu, C.; Wrobleski, S. T.; Lin, J.; Ahmed, G.; Metzger, A.; Wityak, J.; Gilllooly, K. M.; Shuster, D. J.; McIntyre, K. W.; Pitt, S.; Shen, D. R.; Zhang, R. F.; Zhang, H.; Doweyko, A. M.; Diller, D.; Henderson, I.; Barrish, J. C.; Dodd, J. H.; Schieven, G. L.; Leftheris, K. 5-Cyanopyrimidine derivatives as a novel class of potent, selective, and orally active inhibitors of p38α MAP kinase. *J. Med. Chem.* **2005**, *48*, 6261–6270.

24. Hynes, J., Jr.; Dyckman, A. J.; Lin, S.; Wrobleski, S. T.; Wu, H.; Gilllooly, K. M.; Kanner, S. B.; Lonial, H.; Loo, D.; McIntyre, K. W.; Pitt, S.; Shen, D. R.; Shuster, D. J.; Yang, X.; Zhang, R.; Behnia, K.; Zhang, H.; Marathe, P. H.; Doweyko, A. M.; Tokarski, J. S.; Sack, J. S.; Pokross, M.; Kiefer, S. E.; Newitt, J. A.; Barrish, J. C.; Dodd, J.; Schieven, G. L.; Leftheris, K. Design, synthesis, and anti-inflammatory properties of orally active 4-(phenylamino)-pyrrolo[2,1-f][1,2,4]triazine p38α mitogen-activated protein kinase inhibitors. *J. Med. Chem.* **2008**, *51*, 4–16.

25. Hunt, J. T.; Mitt, T.; Borzilleri, R.; Gullo-Brown, J.; Fargnoli, J.; Fink, B.; Han, W.-C.; Mortillo, S.; Vite, G.; Wautlet, B.; Wong, T.; Yu, C.; Zheng, Z.; Bhide, R. Discovery of the pyrrolo[2,1-f][1,2,4]triazine nucleus as a new kinase inhibitor template. *J. Med. Chem.* **2004**, *47*, 4054–4059.

26. Pargellis, C.; Tong, L.; Churchill, L.; Cirillo, P. F.; Gilmore, T.; Graham, A. G.; Grob, P. M.; Hickey, E. R.; Moss, N.; Pav, S.; Regan, J. Inhibition of p38 MAP kinase by utilizing a novel allosteric binding site. *Nat. Struct. Biol.* **2002**, *9*, 268–272.

27. Wrobleski, S. T.; Lin, S.; Hynes, J.; Wu, H.; Pitt, S.; Shen, D. R.; Zhang, R.; Gilllooly, K. M.; Shuster, D. J.; McIntyre, K. W.; Doweyko, A. M.; Kish, K. F.; Tredup, J. A.; Duke, G. J.; Sack, J. S.; McKinnon, M.; Dodd, J.; Barrish, J. C.; Schieven, G. L.; Leftheris, K. Synthesis and SAR of new pyrrolo[2,1-f][1,2,4]triazines as potent p38α MAP kinase inhibitors. *Bioorg. Med. Chem. Lett.* **2008**, *18*, 2739–2744.

28. Das, J.; Moquin, R. V.; Pitt, S.; Zhang, R.; Shen, D. R.; McIntyre, K. W.; Gilllooly, K. M.; Doweyko, A. M.; Sack, J. S.; Zhang, H.; Kiefer, S. E.; Kish, K. F.; McKinnon, M.; Barrish, J. C.; Dodd, J.; Schieven, G. L.; Leftheris, K. Pyrazolo-pyrimidines: a novel heterocyclic scaffold for potent and selective p38α inhibitors. *Bioorg. Med. Chem. Lett.* **2008**, *18*, 2652–2657.

29. Hynes, J.; Wu, H.; Pitt, S.; Shen, D. R.; Zhang, R.; Schieven, G. L.; Gilllooly, K. M.; Shuster, D. J.; Taylor, T. L.; Yang, X.; McIntyre, K. W.; McKinnon, M.; Zhang, H.; Marathe, P. H.; Doweyko, A. M.; Kish, K.; Kiefer, S. E.; Sack, J. S.; Newitt, J. A.; Barrish, J. C.; Dodd, J.; Leftheris, K. The discovery of (R)-2-(sec-butylamino)-N-(2-methyl-5-(methylcarbamoyl)phenyl) thiazole-5-carboxamide (BMS-640994) – A potent and efficacious p38α MAP kinase inhibitor. *Bioorg. Med. Chem. Lett.* **2008**, *18*, 1762–1767.

30. Mavunkel, B. J.; Chakravarty, S.; Perumattam, J. J.; Luedtke, G. R.; Liang, X.; Lim, D.; Xu, Y.-J.; Laney, M.; Liu, D. Y.; Schreiner, G. F.; Lewicki, J. A.; Dugar, S. Indole-based heterocyclic inhibitors of p38α MAP kinase: designing a conformationally restricted analogue. *Bioorg. Med. Chem. Lett.* **2003**, *13*, 3087–3090.

31. Dhar, T. G. M.; Wrobleski, S. T.; Lin, S.; Furch, J. A.; Nirschl, D. S.; Fan, Y.; Todderud, G.; Pitt, S.; Doweyko, A. M.; Sack, J. S.; Mathur, A.; McKinnon, M.; Barrish, J. C.; Dodd, J. H.; Schieven, G. L.; Leftheris, K. Synthesis and SAR of p38α MAP kinase inhibitors based on heterobicyclic scaffolds. *Bioorg. Med. Chem. Lett.* **2007**, *17*, 5019–5024.

32. Boehm, J. C.; Smietana, J. M.; Sorenson, M. E.; Garigipati, R. S.; Gallagher, T. F.; Sheldrake, P. L.; Breadbeer, J.; Badger, A. M.; Laydon, J. T.; Lee, J. C.; Hillegass, L. M.; Griswold, D. E.; Breton, J. J.; Chabot-Fletcher, M. C.; Adams, J. L. 1-Substituted 4-aryl-5-pyridinylimidazoles: a new class of cytokine suppressive drugs with low 5-lipoxygenase and

cyclooxygenase inhibitory potency. *J. Med. Chem.* **1996**, *39*, 3929–3937.

33. Trejo, A.; Arzeno, H.; Browner, M.; Chanda, S.; Cheng, S.; Comer, D. D.; Dalrymple, S. A.; Dunten, P.; Lafargue, J.; Lovejoy, B.; Freire-Moar, J.; Lim, J.; McIntosh, J.; Miller, J.; Papp, E.; Reuter, D.; Roberts, R.; Sanpablo, F.; Saunders, J.; Song, K.; Villasenor, A.; Warren, S. D.; Welch, M.; Weller, P.; Whiteley, P. E.; Zeng, L.; Goldstein, D. M. Design and synthesis of 4-azaindoles as inhibitors of p38 MAP kinase. *J. Med. Chem.* **2003**, *46*, 4702–4713.

34. Dombroski, M. A.; Letavic, M. A.; McClure, K. F.; Barberia, J. T.; Carty, T. J.; Cortina, S. R.; Csiki, C.; Dipesa, A. J.; Elliott, N. C.; Gabel, C. A.; Jordan, C. K.; Labasi, J. M.; Martin, W. H.; Peese, K. M.; Stock, I. A.; Svensson, L.; Sweeney, F. J.; Yu, C. H. Benzimidazolone p38 inhibitors. *Bioorg. Med. Chem. Lett.* **2004**, *14*, 919–923.

35. McClure, K. F.; Letavic, M. A.; Kalgutkar, A. S.; Gabel, C. A.; Audoly, L.; Barberia, J. T.; Braganza, J. F.; Carter, D.; Carty, T. J.; Cortina, S. R.; Dombroski, M. A.; Donahue, K. M.; Elliott, N. C.; Gibbons, C. P.; Jordan, C. K.; Kuperman, A. V.; Labasi, J. M.; LaLiberte, R. E.; McCoy, J. M.; Naiman, B. M.; Nelson, K. L.; Nguyen, H. T.; Peese, K. M.; Sweeney, F. J.; Taylor, T. J.; Trebino, C. E.; Abramov, Y. A.; Laird, E. R.; Volberg, W. A.; Zhou, J.; Bach, J.; Lombardo, F. Structure-activity relationships of triazolopyridine oxazole p38 inhibitors: identification of candidates for clinical development. *Bioorg. Med. Chem. Lett.* **2006**, *16*, 4339–4344.

36. Liu, C.; Lin, J.; Pitt, S.; Zhang, R. F.; Sack, J. S.; Kiefer, S. E.; Kish, K.; Doweyko, A. M.; Zhang, H.; Marathe, P. H.; Trzaskos, J.; McKinnon, M.; Dodd, J. H.; Barrish, J. C.; Schieven, G. L.; Leftheris, K. Benzothiazole based inhibitors of p38α MAP kinase. *Bioorg. Med. Chem. Lett.* **2008**, *18*, 1874–1879.

14

Structure-based design of novel P2-P4 macrocyclic inhibitors of hepatitis C NS3/4A protease

M. Katharine Holloway and Nigel J. Liverton

INTRODUCTION

Approximately 170 million people worldwide are chronically infected with hepatitis C virus (HCV),[1] a (+)-strand RNA virus of the Flaviviridae family, which is spread primarily by direct contact with human blood.[2] HCV causes chronic liver disease, including cirrhosis and hepatocellular carcinoma.[3] At present, HCV is a leading cause of death in HIV co-infected patients[4] and is the most common indication for liver transplantation.[5] In the United States alone, data from death certificates suggest that there are 10,000 to 12,000 deaths annually due to hepatitis C.[6]

Unlike HIV, HCV can be "cured"; that is, patients can achieve a sustained virologic response (SVR), in which the virus remains undetectable after termination of therapy. The current standard of care for the most prevalent genotype 1 infection is a regimen of pegylated interferon (IFN) plus ribavirin for 48 weeks.[7] Due to limited efficacy (only about half of genotype 1 patients are able to achieve SVR at twenty-four weeks post-therapy) and significant side effects (e.g., injection site inflammation, flu-like symptoms, depression, and anemia), many patients discontinue treatment. Thus, there is a significant need to improve efficacy, reduce the duration of treatment, and develop an IFN-free regimen with a more convenient route of administration.

DRUG DESIGN TARGET

Several promising antiviral targets for HCV have emerged in recent years.[8] As with HIV, most efforts have focused on inhibiting the key viral enzymes (see Figure 14.1). Inhibitors of one such target, HCV NS3/4A, have perhaps shown the most dramatic antiviral effects.[9,10] The full-length NS3/4A protein is comprised of an N-terminal trypsin-like serine protease (residues 1–180), a C-terminal NTPase/helicase (residues 189–626), and a fifty-four residue NS4A cofactor. The NS3/4A serine protease is responsible for *cis* cleavage at the NS3/4A junction, as well as *trans* cleavage at the NS4A/4B, NS4B/5A, and NS5A/5B junctions[11] and is essential for viral replication.[12] Clinical proof of concept for NS3/4A protease inhibitors has also been demonstrated, both for rapidly reversible noncovalent protease inhibitors

such as BILN-2061 (**1**)[13] and for slowly reversible covalent serine-trap inhibitors such as VX-950 (telaprevir, **2**),[14] shown in Figure 14.2.

INITIAL MODELING

Examination of published views of a close analog of **1** bound to the 1–180 protease domain of NS3 protease[15] suggests that the P2 thiazolylquinoline portion of the inhibitor lies on a relatively featureless enzyme surface with binding interactions that provide little apparent basis for the dramatic potency derived from that moiety (>30,000-fold) in a related series of tripeptide inhibitors.[16] As the crystal structure of this complex was unavailable, we recapitulated the binding pose by creating a model of **1** in the NS3/4A protease domain active site, based on the published view and employing a previously deposited NS3/4A protease domain crystal structure (PDB identifier 1JXP).[17] Figure 14.3 illustrates the solvent-exposed positioning of the P2 thiazolylquinoline in the model of **1** bound to the NS3/4A protease domain. Based on this view of binding to the relatively shallow, solvent-exposed, protease domain pocket, developing a tight-binding, drug-like inhibitor of NS3/4A protease was once likened to the probability of success of a climber scaling a featureless dome-shaped rock with few, if any, hand- or toe-holds.

In an effort to reconcile the bound pose with the observed structure/activity profile, we chose to model **1** bound to the full-length NS3/4A protein, including the significantly larger helicase domain, to determine what role the helicase might play in inhibitor binding. No full-length NS3/4A structures with inhibitors bound are currently available. Consequently, a published *apo* enzyme structure[18] of a single-chain form of NS3/4A was used as the starting point (Figure 14.4). In this structure, the six C-terminal residues (DLEVVT) of the helicase domain occupy the NS3 protease active site, forming twelve hydrogen bonds and creating a contact surface of ~500Å². To mimic the conformational change required to permit inhibitor binding, these six residues were deleted. Additionally, to accommodate the model of **1**, the crystallographic conformation of some protein side chains (e.g., R155 and Q526)

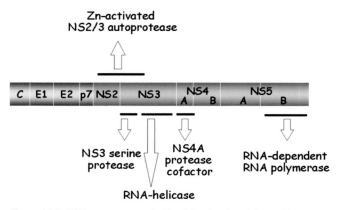

Figure 14.1. HCV genome organization (structural proteins = blue, non-structural proteins = green) with key enzyme targets labeled.

was manually adjusted. During subsequent energy minimization of the complex using the Merck Molecular Force Field (MMFF),[19–23] all side chains within 4Å of any atom of the inhibitor were allowed to relax. The resulting model of **1** bound to full-length NS3/4A is depicted in Figure 14.5.

VIRTUAL DESIGN

Analysis of this model indicated that the helicase domain can provide a surface (shown in blue in Figure 14.5) over the P2 moiety, including a pocket to accommodate the thiazolyl substituent. Specific inhibitor-helicase interactions include His528-carbamate oxygen and Gln526-quinoline. Thus, our working hypothesis was that modeling inhibitors in the full-length NS3/4A crystal structure produced binding poses more consistent with the observed structure/activity pattern and was consequently more relevant to our computer-aided drug design efforts. More importantly, it was apparent from this study that there is space to accommodate a connection between the carbamate cyclopentane and the quinoline ring. Reexamination of the helicase C-terminus from the *apo* structure (Figure 14.6), overlaid with the model of **1**, demonstrates that the side chain of Glu628

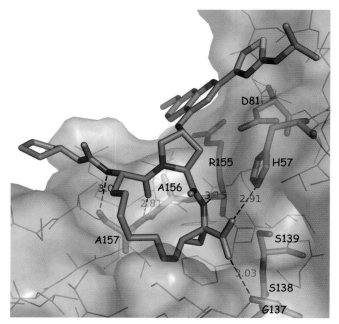

Figure 14.3. Model of **1** (magenta) bound to the protease domain of NS3/4A (green) with a molecular surface and key protein/inhibitor interactions shown. Note the shallowness of the binding pocket and the solvent-exposed face of the inhibitor, in particular the P2 thiazolylquinoline substituent in the upper right-hand quadrant.

occupies the same space as the proposed linker. Together, these observations strongly suggested the possibility of an alternative P4 cyclopentyl – P2 quinoline macrocyclization to form a structurally distinct series of inhibitors.

Initially targeted were carbamate derivatives **3a-3d** (Figure 14.7), in which the P1-P3 macrocyclic linker was disconnected, the proposed P2-P4 linker formed, and a 3-phenylquinoline P2 used to facilitate rapid synthesis of a range of analogs. Models of these proposed inhibitors were derived from the model of **1** bound to the full-length enzyme. The flexibility of the macrocyclic linker in **3a-3d** was explored by generating twenty-five conformers using a distance geometry algorithm.[24,25] Bound poses were energy minimized using the MMFF[19–23] with a distance-dependent dielectric constant ($\varepsilon = 2r$) in the rigid NS3/4A active site defined by selecting all residues within 10Å of any atom of the model of **1**. All titratable enzyme residues were charged and all inhibitors were defined as carboxylates. The pose that resulted in the lowest conformational energy for the ligand was selected and scored based on the corresponding enzyme/ligand energy (E_{inter}) and X-Score[26] in the same active site. The predicted bound poses are shown overlaid in Figure 14.8. Both scoring methods predicted that the 5- and 6-carbon linkers would show greatest activity (Table 14.1).

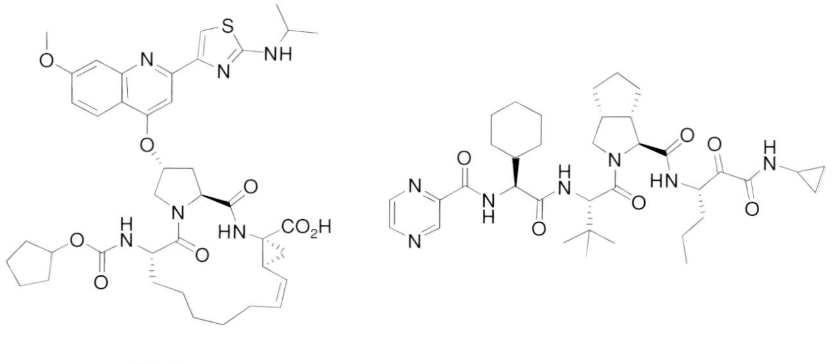

BILN-2061 (**1**)   VX-950 (**2**)

Figure 14.2. NS3/4A protease inhibitors.

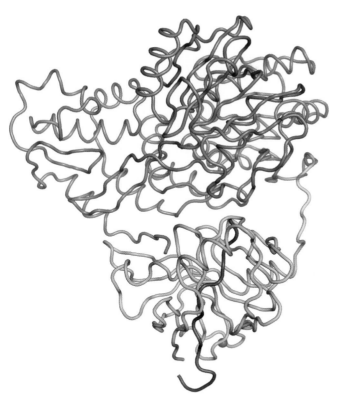

Figure 14.4. X-ray structure of full-length HCV NS3/4A[18] (NS3 protease = green; linking region = yellow; NS3 helicase = blue; NS4A = red; structural Zn = purple). Note that the C-terminus of the NS3 helicase occupies the catalytic site of the NS3 protease, which performs the cleavage at the NS3/4A junction.

PROOF OF CONCEPT

The desired compounds were prepared[27] via a high-yielding ring closing metathesis (RCM) strategy. Compound **3a**, with the three-carbon linker, proved to have very modest activity of 2,000 nM in a genotype 1b NS3/4A enzyme inhibition

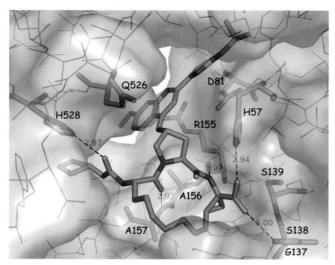

Figure 14.5. Model of **1** (magenta) bound to full-length NS3/4A (protease = green, helicase = blue) with key protein/inhibitor interactions shown.

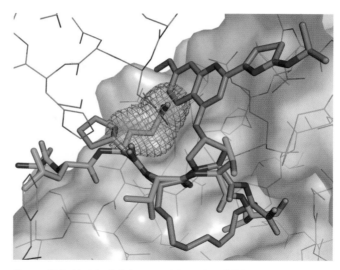

Figure 14.6. Model of **1** (magenta) bound to full-length NS3/4A with the helicase C-terminus (green) restored and the side chain of Glu628 highlighted with a mesh surface (orange). The molecular surface of the helicase domain (blue) has been omitted for better viewing.

assay[28] (Table 14.1). However, in agreement with the modeling study, incremental lengthening of the linker afforded dramatic improvement, with optimized activity of 8.5 nM in the case of the pentyl linker **3c**. A corresponding improvement in genotype 1b cell-based replicon activity[29] was also observed. The point of attachment on the quinoline was shown to be critical through synthesis of the corresponding 5-substituted derivative **4** by an analogous synthetic route, which proved dramatically less active (K_i 4,400 nM). In addition, synthesis of an acyclic analog **5** demonstrated that potency enhancement, particularly in the cell-based replicon assay, could be achieved through macrocyclization.

LEAD OPTIMIZATION

Previous work has established that the carboxylic acid functionality can be effectively replaced with a

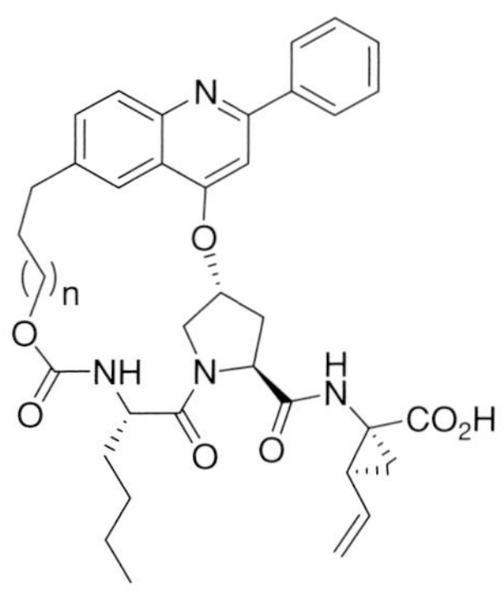

3a n = 1
3b n = 2
3c n = 3
3d n = 4

Figure 14.7. Initial P2–P4 macrocyclic targets **3a–3d**.

Table 14.1. In vitro activity[a]

| Compound | Modeling | | 1b K_i (nM) | 1b replicon IC$_{50}$ (nM) | |
	E_{inter}	X-Score		10% FBS	50% NHS
1			0.3	3	19
2			93	1,100	4,800
3a	−69.5	8.09	2,000	–	–
3b	−70.5	8.26	145	6,100	>100,000
3c	−71.1	8.36	8.5	1,150	5,600
3d	−71.4	8.44	25	1,200	9,100
4			4,400	–	–
5			40	4,800	>100,000
6			<0.016	6.7	26
7			<0.016	13	25
8a			0.07	4.5	14
8b			0.18	8.7	46

[a] Data are geometric averages of three or more determinations.

cyclopropylacylsulfonamide[30] and application of this strategy to **3c** afforded **6**, with subnanomolar inhibition of NS3/4A protease (K_i <0.016 nM). Disappointingly, given the critical need for liver exposure, oral administration of a 5 mg/kg dose of **6** to rats provided low (0.2 μM) compound levels in liver at 4 h with barely detectable plasma exposure (Table 14.2). In contrast, when the P3 *n*-butyl residue was replaced with *t*-butyl, the resultant inhibitor **7**, with a very similar in vitro activity profile, was effectively partitioned into liver with a tissue concentration at 4 h of 3.9 μM,

although plasma levels were unimproved. The dramatic impact of this minor structural change on liver levels strongly suggests that uptake is via an active transporter mediated process.

Having successfully demonstrated that this macrocyclization approach could yield potent compounds with significant liver exposure, we sought to broaden the strategy to include alternative P2 moieties. The use of an isoquinoline P2 to generate potent inhibitors has been reported previously.[31] In addition to potency enhancement, in their unsubstituted form they also offer somewhat reduced molecular weight inhibitors that might lead to improved systemic exposure. To this end, the isoquinoline analogs **8a** and **8b**, possessing the optimal five-carbon macrocycle linker length, were prepared. Both analogs showed very potent inhibition in both in vitro enzyme and replicon assays, but, more importantly, liver exposure was dramatically improved with 4 h liver concentrations of 18.6 and 13.4 μM, respectively, for **8a** and **8b**. Furthermore, drug was now clearly detectable in plasma for both compounds with

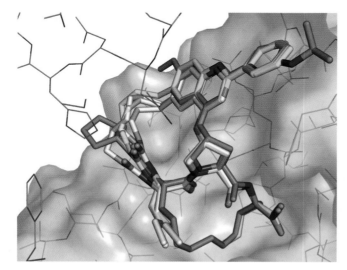

Figure 14.8. Models of P2-P4 macrocycle targets **3a-3d** overlaid with the model of **1** (magenta). The optimum macrocyclic ring in **3c** (yellow) appears to best overlay with **1**, consistent with the scoring results and in vitro activities reported in Table 14.1. The molecular surface of the helicase domain (blue) has been omitted for better viewing.

Table 14.2. Pharmacokinetic profiles of key compounds[a]

Compound	C_{max} (nM)	Plasma AUC 0–4h (μM*h)	4 h liver concentration (μM)
6	7	0.006	0.2
7	6	0.01	3.9
8a	240	0.36	18.6
8b	110	0.27	13.4

[a] Compounds dosed at 5 mg/kg P.O. in PEG400 ($n = 2–3$).

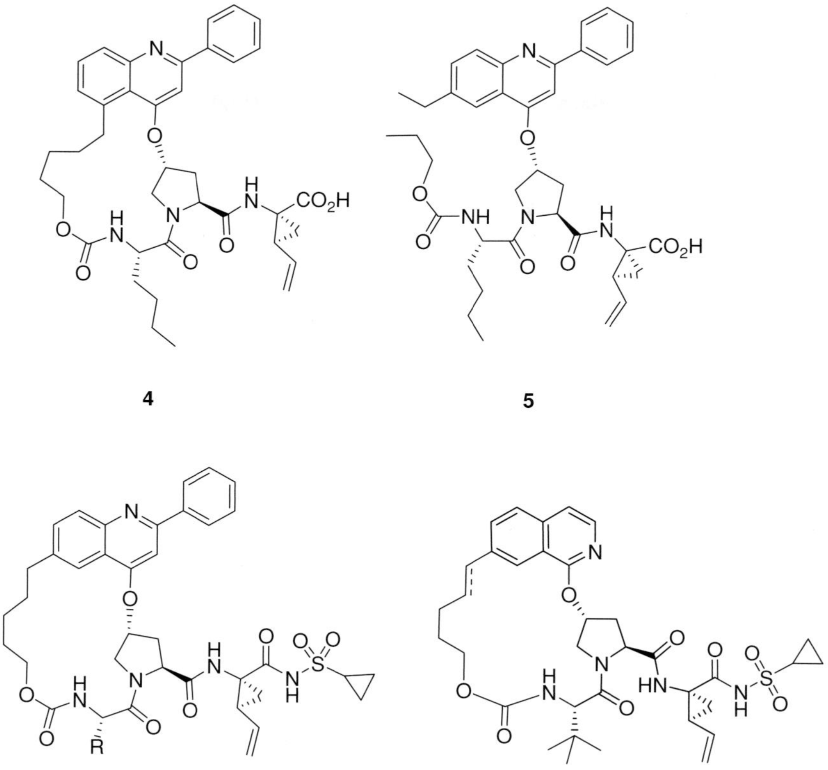

4   **5**

6 R= *n*-Bu   **8a** double bond
7 R= *t*-Bu   **8b** single bond

Figure 14.9. Additional quinoline and isoquinoline based NS3/4A inhibitors, **4–8**.

AUCs of 0.36 and 0.27 μM*h, respectively. Sustained exposure in liver is clearly an important factor for any potential treatment of HCV and high drug levels relative to activity in the replicon assay (500 nM, 35 × replicon EC_{50} in presence of 50% NHS) are maintained in rat liver for 24 h following a 5 mg/kg dose of **8a**.

A detailed evaluation of the more potent analog **8a** revealed no significant activity versus other serine proteases (>50,000-fold selectivity over trypsin and chymotrypsin), hERG binding ($IC_{50} > 30$ μM), or in a broad-based Panlabs screen (>4,000-fold selectivity). Although **8a** has a number of functionalities that might be viewed as potentially susceptible to metabolism, it is primarily excreted in bile as unchanged parent after rat IV dosing.

An additional attraction of this class of macrocycles is the potential to use a range of macrocyclization strategies in any advanced development (including intramolecular Heck or Suzuki reactions, proline amide coupling, or RCM), in contrast to P1-P3 macrocyclic compounds such as **1**, where an RCM step appears unavoidable.[32] Although there are reports of compounds employing a related P2-P4 cyclization strategy,[33,34] the inhibitors had only modest micromolar potencies. Synthesis of the cyclopropylacylsulfonamide analog of one of these compounds had little effect on potency.[27]

CONCLUSION

In summary, molecular modeling of inhibitor-bound full-length NS3/4A protease structures proved to be a key tool in the design of a novel series of potent macrocyclic NS3/4a protease inhibitors **3a-3d** that was optimized to compound **8a**. The in vitro activity and selectivity as well as the rat pharmacokinetic profile of **8a** compare favorably with the data for other NS3/4A protease inhibitors currently in clinical development for the treatment of HCV.

REFERENCES

1. Hepatitis C – global prevalence (update). *Weekly Epidemiology Record* **1999**, *74*, 425–427.
2. Alter, M. J. Epidemiology of hepatitis C. *Hepatology* **1997**, *26*, 62S–65S.
3. Liang, T. J.; Heller, T. VX-950, a novel hepatitis C virus (HCV) NS3-4A protease inhibitor, exhibits potent antiviral activities in HCV replicon cells. *Gastroenterology* **2004**, *127*, S62–S71.
4. Salmon-Ceron, D.; Lewden, C.; Morlat, P.; Bevilacqua, S.; Jougla, E.; Bonnet, F.; Heripret, L.; Costagliola, D.; May, T.; Chene, G. Liver disease as a major cause of death among HIV infected patients: role of hepatitis C and B viruses and alcohol. *J. Hepatol.* **2005**, *42*, 799–805.
5. Brown, R. S. Hepatitis C and liver transplantation. *Nature* **2005**, *436*, 973–978.

6. In *Management of Hepatitis C:* **2002**; National Institutes of Health, 2002. http://consensus.nih.gov/2002/2002HepatitisC2002116html.htm.

7. Poynard, T.; Marcellin, P.; Lee, S. S.; Niederau, C.; Minuk, G. S.; Ideo, G.; Bain, V.; Heathcote, J.; Zeuzem, S.; Trepo, C.; Albrecht, J. Randomised trial of interferon alpha2b plus ribavirin for 48 weeks or for 24 weeks versus interferon alpha2b plus placebo for 48 weeks for treatment of chronic infection with hepatitis C virus. International Hepatitis Interventional Therapy Group (IHIT). *Lancet* **1998**, *352*, 1426–1432.

8. Gordon, C. P.; Keller, P. A. Control of hepatitis C: a medicinal chemistry perspective. *J. Med. Chem.* **2005**, *48*, 1–20.

9. Thomson, J. A.; Perni, R. B. Hepatitis C virus NS3-4A protease inhibitors: countering viral subversion in vitro and showing promise in the clinic. *Curr. Opin. Drug Discov. Devel.* **2006**, *9*, 606–617.

10. Chen, S. H.; Tan, S. L. Discovery of small-molecule inhibitors of HCV NS3-4A protease as potential therapeutic agents against HCV infection. *Curr. Med. Chem.* **2005**, *12*, 2317–2342.

11. Bartenschlager, R.; Ahlborn-Laake, L.; Mous, J.; Jacobsen, H. Nonstructural protein 3 of the hepatitis C virus encodes a serine-type proteinase required for cleavage at the NS3/4 and NS4/5 junctions. *J. Virol.* **1993**, *67*, 3835–3844.

12. Kolykhalov, A. A.; Mihalik, K.; Feinstone, S. M.; Rice, C. M. Hepatitis C virus-encoded enzymatic activities and conserved RNA elements in the 3' nontranslated region are essential for virus replication in vivo. *J. Virol.* **2000**, *74*, 2046–2051.

13. Llinas-Brunet, M.; Bailey, M. D.; Bolger, G.; Brochu, C.; Faucher, A. M.; Ferland, J. M.; Garneau, M.; Ghiro, E.; Gorys, V.; Grand-Maitre, C.; Halmos, T.; Lapeyre-Paquette, N.; Liard, F.; Poirier, M.; Rheaume, M.; Tsantrizos, Y. S.; Lamarre, D. Structure-activity study on a novel series of macrocyclic inhibitors of the hepatitis C virus NS3 protease leading to the discovery of BILN 2061. *J. Med. Chem.* **2004**, *47*, 1605–1608.

14. Perni, R. B.; Almquist, S. J.; Byrn, R. A.; Chandorkar, G.; Chaturvedi, P. R.; Courtney, L. F.; Decker, C. J.; Dinehart, K.; Gates, C. A.; Harbeson, S. L.; Heiser, A.; Kalkeri, G.; Kolaczkowski, E.; Lin, K.; Luong, Y. P.; Rao, B. G.; Taylor, W. P.; Thomson, J. A.; Tung, R. D.; Wei, Y.; Kwong, A. D.; Lin, C. Preclinical profile of VX-950, a potent, selective, and orally bioavailable inhibitor of hepatitis C virus NS3-4A serine protease. *Antimicrob. Agents Chemother.* **2006**, *50*, 899–909.

15. Tsantrizos, Y. S.; Bolger, G.; Bonneau, P.; Cameron, D. R.; Goudreau, N.; Kukolj, G.; LaPlante, S. R.; Llinas-Brunet, M.; Nar, H.; Lamarre, D. Macrocyclic inhibitors of the NS3 protease as potential therapeutic agents of hepatitis C virus infection. *Angew. Chem. Int. Ed. Engl.* **2003**, *42*, 1356–1360.

16. Laplante, R.; Llinas-Brunet, M. Dynamics and Structure-based Design of Drugs Targeting the Critical Serine Protease of the Hepatitis C Virus – From a Peptidic Substrate to BILN 2061. *Curr. Med. Chem. Antiinfect. Agents* **2005**, *4*, 111–132.

17. Yan, Y.; Li, Y.; Munshi, S.; Sardana, V.; Cole, J. L.; Sardana, M.; Steinkuehler, C.; Tomei, L.; De Francesco, R.; Kuo, L. C.; Chen, Z. Complex of NS3 protease and NS4A peptide of BK strain hepatitis C virus: a 2.2 A resolution structure in a hexagonal crystal form. *Protein Sci.* **1998**, *7*, 837–847.

18. Yao, N.; Reichert, P.; Taremi, S. S.; Prosise, W. W.; Weber, P. C. Molecular views of viral polyprotein processing revealed by the crystal structure of the hepatitis C virus bifunctional protease-helicase. *Structure* **1999**, *7*, 1353–1363.

19. Halgren, T. A. Merck Molecular Force Field. I. Basis, form, scope, parameterization, and performance of MMFF94. *J. Comput. Chem.* **1996**, *17*, 490–519.

20. Halgren, T. A. Merck Molecular Force Field. II. MMFF94 van der Waals and electrostatic parameters for intermolecular interactions. *J. Comput. Chem.* **1996**, *17*, 520–552.

21. Halgren, T. A. Merck Molecular Force Field. III. Molecular geometries and vibrational frequencies for MMFF94. *J. Comput. Chem.* **1996**, *17*, 553–586.

22. Halgren, T. A.; Nachbar, R. B. Merck Molecular Force Field. IV. Conformational energies and geometries for MMFF94. *J. Comput. Chem.* **1996**, *17*, 587–615.

23. Halgren, T. A. Merck Molecular Force Field. V. Extension of MMFF94 using experimental data, additional computational data, and empirical rules. *J. Comput. Chem.* **1996**, *17*, 616–641.

24. Crippen, C. M.; Havel, T. F. *Distance Geometry and Molecular Conformation.* New York, NY: John Wiley & Sons; **1988**.

25. Kuszewski, J.; Nilges, M.; Brunger, A. T. Sampling and efficiency of metric matrix distance geometry: a novel partial metrization algorithm. *J. Biomol. NMR* **1992**, *2*, 33–56.

26. Wang, R.; Lu, Y.; Fang, X.; Wang, S. An extensive test of 14 scoring functions using the PDBbind refined set of 800 protein-ligand complexes. *J. Chem. Inf. Comput. Sci.* **2004**, *44*, 2114–2125.

27. Liverton, N. J.; Holloway, M. K.; McCauley, J. A.; Rudd, M. T.; Butcher, J. W.; Carroll, S. S.; DiMuzio, J.; Fandozzi, C.; Gilbert, K. F.; Mao, S. S.; McIntyre, C. J.; Nguyen, K. T.; Romano, J. J.; Stahlhut, M.; Wan, B. L.; Olsen, D. B.; Vacca, J. P. Molecular modeling based approach to potent P2-P4 macrocyclic inhibitors of hepatitis C NS3/4A protease. *J. Am. Chem. Soc.* **2008**, *130*, 4607–4609.

28. Mao, S. S.; DiMuzio, J.; McHale, C.; Burlein, C.; Olsen, D.; Carroll, S. S. A time-resolved, internally quenched fluorescence assay to characterize inhibition of hepatitis C virus nonstructural protein 3-4A protease at low enzyme concentrations. *Anal. Biochem.* **2008**, *373*, 1–8.

29. Migliaccio, G.; Tomassini, J. E.; Carroll, S. S.; Tomei, L.; Altamura, S.; Bhat, B.; Bartholomew, L.; Bosserman, M. R.; Ceccacci, A.; Colwell, L. F.; Cortese, R.; De Francesco, R.; Eldrup, A. B.; Getty, K. L.; Hou, X. S.; LaFemina, R. L.; Ludmerer, S. W.; MacCoss, M.; McMasters, D. R.; Stahlhut, M. W.; Olsen, D. B.; Hazuda, D. J.; Flores, O. A. Characterization of resistance to non-obligate chain-terminating ribonucleoside analogs that inhibit hepatitis C virus replication in vitro. *J. Biol. Chem.* **2003**, *278*, 49164–49170.

30. Tu, Y.; Scola, P., Michael; Good, A., Charles; Campbell, J. A. Bristol-Myers Squibb. Preparation of prolinamide peptides as hepatitis C virus inhibitors: WO 2005054430, **2005**.

31. Wang, X. A.; Sun, L.-Q.; Sit, S.-Y.; Sin, N.; Scola, P. M.; Hewawasam, P.; Good, A. C.; Chen, Y.; Campbell, J. A. Bristol-Myers Squibb Hepatitis C Virus Inhibitors: US 6,995,174, **2006**.

32. Nicola, T.; Brenner, M.; Donsbach, K.; Kreye, P. First Scale-Up to Production Scale of a Ring Closing Metathesis Reaction Forming a 15-Membered Macrocycle as a Precursor of an Active Pharmaceutical Ingredient. *Org. Process Res. Dev.* **2005**, *9*, 513–515.

33. Marchetti, A.; Ontoria, J. M.; Matassa, V. G. Synthesis of Two Novel Cyclic Biphenyl Ether Analogs of an Inhibitor of HCV NS3 Protease. *Synlett* **1999**, S1, 1000–1002.

34. Chen, K. X.; Njoroge, F. G.; Pichardo, J.; Prongay, A.; Butkiewicz, N.; Yao, N.; Madison, V.; Girijavallabhan, V. Potent 7-hydroxy-1,2,3,4-tetrahydroisoquinoline-3-carboxylic acid-based macrocyclic inhibitors of hepatitis C virus NS3 protease. *J. Med. Chem.* **2006**, *49*, 567–574.

15

Purine nucleoside phosphorylases as targets for transition-state analog design

Andrew S. Murkin and Vern L. Schramm

INTRODUCTION

Among the most powerful enzyme-targeted drugs are those that bear a strong resemblance to the transition state of the chemical reaction undergoing catalysis. This chapter illustrates that experimental determination of enzymatic transition-state structure permits chemically stable analogs to be designed. Mimics of these transition states exhibit binding affinities exceeding those of the substrates by factors of greater than 10^6. To appreciate this approach to drug design, it is necessary to understand the nature of transition-state formation and how it relates to the strong binding interactions between enzymes and transition-state analogs.

Enzymatic transition-state formation

All chemical reactions proceed through at least one transition state, an unstable structure of maximal energy along the reaction coordinate. Having a lifetime of under 100 fs (10^{-13} s), the time required for a single bond vibration, the transition state is the most unstable species along a chemical reaction coordinate. In the absence of a catalyst, the probability of transition-state formation is extremely low. Enzymes achieve great catalytic reaction rates by providing appropriately positioned functional groups within the active site, which interact with and distort the substrate toward the transition state by dynamic motions of the complex.

Although the physical means of enzymatic transition-state formation remain the subject of scientific debate, several theories have been proffered. In the early 1940s, Linus Pauling postulated that enzymes bind most optimally not to the normal substrate molecule but rather to the substrate molecule in a strained configuration corresponding to the "activated complex."[1] He suggested that various attractive forces with the enzyme cause the substrate to adopt the strained configuration, thereby favoring the chemical reaction and accounting for the lowered activation energy of the catalyzed reaction. Wolfenden later expanded this theory by considering a thermodynamic equilibrium between the nonenzymatic transition state and the enzyme-bound transition state (Figure 15.1).[2,3] A nonenzymatic reaction proceeds from substrate (S) to products with a rate constant k_{non} via a transition state (S‡), governed by the equilibrium constant $K_{non}^\ddagger$. The corresponding enzymatic process proceeds first through a Michaelis complex (E·S), given by the dissociation constant K_d, followed by the enzymatic transition state (E·S‡), which is given by rate constant k_{enz} and equilibrium constant $K_{enz}^\ddagger$. A hypothetical binding equilibrium ($K_d^\ddagger$) between the enzyme and transition state completes the thermodynamic box. The rate acceleration for the enzyme-catalyzed reaction over the nonenzymatic reaction, k_{enz}/k_{non}, therefore indicates the degree of tightness to which the transition state is bound relative to the substrate, typically between 10^{10} and 10^{15}.

A related factor that may play a role in transition-state formation is ground-state destabilization. In much the same way that the transition-state stabilization model of Wolfenden explains lowering of the activation-energy barrier through stabilizing interactions with the enzyme, Jencks and others have suggested that destabilizing interactions with the bound substrate could promote distortions toward the transition state (Figure 15.2).[4,5] Strategies by which these binding interactions can assist the chemical reaction include desolvation of substrate functional groups, positioning substrates in the active site, and geometrically or electrostatically destabilizing substrates.[6] This third strategy has been proposed for orotidine-5′-phosphate (OMP) decarboxylase,[7] in what Jencks has termed the "Circe effect," whereby the enzyme attracts the substrate by forming energetically favorable binding interactions at one region of the substrate but simultaneously destabilizes the reactive group that undergoes chemical transformation. Richard and coworkers have since observed formation of a carbanion intermediate that OMP decarboxylase stabilizes by at least 14 kcal/mol, suggesting transition-state stabilization is the dominant factor in the 10^{17}-fold rate acceleration by this enzyme.[8] Thus, it is possible that transition-state stabilization and ground-state destabilization function in complementarity to achieve rate enhancements, as is depicted in Figure 15.2.

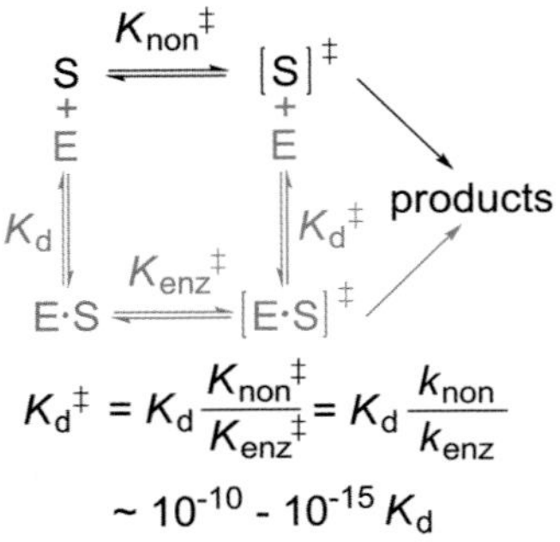

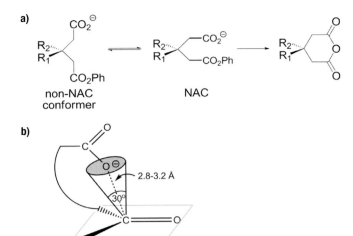

Figure 15.1. Thermodynamic box relating equilibria for nonenzymatic (black) and enzymatic (red) transition-state formation ($K_{non}^{\ddagger}$ and $K_{enz}^{\ddagger}$, respectively), dissociation of substrate from the Michaelis complex (K_d), and the hypothetical dissociation of the transition state from the enzyme ($K_d^{\ddagger}$). Assuming equal transmission coefficients, $K_d^{\ddagger}$ is equal to K_d multiplied by the ratio of the reaction rate constants for nonenzymatic (k_{non}) and enzymatic (k_{enz}) reactions. E = enzyme; S = substrate.

A third explanation for enzymatic transition-state formation involves the substrate's adoption of a reactive conformation. According to Bruice and coworkers, a chemical reaction will occur only with a limited range of substrate conformers, termed *near-attack conformers* (NACs), which are characterized by having a geometric arrangement of reactive functional groups sufficient for formation of a transition state.[9] An example of a NAC is given by the intramolecular cyclization of dicarboxylic acid monoesters to generate five- and six-membered rings [Figure 15.3(a)]. Computational modeling revealed that a NAC existed when the distance between the nucleophilic oxygen and carbonyl carbon was 2.8–3.2Å and the angle of attack was within a 30° cone of the optimal angle of 15° [Figure 15.3(b)].[10] The

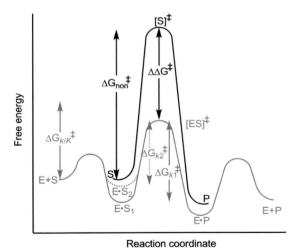

Figure 15.2. Enzyme catalysis by transition-state stabilization and ground-state destabilization. The free-energy profile for the nonenzymatic reaction (black) proceeds from substrate (S) to product (P) via the transition state $[S]^{\ddagger}$ with energetic barrier $\Delta G_{non}^{\ddagger}$. In the enzymatic reaction (red), the transition state $[E \cdot S]^{\ddagger}$ is stabilized by $\Delta\Delta G^{\ddagger}$, resulting in a barrier $\Delta G_{k/K}^{\ddagger}$ on k_{cat}/K_m (that is, from E+S to $[E \cdot S]^{\ddagger}$) and a barrier $\Delta G_{k1}^{\ddagger}$ on k_{cat} (that is, from $E \cdot S_1$ to $[E \cdot S]^{\ddagger}$). With ground-state destabilization on the Michaelis complex ($E \cdot S_2$, dotted line), the barrier on k_{cat}/K_m remains unchanged, but the barrier on k_{cat} is reduced to $\Delta G_{k2}^{\ddagger}$.

Figure 15.3. Proximity effect demonstrated by near-attack conformers (NACs). **(a)** Conformers of dicarboxylic acid monoesters with inappropriate geometry between the reactive groups must rotate into NACs to cyclize. **(b)** Geometric features of NACs for the cyclization reaction in **(a)** include an interatomic distance of 2.8–3.2Å and an angle of approach within 30° from the optimal angle of 15° to the perpendicular to the carbonyl plane. Modified from Lightstone and Bruice.[10]

proximity effect demonstrated by the neighboring-group participation of these compounds, it is argued, is also created in the active sites of enzymes. The greater the population of substrate conformers existing as NACs, the greater the rate of reaction; hence, enzymes accelerate reaction rates, at least in part, by increasing the likelihood that an E·S complex is a NAC.

A recent theory of transition-state formation that has gained support is the coupling of dynamic motions to the reaction coordinate. It has been reasoned that certain discrete atomic vibrations, often called protein-promoting vibrations (PPVs), within the protein work in concert to cause bond cleavage and/or bond formation along the reaction coordinate.[11] These promoting motions are the result of the enzyme's dynamic excursions along the allowed vibrational modes. When PPVs function together, the substrate and enzymatic groups promoting catalysis are pushed toward the transition state as the chemical reaction proceeds. Examples for which there is evidence supporting PPVs include hydrogen-transfer reactions catalyzed by alcohol dehydrogenase,[12] dihydrofolate reductase,[13,14] and lactate dehydrogenase,[11] as well as the phosphate-ribosyl transfer reaction catalyzed by purine nucleoside phosphorylase (PNP),[15] which is the subject of discussion in the remaining sections of this chapter. Figure 15.4 illustrates reaction-coupled dynamic motions located in the His104Arg mutant of PNP, whereby the movement of Arg104 (magenta), a distant residue from catalytic site ligands (green), is coupled to Phe159 (red), which in turn affects the dynamics of the active site residues (orange).[16] It is important to keep in mind that the above theories of transition-state formation are mutually compatible and any or all may be involved to varying degrees.

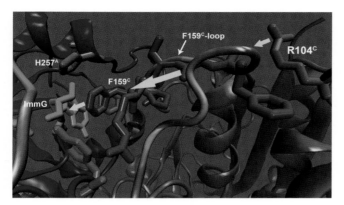

Figure 15.4. Dynamic perturbation of the purine nucleoside phosphorylase reaction coordinate, simulated by molecular dynamics calculations by Saen-Oon et al.[16] The motion of Arg104 (magenta) is coupled to the movement of Phe159 (red), located in a catalytic loop at the interface of two subunits (A, blue and C, tan) in the trimeric protein. Phe159 in turn impinges on the ligands (green) ImmG and phosphate (partially obscured) and surrounding active-site residues (orange) in the adjacent subunit. The vector of dynamic perturbation is shown as yellow arrows. Modified from Saen-Oon et al.[16]

Transition-state mimicry

The various transition-state theories share an essential feature in their description of an enzyme's structure and function: enzymes have evolved to interact most optimally to generate the transition state. This is achieved by strategic placement of appropriate functional groups, which operate collectively to convert the stable substrate molecule into an unstable structure within a relatively short (typically ms) time scale. It has been recognized for many decades that if a chemically stable version of the transition state could be engineered and introduced into the active site, very strong associations with the enzyme would be expected.[2,3,17]

The tight binding of transition-state mimics is best explained by the thermodynamic model of transition-state stabilization (see "Enzymatic transition-state formation"). In the hypothetical binding equilibrium between the enzyme and its transition state (Figure 15.1), the transition state is held more tightly than the substrate by a factor equal to the rate acceleration, k_{enz}/k_{non}, and the energy of this "association" is given by $\Delta\Delta G^{\ddagger}$ (Figure 15.2). Although a *virtual* thermodynamic equilibrium cannot exist because of the subbond vibrational lifetime of the transition state, it is instructive to imagine capturing the system at the moment the transition state is formed. This energetic interaction is approximated by the *real* binding equilibrium with a transition-state analog, which, if it were a perfect mimic, would completely convert the transition-state stabilization energy, $\Delta\Delta G^{\ddagger}$, into binding energy.[18,19]

The dynamic view of transition-state theory explains the tight-binding property of transition state analogs by a conformational collapse of the enzyme around the chemically stable mimic.[20] The chemically inert transition-state analog converts the dynamic excursions found at the transition state to a stable convergence of the enzyme conformation,

Adenosine deaminase

γ-Glutamylcysteine synthetase

Sialidase (Neuroaminidase)

Deoxycoformycin
$K_d = 2.5$ pM

Sulfoximine
$K_d = 39$ nM

Zanamivir
$K_d = 75 - 700$ pM
(Varius influenza virus strains)

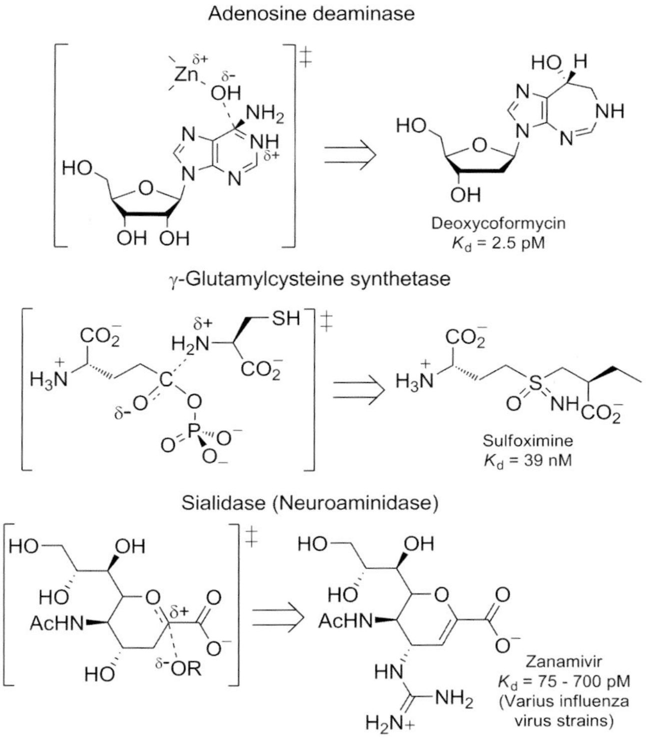

Figure 15.5. Enzymatic transition states and their chemically stable analogs. Dissociation constants for inhibitors of adenosine deaminase,[135] γ-glutamylcysteine synthetase,[136] and sialidase (neuraminidase)[137] are given.

resulting in the conversion of catalytic dynamics into static binding energy.

Regardless of the precise mechanism by which enzymatic transition states are formed, the incredibly potent inhibition exhibited by their analogs – in contrast to substrate and product analogs, for instance – underscores the importance of their development. Figure 15.5 illustrates examples of transition-state analogs from among the hundreds of known enzyme targets.[21] To design transition-state analogs, we must first have knowledge of the structure of the transition state.

Determination of transition-state structure from kinetic isotope effects

Unfortunately, the structure of the transition state cannot be determined by the analytical methods used for stable compounds, including crystallography, nuclear magnetic resonance (NMR), infrared/Raman, ultraviolet/visible spectroscopy, and mass spectrometry. With a lifetime less than a single bond vibration, methods probing the ground state are clearly insufficient. Indirect kinetic methods provide some structural information. For instance, variations in the reactivity of functional groups (e.g., varying pK_a or electron-withdrawing properties, analyzed by Hammett plots) in the substrate have been introduced to examine

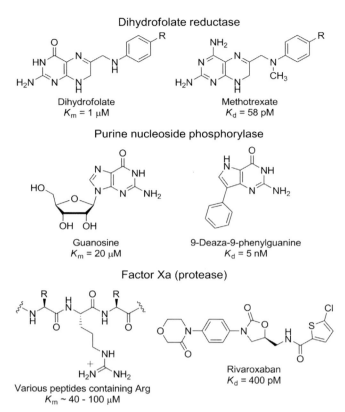

Dihydrofolate reductase

Dihydrofolate
$K_m = 1$ μM

Methotrexate
$K_d = 58$ pM

Purine nucleoside phosphorylase

Guanosine
$K_m = 20$ μM

9-Deaza-9-phenylguanine
$K_d = 5$ nM

Factor Xa (protease)

Various peptides containing Arg
$K_m \sim 40 - 100$ μM

Rivaroxaban
$K_d = 400$ pM

Figure 15.6. Tight-binding inhibitors of dihydrofolate reductase and purine nucleoside phosphorylase that are not transition-state analogs. The substrates and K_m values are given, along with the dissociation constants (K_d) for methotrexate,[138] 9-deaza-9-phenylguanine,[139] and rivaroxaban.[140]

the position of the transition state in the reaction coordinate of chemical reactions.[22,23] Substrate specificity usually limits the utility of this method in enzyme-catalyzed reactions, however. Tight-binding inhibitors, as mentioned above, have also been used to survey transition-state structure, whereby particularly potent inhibition (low nM or pM) is proposed to reflect features of the transition state. However, without direct information on transition-state structure, one cannot be confident that inhibition is due to transition-state mimicry. Tight-binding inhibitors that are not transition-state analogs are well known (Figure 15.6).

Kinetic isotope effects

Features of the transition state, however, can be captured in the vibrational frequencies of atomic stretching and bending modes within the substrate at the transition state relative to those in the ground state. It has long been recognized that isotopic substitution at specific positions in the substrate often result in different reaction rates for the light and heavy species; these phenomena are known as kinetic isotope effects (KIEs; Figure 15.7). When the bonding environment surrounding the atom of interest becomes less restrained at the transition state, the gap in zero point energies (ZPEs) of the bonds to the light and heavy isotopes becomes smaller; thus, the rate constant for the light

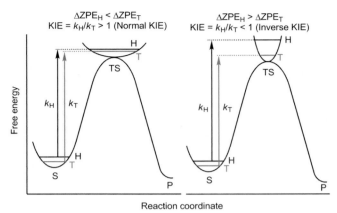

$\Delta ZPE_H < \Delta ZPE_T$
KIE = $k_H/k_T > 1$ (Normal KIE)

$\Delta ZPE_H > \Delta ZPE_T$
KIE = $k_H/k_T < 1$ (Inverse KIE)

Figure 15.7. Origin of normal and inverse kinetic isotope effects (KIEs). Differences in the zero-point energies (ZPEs) of bonds to light (H) and heavy (T) isotopes at the ground state (S) and the transition state (TS) result in differences in the corresponding rate constants, k_H and k_T. For a looser bond at the transition state (left diagram), the ZPEs of the light and heavy isotopes are closer, giving rise to a normal KIE ($k_H/k_T > 1$). In contrast, for a stiffer bond at the transition state (right diagram), the ZPEs are more greatly separated, yielding an inverse KIE ($k_H/k_T < 1$).

species is greater than that for the heavy species, and a normal KIE (i.e., $k_{light}/k_{heavy} > 1$) is obtained. In contrast, when the bonding environment becomes more restrained at the transition state, the difference in ZPEs becomes larger, yielding an inverse KIE (i.e., $k_{light}/k_{heavy} < 1$). The magnitude of the KIE indicates the degree to which the bonding environment has changed between the ground state and the transition state. This information reports on the extent of bond formation/cleavage, as well as geometrical changes at and remote from the reactive center. If KIEs are determined for multiple positions in the substrate, one can deduce a structure for the transition state with the aid of computational modeling.[21,24]

Methods for the measurement of enzymatic KIEs and their interpretation in relation to transition-state structure have been well described in the literature.[25–29] Two major approaches for the measurement of KIEs are the competitive and noncompetitive (direct) methods. The direct approach involves measurement of the reaction kinetics for the light and heavy isotopologs in separate experiments, and the ratio of the rate constants gives the experimental KIE. The competitive method, in contrast, involves a mixture of the heavy (e.g., ^3H) and light (e.g., ^1H with remote ^{14}C) isotopologs, with the remote label acting as an internal standard. A normal KIE will cause an enrichment in the light, faster-reacting isotope (i.e., larger $^{14}C/^3H$ ratio) in the product, whereas the isotopic ratio of unreacted substrate will decrease. Experimental KIEs are calculated from comparison of the ratios before reaction and after partial enzymatic conversion. Because the reaction conditions are always identical for both species in the competitive method, it is an order of magnitude more precise than the direct method and is a superior technique usually employed in transition-state analysis.[26,30]

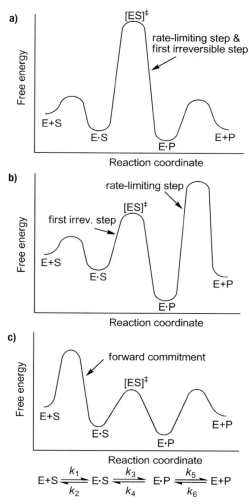

Figure 15.8. Free-energy diagrams for hypothetical enzymatic reactions, illustrating the effect of kinetic complexity on experimental kinetic isotope effects. **(a)** In the simplest scenario, the isotope-sensitive step is both the rate-limiting step and the first irreversible step. The intrinsic KIE will be fully expressed in the V/K KIE. **(b)** If the rate-limiting step occurs after the first irreversible step (which is the same as or follows the isotope-sensitive step), the intrinsic KIE will still be fully expressed in the V/K KIE. **(c)** If the substrate is sticky ($k_3 > k_2$), forward commitment will cause masking of the intrinsic KIE. Modified from Berti and Tanaka.[30]

Intrinsic isotope effects

To establish the transition state for a reaction, it is imperative that the KIEs be *intrinsic*; that is, they must reflect only the chemical step. The simplest case is where the chemical step is both the rate-limiting step and the first irreversible step [Figure 15.8(a)]. However, it is common for enzymatic reactions to involve different rate-limiting and first irreversible steps [Figure 15.8(b)] and to involve additional kinetically significant steps [Figure 15.8(c)]. A feature of the competitive method is that it reflects isotope effects on the enzyme's specificity constant, k_{cat}/K_m (or V_{max}/K_m; these isotope effects are commonly referred to as V/K KIEs) and therefore reports on atomic vibrational frequency changes between the unbound substrate and the first irreversible step. Following the first irreversible step,

the bound species is committed to proceeding to completion and no further isotopic discrimination can occur; thus, situations such as that depicted in Figure 15.8(b) would not interfere with the measurement of V/K KIEs. A possibility that may prevent V/K KIEs from being intrinsic, however, is with a "sticky" substrate, which, once bound to the enzyme, has a greater tendency to partition toward products than to dissociate back into solution [i.e., $k_3 > k_2$ in Figure 15.8(c)]. This occurrence, called "commitment to catalysis" or simply "commitment," causes the magnitude of the observed V/K KIE to always be lower than the intrinsic KIE; as a result, one must choose alternative reaction conditions to reduce or eliminate commitments or conduct additional experiments (e.g., isotope trapping[31]) to quantitate and correct for this effect. It is of interest to note that more catalytically efficient enzymes have increasing commitments to catalysis, with "perfect enzymes" (i.e., $k_{cat}/K_m \sim 10^9$ M^{-1} s^{-1}) being fully committed and therefore exhibiting no KIE.

Computational modeling of transition states

At present, there are no algorithms for generating transition-state structure directly from experimentally determined KIEs. Instead, one relies on iterative computational modeling of predicted structures to calculate KIEs that, when the structure is optimized, match the experimental values. This method requires modeling of both the substrate, whose structure can often be obtained from crystallographic, spectroscopic, or other means, and the transition state. The latter structure can be obtained by iterative model manipulation, such as fixing bond lengths and angles, and frequency calculation of all vibrational modes, with the assistance of structure software applications, such as Gaussian,[32] which can be run on common desktop computers but may require advanced computational capabilities for more complex systems. The vibrational frequencies can be then be analyzed by programs such as QUIVER[33] or ISOEFF98,[34] which are based on equations of the form in Equation (15.1),[35] originally derived in the midtwentieth century by Bigeleisen:[36–38]

$$\frac{k_L}{k_H} = \frac{v_L^{\ddagger}}{v_H^{\ddagger}} \times \prod_i^{3n-6} \frac{u_{iL}^R \sinh\left(u_{iH}^R/2\right)}{u_{iH}^R \sinh\left(u_{iL}^R/2\right)} \times \prod_i^{3n-7} \frac{u_{iH}^{\ddagger} \sinh\left(u_{iL}^{\ddagger}/2\right)}{u_{iL}^{\ddagger} \sinh\left(u_{iH}^{\ddagger}/2\right)},$$

(15.1)

where the subscripts L and H indicate light and heavy isotope, respectively; the superscripts R and ‡ indicate reactant and transition state, respectively; n is the number of atoms in the system; $v^{\ddagger}$ is the imaginary frequency of bond lysis at the transition state; and $u_i = hv_i/k_B T$, where h is Planck's constant, v_i is the frequency of the ith vibrational mode in wave numbers, k_B is Boltzmann's constant, and T is the absolute temperature.[35] Systematic variation of model geometry is necessary to identify the ranges of bond lengths, bond angles, and dihedral angles that would give rise to the observed KIEs, within experimental error. The extent of computational space may be greatly reduced with knowledge of geometries permitted in the active site, which is often available from crystallographic data, especially from bound substrate and substrate analogs.

General approach to transition-state-based inhibitor design

In summary, solving the transition-state structure of an enzymatic reaction requires the following steps:

1. Chemical or biochemical synthesis of substrate molecules containing isotopic labels at specific positions.
2. Determination of experimental conditions wherein intrinsic isotope effects – that is, KIEs reflecting only the chemical step – can be measured.
3. Measurement of KIEs for each position labeled in step 1.
4. Iterative computation of theoretical KIEs from quantum mechanical calculations with model structures until the KIEs match those from experiment in step 3.

The demands of these conditions often limit the enzymatic systems that can be analyzed by this approach to inhibitor design. For instance, unstable or elaborate substrates may render isotopic label incorporation prohibitive. In other cases, the structure of substrates and their transition states may be too simple (e.g., in kinase reactions), such that structural information obtained from transition-state analysis is of no utility for inhibitor design. Additionally, intrinsic KIEs may be obscured by kinetically significant steps other than chemistry; however, alternative substrates, active site mutants, altered pH, and single-turnover analyses have been used to avoid these complications.[21,39] Finally, multiple steps in the enzymatic reaction coordinate, including substrate binding, and multiple chemical steps may contribute to the observed KIE, and these must be separated to establish the intrinsic KIE.[40–42]

Once the transition-state structure has been determined, aspects of its geometric and electrostatic properties can be incorporated into the design of appropriate chemically stable analogs. The remainder of this chapter demonstrates the methods of transition-state structure determination by the example of purine nucleoside phosphorylases and how this approach has led to the development of several generations of tight-binding inhibitors now in clinical trials for the treatment of various diseases.

PURINE NUCLEOSIDE PHOSPHORYLASE

Physiological role and basis for drug targeting

The cleavage of purine nucleosides (i.e., inosine and guanosine) and their 2′-deoxy counterparts is achieved by the phosphorolytic reaction catalyzed by PNP. This reaction forms a purine base (i.e., hypoxanthine or guanine) and (deoxy)ribose 1-phosphate (Figure 15.9) and is an essential process in human nucleoside metabolism and purine salvage. A rare genetic disorder of T-cell immunodeficiency has been attributed to a deficiency of PNP.[43,44] Without PNP, deoxyguanosine (dGuo) accumulates in the blood

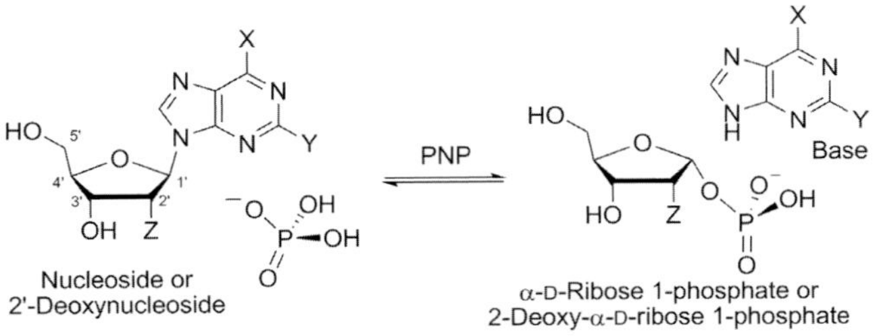

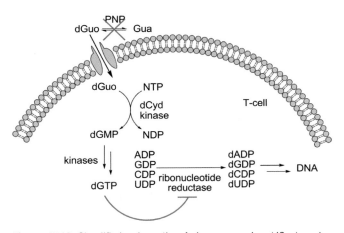

Nucleoside	Base	X	Y	Z
Inosine	Hypoxanthine	OH	H	OH or H
Guanosine	Guanine	OH	NH$_2$	OH or H
Adenosine	Adenine	NH$_2$	H	OH or H

Figure 15.9. Phosphorolysis of the purine nucleosides inosine (Ino), guanosine (Guo), and adenosine (Ado) catalyzed by PNP.

and is phosphorylated to deoxyguanosine monophosphate (dGMP) by deoxycytidine kinase most actively in rapidly dividing T cells (Figure 15.10).[43] Further phosphorylation to deoxyguanosine triphosphate (dGTP) causes inhibition of T-cell proliferation[45] and apoptosis.[46] This T-cell-specific effect has been exploited in the development of pharmaceuticals for the treatment of a variety of T-cell immunodisorders, including T-cell lymphoma, rheumatoid arthritis, lupus, psoriasis, and multiple sclerosis.[21]

Kinetic mechanism

The acid-catalyzed hydrolysis of purine nucleosides proceeds via N-7 protonation of the leaving group, followed by cleavage of the *N*-ribosidic bond to generate an oxacarbenium-ion intermediate, which is immediately

Figure 15.10. Simplified schematic of deoxyguanosine (dGuo) metabolism in human T cells. In the absence of PNP activity, high levels of dGuo are available for entry into T cells. Deoxycytidine (dCyd) kinase phosphorylates dGuo to dGMP, which, unlike the enzyme's normal product dCMP, does not cause product inhibition. Thus, dGMP is available for efficient conversion to dGTP, which allosterically inhibits ribonucleotide reductase-mediated production of deoxynucleosides and ultimately halts DNA synthesis and T-cell replication.

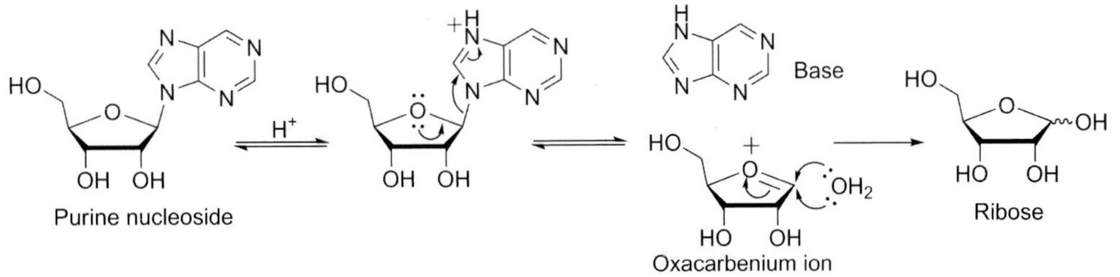

Figure 15.11. Mechanism of acid-catalyzed hydrolysis of purine nucleosides. Protonation at N7 increases the leaving-group ability of the purine base (substituents have been omitted for clarity). Donation of electrons from the ribosyl ring oxygen into the σ^* orbital at C1′ results in cleavage of the C–N glycosidic bond, generating an oxacarbenium ion. Nucleophilic attack by water on either face of the intermediate yields α- and β-ribose.

intercepted by a nucleophilic water molecule (Figure 15.11).[47] The transition-state structure of the acid-catalyzed hydrolysis of dAMP was recently solved, and direct evidence for the oxacarbenium-ion intermediate was obtained.[48] These findings have prompted enzymologists to question whether the PNP-catalyzed phosphorolysis reaction proceeds through a similar S_N1 mechanism.

To approach this problem, it was first necessary to establish the kinetic scheme of substrate and product binding, reaction, and release from the enzyme. Early studies on PNP from human erythrocytes indicated that phosphorolysis proceeds through a ternary complex consisting of phosphate and nucleoside bound to the enzyme,[49] without forming a covalent intermediate.[50] Kinetic studies on PNP from various sources, however, have not resulted in a consistent mechanism. For instance, an ordered Bi-Bi mechanism [Figure 15.12(a)][50] is commonly reported; Lewis and Lowry have proposed a Theorell-Chance mechanism, where phosphate binding, reaction, and release of ribose 1-phosphate occur so rapidly that the effective concentration of ternary complex is zero.[51] Whereas Kim et al.[50] and Lewis and Glantz[52] favored binding of the nucleoside prior to phosphate, Porter[53] and Carlson and Fischer[54] reported the opposite. Kline and Schramm demonstrated unequivocally through kinetic isotope effect determinations of

the arsenolysis reaction catalyzed by PNP that a random mechanism was in effect [Figure 15.12(b)].[55] Structural data provided by Ealick and coworkers supported this conclusion by showing that the active site could accommodate phosphate when inosine was already bound and vice versa but that binding of ribose 1-phosphate precluded the subsequent binding of hypoxanthine.[56] Fluorescence and radioactive binding titrations with hypoxanthine and guanine revealed that the release of nucleobase product, which is the rate-limiting step in steady-state kinetics, is facilitated by the presence of phosphate [Figure 15.12(b)].[57,58]

Transition-state structure of bovine PNP

Synthesis of labeled substrates

Determination of the transition-state structure of PNP required the synthesis of several substrate isotopologs (Figure 15.13).[55,59] The procedure was performed in two stages, each involving several enzymes and substrates in a single reaction mixture. In most cases, an appropriately radiolabeled glucose and/or ^{15}N-substitued adenine is converted to ATP, which is isolated by HPLC. Because H-3 of glucose is lost on formation of ribulose 5-phosphate, [2′-³H]ATP is synthesized from [2′-³H]ribose 5-phosphate

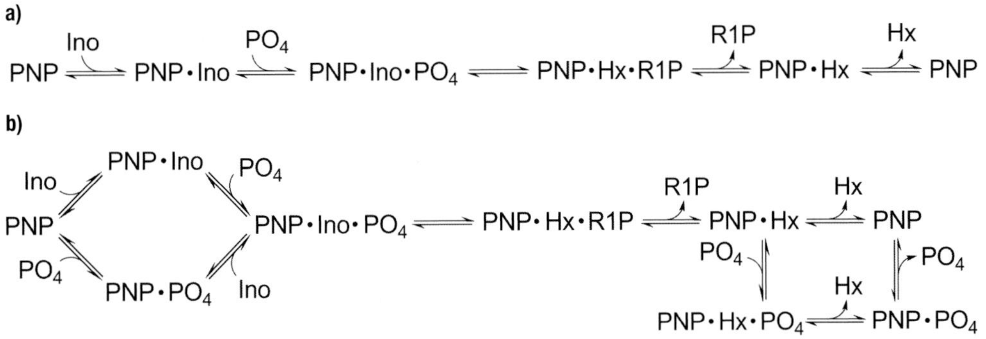

a)

b)

Figure 15.12. Proposed kinetic mechanisms for substrate binding, reaction, and product release from PNP. **(a)** Bi-Bi ordered sequential mechanism proposed by Kim et al.,[50] featuring nucleoside (e.g., inosine, Ino) and nucleobase (e.g., hypoxanthine, Hx) binding to free enzyme in phosphorolysis and synthesis directions, respectively. **(b)** Random sequential mechanism proposed by Kline and Schramm.[55] This mechanism, whose upper path is identical to that in **(a)**, additionally allows for ternary complex formation through binding of phosphate prior to nucleoside and accounts for the observation of looser binding of the nucleobase in the presence of phosphate.[57,58]

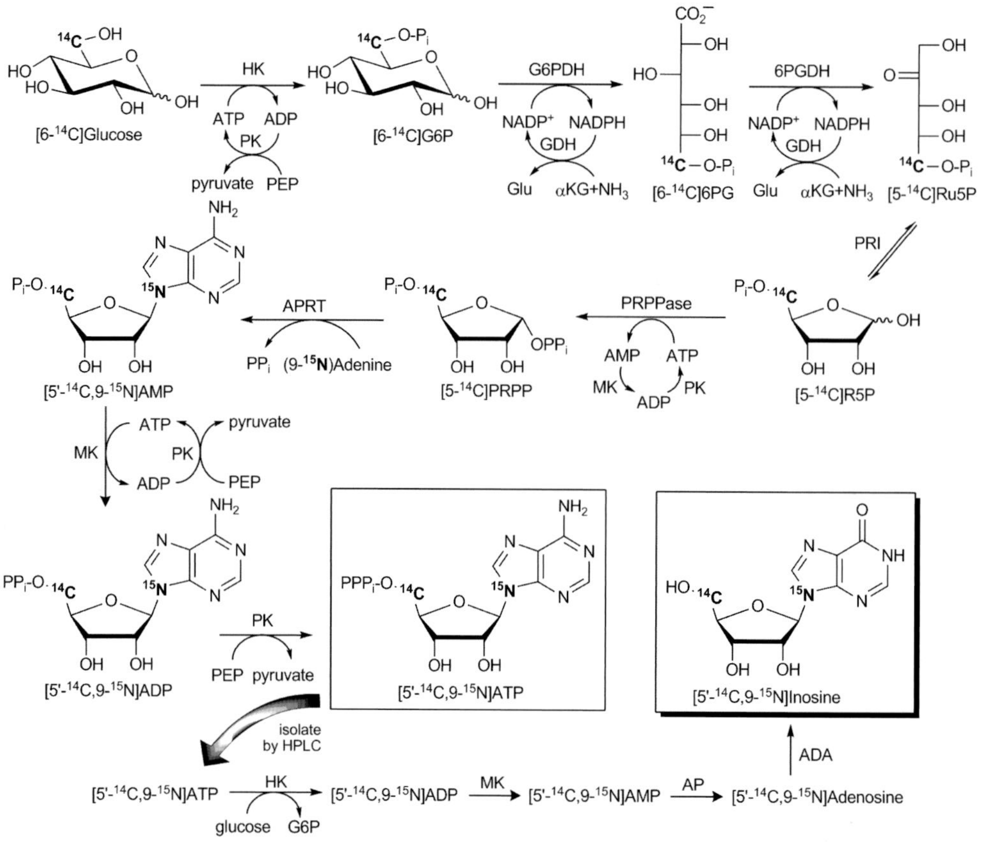

Figure 15.13. Synthetic scheme for the preparation of labeled inosine. In a single reaction mixture, glucose is converted to ATP, which is isolated by chromatography. In a second stage, ATP is dephosphorylated to adenosine, which is deaminated to inosine. Enzyme abbreviations: HK = hexokinase, PK = pyruvate kinase, G6PDH = glucose-6-phosphate dehydrogenase, GDH = glutamate dehydrogenase, 6PGDH = 6-phosphogluconic dehydrogenase, PRI = phosphoriboisomerase, PRPPase = 5-phosphoribosyl-1-pyrophosphate synthetase, MK = myokinase, APRT = adenine phosphoribosyltransferase, AP = alkaline phosphatase, ADA = adenosine deaminase. Chemical abbreviations: PEP = phosphoenolpyruvate, αKG = α-ketoglutarate, Glu = L-glutamate, G6P = D-glucose 6-phosphate, 6PG = 6-phosphogluconate, Ru5P = D-ribulose 5-phosphate, R5P = D-ribose 5-phosphate, PRPP = 5-phosphoribosyl 1-pyrophosphate. [1'-^{14}C]-, [5'-^{14}C]-, [1'-^{3}H]-, [4'-^{3}H]-, and [5'-^{3}H$_2$]inosine can be prepared from [2-^{14}C]-, [6-^{14}C]-, [2-^{3}H]-, [5-^{3}H]-, and [6-^{3}H$_2$]glucose, respectively. Remotely labeled [5'-^{14}C, 9-^{15}N]inosine is made from [6-^{14}C]glucose and (9-^{15}N)adenine (as shown), and [2'-^{3}H]inosine is prepared from [2-^{3}H]R5P, which is derived from the PRI-catalyzed incorporation of tritium from [^{3}H]H$_2$O.[60]

(R5P), prepared by solvent isotope exchange of unlabeled R5P with [^{3}H]H$_2$O catalyzed by phosphoriboisomerase.[60] The purified nucleotides are then dephosphorylated to adenosine, which is converted to inosine by adenosine deaminase.

Measurement of experimental kinetic isotope effects

KIEs for the phosphorolysis of [1'-^{2}H]inosine and [1'-^{2}H] adenosine by *Escherichia coli* PNP[61,62] or of [1'-^{3}H] inosine with *Bos taurus* PNP (BtPNP)[55] indicated masked KIEs, ranging from 1.008 to 1.094 at pH 7.3, with elevated KIEs at higher and lower pH. These findings indicate that events other than ribosidic bond cleavage, such as substrate binding, conformational changes, or product release, dominate at physiological pH. These commitment factors (recall 15.1.3) complicate the interpretation of KIEs, especially for reversible reactions such as this.[39] To minimize

these shortcomings, phosphate was substituted with arsenate, which reacts as a nucleophile to form ribose 1-arsenate, which readily hydrolyzes irreversibly to ribose and arsenate (Figure 15.14).[63] Accordingly, Kline and Schramm examined the transition state of BtPNP by measuring KIEs from the arsenolysis of inosine.[55] The procedure involved incubating the enzyme with a mixture of ^{3}H- and ^{14}C-labeled inosine in the presence of saturating arsenate. For ^{3}H KIE measurements, [5'-^{14}C]inosine served as a remote radiolabel for the ^{1}H species, whereas for ^{14}C or ^{15}N KIEs, [4'-^{3}H]- or [5'-^{3}H]inosine served as a remote radiolabel for the ^{12}C or ^{14}N species. Following about 30% reaction completion, a portion of the mixture was quenched by application to a charcoal column, which binds hypoxanthine and unreacted inosine through hydrophobic interactions while allowing the radiolabeled ribose product to be collected. The remainder of the mixture was allowed to

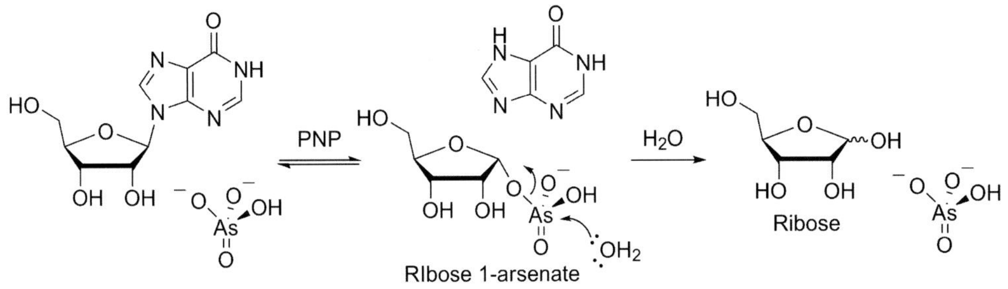

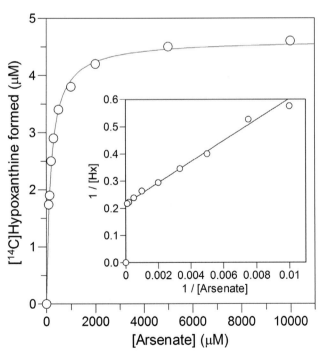

Figure 15.14. Arsenolysis reaction catalyzed by purine nucleoside phosphorylase. Ribose 1-arsenate is unstable and immediately hydrolyzes to ribose on release from the enzyme, rendering the overall reaction irreversible.

react to completion before being applied to a charcoal column. The $^3H/^{14}C$ ratios in the partially (R_p) and completely (R_o) converted samples were determined by scintillation counting, and the experimental V/K KIEs were calculated from Equation (15.2):

$$V/K \text{ KIE} = \frac{\ln(1 - f)}{\ln(1 - fR_p/R_o)}, \qquad (15.2)$$

where f is the fraction conversion of the light isotopolog, determined by the ratio of counts from the remote radio-label in partially versus completely converted samples.[35]

Correcting V/K KIEs for commitment to catalysis

To convert the V/K KIEs to intrinsic KIEs, Kline and Schramm determined the forward commitment for BtPNP

using the isotope-trapping technique described by Rose.[31] The experiment is designed to determine the partitioning of the first substrate in the binary complex reacting toward products versus dissociating into solution [Figure 15.8(c)]. The enzyme was briefly preincubated with [^{14}C]inosine, and this "pulse" solution was introduced into a "chase" solution consisting of varying concentrations of the second substrate, arsenate, and a pool of excess unlabeled inosine. The excess cold reactant ensures that radioactivity in the product results only from enzymatic turnover of the initial binary complex. After several turnovers, the relative amounts of [^{14}C]hypoxanthine product and unreacted [^{14}C]inosine were measured. The amount of [^{14}C]hypoxanthine formed increases hyperbolically with the concentration of arsenate, and the value at saturation indicates the concentration of bound inosine leading to products (Figure 15.15). Thus, by dividing this concentration by the concentration of dissociated inosine, the forward commitment, C_f, was found to be 0.19.[55] This value was used to calculate the intrinsic KIEs from the V/K KIEs by Equation (15.3), derived by Northrop:[39]

$$^3(V/K) = \frac{^3k + C_f + C_r{}^3K_{eq}}{1 + C_f + C_r} = \frac{^3k + C_f}{1 + C_f}, \qquad (15.3)$$

where $^3(V/K)$ is the experimental V/K KIE (tritium in this example), ^3k is the intrinsic KIE, $^3K_{eq}$ is the equilibrium isotope effect (EIE), and C_r is the reverse commitment, representing the partitioning of products returning to reactants versus dissociating from the enzyme. The rapid release of ribose 1-arsenate together with its irreversible hydrolysis was presumed to make C_r negligible,[55] thereby simplifying the equation as indicated. Equation (15.3) is valid only when there are no isotopically sensitive steps prior to chemistry. As will be discussed later in the chapter, however, this assumption is not always true, as in the case of isotope effects on binding.

Interpretation of KIEs for inosine arsenolysis

The magnitudes of [$1'$-^{14}C]-, [9-^{15}N]-, and [$1'$-^3H]inosine isotope effects are diagnostic for the degree of nucleophile association and leaving group dissociation at the transition state of the PNP reaction. At one extreme is the concerted, associative A_ND_N (S_N2) mechanism, which is characterized by synchronous nucleophile bond formation and

Figure 15.15. Determination of forward commitment by isotope trapping of the PNP·inosine binary complex. The pulse solution contained BtPNP and [8–^{14}C]inosine, and the chase solution contained excess unlabeled inosine and varying sodium arsenate concentrations from 0.1 to 10 mM. (Inset) double-reciprocal plot, whose y-intercept indicates the concentration of [^{14}C]hypoxanthine resulting from the trapped inosine. Modified from Kline and Schramm.[55]

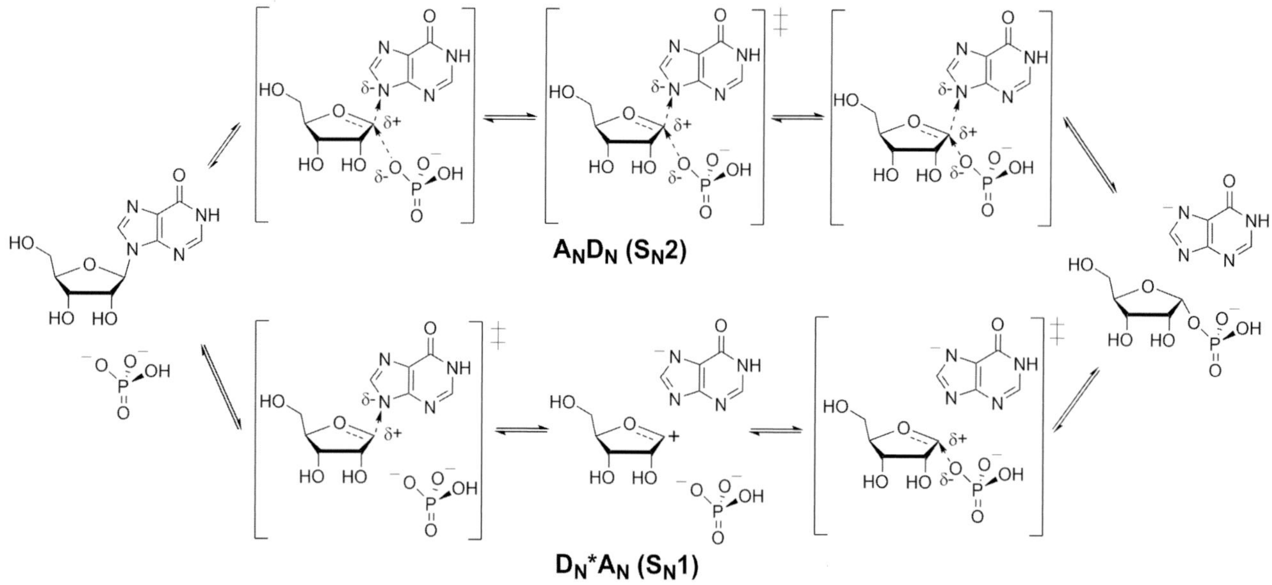

Figure 15.16. Possible mechanisms for the phosphorolysis (arsenolysis) of inosine. An A_ND_N mechanism (upper pathway) involves a single transition state characterized by concerted phosphate association and hypoxanthine dissociation. In a synchronous A_ND_N reaction (S_N2), the association and dissociation events are exactly balanced, and the transition state exists when the bond order to each group is equal, as in the middle structure. A $D_N{}^*A_N$ mechanism (S_N1, lower pathway) involves two distinct steps with two transition states; dissociation of hypoxanthine generates an oxacarbenium-ion intermediate (middle structure), and association of phosphate yields the ribose 1-phosphate product. In a D_NA_N reaction, the degree of dissociation exceeds the degree of association, and the transition state exists with unequal bond order to each group; because of the highly dissociative nature of this mechanism, it is also sometimes referred to as S_N1-like (differing from "true" S_N1 in the number of steps and transition states). Modified from Berti and McCann.[109]

leaving-group bond cleavage such that the net bond order to the reaction center (C-1′) is conserved (Figure 15.16). At the other extreme is the stepwise, dissociative $D_N{}^*A_N$ (S_N1) mechanism, in which the bond to the leaving group is completely broken to give a carbocationic intermediate, to which the nucleophile forms a bond in a second step. Many enzymatic substitution reactions lie somewhere between these two extremes as D_NA_N mechanisms,[64] having varying degrees of bond order to both groups throughout the reaction, with nucleophile bond formation trailing leaving-group departure. The 1′-^{14}C KIEs for A_ND_N and D_NA_N mechanisms vary inversely with the degree of dissociation, in the range 1.025–1.16, with highly synchronous reactions near the upper limit[65] and highly dissociative reactions near the lower limit.[60,66–79] $D_N{}^*A_N$ mechanisms, however, result in near-unity 1′-^{14}C KIEs, ranging around 0.99–1.02.[59,73,80–84] The 9-^{15}N KIEs increase as the N-ribosidic bond order decreases, ranging between 1.00 and 1.04 for zero and complete dissociation, respectively. The α-secondary KIEs resulting from hydrogen labeling at C-1′ are typically large (1.15–1.34) for both $D_N{}^*A_N$ and D_NA_N mechanisms, due to the change in orbital hybridization from sp^3 to sp^2 and the decrease in steric crowding that would otherwise dampen the out-of-plane bending mode of the C1′–H1′ bond at the transition state. In contrast, a synchronous A_ND_N mechanism would yield a low or inverse 1′-^{3}H KIE due to restricted bending resulting from increased steric crowding from

nucleophile and leaving-group participation at the transition state.

The experimental V/K and intrinsic KIEs for the arsenolysis of inosine by BtPNP are given in Table 15.1. The 1′-^{14}C KIE of 2.6% and 1′-^{3}H KIE of 14.1% are consistent with a dissociative A_ND_N mechanism. The 9-^{15}N KIE of

Table 15.1. Kinetic isotope effects for inosine arsenolysis catalyzed by bovine PNP

Isotope	Remote label	V/K KIE	Intrinsic KIE[a]
1′-^{14}C	5′-^{3}H	1.022 ± 0.005[d]	1.026 ± 0.006
9-^{15}N, 5′-^{14}C[b]	5′-^{3}H	1.009 ± 0.004[d]	1.010 ± 0.005
1′-^{3}H	5′-^{14}C[c]	1.118 ± 0.003	1.141 ± 0.004
2′-^{3}H	5′-^{14}C[c]	1.128 ± 0.003	1.152 ± 0.003
4′-^{3}H	5′-^{14}C[c]	1.007 ± 0.003	1.008 ± 0.004
5′-^{3}H	5′-^{14}C[c]	1.028 ± 0.004	1.033 ± 0.005

Notes: Reactions were in presence of 50 mM sodium arsenate at pH 7.5. Data adapted from Kline and Schramm.[55]

[a] Intrinsic KIEs were corrected from V/K KIEs using Equation (15.3) and $C_f = 0.19$.

[b] ^{14}C serves as a remote radiolabel for ^{15}N.

[c] The 5′-^{14}C KIE is assumed to be 1.

[d] Due to the KIE from the remote label, the V/K KIEs were corrected by multiplying by the 5′-^{3}H KIE.

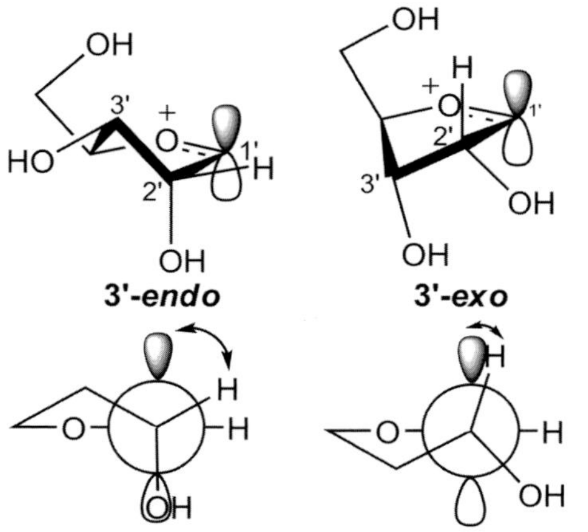

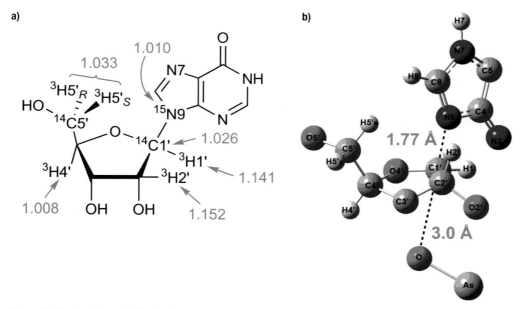

Figure 15.17. 3'-*Endo* and 3'-*exo* conformations of a ribooxacarbenium-ion transition state. Hyperconjugation between the 2'-C–H σ bond and the adjacent *p* orbital at C-1' is greater for the 3'-*exo* conformation due to better orbital overlap, as can be seen in the Newman projections (bottom). This generates a larger 2'-³H KIE.

1.0%, however, is very low for a highly dissociative mechanism as depicted in Figure 15.16. To account for this, it is proposed that hypoxanthine departs as the neutral, N7H tautomer rather than the anion during transition-state formation. N7 protonation enhances the leaving group ability of hypoxanthine and causes a decrease in C8–N9 bond order, which in turn results in a decreased 9-¹⁵N KIE.

The remaining isotope effects in the ribosyl moiety provide information on the ribose conformation at the transition state. Of these, the most important is the 2'-³H KIE, which results from hyperconjugation between the 2'-C–H σ-bond and the *p* orbital developing at C-1'. This electron donation serves to stabilize the oxacarbenium-ion transi-

tion state but weakens the C–H bond, resulting in a less restricted vibrational environment and therefore a fairly large, normal KIE. The extent of hyperconjugation and consequently the magnitude of the KIE are related to the geometry of orbital overlap, being maximal at 0° and minimal at 90°. Thus, a KIE >10% is typically indicative of a 3'-*exo* conformation, whereas a KIE <5%, is consistent with a 3'-*endo* conformation (Figure 15.17). The large 15.2% 2'-³H KIE observed for BtPNP clearly indicates that a 3'-*exo* conformation is assumed at the transition state. Being three and four bonds removed from the reaction center, respectively, the 4'-³H and 5'-³H KIEs would be expected to be close to unity, and this is observed for the former but not the latter. The significant 5'-³H KIE of 3.3% cannot be explained simply by effects within the substrate alone; rather, it reflects contributions from interactions with the enzyme, a finding that is common among many nucleoside transferases and hydrolases,[59,60,65–71,80] and this will be described in more detail in later sections of this chapter.

Computational modeling enabled Kline and Schramm to assemble the structure of the BtPNP-catalyzed transition state for inosine arsenolysis (Figure 15.18). The ground-state model of inosine was taken from crystallographic coordinates,[85] and this was compared by bond-vibrational analysis to varied approximations of the transition state until calculated KIEs best matched experimental values. The transition state occurs early in the reaction coordinate, as indicated by the significant C1'–N9 bond (1.77Å; bond order = 0.38) that still exists to the leaving group. The 3.0Å distance between C-1' and the nucleophilic oxygen of arsenate indicates that essentially no bonding has yet formed at the transition state.

With characteristics of the transition state in hand, it was possible to design and evaluate various stable analogs

Figure 15.18. Experimental KIEs for the arsenolysis of inosine **(a)** and transition-state geometry **(b)**. Only the atoms used in the computational analysis by Kline and Schramm are shown.[55]

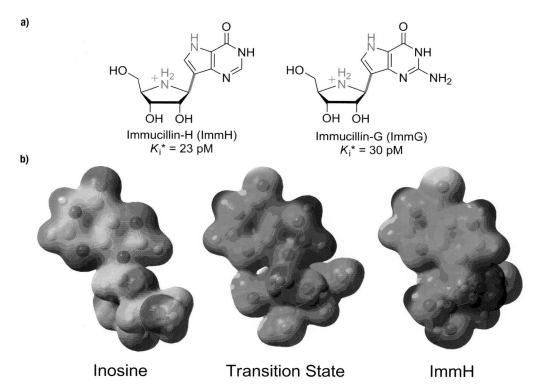

Figure 15.19. Immucillin-H (ImmH) and Immucillin-G (ImmG). **(a)** Structures of ImmH and ImmG with features based on the transition state shown in red. **(b)** Molecular electrostatic potential (MEP) surfaces for ground-state inosine, BtPNP transition state, and ImmH calculated using Gaussian03 and visualized with GaussView at a density of 0.008 electrons/bohr^3. Ball-and-stick models are superimposed with the surfaces. The color scale indicates regions that are electron rich (red) and electron deficient (blue). Positive-charge character can clearly be seen at N7 of the transition state and at the 4′-position of the ring in the analog, but these regions are electron rich in the reactant state.

incorporating these chemical features. The next section describes the first series of such analogs developed as potent inhibitors against BtPNP.

FIRST-GENERATION TRANSITION-STATE ANALOGS OF PNP: IMMUCILLINS

Immucillins as mimics of bovine PNP transition state

Comparison of ImmH with bovine PNP transition state

The key features of the BtPNP transition state that would be desirable to be included in the design of an analog include a partially charged ribooxacarbenium ion with significant bonding to the leaving group, protonation at N7 of hypoxanthine, and van der Waals contact to phosphate. Accordingly, Schramm and coworkers developed Immucillin-H (ImmH) and Immucillin-G (ImmG) [Figure 15.19(a)].[86] These compounds possess an imino group with a pK_a of 6.9,[87] providing some positive charge character at physiological pH. The replacement of N9 with a carbon provided a C–C ribosidic linkage, preventing the susceptibility to hydrolysis or phosphorolysis exhibited by substrates. This modification also altered the conjugation in the imidazole ring such that the pK_a of N7 was elevated

from ~2 in inosine and guanosine to ~9 in ImmH and ImmG.[88] Although the pK_a of N7 at the transition state is not known, it has been estimated to be ≥7 as the ribosidic bond becomes cleaved. The effect of including a proton at N7 is similar to that observed with N7-methyl derivatives of inosine and guanosine,[89] which function as substrates with enhanced reactivity, due to their ability to assist the purine to accept electrons from the ribosidic bond.

Although the modifications introduced into ImmH impose no steric alterations relative to inosine, they do result in a major change in the molecular electrostatic potential (MEP) surface [Figure 15.19(b)]. Whereas the reactant state bears an abundance of electron density at the ring oxygen and at N7, the transition state and ImmH exhibit a great reduction in electron density in these regions. The MEP similarity shared between a transition state and its analog has been demonstrated for several enzymes to correlate with the observed affinity of the enzyme for the inhibitor.[90,91] Thus, ImmH was expected to be a potent transition-state inhibitor of PNP.

Synthesis of Immucillins

ImmH and ImmG were first synthesized by a linear scheme of over twenty steps (Figure 15.20, Path A).[92] Although this provided proof of concept, this method is impractical for

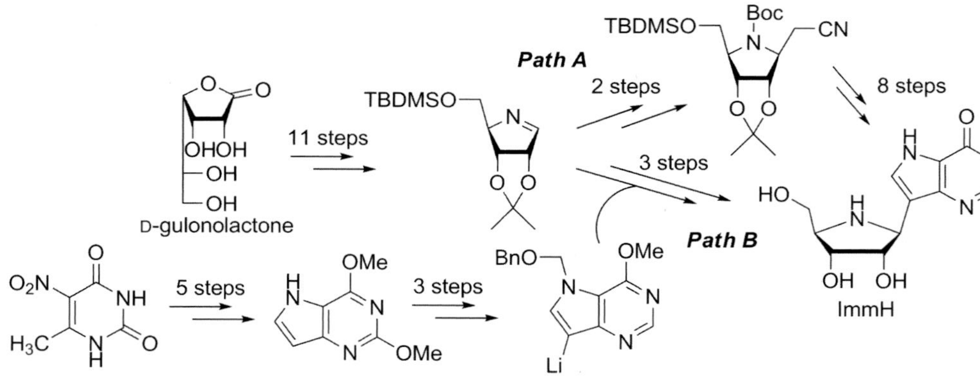

Figure 15.20. Synthesis of ImmH by linear (Path A) and convergent (Path B) strategies.

large-scale production. Evans et al. reconfigured the preparation as a convergent synthesis (Figure 15.20, Path B), enabling efficient scale-up for use in biological and pharmaceutical studies.[93]

Inhibition of bovine PNP by Immucillins

Determination of dissociation constants for slow-onset inhibition

As mimics of the transition state, ImmH and ImmG bind competitively versus substrate to the active site of PNP. The PNP-catalyzed phosphorolysis of inosine in the presence of these analogs was monitored by coupling the hypoxanthine product to xanthine oxidase, converting it to uric acid, which provides a chromophoric species for continuous UV detection [Figure 15.21(a)].[86] Following a brief period of moderate inhibition, a second, strongly inhibited stage was observed in inhibited samples [Figure 15.21(b)]. These characteristics are common to slow-onset, tight-binding inhibitors, which bind reversibly as competitive inhibitors during the first stage, but then a slow conformational change in the enzyme increases binding and restricts their dissociation [Figure 15.21(a)]. Fitting initial and final rates to the equation for competitive inhibition [Equation (15.4)] enabled the determination of K_i and K_i^*, the dissociation constants for the initial, weakly bound complex and the final, tightly bound complex, respectively [Figure 15.21(c)]:

$$v_i = \frac{v_o [S]}{[S] + K_m (1 + [I]/K_i)}, \qquad (15.4)$$

where v_i and v_o are rates in the presence and absence of inhibitor, respectively, and K_m is the Michaelis constant. Equation (15.4) is valid when the concentration of inhibitor is at least tenfold greater than the concentration of enzyme; otherwise, the concentration of free inhibitor must be corrected for the amount bound to the enzyme [Equation (15.5)]:

$$[I]_{free} = [I]_{total} - (1 - v_i/v_o) \times [E]. \qquad (15.5)$$

ImmH was found to be a potent inhibitor having a K_i of 41 nM and K_i^* of 23 pM.[86] Thus, ImmH binds 740,000 times more tightly to PNP than inosine, as indicated by the K_m / K_i^* ratio. The rate of conformational rearrangement leading to the 2,000-fold increase in affinity from E·I to E*·I was calculated to be governed by a rate constant of formation, k_5, of 0.06 s^{-1} and of release, k_6, of only 0.000 04 s^{-1}, corresponding to a $t_{1/2}$ of 4.8 h.

Stoichiometry of transition-state analog binding

The active form of mammalian PNPs consists of a homotrimer of 32-kDa subunits,[94] and the stoichiometry of transition-state analog binding was determined. Following an incubation period of 3–4 h in the presence of phosphate, mixtures of BtPNP and ImmH or ImmG at varying ratios were mixed with inosine and assayed for activity. A plot of initial rate versus moles of inhibitor per mole of trimer revealed that binding of only one molecule per trimer gives complete inhibition (Figure 15.22). The one-third-the-sites inhibition indicates cooperativity between subunits, whereby occupation of one subunit is sufficient to prevent catalysis at all three sites. This conclusion is additionally supported by the observation that, in the absence of phosphate, one PNP trimer hydrolyzes one molecule of inosine, resulting in the formation of a tightly bound hypoxanthine ($K_d = 1.3$ pM) at one of the subunits.[58] Occupation of one of the three active sites precludes reactivity with a second molecule of inosine. Earlier kinetic studies and x-ray structures had revealed that various ligands, including substrates, products, and inhibitors, bind symmetrically at all three sites.[95] It is apparent, therefore, that the binding sites exhibit differing ligand affinities depending on occupancy, with the first site filling with the tightest affinity (i.e., picomolar), followed by the second and third sites with much weaker binding (i.e., micromolar).[88,96]

Crystal structure of bovine PNP with ImmH

Bovine PNP was crystallized in the presence of excess ImmH and phosphate to ensure symmetric occupancy of the three subunits of the trimer.[97] Comparisons of the 1.5Å structure to previously solved structures of PNP complexes

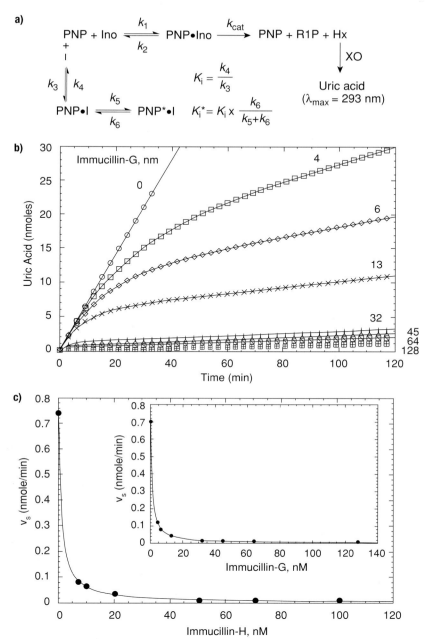

Figure 15.21. Kinetics of slow-onset inhibition of PNP by ImmH and ImmG. **(a)** In the kinetic scheme, I = inhibitor, Ino = inosine, R1P = ribose 1-phosphate, Hx = hypoxanthine, PNP* = tight-binding conformation of PNP, XO = xanthine oxidase. Phosphate is present at all steps but has been omitted for clarity. Equations in terms of rate constants are given for K_i, the dissociation constant for the initial weakly bound complex, and K_i^*, the dissociation constant for the tightly bound complex. **(b)** Slow-onset inhibition kinetic profiles measured for BtPNP in the presence of ImmH at the concentrations indicated. Hypoxanthine formation is monitored by conversion to uric acid by xanthine oxidase. **(c)** The rate during the second stage of inhibition (v_s) is plotted against the inhibitor concentration to calculate the dissociation constant, K_i^*. Graphs are from Miles et al.[86]

introduced or made stronger in the PNP·ImmH·PO$_4$ complex [Figure 15.23(b)] compared to the PNP·inosine·SO$_4$ complex (Figure 15.23). Additionally, the nucleophilic oxygen of the phosphate has been brought nearly 1Å closer to C-1′ and forms an ion pair with the cationic N-4′. The 3.2Å distance between the nucleophile and the anomeric carbon of ImmH is consistent with the structure for the early dissociative transition state determined by Kline and Schramm.[55] Continued progress to products is accompanied with relaxation of nine atomic contacts with the enzyme [Figure 15.23(c)].

Of particular interest from the structural comparisons is the discovery of unprecedented motion in the reaction coordinate. First, the protein immobilizes the phosphate and hypoxanthine groups within the active site through a network of hydrogen bonds. Then, generation of the ribooxacarbenium-ion transition state occurs as the enzyme brings the 5′-hydroxyl and nucleophilic oxygen of the phosphate into alignment with the ring oxygen (nitrogen in ImmH) in an "oxygen stack" (Figure 15.24).[24] Dynamic vibrational compression of the three oxygen atoms introduces localized electron density that increases the leaving-group ability of the purine base through stabilization of the developing oxacarbenium-ion transition state. This hypothesis is further supported by quantum mechanical/molecular mechanical calculations, which demonstrated a correlation between catalysis and the motions of O-5′ and O$_P$ toward O-4′.[15] The negative charge that this stack motion introduces into the purine ring is neutralized by the stronger H-bond interactions to N1, O6, and N7 observed in the transition-state analog complex. The nucleophilic phosphate anion, located directly below the anomeric carbon, attracts electrophile migration to form the phosphate ester bond. The positions of the phosphate and of the 5′-end of the ribooxacarbenium ion remain fixed during the 1.7Å movement of C-1′, which is best visualized by a superposition of the transition-state analog and ribose 1-phosphate (Figure 15.25). As there are no enzyme residues in proximity of the anomeric carbon, this migration occurs without the need for protein motion. This "nucleophilic displacement by electrophile migration" mechanism, as it has been termed,[97] is common to many N-ribosyltransferases including PNPs from other species, purine phosphoribosyltransferases,[64,98–100] orotate

with inosine and ribose 1-phosphate[95] reveal important structural changes that occur as the enzyme progresses from the Michaelis complex, through the transition state, to products. In particular, six hydrogen bonds were either

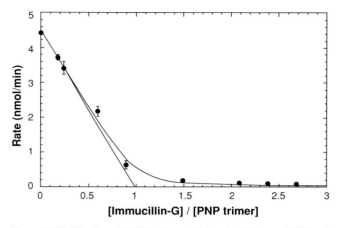

Figure 15.22. Titration of BtPNP trimer with ImmG. Mixtures of PNP and varying concentrations of inhibitor were preincubated for 3–4 h, inosine was added, and production of hypoxanthine was monitored by the xanthine oxidase coupled assay. Initial reaction rates are plotted against the ratio of moles of ImmG to moles of PNP trimer.

phosphoribosyltransferase (OPRT),[101] sirtuins,[102] DNA-uracil glycosylase,[82,103] and lysozyme.[104]

Protein dynamics with bound ImmH

As indicated by the slow-onset, tight-binding nature of inhibition, the association of ImmH in PNP's active site induces a conformational change that causes the protein to condense around the transition-state analog in a relatively static, stable complex. This structure not only greatly restricts release of inhibitor from its active site but also hinders access from solvent.

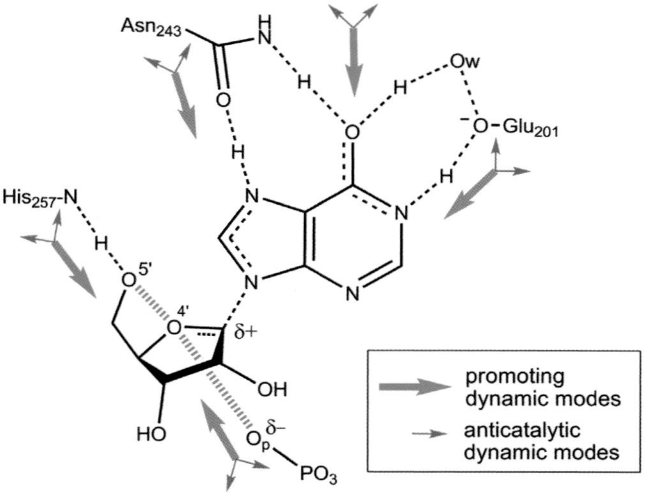

Figure 15.24. Dynamic vibrational modes leading to generation of the transition state. Reaction-promoting motions are represented by the larger, green arrows, while examples of anticatalytic vibrational modes are shown as smaller, red arrows. Localized electron density generated from dynamic compression (green dashed lines) of the "oxygen stack," consisting of O-5′ and O-4′ of inosine and O_P of the phosphate nucleophile, stabilizes the developing oxacarbenium ion and introduces electron density into the purine leaving group. Neighboring enzymatic residues stabilize this negative charge density by the formation of hydrogen bonds, which were either much weaker or nonexistent in the Michaelis complex. Modified from Schramm.[24]

The limited dynamic motion in the transition-state analog-bound enzyme was revealed in a hydrogen/deuterium (H/D) solvent exchange study by Wang and coworkers.[96] Introduction of a protein sample into D_2O causes deuterium incorporation into the solvent-accessible

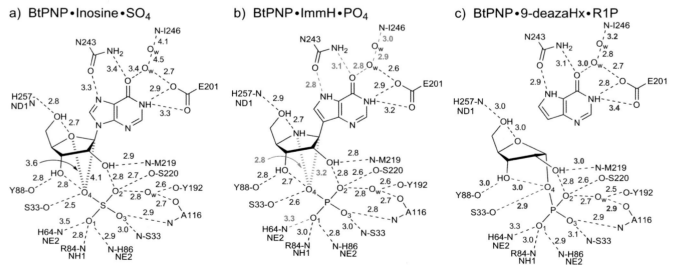

Figure 15.23. Structures of BtPNP complexed with **(a)** substrate analogs (inosine and SO_4), **(b)** transition-state analog (ImmH and PO_4), and **(c)** product analogs (9-deazahypoxanthine and ribose 1-phosphate), based on atomic positions in the x-ray crystal structures (PDB IDs 1A9S,[95] 1B80,[97] and 1A9T,[95] respectively). Hydrogen-bond distances are indicated in angstroms. Conversion from the reactant state to the transition state introduces six stronger H-bonds and closer contacts (red). Once past the transition state, nine H-bonds and contacts relax (blue) in the product complex. Modified from Fedorov et al.[97]

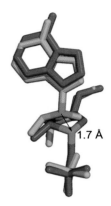

1.7 Å

Figure 15.25. Electrophile migration in the mechanism of inosine phosphorolysis by PNP. The crystal structures of the PNP·ImmH·PO$_4$ and PNP·hypoxanthine·ribose 1-phosphate complexes were overlaid; shown are only the ligands ImmH/PO$_4$ (cyan) and Hx/R1P (red). C-1′ is indicated in green.

backbone amides. Although surface amides exchange readily, on the order of seconds or faster, those buried in the hydrophobic protein interior do not exchange without treatment with denaturants. Intermediate residues exchange slowly, on the order of minutes to hours, requiring motion of the protein for solvent exposure; it is these dynamically accessible amides that may be distinguished when comparing H/D exchange of various enzyme/ligand complexes. The BtPNP apoprotein was found to exchange 122 of its amides rapidly, followed by a slower exchange of fifty additional positions (Figure 15.26). Introduction of formycin B, a substrate analog, or hypoxanthine blocked the exchange of ten of these amides, but in the presence of ImmH, thirty-two protons were protected. Although formycin B and ImmH are isosteric, it is apparent that the

Table 15.2. Kinetic isotope effects for inosine arsenolysis catalyzed by human PNP

Isotope	Remote label	V/K KIE	Intrinsic KIE[a]
1′-^{14}C	4′-^{3}H	1.002 ± 0.006[d]	1.002 ± 0.006
9-^{15}N, 4′-^{3}H[b]	5′-^{14}C	1.025 ± 0.006[d]	1.029 ± 0.006
1′-^{3}H	5′-^{14}C[c]	1.160 ± 0.004	1.184 ± 0.004
2′-^{3}H	5′-^{14}C[c]	1.024 ± 0.004	1.031 ± 0.004
4′-^{3}H	5′-^{14}C[c]	1.021 ± 0.003	1.024 ± 0.003
5′-^{3}H	5′-^{14}C[c]	1.054 ± 0.002	1.062 ± 0.002

Notes: Reactions were in presence of 50 mM sodium arsenate at pH 7.5. Data adapted from Lewandowicz and Schramm.[59]
[a] Intrinsic KIEs were corrected from V/K KIEs using Equation (15.3) and $C_f = 0.147$; errors do not include error from C_f.
[b] ^{3}H serves as a remote radiolabel for ^{15}N.
[c] The 5′-^{14}C KIE is assumed to be 1.
[d] Due to the KIE from the remote label, the V/K KIEs were corrected by multiplying by the 4′-^{3}H KIE.

10^6-fold difference in their binding affinities accounts for the observed differences in H/D exchange. Thus, this study demonstrated that formation of the Michaelis complex results in some degree of restricted protein motion but that binding of transition-state analogs captures the enzyme in a collapsed state with greatly reduced dynamics.

HUMAN PNP AND SECOND-GENERATION TRANSITION-STATE ANALOGS: DADME-IMMUCILLINS

Human PNP

The transition-state structure analysis with bovine PNP and development of the Immucillin inhibitors served as a confirmation of the principles relating enzymatic transition-state formation to tight-binding interactions with transition-state analogs. As indicated earlier (see "Physiological role and basis for drug targeting"), PNP has been linked to a rare T-cell immunodeficiency and consequently has been implicated as a drug target for T-cell lymphoma and various autoimmune diseases. Thus, in the context of drug development, it is essential to establish that the transition-state analog methodology extends to the human ortholog of PNP.

Human PNP transition state

Human PNP (HsPNP) shares 87% amino acid sequence identity with BtPNP, with active-site residues being almost completely conserved. Despite this strong similarity, though, the transition states of the two orthologs were found to be different. As before, arsenolysis of labeled inosines was used to measure kinetic isotope effects for HsPNP (Table 15.2).[59] The most diagnostic of these KIEs is that from the anomeric carbon. A 1′-^{14}C KIE of

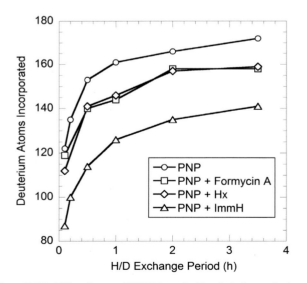

Figure 15.26. H/D exchange of BtPNP bound with substrate, product, and transition-state analogs. The number of deuterium atoms introduced into each protein complex in D$_2$O as a function of time was determined by electrospray ionization mass spectrometry (ESI-MS). Hx = hypoxanthine; formycin B = 8-aza-9-deazainosine. Modified from Wang et al.[96]

0.2% is consistent with a $D_N{}^*A_N$ mechanism, wherein a discrete oxacarbenium-ion intermediate is generated, whose corresponding transition state bears complete dissociation of the leaving group and no significant bond order to the nucleophile; both groups are only in van der Waals contact (>3.0Å) with the ribooxacarbenium ion (Figure 15.27). The relatively large KIEs for $1'$-^{3}H (18.4%) and 9-^{15}N (2.9%) lend additional support for this S_N1 mechanism. These values are both larger than those found in BtPNP, where a Pauling bond order of 0.4 was found for the ribosidic bond at the transition state. Furthermore, a $2'$-^{3}H KIE of 3.1% established that, in contrast to BtPNP, the ribosyl moiety adopts a 3-*endo* conformation, placing the 2-C–H bond at a dihedral angle of 57.3° to the empty p orbital at C-1.

Comparing bovine and human PNP transition states indicates that BtPNP has the earlier transition state, closer to reactants than to products, while HsPNP has a later transition state, resembling a fully developed ribooxacarbenium-ion intermediate (Figure 15.28). According to transition-state theory, this distinction in transition-state structure between the two enzymes may be manifested in inhibition with analogs designed with specific features of the transition state.

Inhibition of Human PNP with Immucillins

When the transition state of HsPNP was solved in 2004, a family of Immucillin-based inhibitors with substitutions and small modifications in the iminoribitol and deazahypoxanthine moieties had been characterized with BtPNP (Figure 15.29).[105,106] Along with the parent compounds ImmH and ImmG, these analogs were tested as inhibitors for both BtPNP and HsPNP. Most of these compounds exhibited the slow-onset, tight-binding inhibition profiles familiar for ImmH and ImmG, resulting in picomolar or low nanomolar inhibition constants. In all cases, the final dissociation constants, K_i^*, were higher with HsPNP than with BtPNP. With ImmH and ImmG, for example, K_i^* values of 58 and 42 pM, respectively, were measured, but with BtPNP, the corresponding values were 23 and 30 pM.[41,106,107] This trend in dissociation constant differences between the two PNP enzymes suggested that the degree of inhibition is correlated to the structural similarity between the transition state and its mimics.

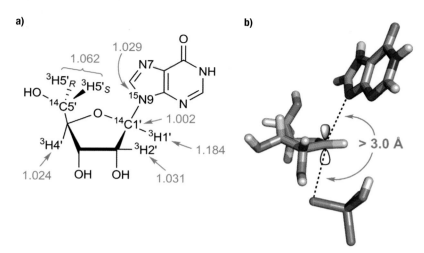

Figure 15.27. Experimental KIEs for inosine arsenolysis by human PNP **(a)** and computationally determined transition-state geometry **(b)**. The unity $1'$-^{14}C KIE indicates complete dissociation of hypoxanthine and no significant bond order to arsenate; thus, these groups are only in van der Waals contact (> 3.0Å) with the ribooxacarbenium ion. The 2'-C–H bond makes a 57.3° dihedral angle with the p orbital at C-1'. This angle places the ribosyl ring in a 3-*endo* conformation.

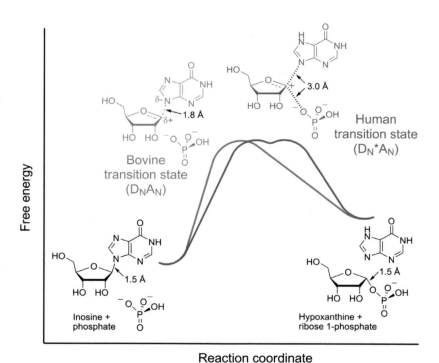

Figure 15.28. Comparison of the reaction coordinates for the reactions catalyzed by bovine and human PNPs. The BtPNP-catalyzed reaction (D_NA_N, red) proceeds through an early transition state, resembling reactants more than products, with a C–N distance of 1.8Å. The HsPNP-catalyzed reaction ($D_N{}^*A_N$, green) proceeds through an oxacarbenium ion intermediate, with > 3.0Å separation from both leaving group and nucleophile. The transition state resembles the intermediate (either just before or after), occurring later in the reaction coordinate than that of BtPNP. Adapted from Taylor Ringia and Schramm.[141]

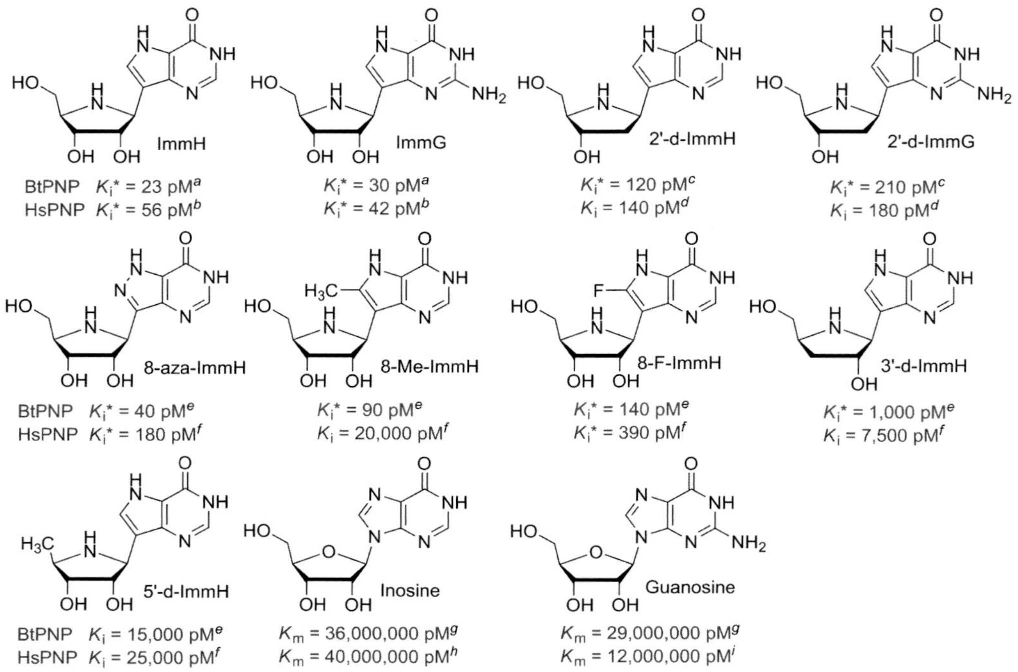

Figure 15.29. Selected Immucillin inhibitors and dissociation constants for bovine and human PNPs. The tightest values are reported – K_i^* in cases of slow-onset inhibition, K_i in other cases. *Sources:* [a] Miles et al.,[86] [b] Evans et al.,[106] [c] Taylor Ringia et al.,[114] [d] Lewandowicz et al.,[117] [e] Kicska et al.,[105] [f] Kicska et al.,[142] [g] Barsacchi et al.,[143] [h] Erion et al.,[56] [i] Stoeckler et al.[144]

DADMe-Immucillins

Comparison of DADMe-ImmH with human PNP transition state

To establish the most powerful inhibitors for human PNP, distinct features of its transition state need to be exploited. A good HsPNP transition-state mimic should include a cationic ribose analog with chemical stability at the anomeric position and only van der Waals contact to phosphate. Distinct from the BtPNP transition-state analog the distance from the leaving group to the 1′-carbocation is greater for HsPNP and needs to be increased in analogs specific for this enzyme. DADMe-Immucillin-H (DADMe-ImmH, abbreviated from 4′-Deaza-1′-Aza-2′-Deoxy-1′,9-Methylene-ImmH) and DADMe-Immucillin-G (DADMe-ImmG) were prepared as second-generation transition-state analogs specific for HsPNP [Figure 15.30(a)]. DADMe-ImmH and DADMe-ImmG were found to inhibit HsPNP with K_i^* values of 11[41] and 7 pM,[107] respectively, corresponding to 2,000,000- to 3,600,000-fold tighter binding than substrates, based on K_m/K_d values. These inhibition values are five- to tenfold lower than the corresponding ImmH and ImmG values with the human enzyme, indicating that HsPNP transition-state features are better captured by these second-generation inhibitors.

The DADMe-Immucillins possess an *N*-substituted hydroxymethylpyrrolidine ring, which is known to have a pK_a near 10 and therefore is nearly fully protonated at

physiological pH values.[108] The nitrogen cationic mimic of the carbocation was moved from the 4′ position to the anomeric position, which has been demonstrated to be the center in the ribooxacarbenium ion that bears the greatest positive charge.[30,109] Placing nitrogen at this position of the nucleoside analog creates chemical instability in the presence of an α-alcohol group. Because 2′-deoxy derivatives of nucleosides (i.e., deoxyinosine and deoxyguanosine) are good substrates for PNP, chemical instability is avoided by preparing these modified Immucillin analogs as 2′-deoxy compounds. Another significant alteration to the Immucillin structure is the introduction of a methylene linker between N-1′ and C-9. The result of this modification is to increase the distance to the leaving group from 1.5Å in ImmH to 2.5Å in DADMe-ImmH.

The electronic impact of the alterations is illustrated in the MEPs for DADMe-ImmH [Figure 15.30(b)]. Both ImmH and DADMe-ImmH capture electrostatic features of the transition state much more than inosine because of the iminoribitol ring. A major distinction between the two analogs is the location of the positive charge; DADMe-ImmH, as in the oxacarbenium-ion transition state, places this charge at the 1′ position, making it a better match to the transition state for HsPNP.

Synthesis of DADMe-Immucillins

DADMe-ImmH and DADMe-ImmG were first synthesized by an extension of the methods used for preparation

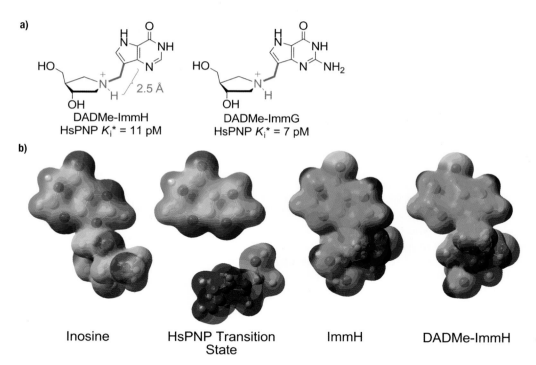

Figure 15.30. DADMe-Immucillin-H (DADMe-ImmH) and DADMe-Immucillin-G (DADMe-ImmG). **(a)** Structures of DADMe-ImmH and DADMe-ImmG with features based on the transition state shown in red. Dissociation constants are indicated for BtPNP and HsPNP. *Sources*: DADMe-ImmH, Murkin et al.[41]; DADMe-ImmG, Lewandowicz et al.[107] **(b)** Molecular electrostatic potential (MEP) surfaces for ground-state inosine, HsPNP transition state, ImmH, and DADMe-ImmH, calculated using Gaussian03 and visualized with GaussView at a density of 0.008 electrons/bohr^3. Positive-charge character found at C-1 of the ribooxacarbenium-ion transition state, though close to this vicinity in ImmH, is found at this position in DADMe-ImmH.

of ImmH and ImmG. The lithium-protected purine (Figure 15.20) was formylated to the aldehyde, which was reductively aminated with (3R,4R)-3-hydroxy-4-(hydroxymethyl) pyrrolidine and deprotected to give DADMe-ImmH (Figure 15.31, Path A).[110] This method required the convergent synthesis of the pyrrolidine (thirteen steps) and aldehyde (nine steps) and was therefore of similar efficiency

as the preparation of ImmH. A more elegant method was achieved through the formaldehyde-mediated Mannich reaction between the pyrrolidine and 9-deazahypoxanthine (Figure 15.31, Path B).[111] This mild reaction, complete in a single step with no need for protecting groups, shortened the synthesis by six steps before the Mannich condensation step.[112]

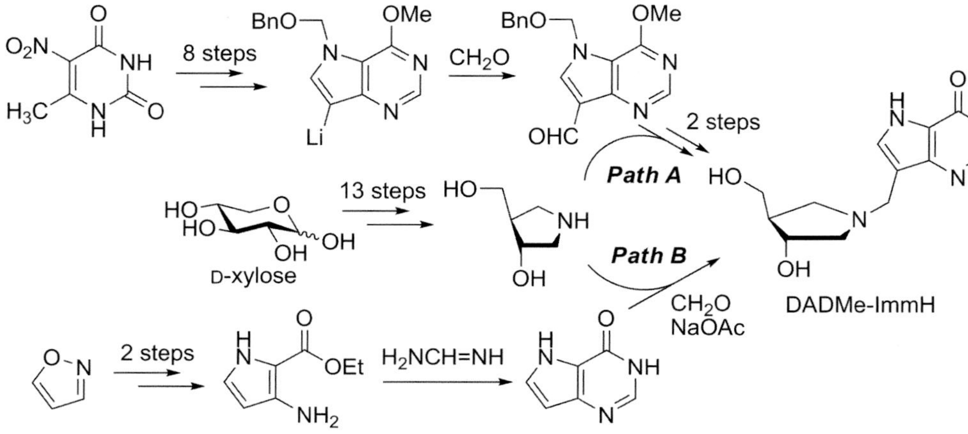

Figure 15.31. Synthesis of DADMe-ImmH by reductive amination (Path A) or Mannich reaction (Path B). Synthesis by the Mannich reaction is more efficient by seven steps. The pyrrolidine nitrogen of DADMe-ImmH becomes protonated when dissolved in aqueous solutions at pH < 10.

Crystal structure of human PNP with DADMe-ImmH

Human PNP was crystallized in the presence of DADMe-ImmH and sulfate (PDB 1RSZ), mimics of the oxacarbenium-ion transition state and phosphate.[41] For comparison, the human enzyme was crystallized with ImmH and phosphate (PDB 1RR6) or sulfate (1RT9); the structures are nearly identical to that of bovine PNP described earlier. The fold of the HsPNP protein structure is unchanged by substitution of DADMe-ImmH in place of ImmH [Figure 15.32(a)]. Close examination of the active site reveals that the hydrogen-bond network is tightened in the complex with DADMe-ImmH [Figure 15.32(b) and 15.32(c)]. In particular, three hydrogen bonds to the 9-deazahypoxanthine moiety have become 0.2 to 0.6Å shorter, and the phenolic oxygen of Tyr88 has moved 0.3Å closer to O-3'. The absence of the 2'-hydroxyl group in DADMe-ImmH, which is H-bonded only to O_3 of phosphate in the ImmH complex, permits a water molecule to occupy this site and to form hydrogen bonds with N-1' and O-3' of DADMe-ImmH and O_4 and O_3 of sulfate. These bridging H-bonds are proposed to compensate for losses due to the absence of the 2'-hydroxyl group.

The ion-pair interaction between the transition-state analog and phosphate (sulfate) is also of significance. Placing the cationic atom of DADMe-ImmH at the 1' position in addition to insertion of the methylene group results in closer proximity of the pyrrolidine cation toward the nucleophilic anion. The C-1'–O_4 distance in the HsPNP·ImmH·PO_4 complex is 3.5Å, while the N-1'–O_4 distance in the HsPNP·DADMe-ImmH·SO_4 complex is 3.0Å. The presence of a methylene bridge linking the pyrrolidine and deazahypoxanthine groups introduces a geometric change to separate these moieties by 1.0Å relative to ImmH, enabling them to interact more favorably with enzymatic residues and the nucleophile. ImmH is cationic in the active site of HsPNP[87] and forms a 3.5Å ion pair with phosphate [green dashed line in Figure 15.32(b)]. DADMe-ImmH establishes a 3.0Å ion pair [green dashed line in Figure 15.32(c)]. A similarly improved ion-pair association was also observed for these ligands with PNP from *Mycobacterium tuberculosis*.[113] According to Coulomb's law, the tighter ion pair could stabilize the binding energy by as much as 15.7 kcal/mol (assuming a dielectric constant of 1).

MECHANISTIC IMPLICATIONS FROM TWO GENERATIONS OF PNP INHIBITORS

Transition-state discrimination by selective inhibition of PNPs

Transition-state studies with bovine and human PNPs established that the same chemical reaction can be altered through subtle differences in enzyme/substrate interactions. The BtPNP-catalyzed reaction proceeds through a $D_N A_N$ mechanism, with transition-state formation early in the reaction coordinate and significant bond order to the leaving group (Figure 15.28). Despite the 87% sequence identity between the enzymes, HsPNP uses a stepwise D_N*A_N mechanism, in which the transition state occurs later in the reaction coordinate, closely resembling the ribooxacarbenium-ion/hypoxanthine intermediate.

Transition-state theory predicts that differences in transition-state structure should be manifested in the tightness of binding of transition-state analogs. This hypothesis was probed by exploring the relative affinities of BtPNP and HsPNP for various representatives from the Immucillin and DADMe-Immucillin families.[114] The Immucillins were modeled after the BtPNP transition state, with the key features being a short iminoribitol-base distance, iminoribocationic character, and N7 protonation. The DADMe-Immucillins incorporated aspects of the more dissociative HsPNP transition state, including greater pyrrolidine-base separation and relocation of the positively charged nitrogen to the 1'-position. When tested against BtPNP, ImmH is a stronger inhibitor than DADMe-ImmH, with dissociation constants of 23 and 110 pM, respectively (Table 15.3). However, HsPNP has opposite affinities for these inhibitors, with K_i^* values of 58 and 11 pM, respectively. A similar inhibition pattern was observed with ImmG and DADMe-ImmG. 2'-Deoxy-ImmH and 2'-deoxy-ImmG were tested against the enzymes to assess the contribution of the 2'-hydroxyl. Both compounds bound less tightly ($K_i^* = $ 120–210 pM) to BtPNP and HsPNP than their 2'-hydroxy counterparts without preference for human or bovine PNPs. Finally, ImmH and DADMe-ImmH analogs without pyrrolidine hydroxyl groups were tested against the two enzymes. Although removal of the hydroxyls elevated the dissociation constants into the nanomolar range, geometric differences between these compounds were sufficient to show preferential binding of the ImmH analog to BtPNP and of the DADMe-ImmH analog to HsPNP.

Enantiomers of ImmH and DADMe-ImmH

Many pharmaceutically active sugars and nucleosides maintain potency in their enantiomeric forms. For instance, 2'-deoxy-L-cytidine and other L-nucleoside derivatives have shown potent, selective inhibition of replication of the hepatitis B virus, and Levovirin exhibits different antiviral activity and improved safety characteristics compared to its D-enantiomer, Ribavirin (Figure 15.33). ImmH and DADMe-ImmH were synthesized as L-nucleoside analogs, having inverted stereochemistry at all stereocenters relative to the familiar D counterparts.[115] When these enantiomeric analogs were tested against inosine phosphorolysis by HsPNP, they were found to be inhibitors with dissociation constants of 12 nM for L-ImmH and 380 pM for L-DADMe-ImmH (Table 15.4).[116] Although these compounds are 210- and 35-fold less effective than their D counterparts, their binding affinity is remarkable considering that many ImmH and DADMe-ImmH derivatives exhibit high nanomolar-to-micromolar dissociation constants.[117]

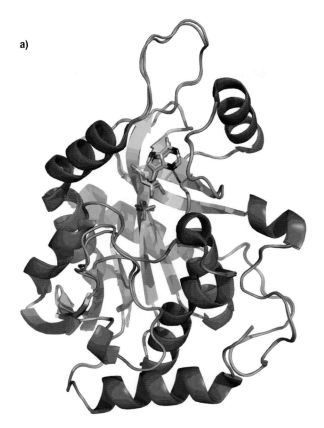

a)

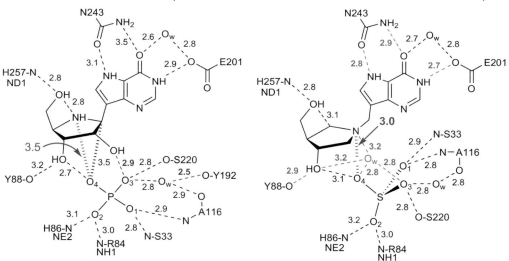

b) HsPNP•ImmH•PO₄

c) HsPNP•DADMe-ImmH•SO₄

Figure 15.32. Structures of HsPNP complexed with ImmH and DADMe-ImmH. **(a)** Overlaid x-ray crystal structures of HsPNP·ImmH·PO₄ (ImmH in green; PDB ID 1RR6) and HsPNP·DADMe-ImmH·SO₄ (DADMe-ImmH in cyan; PDB ID 1RSZ).[41] **(b)** Hydrogen bonds and closest contacts for ImmH **(b)** and DADMe-ImmH **(c)** complexes, with distances indicated in angstroms. Significantly stronger hydrogen bonds have been indicated in red, along with a new water molecule in the DADMe-ImmH complex. Hydrogen bonds present in the ImmH complex but not in the DADMe-ImmH complex are in blue. The ion-pair interactions and distances are in green.

Table 15.3. Dissociation constants for various Immucillins and DADMe-Immucillins with bovine and human PNPs

Compound	Structure	Dissociation constant (K_d)	
		HsPNP (pM)	BtPNP (pM)
ImmH		57.9 ± 1.5[a]	23 ± 5[b]
DADMe-ImmH		10.7 ± 1.1[a]	110 ± 10[c]
ImmG		42 ± 6[d]	30 ± 6[b]
DADMe-ImmG		7 ± 1[e]	23 ± 5[c]
2′-D-ImmH		140 ± 10[f]	120 ± 20[c]
2′-D-ImmG		180 ± 10[f]	210 ± 40[c]
9-(pyrrolidin-2-yl)-9-deazaHx		$840,000 \pm 110,000$[c]	$380,000 \pm 20,000$[c]
9-(pyrrolidin-1-ylmethyl)-9-deazaHx		$5,500 \pm 900$[c]	$21,000 \pm 3,000$[c]

Notes: Dissociation constants represent final, equilibrium values following slow-onset inhibition when applicable (all cases with $K_d < 10$ nM).

[a] Data from Murkin et al.[41]
[b] Data from Miles et al.[86]
[c] Data from Taylor Ringia et al.[114]
[d] Data from Evans et al.[106]
[e] Data from Evans et al.[110]
[f] Data from Lewandowicz et al.[117]

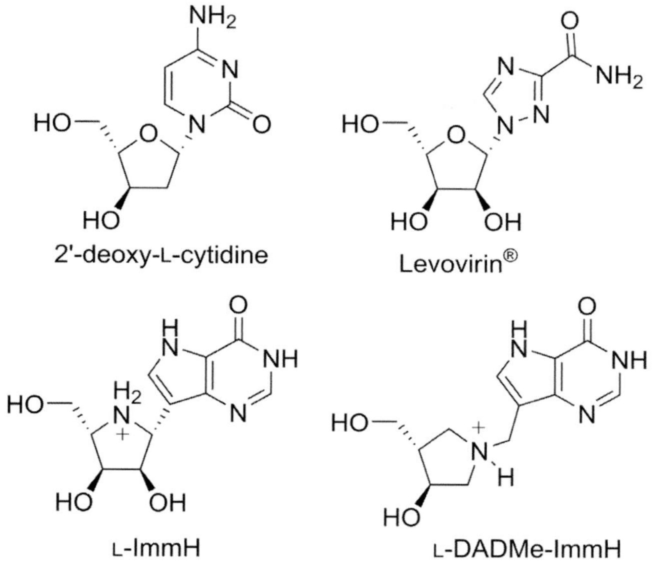

Figure 15.33. L-Enantiomers of pharmaceutically active nucleosides, including ImmH and DADMe-ImmH.

Enzyme/inhibitor interactions that permit L-enantiomer Immucillin binding were determined by cocrystallization with HsPNP and phosphate.[116] The x-ray crystal structures (L-ImmH, PDB 2Q7O; L-DADMe-ImmH, PDB 3BGS), although nearly identical in overall protein structure to the corresponding complexes with the D-nucleoside analogs, revealed differences in H-bonding patterns and ionic interactions. Comparison of the enzyme-bound configurations of L- and D-ImmH shows that the bases bind in the same manner, but the plane of the iminoribitol ring is rotated 180° about the C1'–C9 bond [Figures 15.34(a) and 15.34(b)]. This geometry prevents the 2'-, 3'-, and 5'-OH groups of L-ImmH from forming the same favorable H-bonds as with D-ImmH; in particular, a hydrogen bond between His257 and the 5'-OH has been shown by mutational analysis to be critical for the tight-binding inhibition exhibited by D-ImmH (see "Remote interactions important in transition-state formation and potent inhibition by Immucillins"),[41]

but this important interaction is lost with the L-isomer. Comparison of the D- and L-DADMe-ImmH structures indicates only small deviations in the positions of the 3'- and 5'-OH groups (Figures 15.34(c) and 15.34(d)). A significant structural deviation is that the phosphate in the L-DADMe-ImmH complex has rotated such that the N1'–O4 distance is increased from 3.0Å to 3.9Å, resulting in a weaker ion-pair interaction. Although disruption of some of the H-bonding and ionic interactions found in the D-enantiomer transition-state analog complexes results in moderately compromised binding affinities with the L-enantiomers, these compounds are capable of some structural compensation. In the case of L-ImmH, the altered iminoribitol geometry allows for alternative hydrogen bonds to the 2'-OH (from phosphate and water) and to the 3'-OH (from N_{ϵ} of His257). In the case of L-DADMe-ImmH, flexibility imparted from the methylene bridge enables spatial adjustment of the pyrrolidine ring, placing the 3'- and 5'-OH groups in nearly the same location as with the D isomer and maintaining their hydrogen bonds. This characteristic of the D- and L-DADMe-ImmH compounds likely accounts for the smaller reduction in binding affinity compared to D- and L-ImmH (35-fold vs. 210-fold, respectively).

Remote interactions important in transition-state formation and potent inhibition by Immucillins

Isotope effect studies with bovine and human PNPs revealed significant $5'-^3H$ V/K KIEs for the arsenolysis of inosine (2.8% and 5.4%, respectively). The 5'-position of the substrate is not directly involved in the reaction chemistry, and the surprisingly large isotope effects reflect enzyme/substrate interactions in the molecule on binding and/or at the transition state. The 5'-hydroxyl of inosine is involved in a hydrogen bond to His257, and this residue was mutated to assess the importance of this interaction on transition-state formation and the binding of ImmH and DADMe-ImmH.[41]

The mutants His257Phe, His257Gly, and His257Asp exhibited intrinsic $5'-^3H$ KIEs differing from those of the native enzyme (Table 15.5). His257Phe and His257Gly yielded inverse KIEs of −3.2% and −14.1%, respectively, while the native enzyme and His257Asp gave normal KIEs of 4.6% and 6.9%. These findings divided the variants into two groups: those incapable of 5'-hydroxyl hydrogen bonding and those capable of forming a hydrogen bond to the 5'-hydroxyl. H-bonding polarizes the 5'-OH, thereby loosening the adjacent 5'-C–H bonds through hyperconjugation, resulting in a normal KIE. Thus, the $5'-^3H$ KIE is sensitive to the H-bonding environment at the transition state and underscores the importance of His257 in development of the transition state. Recall that O-5' participates in an "oxygen stack" with O-4' and O_P (Figure 15.24), providing electron density to stabilize the incipient oxacarbenium ion and to assist cleavage of the ribosidic bond. This action is

Table 15.4. Dissociation constants for D- and L-Immucillins and DADMe-Immucillins

Compound	Dissociation constants		
	K_i (nM)	K_i^* (nM)	L/D K_d ratio[a]
D-ImmH	3.3 ± 0.2[b]	0.0579 ± 0.0015[c]	210
L-ImmH	190 ± 30[d]	12 ± 2[d]	
D-DADMe-ImmH	1.10 ± 0.12[b]	0.0107 ± 0.0011[c]	35
L-DADMe-ImmH	0.38 ± 0.03[d]	Not observed	

[a] For ImmH, K_i^*/K_i^* was used and for DADMe-ImmH, K_i/K_i^* was used.
[b] Data adapted from Evans et al.[110]
[c] Data adapted from Murkin et al.[41]
[d] Data adapted from Rinaldo-Matthis et al.[116]

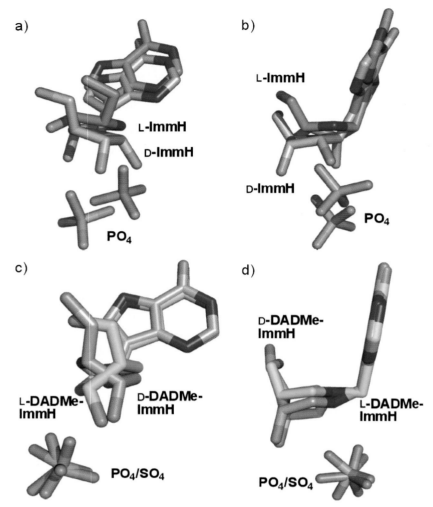

Figure 15.34. Overlapping views of enantiomers of ImmH and DADMe-ImmH from overlayed structures of their respective complexes with HsPNP. In **(a)** and **(b)**, D-ImmH is in gray and L-ImmH is in magenta. In **(c)** and **(d)**, D-DADMe-ImmH is in gray and L-DADMe-ImmH is in yellow. Phosphates are shown in orange and red, and sulfate (from the D-DADMe-ImmH structure) is shown in tan and red. Modified from Rinaldo-Matthis et al.[116]

Table 15.5. $5'$-^{3}H KIEs for inosine arsenolysis catalyzed by His257 mutants of human PNP

	V/K KIE		Intrinsic KIE	
PNP variant	KIE	%	KIE	%
Native	1.054 ± 0.002^a	5.4% (Normal)	1.046 ± 0.004	4.6% (Normal)
His257Asp	1.046 ± 0.004	4.6% (Normal)	1.069 ± 0.007	6.9% (Normal)
His257Phe	0.992 ± 0.003	−0.8% (Inverse)	0.968 ± 0.005	−3.2% (Inverse)
His257Gly	0.925 ± 0.005	−7.5% (Inverse)	0.859 ± 0.007	−14.1% (Inverse)

Notes: The intrinsic KIE was calculated from the V/K KIE after correcting for forward commitment and a $5'$-^{3}H binding isotope effect; see Murkin et al. for full details.[41] All values except the following are from Murkin et al.[41]

^{a} Lewandowicz and Schramm.[59]

proposed to be dynamically driven by motion from enzyme residues including His257.[16,118]

It was reasoned that if mutation of His257 affects transition-state formation, it would also interfere with the binding of the transition-state analogs. Binding of DADMe-ImmH resulted in subnanomolar inhibition of all PNP mutants (Table 15.6), which, after accounting for differing K_m values, gave K_m/K_d values ranging from 337,000 to 2,800,000. These values are within a factor of 11 of the native value; therefore, binding of DADMe-ImmH is relatively unaffected by alteration of His257. In contrast, these mutants bound ImmH more poorly than native PNP, yielding as much as 370-fold lower K_m/K_d values. Mutation also abolished the slow-onset inhibition characteristic of ImmH. Thus, His257 is most important in early stages of the reaction coordinate, where significant bond order still remains to the leaving group, as it is better mimicked by the first-generation analog. In later stages of the reaction coordinate, which are better mimicked by the second-generation inhibitor, DADMe-ImmH, His257 serves a diminished role, and interactions at the reaction center dominate.

Transition-state features from binding isotope effects of ImmH and DADMe-ImmH

Mutations at His257 highlighted the important role of enzymatic interactions at the $5'$-end of the transition state and its analogs. The $5'$-^{3}H KIEs for the arsenolysis of inosine indicate the degree of vibrational bond distortion as the substrate proceeds from solution to the enzymatic transition state. Murkin et al. examined the extent of $5'$-hydroxyl group distortions that occur on binding of the transition-state analogs ImmH and DADMe-ImmH.[119] Chemical synthesis afforded [$5'$-^{3}H]ImmH and [$5'$-^{3}H]DADMe-ImmH, as well as the remotely labeled isotopologs [5-^{14}C]ImmH and [methylene-^{14}C]DADMe-ImmH (Figure 15.35). Mixtures of each ^{3}H/^{14}C pair were separately incubated with HsPNP and phosphate to establish an equilibrium between free and tightly bound inhibitor.

Different bond vibrational environments between unbound and bound states gives rise to an equilibrium binding isotope effect (BIE), in much the same way that a difference between the ground state and

Table 15.6. Dissociation constants of transition-state analogs with HsPNP and His257 mutants

PNP variant	DADMe-ImmH			ImmH		
	K_d	K_m/K_d value	x-fold change	K_d	K_m/K_d value	x-fold change
Native	10.7 pM	3,700,000	1	57.9 pM	690,000	1
His257Asp	900 nM	1,500,000	2	86 nM	15,700	45
His257Phe	950 nM	337,000	11	172 nM	1,860	370
His257Gly	270 nM	2,800,000	1	11.0 nM	68,100	10

Notes: These dissociation constants are final, equilibrium constants after any slow-onset phase of inhibition, if applicable (those where $K_d < 1$ nM). Data adapted from Murkin et al.[41]

transition state generates a KIE. ImmH was found to yield a $5'$-^{3}H BIE of 12.6%, and DADMe-ImmH gave an unprecedented, large 29.2% BIE (Table 15.7).[119] These values dwarf the 1.5% and 4.6% isotope effects resulting from binding of the substrate and from formation of the transition state, respectively.[41] Thus, much greater bond distortional forces are operative with the binding of transition-state analogs than in formation of the actual transition state.

These BIEs provide some insight regarding the nature of transition-state formation. In the thermodynamic model of transition-state theory, the transition state is viewed – at least conceptually – in equilibrium with the enzyme, to which it binds tightly. This theory would predict the magnitude of the transition-state analog BIEs to be similar to that of the KIE for formation of the transition state ($\sim$5%). A dynamic model of transition-state formation explains tight binding of analogs by a conversion of dynamic transition-state excursions into a more stable protein structure condensed around the chemically inert transition-state mimic. It is conceivable that this effect captures the ligand in a more bond-distorted form, giving rise to larger BIEs.

PHARMACOLOGICAL APPLICATIONS OF IMMH AND DADME-IMMH

The rare genetic PNP deficiency is associated with T-cell immunodeficiency due to an accumulation of dGuo in blood, which ultimately causes inhibition of DNA replication through the inhibition of ribonucleotide reductase by dGTP in dividing T cells (Figure 15.10). PNP inhibitors such as the Immucillins could exploit this behavior in proliferative T-cell disorders by causing arrest of cell division specifically in T cells. Ongoing efforts have been made to study the in vivo effects of these potent PNP inhibitors.

In vivo studies with ImmH

Effects of ImmH on cultured human T cells

The effects of ImmH on the growth of the human T-cell culture lines CCRF-CEM and MOLT-4 were evaluated by treat-

ment with varying concentrations of ImmH in the presence and absence of dGuo.[120] Inclusion of dGuo is required for the cellular accumulation of dGTP that occurs with PNP deficiency. Proliferation of both cell lines was selectively blocked by ImmH (IC$_{50}$ = 0.4–5 nM) and only in the presence of dGuo (Figure 15.36). Inhibition of DNA synthesis by ImmH was also demonstrated by the reduced incorporation of [^{3}H]thymidine in its presence [Figure 15.36(b)]. At concentrations up to 50 μM, ImmH exhibited no toxic effects on a variety of non-T-cell tumors from

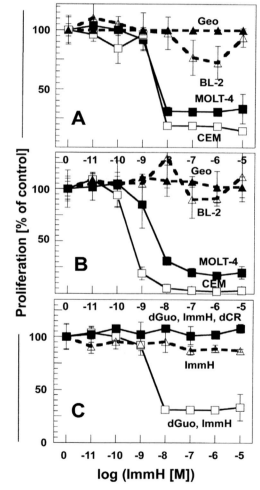

Figure 15.35. Inhibition of human T-cell leukemia cell lines by the joint action of ImmH and dGuo. Geo and BL-2 are human colon carcinoma and B-cell leukemia cell lines, respectively, while MOLT-4 and CEM are human T-cell leukemia cell lines. Cell lines were incubated with 20 μM dGuo and varying concentrations of ImmH and were analyzed for cell viability by (A) WST-1 and (B) incorporation of [^{3}H]thymidine. (C) Inhibition of proliferation only occurs when ImmH is treated in the presence of dGuo, but the activity can be regained by deoxycytidine (dCyd) rescue (dCR); dCyd, the preferred substrate for dCyd kinase, is converted to dCMP which inhibits the phosphorylation of dGuo, thereby preventing inhibition of ribonucleotide reductase by dGTP (see Figure 15.10). Reproduced from Kicska et al.[120]

Table 15.7. $5'$-^{3}H binding isotope effects for substrate and transition-state analogs with human PNP

Ligands	K_d or K_m	BIE/KIE Type of IE	Isotope effect
$[5'$-^{3}H]-, $[5'$-^{14}C]Inosine	40 μM	BIE[a]	1.015 ± 0.003 (9)[b]
		Intrinsic KIE	1.046 ± 0.004 (9)[b]
$[5'$-^{3}H]-, $[5$-^{14}C]ImmH	58 pM	BIE	1.126 ± 0.005 (32)[c]
$[5'$-^{3}H]-, $[^{14}$C]DADMe-ImmH	11 pM	BIE	1.292 ± 0.012 (27)[c]

Notes: The BIE (or intrinsic KIE) is expressed as ± standard error with the number of replicates in parentheses.
[a] BIE measurements with inosine were performed using sulfate as a substrate analog in place of phosphate.
[b] Data adapted from: Murkin et al.[41]
[c] Data adapted from: Murkin et al.[119]

various tissues, further supporting the inhibitor's T-cell-specific mode of action.

The effect of ImmH on normal human T cells was investigated in the presence of dGuo with and without cell-division stimulants.[120] Without stimulation, T cells were unaffected; however, rapid cell division caused by the introduction of monocytic cells and interleukin-2 was greatly reduced by increasing doses of ImmH (IC$_{50}$ = 5 nM; Figure 15.37). These findings, together with direct observation of elevated levels of dGTP, demonstrated that inhibition of PNP by ImmH causes dGTP-mediated apoptosis specifically in rapidly dividing T cells.

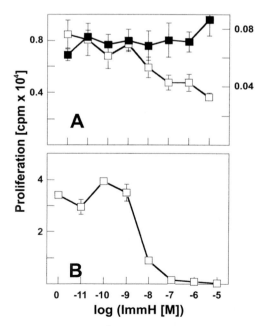

Figure 15.36. Inhibition of [^{3}H]thymidine incorporation in activated human T-cells by ImmH. Proliferation was determined with no stimulation (■, A), with physiological levels of interleukin-2 (IL-2, □, upper panel), or with excess IL-2 and monocytic cells (□, B). Reproduced from Kicska et al.[120]

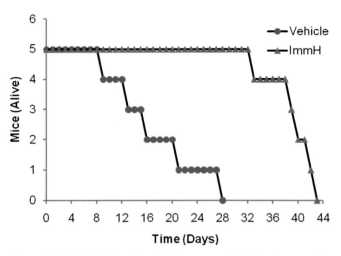

Figure 15.37. Effect of ImmH on SCID mouse survival following engraftment with human peripheral blood lymphocytes. Treated mice were given 20 mg/kg ImmH orally for five days prior to engraftment to boost levels of dGuo. Dosing then continued until the animals died. Modified from Bantia et al.[121]

Effects of ImmH on mice and human T-cell xenografts

The whole-organism effectiveness of ImmH as a potential therapeutic agent for autoimmune disorders was tested in immunologically compromised mice.[121] A single dose of 10 mg/kg ImmH caused dGuo to accumulate up to 5 μM in the blood, where it is normally present at undetectable levels in both mice and humans. Similar levels (3 to 17 μM) of dGuo accumulate in the plasma of humans afflicted with genetic PNP deficiency.

A similar protocol with severe combined immunodeficient (SCID) mice grafted with human peripheral blood lymphocytes (hPBLs) served as a model for human immune transplantation rejection.[121] Host antigens stimulate division of the hPBLs, causing death of the SCID mice due to xenogeneic graft-versus-host disease. Mice treated with ImmH had a doubled lifespan (Figure 15.38). The mouse xenograft study established that ImmH provides sufficient total-organism PNP inhibition to maintain elevated levels of dGuo.

Clinical trials with ImmH (aka Forodesine)

Human patient clinical trials with ImmH have been initiated by BioCryst Pharmaceuticals Inc. under the trade name Forodesine (initially as BCX-1777). Intravenous and oral formulations have been administered to patients suffering from various T-cell and B-cell lymphomas and leukemias, as well as from solid tumors.[122–129] Early trials demonstrated that ImmH has a good safety profile, with few serious adverse effects, and is effective physiologically. Phase IIa trials in patients with advanced T-cell leukemia resulted in a 35% overall response rate (22% complete response, 13% partial response) when treated once daily over a 5-day-per-week cycle. ImmH is reported to be in clinical trials for other leukemias and lymphomas.[130]

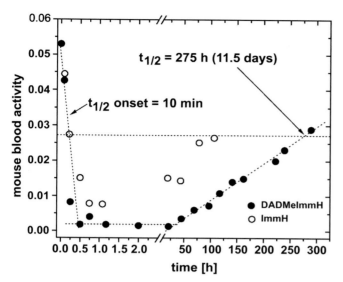

Figure 15.38. Oral availability and inhibition of mouse blood PNP by ImmH and DADMe-ImmH. $t_{1/2}$ onset is the time following oral administration that 50% of PNP activity remains. The $t_{1/2}$ for activity recovery is 100 h for ImmH (○) and 275 h for DADMe-ImmH (●). Reproduced from Lewandowicz et al.[107]

In vivo studies with DADMe-ImmH

The in vivo inhibition of mouse PNP by DADMe-ImmH was used to determine inhibitor bioavailability and physiological response.[107] Oral administration of 0.8 mg/kg ImmH or DADMe-ImmH caused blood PNP activity to drop rapidly, reaching 50% in 14 and 10 min, respectively (Figure 15.39). Both analogs are orally available and associate with blood PNP faster than they can be excreted or metabolized. Continued monitoring of blood PNP activity indicated that after 100 h (4 days) with ImmH, 50% of the original level had been recovered, but DADMe-ImmH required 275 h (11.5 days) to

reach this point. This long recovery time reflects replacement of blood cells with new erythrocytes. As the lifespan of mouse erythrocytes is approximately 25 days, in the 11.5 days for half-recovery, 46% of the blood cells would have been replaced. This mouse model suggests that DADMe-ImmH attains the ultimate physiological goal in inhibitor design. A single oral dose results in inhibition of the target enzyme for the lifetime of the cell.

THIRD-GENERATION PNP TRANSITION-STATE ANALOGS AND BEYOND

Acyclic and achiral Immucillins

DATMe-ImmH

The Immucillin and DADMe-Immucillin generations of PNP transition-state analogs have proven effective both in vitro and in vivo. However, the chemical structures of the purine base and iminoribitol and pyrrolidine rings demand significant synthetic effort. A third generation of PNP inhibitors was designed to replace the pyrrolidine present in the DADMe series with an acyclic hydroxylated amine.

Acyclic DADMe-based compounds, 3′,4′-seco-DADMe-ImmH and its 5′-truncated analogs, had the C3′–C4′ bond removed and were modest inhibitors of HsPNP, with K_i values between 120 and 1.3 nM (Figure 15.40).[117,131] Alterations in the aminoalcohol group gave an array of dissociation constants with many in the low-nanomolar to picomolar range.[132] Derivatives with a secondary amine gave the best binding to PNP (compare second and third rows to first row in Figure 15.40). The tightest binding secondary amines possessed three alcohol groups. One of

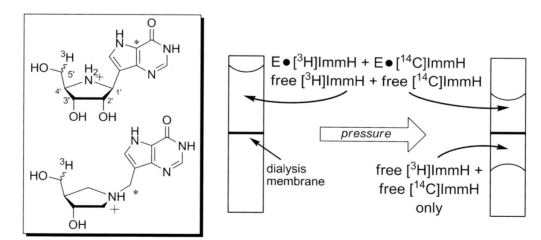

Figure 15.39. Schematic diagram of the measurement of binding isotope effects (BIEs) by ultrafiltration. The inset shows the locations of the radioisotope labels in the transition-state analogs ImmH and DADMe-ImmH. A mixture of HsPNP, phosphate, and $^3H/^{14}C$ labeled inhibitor was added to the top chamber in an ultrafiltration apparatus. After applying pressure, solution containing only unbound inhibitor passed through the dialysis membrane to the bottom chamber, leaving a mixture of bound and unbound inhibitor (of equal concentration to that below) above. Equal-volume aliquots were removed, and radioactivity was measured by scintillation counting.

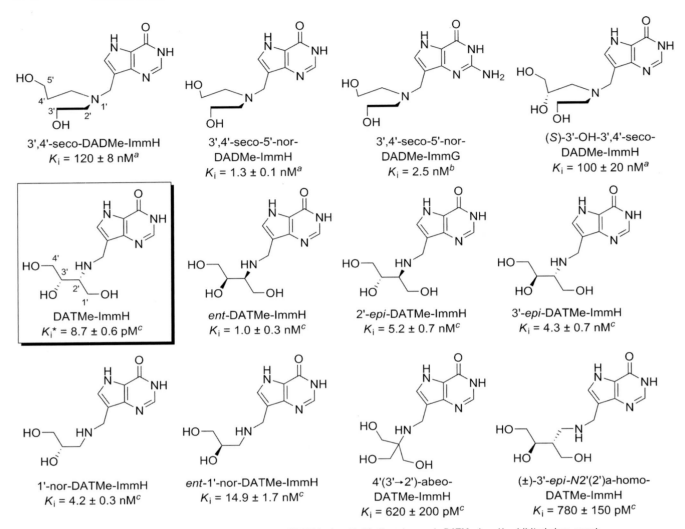

Figure 15.40. Examples of acyclic analogs of DADMe-ImmH. Of all analogs only DATMe-ImmH exhibited slow-onset inhibition, and the dissociation constant (K_i^*) for the final, tight complex is given. Compound names do not follow IUPAC standards but are used to indicate changes relative to the parent compounds DADMe-ImmH and DATMe-ImmH. Numbering is maintained from the parent; in the case of DATMe-ImmH, the amino-substituted carbon is given the lowest locant (i.e., 2′); prefixes as defined by IUPAC are as follows: seco = bond breakage in a ring; nor = methylene removal; homo = methylene insertion; abeo = bond migration; ent = enantiomer, epi = epimer. *Sources*: [a] Lewandowicz et al.,[117] [b] Semeraro et al.,[131] [c] Taylor et al.[132]

these trihydroxy secondary amines, DATMe-ImmH,[133] gave tight, slow-onset inhibition of HsPNP. With a K_i^* of 8.7 pM, DATMe-ImmH is more potent than ImmH and DADMe-ImmH, yet requires fewer synthetic steps. Seemingly minor stereochemical modifications of DATMe-ImmH (second row of Figure 15.40) abolish the slow-onset inhibitory behavior and result in weaker affinity. Crucial binding interactions may be revealed by protein structural studies with these new inhibitors.

Achiral Immucillins

The recent discovery of potent inhibition by the third generation of PNP transition-state analogs provides promise for the further development of synthetically accessible inhibitors. Particularly desirable are analogs lacking stereocenters to permit facile preparation from readily available

precursors. Removal of the C3′–C4′ bond of the DADMe-pyrrolidine ring destroys the stereogenicity at these two carbons, as exemplified by the first three compounds in Figure 15.40. One of the DATMe-ImmH derivatives, 4′(3′→2′)-abeo-DATMe-ImmH, contains Tris base as its trihydroxyalkylamine group. Further elaboration on this small family of PNP transition-state analogs may uncover picomolar inhibitors that would be suitable for pharmaceutical undertakings.

Conclusions

Scrutiny of the mammalian PNPs has led to novel insights for enzymatic reaction mechanisms, transition-state structure, and inhibitor design. The PNPs catalyze ribosyl transfer chemistry via migration of the anomeric carbon between the purine leaving group and the anionic nucleophile. This mechanism was first described for PNP and has since been shown to apply to other glycosyltransferases. With fixed nucleophiles in the catalytic site, a ribooxacarbenium-ion transition state is formed at some point during the ribosyl migration. The exact nature of PNP transition states is dictated by the migration distance and protein vibrational modes that form the transition state. Remarkable differences in transition-state structure can occur with nearly identical protein structures. These differences can guide the design of transition-state analogs that demonstrate specificity for enzyme variants from different species. Knowledge of the transition-state structures has permitted access to picomolar compounds with favorable pharmokinetic properties. Two of these have entered clinical trials for T-cell disease. PNP has also served as one of the first enzymes for exploration of catalytic-site-induced substrate distortions by binding isotope effects. These results are providing new insights into the fundamental notions of enzymatic catalysis, induced fit, and transition-state structure.

REFERENCES

1. Pauling, L. Molecular architecture and biological reactions. *Chem. Eng. News* **1946**, *24*, 1375–1377.
2. Wolfenden, R. Transition state analogues for enzyme catalysis. *Nature* **1969**, *223*, 704–705.
3. Wolfenden, R. Analog approaches to the structure of the transition state in enzyme reactions. *Acc. Chem. Res.* **1972**, *5*, 10–18.
4. Jencks, W. Binding energy, specificity, and enzymic catalysis: the Circe effect. *Adv. Enzymol. Relat. Areas Mol. Biol.* **1975**, *43*, 219–410.
5. Anderson, V. Ground state destabilization. In: *Encyclopedia of Life Sciences*. Chichester: John Wiley & Sons, Ltd.; **2001**, 1–5.
6. Shih, I.; Been, M. Catalytic strategies of the hepatitis delta virus ribozymes. *Annu. Rev. Biochem.* **2002**, *71*, 887–917.
7. Wu, N.; Mo, Y.; Gao, J.; Pai, E. Electrostatic stress in catalysis: structure and mechanism of the enzyme orotidine monophosphate decarboxylase. *Proc. Natl. Acad. Sci. U.S.A.* **2000**, *97*, 2017–2022.
8. Amyes, T. L.; Wood, B. M.; Chan, K.; Gerlt, J. A.; Richard, J. P. Formation and stability of a vinyl carbanion at the active site of orotidine 5′-monophosphate decarboxylase: pKa of the C-6 proton of enzyme-bound UMP. *J. Am. Chem. Soc.* **2008**, *130*, 1574–1575.
9. Bruice, T. C.; Lightstone, F. C. Ground state and transition state contributions to the rates of intramolecular and enzymatic reactions. *Acc. Chem. Res.* **1999**, *32*, 127–136.
10. Lightstone, F. C.; Bruice, T. C. Ground state conformations and entropic and enthalpic factors in the efficiency of intramolecular and enzymatic reactions. 1. Cyclic anhydride formation by substituted glutarates, succinate, and 3,6-endoxo-Δ4-tetrahydrophthalate monophenyl esters. *J. Am. Chem. Soc.* **1996**, *118*, 2595–2605.
11. Antoniou, D.; Basner, J.; Núñez, S.; Schwartz, S. Computational and theoretical methods to explore the relation between enzyme dynamics and catalysis. *Chem. Rev.* **2006**, *106*, 3170–3187.
12. Kohen, A.; Cannio, R.; Bartolucci, S.; Klinman, J. Enzyme dynamics and hydrogen tunnelling in a thermophilic alcohol dehydrogenase. *Nature* **1999**, *399*, 496–499.
13. Agarwal, P.; Billeter, S.; Rajagopalan, P.; Benkovic, S.; Hammes-Schiffer, S. Network of coupled promoting motions in enzyme catalysis. *Proc. Natl. Acad. Sci. U.S.A.* **2002**, *99*, 2794–2799.
14. Wong, K.; Selzer, T.; Benkovic, S.; Hammes-Schiffer, S. Impact of distal mutations on the network of coupled motions correlated to hydride transfer in dihydrofolate reductase. *Proc. Natl. Acad. Sci. U.S.A.* **2005**, *102*, 6807–6812.
15. Nunez, S.; Antoniou, D.; Schramm, V. L.; Schwartz, S. D. Promoting vibrations in human purine nucleoside phosphorylase: a molecular dynamics and hybrid quantum mechanical/molecular mechanical study. *J. Am. Chem. Soc.* **2004**, *126*, 15720–15729.
16. Saen-Oon, S.; Ghanem, M.; Schramm, V.; Schwartz, S. Remote mutations and active site dynamics correlate with catalytic properties of purine nucleoside phosphorylase. *Biophys. J.* **2008**, *94*(10), 4078-4088.
17. Lienhard, G. Enzymatic catalysis and transition-state theory. *Science* **1973**, *180*, 149–154.
18. Wolfenden, R.; Kati, W. M. Testing the limits of protein-ligand binding discrimination with transition-state analogue inhibitors. *Acc. Chem. Res.* **1991**, *24*, 209–215.
19. Wolfenden, R. Conformational aspects of inhibitor design: enzyme-substrate interactions in the transition state. *Bioorg. Med. Chem.* **1999**, *7*, 647–652.
20. Schramm, V. Enzymatic transition state theory and transition state analogue design. *J. Biol. Chem.* **2007**, *282*, 28297–28300.
21. Schramm, V. Enzymatic transition states and transition state analog design. *Annu. Rev. Biochem.* **1998**, *67*, 693–720.
22. Hammond, G. S. A correlation of reaction rates. *J. Am. Chem. Soc.* **1955**, *77*, 334–338.
23. Jencks, W. In: *Catalysis in Chemistry and Enzymology*. Dover: New York, **1987**, 170–182.
24. Schramm, V. Enzymatic transition states: thermodynamics, dynamics and analogue design. *Arch. Biochem. Biophys.* **2005**, *433*, 13–26.
25. Cleland, W. Isotope Effects: Determination of enzyme transition state structure. *Methods Enzymol.* **1995**, *249*, 341–373.
26. Parkin, D. W. In: *Enzyme Mechanism from Isotope Effects*, Cook, P. F.; Ed. Boca Raton: CRC Press; **1991**, 269–290.
27. Rodgers, J.; Femec, D. A.; Schowen, R. L. Isotopic mapping of transition-state structural features associated with enzymic catalysis of methyl transfer. *J. Am. Chem. Soc.* **1982**, *104*, 3263–3268.
28. Sunhel, J.; Schowen, R. In: *Enzyme Mechanism from Isotope Effects*, Cook, P. F.; Ed. Boca Raton: CRC Press; **1991**, 3–36.
29. Huskey, W. In: *Enzyme Mechanism from Isotope Effects*, Cook, P. F.; Ed. Boca Raton: CRC Press; **1991**, 37–72.
30. Berti, P. J.; Tanaka, K. S. E. Transition state analysis using multiple kinetic isotope effects: mechanisms of enzymatic and non-enzymatic glycoside hydrolysis and transfer. *Adv. Phys. Org. Chem.* **2002**, *37*, 239–314.
31. Rose, I. The isotope trapping method: desorption rates of productive e.s complexes. *Methods Enzymol.* **1980**, *64*, 47–59.
32. Frisch, M. J.; Trucks, G. W.; Schlegel, H. B.; Scuseria, G. E.; Robb, M. A.; Cheeseman, J. R.; Zakrzewski, V. G.; Montgomery, J.; Stratmann, R. E.; Burant, J. C.; Dapprich, S.; Millam, J. M.; Daniels, A. D.; Kudin, K. N.; Strain, M. C.; Farkas, O.; Tomasi, J.; Barone, V.; Cossi, M.; Cammi, R.; Mennucci, B.; Pomelli, C.; Adamo, C.; Ochterski, J.; Petersson, G. A.; Ayala,

P. Y.; Cui, Q.; Morokuma, K.; Rega, N.; Salvador, P.; Dannenberg, J. J.; Malick, D. K.; Rabuck, A. D.; Raghavachari, K.; Foresman, J. B.; Cioslowski, J.; Ortiz, J. V.; Baboul, A. G.; Stefanov, B. B.; G. Liu, A. L.; Piskorz, P.; Komaromi, I.; Gomperts, R.; Martin, R. L.; Fox, D. J.; Keith, T.; Al-Laham, M. A.; Peng, C. Y.; Nanayakkara, A.; Challacombe, M.; Gill, P. M. W.; Johnson, B.; Chen, W.; Wong, M. W.; Andres, J. L.; Gonzalez, C.; Head-Gordon, M.; Replogle, E. S.; Pople, J. A.; Revision A.11.2 ed.; Gaussian, Inc.: Pittsburgh, PA, **2001**.

33. Saunders, M.; Laidig, K. E.; Wolfsberg, M. Theoretical calculation of equilibrium isotope effects using ab initio force constants: application to NMR isotope perturbation studies. *J. Am. Chem. Soc.* **1989**, *111*, 8989–8994.

34. Anisimov, V.; Paneth, P. ISOEFF98: a program for studies of isotope effects using hessian modifications. *J. Math. Chem.* **1999**, *26*, 75–86.

35. Melander, L.; Saunders, W. H., Jr. *Reaction Rates of Isotopic Molecules.* New York, NY: Wiley & Sons; **1980**.

36. Bigeleisen, J. The relative reaction velocities of isotopic molecules. *J. Chem. Phys.* **1949**, *17*, 675–678.

37. Bigeleisen, J.; Wolsberg, M. Theoretical and experimental aspects of isotope effects in chemical kinetics. *Adv. Chem. Phys.* **1958**, *1*, 15–76.

38. Streitwieser, A.; Jagow, R. H.; Fahey, R. C.; Suzuki, S. Kinetic isotope effects in the acetolyses of deuterated cyclopentyl tosylates. *J. Am. Chem. Soc.* **1958**, *80*, 2326–2332.

39. Northrop, D. The expression of isotope effects on enzyme-catalyzed reactions. *Annu. Rev. Biochem.* **1981**, *50*, 103–131.

40. Birck, M.; Schramm, V. Binding causes the remote [5′-³H]thymidine kinetic isotope effect in human thymidine phosphorylase. *J. Am. Chem. Soc.* **2004**, *126*, 6882–6883.

41. Murkin, A. S.; Birck, M. R.; Rinaldo-Matthis, A.; Shi, W. X.; Taylor, E. A.; Almo, S. C.; Schramm, V. L. Neighboring group participation in the transition state of human purine nucleoside phosphorylase. *Biochemistry* **2007**, *46*, 5038–5049.

42. Ruszczycky, M.; Anderson, V. Interpretation of V/K isotope effects for enzymatic reactions exhibiting multiple isotopically sensitive steps. *J. Theor. Biol.* **2006**, *243*, 328–342.

43. Giblett, E. R.; Ammann, A. J.; Wara, D. W.; Sandman, R.; Diamond, L. K. Nucleoside-phosphorylase deficiency in a child with severely defective T-cell immunity and normal B-cell immunity. *Lancet* **1975**, *1*, 1010–1013.

44. Markert, M.; Finkel, B.; McLaughlin, T.; Watson, T.; Collard, H.; McMahon, C.; Andrews, L.; Barrett, M.; Ward, F. Mutations in purine nucleoside phosphorylase deficiency. *Hum. Mutat.* **1997**, *9*, 118–121.

45. Markert, M. Purine nucleoside phosphorylase deficiency. *Immunodef. Rev.* **1991**, *3*, 45–81.

46. Oliver, F.; Collins, M.; López-Rivas, A. dNTP pools imbalance as a signal to initiate apoptosis. *Experientia* **1996**, *52*, 995–1000.

47. Zoltewicz, J.; Clark, D.; Sharpless, T.; Grahe, G. Kinetics and mechanism of the acid-catalyzed hydrolysis of some purine nucleosides. *J. Am. Chem. Soc.* **1970**, *92*, 1741–1749.

48. McCann, J.; Berti, P. Transition state analysis of acid-catalyzed dAMP hydrolysis. *J. Am. Chem. Soc.* **2007**, *129*, 7055–7064.

49. Krenitsky, T. Purine nucleoside phosphorylase: kinetics, mechanism, and specificity. *Mol. Pharmacol.* **1967**, *3*, 526–536.

50. Kim, B.; Cha, S.; Parks, R. J. Purine nucleoside phosphorylase from human erythroyctes. II. Kinetic analysis and substrate-binding studies. *J. Biol. Chem.* **1968**, *243*, 1771–1776.

51. Lewis, A.; Lowy, B. Human erythrocyte purine nucleoside phosphorylase: molecular weight and physical properties: a Theorell-Chance catalytic mechanism. *J. Biol. Chem.* **1979**, *254*, 9927–9932.

52. Lewis, A.; Glantz, M. Bovine brain purine-nucleoside phosphorylase purification, characterization, and catalytic mechanism. *Biochemistry* **1976**, *15*, 4451–4457.

53. Porter, D. Purine nucleoside phosphorylase: kinetic mechanism of the enzyme from calf spleen. *J. Biol. Chem.* **1992**, *267*, 7342–7351.

54. Carlson, J.; Fischer, A. Thyroid purine nucleoside phosphorylase. II. Kinetic model by alternate substrate and inhibition studies. *Biochim. Biophys. Acta* **1979**, *566*, 259–265.

55. Kline, P.; Schramm, V. Purine nucleoside phosphorylase: catalytic mechanism and transition-state analysis of the arsenolysis reaction. *Biochemistry* **1993**, *32*, 13212–13219.

56. Erion, M. D.; Stoeckler, J. D.; Guida, W. C.; Walter, R. L.; Ealick, S. E. Purine nucleoside phosphorylase. 2. Catalytic mechanism. *Biochemistry* **1997**, *36*, 11735–11748.

57. Ghanem, M.; Saen-Oon, S.; Zhadin, N.; Wing, C.; Cahill, S.; Schwartz, S.; Callender, R.; Schramm, V. Tryptophan-free human PNP reveals catalytic site interactions. *Biochemistry* **2008**, *47*, 3202–3215.

58. Kline, P.; Schramm, V. Purine nucleoside phosphorylase: inosine hydrolysis, tight binding of the hypoxanthine intermediate, and third-the-sites reactivity. *Biochemistry* **1992**, *31*, 5964–5973.

59. Lewandowicz, A.; Schramm, V. Transition state analysis for human and *Plasmodium falciparum* purine nucleoside phosphorylases. *Biochemistry* **2004**, *43*, 1458–1468.

60. Rising, K. A.; Schramm, V. L. Transition state analysis of NAD⁺ hydrolysis by the cholera toxin catalytic subunit. *J. Am. Chem. Soc.* **1997**, *119*, 27–37.

61. Stein, R.; Cordes, E. Kinetic alpha-deuterium isotope effects for *Escherichia coli* purine nucleoside phosphorylase-catalyzed phosphorolysis of adenosine and inosine. *J. Biol. Chem.* **1981**, *256*, 767–772.

62. Lehikoinen, P.; Sinnott, M.; Krenitsky, T. Investigation of alpha-deuterium kinetic isotope effects on the purine nucleoside phosphorylase reaction by the equilibrium-perturbation technique. *Biochem. J.* **1989**, *257*, 355–359.

63. Parks, R. E., Jr.; Agarwal, R. P. In: *The Enzymes*, Boyer, P. D.; Ed. New York, NY: Academic Press; **1972**, Vol. 7, 483–514.

64. Schramm, V.; Shi, W. Atomic motion in enzymatic reaction coordinates. *Curr. Opin. Struct. Biol.* **2001**, *11*, 657–665.

65. Birck, M.; Schramm, V. Nucleophilic participation in the transition state for human thymidine phosphorylase. *J. Am. Chem. Soc.* **2004**, *126*, 2447–2453.

66. Kline, P.; Schramm, V. Pre-steady-state transition-state analysis of the hydrolytic reaction catalyzed by purine nucleoside phosphorylase. *Biochemistry* **1995**, *34*, 1153–1162.

67. Horenstein, B.; Parkin, D.; Estupiñán, B.; Schramm, V. Transition-state analysis of nucleoside hydrolase from *Crithidia fasciculata*. *Biochemistry* **1991**, *30*, 10788–10795.

68. Scheuring, J.; Berti, P.; Schramm, V. Transition-state structure for the ADP-ribosylation of recombinant gialpha1 subunits by pertussis toxin. *Biochemistry* **1998**, *37*, 2748–2758.

69. Scheuring, J.; Schramm, V. Kinetic isotope effect characterization of the transition state for oxidized nicotinamide adenine dinucleotide hydrolysis by pertussis toxin. *Biochemistry* **1997**, *36*, 4526–4534.

70. Scheuring, J.; Schramm, V. Pertussis toxin: transition state analysis for ADP-ribosylation of G-protein peptide alphai3C20. *Biochemistry* **1997**, *36*, 8215–8223.

71. Berti, P. J.; Blanke, S. R.; Schramm, V. L. Transition state structure for the hydrolysis of NAD⁺ catalyzed by diphtheria toxin. *J. Am. Chem. Soc.* **1997**, *119*, 12079–12088.

72. Parkin, D. W.; Leung, H. B.; Schramm, V. L. Synthesis of nucleotides with specific radiolabels in ribose: primary 14C and secondary 3H kinetic isotope effects on acid-catalyzed glycosidic bond hydrolysis of AMP, dAMP, and inosine. *J. Biol. Chem.* **1984**, *259*, 9411–9417.

73. Parkin, D. W.; Schramm, V. L. Effects of allosteric activation on the primary and secondary kinetic isotope effects for three AMP nucleosidases. *J. Biol. Chem.* **1984**, *259*, 9418–9425.

74. Parkin, D.; Schramm, V. Catalytic and allosteric mechanism of amp nucleosidase from primary, beta-secondary, and multiple heavy atom kinetic isotope effects. *Biochemistry* **1987**, *26*, 913–920.

75. Parikh, S.; Schramm, V. Transition state structure for ADP-ribosylation of eukaryotic elongation factor 2 catalyzed by diphtheria toxin. *Biochemistry* **2004**, *43*, 1204–1212.

76. Parkin, D.; Mentch, F.; Banks, G.; Horenstein, B.; Schramm, V. Transition-state analysis of a Vmax mutant of AMP nucleosidase by the application of heavy-atom kinetic isotope effects. *Biochemistry* **1991**, *30*, 4586–4594.

77. Hunt, C.; Gillani, N.; Farone, A.; Rezaei, M.; Kline, P. Kinetic isotope effects of nucleoside hydrolase from *Escherichia coli*. *Biochim. Biophys. Acta* **2005**, *1751*, 140–149.

78. Singh, V.; Schramm, V. Transition-state structure of human 5′-methylthioadenosine phosphorylase. *J. Am. Chem. Soc.* **2006**, *128*, 14691–14696.

79. Singh, V.; Luo, M.; Brown, R.; Norris, G.; Schramm, V. Transition-state structure of *Neisseria meningitides* 5′-methylthioadenosine/S-adenosylhomocysteine nucleosidase. *J. Am. Chem. Soc.* **2007**, *129*, 13831–13833.

80. Chen, X. Y.; Berti, P. J.; Schramm, V. L. Ricin A-chain: kinetic isotope effects and transition state structure with stem-loop RNA. *J. Am. Chem. Soc.* **2000**, *122*, 1609–1617.

81. Chen, X. Y.; Berti, P. J.; Schramm, V. L. Transition-state analysis for depurination of DNA by ricin A-chain. *J. Am. Chem. Soc.* **2000**, *122*, 6527–6534.

82. Werner, R.; Stivers, J. Kinetic isotope effect studies of the reaction catalyzed by uracil DNA glycosylase: evidence for an oxocarbenium ion-uracil anion intermediate. *Biochemistry* **2000**, *39*, 14054–14064.

83. Singh, V.; Lee, J.; Núñez, S.; Howell, P.; Schramm, V. Transition state structure of 5′-methylthioadenosine/S-adenosylhomocysteine nucleosidase from *Escherichia coli* and its similarity to transition state analogues. *Biochemistry* **2005**, *44*, 11647–11659.

84. Singh, V.; Schramm, V. Transition-state analysis of *S. pneumoniae* 5′-methylthioadenosine nucleosidase. *J. Am. Chem. Soc.* **2007**, *129*, 2783–2795.

85. Munns, A.; Tollin, P. The crystal and molecular structure of inosine. *Acta Crystallogr. B* **1970**, *26*, 1101–1113.

86. Miles, R. W.; Tyler, P. C.; Furneaux, R. H.; Bagdassarian, C. K.; Schramm, V. L. One-third-the-sites transition-state inhibitors for purine nucleoside phosphorylase. *Biochemistry* **1998**, *37*, 8615–8621.

87. Sauve, A.; Cahill, S.; Zech, S.; Basso, L.; Lewandowicz, A.; Santos, D.; Grubmeyer, C.; Evans, G.; Furneaux, R.; Tyler, P.; McDermott, A.; Girvin, M.; Schramm, V. Ionic states of substrates and transition state analogues at the catalytic sites of N-ribosyltransferases. *Biochemistry* **2003**, *42*, 5694–5705.

88. Schramm, V. L. Development of transition state analogues of purine nucleoside phosphorylase as anti-T-cell agents. *Biochim. Biophys. Acta* **2002**, *1587*, 107–117.

89. Bzowska, A.; Kulikowska, E.; Darzynkiewicz, E.; Shugar, D. Purine nucleoside phosphorylase. structure-activity relationships for substrate and inhibitor properties of N-1-, N-7-, and C-8-substituted analogues; differentiation of mammalian and bacterial enzymes with N-1-methylinosine and guanosine. *J. Biol. Chem.* **1988**, *263*, 9212–9217.

90. Bagdassarian, C. K.; Schramm, V. L.; Schwartz, S. D. Molecular electrostatic potential analysis for enzymatic substrates, competitive inhibitors, and transition-state inhibitors. *J. Am. Chem. Soc.* **1996**, *118*, 8825–8836.

91. Braunheim, B.; Miles, R.; Schramm, V.; Schwartz, S. Prediction of inhibitor binding free energies by quantum neural networks: nucleoside analogues binding to trypanosomal nucleoside hydrolase. *Biochemistry* **1999**, *38*, 16076–16083.

92. Evans, G. B.; Furneaux, R. H.; Gainsford, G. J.; Schramm, V. L.; Tyler, P. C. Synthesis of transition state analogue inhibitors for purine nucleoside phosphorylase and N-riboside hydrolases. *Tetrahedron* **2000**, *56*, 3053–3062.

93. Evans, G.; Furneaux, R.; Hutchison, T.; Kezar, H.; Morris, P. J.; Schramm, V.; Tyler, P. Addition of lithiated 9-deazapurine derivatives to a carbohydrate cyclic imine: convergent synthesis of the aza-C-nucleoside Immucillins. *J. Org. Chem.* **2001**, *66*, 5723–5730.

94. Ealick, S.; Rule, S.; Carter, D.; Greenhough, T.; Babu, Y.; Cook, W.; Habash, J.; Helliwell, J.; Stoeckler, J.; Parks, R. J. Three-dimensional structure of human erythrocytic purine nucleoside phosphorylase at 3.2 Å resolution. *J. Biol. Chem.* **1990**, *265*, 1812–1820.

95. Mao, C.; Cook, W. J.; Zhou, M.; Federov, A. A.; Almo, S. C.; Ealick, S. E. Calf spleen purine nucleoside phosphorylase complexed with substrates and substrate analogues. *Biochemistry* **1998**, *37*, 7135–7146.

96. Wang, F.; Miles, R. W.; Kicska, G.; Nieves, E.; Schramm, V. L.; Angeletti, R. H. Immucillin-H binding to purine nucleoside phosphorylase reduces dynamic solvent exchange. *Protein Sci.* **2000**, *9*, 1660–1668.

97. Fedorov, A.; Shi, W.; Kicska, G.; Fedorov, E.; Tyler, P.; Furneaux, R.; Hanson, J.; Gainsford, G.; Larese, J.; Schramm, V.; Almo, S. Transition state structure of purine nucleoside phosphorylase and principles of atomic motion in enzymatic catalysis. *Biochemistry* **2001**, *40*, 853–860.

98. Shi, W.; Li, C.; Tyler, P.; Furneaux, R.; Cahill, S.; Girvin, M.; Grubmeyer, C.; Schramm, V.; Almo, S. The 2.0 Å structure of malarial purine phosphoribosyltransferase in complex with a transition-state analogue inhibitor. *Biochemistry* **1999**, *38*, 9872–9880.

99. Shi, W.; Li, C.; Tyler, P.; Furneaux, R.; Grubmeyer, C.; Schramm, V.; Almo, S. The 2.0 Å structure of human hypoxanthine-guanine phosphoribosyltransferase in complex with a transition-state analog inhibitor. *Nat. Struct. Biol.* **1999**, *6*, 588–593.

100. Héroux, A.; White, E.; Ross, L.; Davis, R.; Borhani, D. Crystal structure of *Toxoplasma gondii* hypoxanthine-guanine phosphoribosyltransferase with XMP, pyrophosphate, and two Mg(2+) ions bound: insights into the catalytic mechanism. *Biochemistry* **1999**, *38*, 14495–14506.

101. Tao, W.; Grubmeyer, C.; Blanchard, J. Transition state structure of *Salmonella typhimurium* orotate phosphoribosyltransferase. *Biochemistry* **1996**, *35*, 14–21.

102. Sauve, A.; Wolberger, C.; Schramm, V.; Boeke, J. The biochemistry of sirtuins. *Annu. Rev. Biochem.* **2006**, *75*, 435–465.

103. Bianchet, M.; Seiple, L.; Jiang, Y.; Ichikawa, Y.; Amzel, L.; Stivers, J. Electrostatic guidance of glycosyl cation migration along the reaction coordinate of uracil DNA glycosylase. *Biochemistry* **2003**, *42*, 12455–12460.

104. Vocadlo, D.; Davies, G.; Laine, R.; Withers, S. Catalysis by hen egg-white lysozyme proceeds via a covalent intermediate. *Nature* **2001**, *412*, 835–838.

105. Kicska, G. A.; Tyler, P. C.; Evans, G. B.; Furneaux, R. H.; Shi, W. X.; Fedorov, A.; Lewandowicz, A.; Cahill, S. M.; Almo, S. C.; Schramm, V. L. Atomic dissection of the hydrogen bond network for transition-state analogue binding to purine nucleoside phosphorylase. *Biochemistry* **2002**, *41*, 14489–14498.

106. Evans, G.; Furneaux, R.; Lewandowicz, A.; Schramm, V.; Tyler, P. Exploring structure-activity relationships of transition state analogues of human purine nucleoside phosphorylase. *J. Med. Chem.* **2003**, *46*, 3412–3423.

107. Lewandowicz, A.; Tyler, P. C.; Evans, G. B.; Furneaux, R. H.; Schramm, V. L. Achieving the ultimate physiological goal in transition state analogue inhibitors for purine nucleoside phosphorylase. *J. Biol. Chem.* **2003**, *278*, 31465–31468.

108. Jiang, Y.; Ichikawa, Y.; Stivers, J. Inhibition of uracil DNA glycosylase by an oxacarbenium ion mimic. *Biochemistry* **2002**, *41*, 7116–7124.

109. Berti, P.; McCann, J. Toward a detailed understanding of base excision repair enzymes: transition state and mechanistic analyses of N-glycoside hydrolysis and N-glycoside transfer. *Chem. Rev.* **2006**, *106*, 506–555.

110. Evans, G.; Furneaux, R.; Lewandowicz, A.; Schramm, V.; Tyler, P. Synthesis of second-generation transition state analogues of human purine nucleoside phosphorylase. *J. Med. Chem.* **2003**, *46*, 5271–5276.

111. Evans, G.; Furneaux, R.; Tyler, P.; Schramm, V. Synthesis of a transition state analogue inhibitor of purine nucleoside phosphorylase via the mannich reaction. *Org. Lett.* **2003**, *5*, 3639–3640.

112. Furneaux, R.; Tyler, P. Improved syntheses of 3H,5H-pyrrolo[3,2-d]pyrimidines. *J. Org. Chem.* **1999**, *64*, 8411–8412.

113. Lewandowicz, A.; Shi, W. X.; Evans, G. B.; Tyler, P. C.; Furneaux, R. H.; Basso, L. A.; Santos, D. S.; Almo, S. C.; Schramm, V. L. Over-the-barrier transition state analogues and crystal structure with mycobacterium tuberculosis purine nucleoside phosphorylase. *Biochemistry* **2003**, *42*, 6057–6066.

114. Taylor Ringia, E. A.; Tyler, P. C.; Evans, G. B.; Furneaux, R. H.; Murkin, A. S.; Schramm, V. L. Transition state analogue discrimination by related purine nucleoside phosphorylases. *J. Am. Chem. Soc.* **2006**, *128*, 7126–7127.

115. Clinch, K.; Evans, G.; Fleet, G.; Furneaux, R.; Johnson, S.; Lenz, D.; Mee, S.; Rands, P.; Schramm, V.; Taylor Ringia, E.; Tyler, P. Syntheses and bio-activities of the L-enantiomers of two potent transition state analogue inhibitors of purine nucleoside phosphorylases. *Org. Biomol. Chem.* **2006**, *4*, 1131–1139.

116. Rinaldo-Matthis, A.; Murkin, A.; Ramagopal, U.; Clinch, K.; Mee, S.; Evans, G.; Tyler, P.; Furneaux, R.; Almo, S.; Schramm, V. L-enantiomers of transition state analogue inhibitors bound to human purine nucleoside phosphorylase. *J. Am. Chem. Soc.* **2008**, *130*, 842–844.

117. Lewandowicz, A.; Ringia, E.; Ting, L.; Kim, K.; Tyler, P.; Evans, G.; Zubkova, O.; Mee, S.; Painter, G.; Lenz, D.; Furneaux, R.; Schramm, V. Energetic mapping of transition state analogue interactions with human and *Plasmodium falciparum* purine nucleoside phosphorylases. *J. Biol. Chem.* **2005**, *280*, 30320–30328.

118. Nunez, S.; Wing, C.; Antoniou, D.; Schramm, V. L.; Schwartz, S. D. Insight into catalytically relevant correlated motions in human purine nucleoside phosphorylase. *J. Phys. Chem. A* **2006**, *110*, 463–472.

119. Murkin, A.; Tyler, P.; Schramm, V. Transition-state interactions revealed in purine nucleoside phosphorylase by binding isotope effects. *J. Am. Chem. Soc.* **2008**, *130*, 2166–2167.

120. Kicska, G.; Long, L.; Hörig, H.; Fairchild, C.; Tyler, P.; Furneaux, R.; Schramm, V.; Kaufman, H. Immucillin H, a powerful transition-state analog inhibitor of purine nucleoside phosphorylase, selectively inhibits human T lymphocytes. *Proc. Natl. Acad. Sci. U.S.A.* **2001**, *98*, 4593–4598.

121. Bantia, S.; Miller, P. J.; Parker, C. D.; Ananth, S. L.; Horn, L. L.; Kilpatrick, J. M.; Morris, P. E.; Hutchison, T. L.; Montgomery, J. A.; Sandhu, J. S. Purine nucleoside phosphorylase inhibitor BCX-1777 (Immucillin-H) – a novel potent and orally active immunosuppressive agent. *Int. Immunopharmacol.* **2001**, *1*, 1199–1210.

122. Galmarini, C. Drug evaluation: forodesine – PNP inhibitor for the treatment of leukemia, lymphoma and solid tumor. *IDrugs* **2006**, *9*, 712–722.

123. Larson, R. A. Three new drugs for acute lymphoblastic leukemia: nelarabine, clofarabine, and forodesine. *Semin. Oncol.* **2007**, *34*, S13–20.

124. Korycka, A.; Blonski, J. Z.; Robak, T. Forodesine (BCX-1777, Immucillin H) – a new purine nucleoside analogue: mechanism of action and potential clinical application. *Mini Rev. Med. Chem.* **2007**, *7*, 976–983.

125. Gore, L.; Stelljes, M.; Quinones, R. Forodesine treatment and post-transplant graft-versus-host disease in two patients with acute leukemia: facilitation of graft-versus-leukemia effect? *Semin. Oncol.* **2007**, *34*, S35–39.

126. Gandhi, V.; Balakrishnan, K. Pharmacology and mechanism of action of forodesine, a T-cell targeted agent. *Semin. Oncology* **2007**, *34*, S8–S12.

127. Furman, R. R.; Hoelzer, D. Purine nucleoside phosphorylase inhibition as a novel therapeutic approach for B-cell lymphoid malignancies. *Semin. Oncol.* **2007**, *34*, S29–S34.

128. Duvic, M.; Foss, F. M. Mycosis fungoides: pathophysiology and emerging therapies. *Semin. Oncol.* **2007**, *34*, S21–28.

129. Duvic, M. Systemic monotherapy vs combination therapy for ctcl: rationale and future strategies. *Oncology* **2007**, *21*, 33–40.

130. BioCryst Pharmaceuticals Inc., Forodesine, October 7, 2009, http://www.biocryst.com/forodesine.

131. Semeraro, T.; Lossani, A.; Botta, M.; Ghiron, C.; Alvarez, R.; Manetti, F.; Mugnaini, C.; Valensin, S.; Focher, F.; Corelli, F. Simplified analogues of Immucillin-G retain potent human purine nucleoside phosphorylase inhibitory activity. *J. Med. Chem.* **2006**, *49*, 6037–6045.

132. Taylor, E.; Clinch, K.; Kelly, P.; Li, L.; Evans, G.; Tyler, P.; Schramm, V. Acyclic ribooxacarbenium ion mimics as transition state analogues of human and malarial purine nucleoside phosphorylases. *J. Am. Chem. Soc.* **2007**, *129*, 6984–6985.

133. Acronym for 2′-Deoxy-2′-Amino-Tetritol-N-(9-Methylene)-ImmH but the IUPAC name is 9-deaza-9-[[(2R,3S)-1,3,4-trihydroxybutan-2-ylamino]methyl]hypoxanthine. This acronym first appeared in Taylor et al., but as an oversight, was never defined; DATMe-ImmH is compound 19 in that manuscript.

134. Taylor, E. A.; Rinaldo-Matthis, A.; Li, L.; Ghanem, M.; Hazleton, K. Z.; Cassera, M. B.; Almo, S. C.; Schramm, V. L. *Anopheles gambiae* purine nucleoside phosphorylase: catalysis, structure, and inhibition. *Biochemistry* **2007**, *46*, 12405–12415.

135. Agarwal, R.; Spector, T.; Parks, R. J. Tight-binding inhibitors. IV. Inhibition of adenosine deaminases by various inhibitors. *Biochem. Pharmacol.* **1977**, *26*, 359–367.

136. Tokutake, N.; Hiratake, J.; Katoh, M.; Irie, T.; Kato, H.; Oda, J. Design, synthesis and evaluation of transition-state analogue inhibitors of *Escherichia coli* gamma-glutamylcysteine synthetase. *Bioorg. Med. Chem.* **1998**, *6*, 1935–1953.

137. von Itzstein, M.; Wu, W.; Kok, G.; Pegg, M.; Dyason, J.; Jin, B.; Van Phan, T.; Smythe, M.; White, H.; Oliver, S. Rational design of potent sialidase-based inhibitors of influenza virus replication. *Nature* **1993**, *363*, 418–423.

138. Bolin, J.; Filman, D.; Matthews, D.; Hamlin, R.; Kraut, J. Crystal structures of *Escherichia coli* and *Lactobacillus casei* dihydrofolate reductase refined at 1.7 Å resolution. I. General features and binding of methotrexate. *J. Biol. Chem.* **1982**, *257*, 13650–13662.

139. Kimble, E.; Hadala, J.; Ludewig, R.; Peters, P.; Greenberg, G.; Xiao, G.; Guida, W.; McQuire, L.; Simon, P. The biochemical and pharmacological activity of 9-benzyl-9-deazaguanine, a potent purine nucleoside phosphorylase (PNP) inhibitor. *Inflamm. Res.* **1995**, *44*(suppl. 2), S181–S182.

140. Perzborn, E.; Strassburger, J.; Wilmen, A.; Pohlmann, J.; Roehrig, S.; Schlemmer, K. H.; Straub, A. In vitro and in vivo studies of the novel antithrombotic agent bay 59–7939 – an oral, direct factor Xa inhibitor. *J. Thromb. Haemost.* **2005**, *3*, 514–521.

141. Taylor Ringia, E. A.; Schramm, V. L. Transition states and inhibitors of the purine nucleoside phosphorylase family. *Curr. Top. Med. Chem.* **2005**, *5*, 1237–1258.

142. Kicska, G. A.; Tyler, P. C.; Evans, G. B.; Furneaux, R. H.; Kim, K.; Schramm, V. L. Transition state analogue inhibitors of purine nucleoside phosphorylase from *Plasmodium falciparum*. *J. Biol. Chem.* **2002**, *277*, 3219–3225.

143. Barsacchi, D.; Cappiello, M.; Tozzi, M.; Del Corso, A.; Peccatori, M.; Camici, M.; Ipata, P.; Mura, U. Purine nucleoside phosphorylase from bovine lens: purification and properties. *Biochim. Biophys. Acta* **1992**, *1160*, 163–170.

144. Stoeckler, J. D.; Poirot, A. F.; Smith, R. M.; Parks, R. E.; Ealick, S. E.; Takabayashi, K.; Erion, M. D. Purine nucleoside phosphorylase. 3. Reversal of purine base specificity by site-directed mutagenesis. *Biochemistry* **1997**, *36*, 11749–11756.

16

GPCR 3D modeling

Frank U. Axe

INTRODUCTION

G-protein-coupled receptors (GPCRs) are a superfamily of membrane proteins that provide cells with the ability to communicate with each other and their environment.[1,2] The core feature of these proteins is their seven transmembrane helices (7TM) that form a bundle located in the cell membrane (Figure 16.1). The seven helices are linked together by three extracellular loops (ECLs) and three intracellular loops (ICLs) and also include N- and C-terminal regions. This 7TM region is responsible for receiving a wide range of signals from small-molecule amines, peptides, proteins, small odorant and taste molecules, and light, which either bind in the interior of the 7TM bundle or to its extracellular surface or interact with chromophores located in its interior. These external signals trigger the coupling of the ICLs (in particular ICL5) with the heterotrimeric G-protein transducin, which in turn initiates a cascade of signaling events that lead to proliferation, differentiation, development, cell survival, angiogenesis, and hypertrophy.[1,2] In light of these facts it is not surprising to find that GPCRs are implicated as targets in a wide range of indications, including heart disease, allergies, depression, mental illness, cognition, and hypertension.[1-3]

The estimated number of GPCRs in humans is ~1,000 members or ~1% of the genome. There are five major classes of GPCRs that are defined by their sequence homology and the type of endogenous ligand.[1,2] The most important of these classes are A, B, and C. GPCRs are dysfunctional or dysregulated in many diseases making them the target of drug therapies.

Many of today's approved drugs target GPCRs and account for somewhere between 30 and 40% of the revenues from pharmaceutical sales.[3] This amounts to over (U.S.)$23.5 billion in sales annually.[3] Many of the well-known blockbuster drugs in use today like Zyrtec, Claritin, Singulair, and Risperdal target GPCRs.[3] So it is clear that many of the future drug treatments of existing and new diseases will involve GPCRs as targets for those therapies. As a result there is an ever-growing need to streamline the discovery process while leveraging all available resources to bring these new drug therapies to market.

Structure-based drug design is an integral part of the drug discovery process today and has played an essential role in the discovery of new pharmaceutical medicines.[4-7] In the past modeling of GPCR-based therapeutics more often than not involved traditional approaches like 2D searches (similarity, substructure),[6] quantitative structure activity relationships (QSAR),[6] pharmacophore,[8] and shape[9] analysis due to the absence of experimental structures of compounds bound to GPCRs. These methods can pinpoint new compound series or identify essential features for recognition by the receptor; however, they cannot predict outside the range of the probe or training set of molecule(s)[4] used in the analysis. Three dimensional (3D) modeling involving the target can enable the identification and refinement of leads without the necessity of a large set of active and inactive compounds.[5-7]

Since the year 2000 three new crystal structures of GPCRs have been published.[10-14] These structures have helped advance the state of the art of 3D modeling of GPCRs. This chapter reviews these new advances as well as the past literature on 3D modeling of GPCR drug interactions, including the current experimental structural information, techniques for building GPCR models, docking and virtual screening methods, and molecular dynamics studies. In addition future directions in 3D GPCR modeling are discussed.

CRYSTAL STRUCTURES

The experimental structural characterization of the 7TM bundle has proved elusive for several reasons, including conformational flexibility, purity, and solubility.[10-14] Thus, there is a paucity of crystal structures available for drug design work, especially when compared to what is available for enzyme targets. An essential ingredient to any target-based drug discovery project is a crystal structure of the target or one that is homologous to the target of interest.[4,5] In 2000 the first complete crystal structure of the mammalian GPCR, bovine rhodopsin, was solved.[10,11]

Rhodopsin is a light-activated GPCR in which 11-*cis*-retinal acts as a chromophore absorbing light, causing it to change conformation in the binding pocket and triggering a conformational change of the 7TM region. This initial

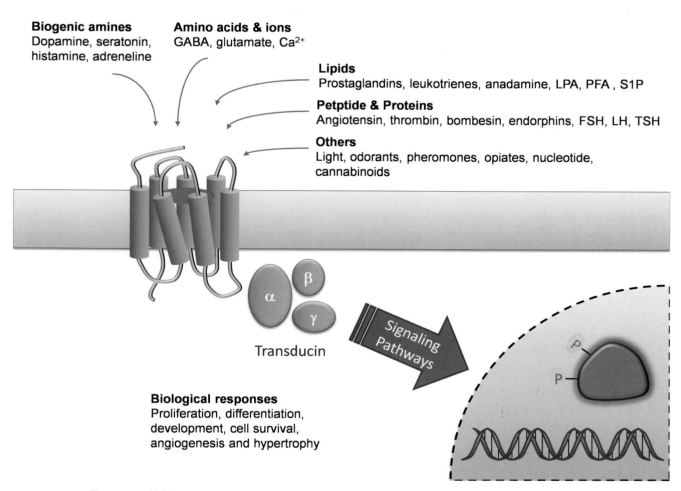

Figure 16.1. GPCR structure, stimuli, and function. GPCRs receive messages from endogenous ligands that can vary significantly. The receptor activates the G-protein (Transducin) and signals gene expression resulting in a full array of biological responses.

structure corresponds to the inactive form of the receptor. The structure revealed that the seven helices are arranged antiparallel and that the retinal molecule was covalently linked to an amino acid side chain (LYS 296) in an interior binding pocket that had little access to the intra- and extracellular and membrane regions. There are also a number of kinks found in several helices, which are initiated by proline residues and may be involved in conformational changes that take place when the receptor is activated.

More recently the crystal structure of the β_2-andrenergic receptor was solved in two ways. First, with the aid of an antibody complexed to helices 5 and 6 and, second, as an engineered fusion protein in which the intracellular loop between helices 5 and 6 was replace with a T4-lysozyme protein. Each of these modifications served a similar function: to stabilize helices 5 and 6 and provide a more polar environment for crystallization.[12–14]

The qualitative arrangement of the 7TM bundle is very similar for the two types of GPCR structures (rhodopsin and β_2-AR) as evidenced visually in Figure 16.2. Specifically all seven helices have similar positions and tilts relative to each other (Figure 16.2). A noticeable difference in the two structures is in the loops on the extracellular side of each protein between helices 4 and 5. In rhodopsin there exists a beta-sheet structure that seals off the active site from the extracellular solvent, while in β_2-AR there is an additional small helical structure making the binding pocket more accessible. These differences underscore the variation that can occur in homologous proteins and is undoubtedly important when building homology model (vida infra). Finally, the structure of β_2-AR contains the surrogate T4-lysozyme (T4L) protein for the ECL between helices 5 and 6. Because this structure has a bound inverse-agonist then T4L could be construed as stabilizing the inactive form of the receptor.

The ligand-binding sites in both rhodopsin and β_2-AR are in very similar locations within the 7TM bundle and occupy roughly the same size and shape. The 11-*cis*-retinal

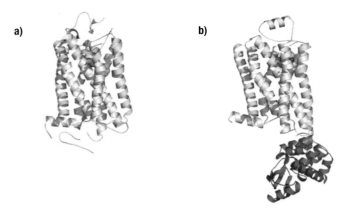

a)   b)

Figure 16.2. Crystal structures of bovine rhodopsin (1F88) **(a)** and β₂-andrenergic (2RH1) **(b)** receptors shown parallel to the lipid membrane. The 11-*cis*-retinal chromophore of rhodopsin and the inverse-agonist carazolol of β₂-AR are shown in green and orange, respectively. The T-4 lysozyme domain of β₂-AR is highlighted in red. Images were created with PYMOL 0.99 (http://pymol.sourceforge.net/).

and carazolol molecules occupy very similar regions of space within the two receptors as evidenced by the structures of the two proteins viewed from similar vantage points (Figure 16.3).

Not surprisingly the carazolol ligand bound to β₂-AR is found to make a key salt-bridging interaction with its basic amine and Asp113 on helix 3. The 2-hydroxyl group of the propyl chain makes hydrogen-bonding interactions with Asn312 on helix 7 (Figure 16.3). Finally, the HN group of the carbazole ring is within hydrogen bond distance of Ser203 on helix 5. All of these interactions were determined to be important for the binding of adrenalin and noradrenalin as well and are believed to be an important part of antagonist binding in general.[5] The encumbrance of ECL2 in rhodopsin is clearly visible (Figure 16.3).

3D STRUCTURE MODELING

Essentially all GPCR drug targets have no known structure, so one has to be constructed based on the available sequence data and the structure of a homologously related protein(s) or construct a model from first principles.[5,15] Before the bovine rhodopsin structure was available homology models were based on the structure of bacterial rhodopsin,[16–20] the C_α coordinates of bovine rhodopsin,[21] or even the low-resolution crystal data on bovine rhodopsin.[22,23] These structural data were used to construct the first full models of GPCRs.[24–27] Many of these models were guided only by these structures and in some cases early de novo approaches were employed.[24–27]

Homology modeling

When the structure of a target of interest is unknown often a suitable model of that target structure can be built if there exists at least one closely related structure. This homology relationship has been exploited by modelers for some time.[15] Until very recently all of the homology models of GPCRs relied exclusively on bovine rhodopsin[28–30] for building a homology model. This limits the amount of variation of structural information going into building a homology model and also suggests that GPCRs belonging to more remote classes (i.e., B and C) will not be as good a match. When the recent crystal structures of β₂-AR[12–14] are compared with bovine rhodopsin,[10,11] both class A GPCRs, there is good structural correspondence between the two receptors, which strengthens the opinion that homology models based on bovine rhodopsin should be reasonable especially for class A GPCRs; however, there are differences. The number of homology models based on rhodopsin is extensive and they were primarily developed for the purpose

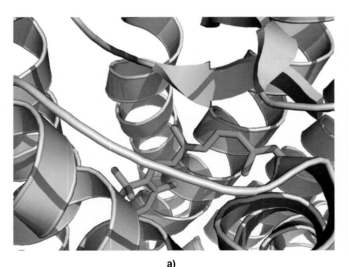

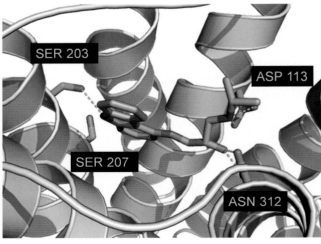

a)   b)

Figure 16.3. The ligand binding sites in the crystal structures of bovine rhodopsin (left) with 11-*cis*-retinal bound (1F88) and β₂-andrenergic (right) with carazolol bound (2RH1) viewed from similar vantage points. Images were created with PYMOL 0.99 (http://pymol.sourceforge.net/).

of ligand docking and refinement as well as site-directed mutagenesis.[31–35]

A recent publication compares a homology model of β_2-AR based on bovine rhodopsin with the new β_2-AR crystal structures.[36] Two models were created, one with the rhodopsin-like second ECL and the other had the second ECL built de novo, and the inverse-agonist carazolol was docked into each of these models. In the former of the two structures the ECL interfered with binding of carazolol, whereas in the later of the two models the ECL did not affect the binding of carazolol. These results are consistent with the experimental differences in the second ECL (Figures 16.2 and 16.3) for rhodopsin and β_2-AR.

De novo structure prediction

The inherent limitations of homology modeling and the unique structural template of the GPCR 7TM region has prompted several groups to develop de novo-based approaches to generating GPCR models that may be applied to receptors in families other than Family A, which have more remote homology with the bovine rhodopsin template.

Two de novo methods have emerged lately that are very similar in their approach to constructing a GPCR model structure, which are the PREDICT[37,38] and MEMBSTRUK[39–41] methods. The protocol for predicting GPCR structures by these methods consists of roughly the following steps: (1) predict the TM regions using hydrophobicity analysis and other sequence analysis techniques; (2) construct the individual helices and pack them together; (3) have each putative structure in the previous step undergo coarse grain optimization; and (4) perform full optimizations of the structures.

Validation of the structures predicted by these methods was twofold. First, for the structure of bovine rhodopsin built by these techniques, a direct comparison with the crystal structure was made and found to be in close agreement. Second, for models in which there is no experimental crystal structure, the docking and assessment of ligand-binding energies was performed and found to be consistent with experimental values. Furthermore, some of these docked structures provided useful insights regarding the nature of the ligand binding interactions.[37–41]

DOCKING STUDIES

Manual docking

Molecular docking is perhaps one of the most illuminating and sublime procedures used by computational chemists.[4–7] It has the ability to reveal aspects of ligand binding that are neither obvious nor trivial and cannot be ascertained from the ligands alone. The literature is filled with numerous studies in which the binding of small molecules and peptides was examined.[43–52] This usually involved a homology model of the receptor and the docking

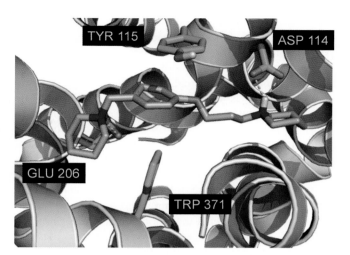

Figure 16.4. Histamine H_3 antagonist docked in the binding site of a homology model followed by 200 ps of molecular dynamics simulation.[36] Image was created with PYMOL 0.99 (http://pymol.sourceforge.net/).

of the ligand was either manual and/or semiautomated. Moreover, site-directed mutagenesis data were often used to determine key residues responsible for endogenous ligand activity as well as antagonist activity too.

For example, homology models have been used to study ligand binding in several types of aminoergic receptors, including dopamine,[44,45] histamine,[33,36] β-andrenergic,[34,43,44] and serotonin.[45] Several docking studies involving the β-andrenergic receptors and antagonists and their natural ligand[34,43,44] usually include the basic amine interaction with the aspartic acid side chain on helix 3 (D3.32), which is consistent with the β_2-AR structure with carazolol bound (Figure 16.3). In addition, the catachol hydroxyl groups make hydrogen bonding interactions with the two serine side chains on helix 5 (S5.42 and S5.46).

Other examples of docking include the histamine receptors.[33,36] Currently, there are four known histamine subtypes (H_1, H_2, H_3 and H_4).[36] Antagonists of H_1 and H_2 comprise some of the better known "blockbuster" drugs on the market today. Like all aminoergic receptors there is a highly conserved aspartic acid on helix 3 (D3.32)[5] that interacts with the basic amine of the natural ligand histamine as well as exogenous antagonists and antagonists (Figure 16.4).

In the H_3 docking model there is an additional basic amine that is based on the model and existing structure/activity relationships are postulated to interact with a glutamic acid (GLU 206) side chain on helix 5.

Fast docking and virtual screening

There is an ever-increasing use of 3D drug targets to rapidly dock compound collections into their active site to discover novel leads for that target especially when no lead compounds are known.[6,7] Several studies involving this type of virtual screening applied to GPCRs has appeared in the literature.[46–52] Most of these studies relied on homology models built from the bovine rhodopsin structure or newer de novo methods. However, because of the advent of the β_2-AR structures there are some new virtual screening studies reported in the literature as well.

Three-dimensional virtual screening applications using homology models of the GPCR based on the bovine rhodopsin structure are plentiful.[46–49] In a systematic study of the dopamine (D3), muscarinic (M1), and vasopressin (V1a) receptors by Bissantz et al., three different docking methods with seven scoring functions were used.[46] The binding sites of the GPCR models were preoptimized to be able to accommodate antagonists better. Each model was then used to dock a randomly chosen set of 990 drug-like molecules plus ten known antagonists for each receptor. The hit rates from these procedures ranged between 5 and 40%. Another systematic study employing PREDICT built models for five different receptors, including biogenic amine, peptide, and chemokine receptors.[38] One docking method and multiple scoring functions were used to screen ~1.6 million druglike compounds available from >20 vendors worldwide. Hits rates between 12 and 21% were achieved for the five receptors, and in most cases the best hit was a novel and potent (1–100 nM) compound. A recent study of the melanin-concentrating hormone receptor identified six novel chemotypes of 187,084 drug-like compounds screened, which amounted to a tenfold improvement over random high-throughput screening.[47] In a final 3D virtual screening study on the histamine H_4 receptor, close to nine million compounds that were available commercially were screened in silico, of which 255 compounds were ordered and 16 were considered active.[48]

Another common technique is to use a hierarchical approach in which a large compound collection is first screened using pharmacophores and the compounds obtained from that filtering process are then docked in the receptor active site.[50,51] This approach takes advantage of the speed and well-established success of pharmacophore searching while potentially eliminating many hits that match the pharmacophore but are poor candidates for the target due to steric clashes with the protein target.

In a recent article, the newly published β_2-AR structure was used to test the ability to dock β_2-AR antagonists in to the binding site.[52] First, a series of seven known β_2-AR antagonists were docked and compared with the experimentally bound carazolol compound. The docked structures of the seven beta-blockers, which included carazolol, were in very good agreement with the binding mode adopted by carazolol in the crystal structure. Similar interactions with the conserved aspartic acidic group on helix 3 and hydrogen bond donor/acceptor groups on helix 5 were achieved. Also, the placement of hydrophobic groups that extended beyond the region of the carbazol macrocycle were reasonable. Next, high-throughput docking with an in-house proprietary (~400,000 compounds) database was performed. In the top 30 compounds, 11 known beta-blockers were found. Finally, a second high-throughput docking experiment involving 4 million compounds was performed. The docking identified compounds that appear to bind in two very different parts of the binding site. One binding region is the traditional site occupied by the known antagonists like carazolol; the second is a region near one of the extracellular loops. Many of the compounds predicted to bind in the second region are unique chemotypes for β_2-AR antagonists. This second binding site is in the loop region of the β_2-AR structure that differs from the bovine rhodopsin structure (Figure 16.2). So it is unlikely that these compounds would be found in a virtual screening of a rhodopsin-based homology model. The experimental results of these new findings are not yet published; however, the ability to make very novel predictions like this is the single most important advantage of the 3D structure-based approach.

MOLECULAR DYNAMICS SIMULATIONS

Molecular dynamics (MD) simulation is an important tool for studying the flexibility, stability, and large-scale motions of molecules often in a condensed-phase environment.[4] These approaches are still very computationally intensive and are still not used routinely in industry for drug discovery. However, these methods are often needed to predict properties of a system that an individual structure cannot provide such as average properties like structure and thermodynamic properties like binding energies.[4] Two ways of carrying out these calculations[4] are (1) to surround the protein system with explicit solvent and impose a periodic boundary condition and (2) to use continuum methods like the generalized Born model. MD has also become a very important technique used to construct and anneal model structures.[4]

Explicit bilayer and solvent

Simulation of protein/ligand interactions are often greatly influenced by the environment in which a protein system resides. This is particularly true for GPCRs that straddle two very different physical regions that have different hydrophilic/hydrophobic properties, namely water and lipid.

In a recent article[53] a 40 ns simulation on the bovine rhodopsin structure examined the average structure of the protein, the average structure of the retinal binding site, the large-scale motions, and the lipid/water interactions. During the simulation the structure of the protein was well maintained, especially the helices. There were larger deviations in the loop and N- and C-terminal regions. A change was observed in the hydrogen bonding near the retinal chromophore that leads to some shifts in the tilts of several helices. This was hypothesized to be important for the reaction cycle of the receptor.

Simulations of β_2-AR with epinephrine and butoxamine bound were run using a de novo model.[54] Butox amine

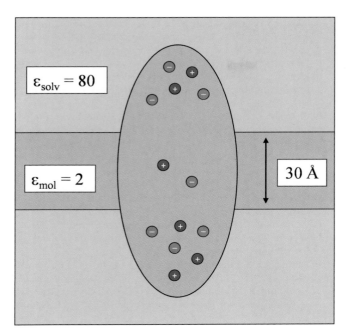

Figure 16.5. Schematic representation of the continuum dielectric regions used in a generalized Born model approach to modeling a GPCR embedded in a lipid bilayer.

maintained a stable complex in the binding site between the residues of helices 3 and 5. However, in the case of epinephrine, an agonist, water molecules during the simulation inserted themselves into the hydrogen bonds of the catechol groups and serine residue side chains on helix 5. This result implies that the model GPCR structure corresponds to the inactive form of the receptor.

A study of the cholecysokinin receptor and its natural ligand the nonapeptide CCK9 was simulated for 31 ns.[55] The structure of the GPCR was well preserved, especially the in the helical regions and there were larger motions in the loop regions. Water-mediated interactions are shown to be involved in the binding. Free-energy perturbation calculations were performed in which several different amino acids of CCK9 were mutated. The calculated relative free energies were in good agreement with experiment. These results offer some validation of the docking model of the ligand.

Finally MD simulations of the CXCR4 receptor with an inverse-agonist T140, a peptide, and a partial agonist AMD3100, a small molecule, were published.[56] T140 was predicted to bind in the ECL region, while AMD3100 was predicted to bind more inside the helical bundle.

Implicit bilayer and solvent

Performing simulations of the GPCR 7TM region using an explicit membrane are computationally demanding; therefore methods that treat the solvents around a protein as a continuum have been extended to include a protein embedded in a lipid membrane.[57,58] These methods have the advantage of being computationally faster and a more straightforward way to analyze results and making it much

easier to manage the calculation. These approaches use an extension of the Born model for solvation[59] that is implemented by considering the membrane region and the protein embedded in it to be a low dielectric region and the surrounding aqueous regions, corresponding to the intra- and extracellular regions, to be high dielectric regions (Figure 16.5).[57] In addition to the electrostatic treatment of these two regions there is an empirical hydrophobic term based on surface area.[57,58]

One of the first applications of this implicit membrane model method was on bovine rhodopsin.[57] This study was primarily aimed at validating the newly developed method. The orientation of the rhodopsin crystal structure in the implicit membrane was first tested in the implicit membrane model. The 7TM bundle was systematically varied relative to the membrane region through rigid-body translations and rotations. The energy function predicted an orientation of the 7TM helices that are perpendicular to the bilayer region. The model also predicted the central part of the GPCR with its hydrophobic side chains well localized in the hydrophobic bilayer region, while hydrophilic side chains of the loop regions preferred the high dielectric region corresponding to aqueous solution.

The implicit bilayer model was applied to the study of several antagonists in the binding site of a histamine H_3 receptor model.[36] The antagonists were manually docked into the binding site that is in close proximity to where 11-*cis*-retinal binds in rhodopsin. The key amino acid residues responsible for binding were previously determined by site-directed mutagenesis for the histamine receptors and they are analogous to the key residues involved in ligand binding in aminoergic GPCRs (vida supra).[36] Over the course of a 200-ps molecular dynamics simulation the helices of the receptor remained embedded in the membrane slab while the intra- and extracellular loops remained in the aqueous regions of the model (Figure 16.4).

Model building

Another use of molecular dynamics methods is for building a model of the active state of GPCRs from the inactive rhodopsin structure.[60,61] Several groups have used experimentally determined constraints for active forms of the receptor and applied them during the course of MD simulations to coerce the receptor structure into its active state. Recently a crystal structure corresponding to the active form of rhodopsin was determined and compared to the inactive form and these models. The initial finding is that the changes in going to the active state in the crystal are smaller than what is implied by the experimental distance constraints.[62]

FRAGMENT-BASED METHODS

The consistent success of 3D modeling of GPCRs in homology and docking suggests that these approaches could also be useful for fragment-based discovery.[63,64] That is small fragments, which by themselves are weak binders, are determined to bind to specific regions of the active site. These fragments are generally very weak binders in that they do not constitute leads in and of themselves; however, they may be linked together to form a significantly more active compound. These methods offer the ability to virtually screen weak binders and provide the mechanism to link them together. If experimental data pertaining to the binding location are available then the GPCR models can be used.

CONCLUSIONS

Over the course of this decade there have been significant advances in the experimental structural characterization of GPCRs, namely the bovine rhodopsin and, more recently, the β_2-AR crystal structures. These structures have in turn propelled the development of homology models of GPCRs in a wide range of studies. In addition advances in docking technology, in particular rapid methods, have made the in silico screening of large libraries now possible. These methods are now poised to give a greater impact in the discovery of new GPCR ligands.

The use of bovine rhodopsin to produce homology models of GPCRs since 2000 has been shown to be reasonable. The ability of these models to provide insights regarding ligand/receptor interactions lends credence to their accuracy and reliability at least for class A receptors. The new crystal structures of β_2-AR with a ligand bound not only provides confirmation of past modeling approaches involving homology models followed by ligand docking but also provides additional information that will improve on this established modeling approach in the future.

More crystal structures of GPCRs are needed to improve homology modeling, our overall understanding of how GPCRs work, how they interact with ligands and drugs, and how they differ among the various classes. There is a need for more crystal structures of GPCRs with ligands that bind in the helices and in the extracellular region, involving GPCRs of different classes, in active and inactive states.

Virtual screening studies have demonstrated the ability of GPCR models and docking calculations to identify leads for drug discovery with hit rates comparable to what is seen for enzyme targets. A new virtual screening study for the β_2-AR receptor has identified very novel ligands that previously have not been reported. Some of these ligands bind in nontraditional regions of the binding site. This is certainly very encouraging and what one would anticipate virtual screening to afford; however, the jury is still out on the ultimate outcome of the predicted results.

REFERENCES

1. Filmore, D. It's a GPCR world *Mod. Drug Discov.* **2004**, *7*, 47–48.
2. Bockaert, J.; Pin, J. P. Molecular tinkering of G protein-coupled receptors: an evolutionary success. *EMBO J.* **1999**, *18*, 1723.
3. Wise, A.; Gearing, K.; Rees, S. Target validation of G-protein coupled receptors. *Drug Discov. Today* **2002**, *7*, 235.
4. Leach, A. R. *Molecular Modeling Principles and Applications.* Essex, UK: Prentice Hall; **2001**.
5. Müller, G. Towards 3D Structures of G Protein-Coupled Receptors: A Multidisciplinary Approach. *Curr. Med. Chem.* **2000**, *7*, 861.
6. Bleicher, K. H.; Green, L. G.; Martin, R. E.; Rogers-Evans, M. Ligand identification for G-protein-coupled receptors: a lead generation perspective. *Curr. Opin. Chem. Biol.* **2004**, *8*, 287.
7. Walters W. P.; Stahl, M. T.; Murcko, M. A. Virtual screening – an overview. *Drug Discov. Today* **1998**, *3*, 160.
8. Hawkins, P. C. D.; Skillman, A.G.; Nicholls, A. Comparison of Shape-Matching and Docking as Virtual Screening Tools. *J. Med. Chem.* **2007**, *50*, 74.
9. Clement, O.; Mehl, A.T. In: *Pharmacophore Preception, Development, and Use in Drug Design*, O. F. Guner, Ed.; La Jolla, CA: International University Line; **2000**, 71.
10. Palczewski, K.; Kumasaka, T.; Hori, T.; Behnke, C. A.; Motoshima, H.; Fox, B. A.; Le Trong, I.; Teller, D. C.; Okada, T.; Stenkamp, R. E.; Yamamoto, M.; Miyano, M. Crystal Structure of Rhodopsin: A G Protein-Coupled Receptor. *Science* **2000**, *289*, 739.
11. Stenkamp, R. E.; Teller, D. C.; Palczewski, K. Crystal Structure of Rhodopsin: A G-Protein-Coupled Receptor. *ChemBioChem* **2002**, *3*, 963.
12. Rasmussen, S. G. F.; Choi, H. J.; Rosenbaum, D. M.; Kobilka, B. K.; Thian, F. S.; Edwards, P. C.; Burghammer, M.; Ratnala, V. R. P.; Sanishvili, R.; Fischetti, R. F.; Schertler, G. F. X.; Weis, W. I.; Kobilka, T. S. Crystal structure of the human β_2 adrenergic G-protein-coupled receptor. *Nature* **2007**, *450*, 383.
13. Cherezov, V.; Rosenbaum, D. M.; Hanson, M. A.; Rasmussen, S. G. F.; Thian, F. S.; Kobilka, T. S.; Choi, H. J.; Kuhn, P.; Weis, W. I.; Kobilka, B. K.; Stevens, R. C. High-Resolution Crystal Structure of an Engineered Human β_2-Adrenergic G Protein-Coupled Receptor. *Science* **2007**, *318*, 1258.
14. Rosenbaum, D. M.; Cherezov, V.; Hanson, M. A.; Rasmussen, S. G. F.; Thian, F. S.; Kobilka, T. S.; Choi, H. J.; Yao, X. J.; Weis, W. I.; Stevens, R. C.; Kobilka, B. K. GPCR Engineering Yields High-Resolution Structural Insights into β_2-Adrenergic Receptor Function. *Science* **2007**, *318*, 1266.
15. Greer, J. Comparative modeling methods: application to the family of the mammalian serine proteases. *Proteins* **1990**, *7*, 317.
16. Lanyi, J.; Luecke, H. Bacteriorhodopsin. *Curr. Opin. Struc. Biol.* **2001**, *11*, 415.
17. Lanyi, J. K. Bacteriorhodopsin. *Annu. Rev. Physiol.* **2004**, *66* 665.
18. Pebay-Peyroula, E.; Rummel, G.; Rosenbusch, J. P; Landau, E. M. X-ray Structure of Bacteriorhodopsin at 2.5 Angstroms from Microcrystals Grown in Lipidic Cubic Phases. *Science*, **1997**, *277*, 1676.
19. Luecke, H.; Richter, H. T.; Lanyi, J. K. Proton transfer pathways in bacteriorhodopsin at 2.3 angstrom resolution. *Science*, **1998**, *280*, 1934.
20. Luecke, H.; Schobert, B.; Richter, H. T.; Cartailler, J. P.; Lanyi, J. K. Structure of Bacteriorhodopsin at 1.55 Å Resolution. *J. Mol. Biol.*, **1999**, *291*, 899.
21. Baldwin, J. M. The probable arrangement of the helices in G protein-coupled receptors. *EMBO J.* **1993**, *12* 1693.
22. Unger, V. M.; Schertler, G. F. X. Low resolution structure of bovine rhodopsin determined by electron cryo-microscopy. *Biophys. J.* **1995**, *68*, 1776.

23. Schertler, G. F.; Villa, C.; Henderson, R. Projection structure of rhodopsin. *Nature* **1993**, *362*, 770.

24. Pardo, L.; Ballesteros, J. A.; Osman, R.; Weinstein, H. On the use of the transmembrane domain of bacteriorhodopsin as a template for modeling the three-dimensional structure of guanine nucleotide-binding regulatory protein-coupled receptors. *Proc. Natl. Acad. Sci. U.S.A.* **1992**, *89*, 4009.

25. Hibert, M. F.; Trumpp-Kallmeyer, S.; Bruinvels, A.; Hofloack, J. Three-dimensional models of neurotransmitter G-binding protein-coupled receptors. *Mol. Pharmacol.* **1991**, *40*, 8.

26. MaloneyHuss, K.; Lybrand, T. P. Three-dimensional structure for the β_2 adrenergic receptor protein based on computer modeling studies. *J. Mol. Biol.* **1992**, *225*, 859.

27. Alorta, I.; Loew, G. H. A 3D model of the ö opioid receptor and ligand-receptor complexes. *Protein Eng.* **1996**, *9*, 573.

28. Archer, E.; Maigret, B.; Escrieut, C.; Pradayrol, L.; Fourmy, D. Rhodopsin crystal: new template yielding realistic models of G-protein-coupled receptors? *Trends Pharmacol. Sci.* **2003**, *24*, 36.

29. Hubbell, W. L.; Altenbach, C.; Hubbell, C. M.; Khorana, H.G. Rhodopsin structure, dynamics, and activation: a perspective from crystallography, site-directed spin labeling, sulfhydryl reactivity, and disulfide cross-linking. *Adv. Protein Chem.* **2003**, *63*, 243.

30. Kobilka, B.; Schertler, F. X. New G-protein-coupled receptor crystal structures: insights and limitations. *Trends Pharmacol. Sci.* **2008**, *29*, 79.

31. Oliveira L.; Hulsen T.; Lutje Hulsik D.; Paiva A. C.; Vriend G. Heavier-than-air flying machines are impossible. *FEBS Lett.* **2004** *564*, 269.

32. Hibert, M. F. Protein homology modeling and drug discovery. In: *The Practice of Medicinal Chemistry.* New York, NY: Academic Press; **1996**, 523–546.

33. Kiss, R.; Kori, Z.; Keserū, G. M. Homology modeling and binding site mapping of the human histamine H1 receptor Eur. *J. Med. Chem.* **2004**, *39*, 959.

34. Furse, K. E.; Lybrand, T. P. Three-Dimensional Models for β-Adrenergic Receptor Complexes with Agonists and Antagonists. *J. Med. Chem.* **2003**, *46*, 4450.

35. Evers, A; Klabunde, T. Structure-based Drug Discovery Using GPCR Homology Modeling: Successful Virtual Screening for Antagonists of the Alpha1A Adrenergic Receptor. *J. Med. Chem.* **2005**, *48*, 1088.

36. Axe, F. U.; Bembenek, S. D.; Szalma, S. Three-dimensional models of histamine H_3 receptor antagonist complexes and their pharmacophore. *J. Mol. Graph. Model.* **2006**, *24*, 456.

37. Costanzi, S. On the Applicability of GPCR Homolgy Models to Computer-Aided Drug Discovery: A Comparison between In Silico and Crystal Structures of the β_2-Adrenergic Receptor. *J. Med. Chem.* **2008**, *51*, 2907.

38. Becker, O. M.; Marantz, Y.; Shacham, S.; Inbal, B.; Heifetz, A.; Kalid, O.; Bar-Haim, S.; Warshaviak, D.; Fichman, M.; Noiman, S. G Protein-coupled receptors: In silico drug discovery in 3D. *Proc. Natl. Acad. Sci. U.S.A.* **2004**, *101*, 11304.

39. Shacham, S.; Marantz, Y.; Bar-Haim, S.; Kalid, O.; Warshaviak, D.; Avisar, N.; Inbal, B.; Heifetz, A.; Fichman, M.; Topf, M.; Naor, Z.; Noiman, S.; Becker, O.M. PREDICT Modeling and In-Silico Screening for G-Protein Coupled Receptors. *Proteins* **2004**, *57*, 51.

40. Vaidehi, N.; Floriano, W. B.; Trabanino, R.; Hall, S. E.; Freddolino, P.; Choi, E. J.; Zamanakos, G.; Goddard, W. A. Prediction of structure and function of G protein-coupled receptors. *Proc. Natl. Acad. Sci. U.S.A.* **2002**, *99*, 12627.

41. Floriano, W. B.; Vaidehi, N.; Goddard, W. A.; Singer, M. S.; Shepherd, G. M. Molecular mechanisms underlying differential odor responses of a mouse olfactory receptor. *Proc. Natl. Acad. Sci. U.S.A.* **2000**, *97*, 10712.

42. Li, Y.; Goddard, W. A. Prediction of the Structure of G-Protein Coupled Receptor with Application for Drug Design. *Pac. Symp. Biocomput.* **2008**, *13*, 344.

43. Kontoyianni, M.; DeWeese, C.; Penzotti, J. E.; Lybrand, T. P. Three-Dimensional Models for Agonist and Antagonist Complexes with β_2 Agrenergic Receptor. *J. Med. Chem.* **1996**, 4406.

44. Xhaard, H.; Rantanen, V. V.; Nyrönen, T.; Johnson, M. S. Molecular Evolution of Adrenoceptors and Dopamine Receptors: Implications for the Binding of Catecholamines. *J. Med. Chem.* **2006**, *49*, 1706.

45. Trumpp-Kallmeyer, S.; Hoflack, J.; Bruinvels, A.; Hibert, M. Modeling of G-Protein-Coupled Receptors: Application to Dopamine, Adrenaline, Serotonin, Acetylcholine, and Mammalian Opsin Receptors. *J. Med. Chem.* **1992**, *35*, 3448.

46. Bissantz, C.; Bernard, P.; Hibert, M.; Rognan, D. Protein-Based Virtual Screening of Chemical Databases. II. Are Homology Models of G-Protein Coupled Receptors Suitable Targets? *Proteins* **2003**, *50*, 5.

47. Cavasotto, C. N.; Orry, A. J. W.; Murgolo, N. J.; Czarniecki, M. F.; Kocsi, S. A.; Hawes, B. E.; O'Neill, K. A.; Hine, H.; Burton, M. S.; Voigt, J. H.; Abagyan, R. A.; Bayne, M. L.; Monsma, F. J. Discovery of Novel Chemotypes to a G-Protein-Coupled Receptor through Ligand-Steered Homology Modeling and Structure-Based Virtual Screening. *J. Med. Chem.* **2008**, *51*, 581.

48. Kiss, R.; Kiss, B.; Könczöl, A.; Szalai, F.; Jelinek, I.; László, V.; Noszál, B.; Falus, A.; Keserū, G. M. Discovery of Novel Human Histamine H4 Receptor Ligands by Large-Scale Structure-Based Virtual Screening. *J. Med. Chem.* **2008**, *51*, 3145.

49. Cavasotto, C. N.; Orry, A. J. W.; Abagyan, R. A. Structure-Based Identification of Binding Sites, Native Ligands and Potential Inhibitors for G-Protein Coupled Receptors. *Proteins* **2008**, *51*, 423.

50. Varady, J.; Wu, X.; Fang, X.; Min, J.; Hu, Z.; Levant, B.; Wang, S. Molecular Modeling of the Three-Dimensional Structure of Dopamine 3 (D_3) Subtype Receptor: Discovery of Novel and Potent D_3 Ligands through a Hybrid Pharmacophore- and Structure-Based Database Screening Approach. *J. Med. Chem.* **2003**, *46*, 4377.

51. Kellenberger, E.; Springael, J. Y.; Parmentier, M.; Hachet-Haas, M.; Galzi, J. L.; Rognan, D. Identification of Nonpeptide CCR5 Receptor Agonists by Structure-based Virtual Screening. *J. Med. Chem.* **2007**, *50*, 1294.

52. Topiol, S.; Sabio, M. Use of the X-ray structure of the Beta2-adrenergic receptor for drug discovery. *Bioorg. Med. Chem. Lett.* **2008**, *18*, 1598.

53. Crozier, P. S.; Stevens, M. J.; Forrest, L. R.; Woolf, T. B. Molecular Dynamics Simulation of Dark-adapted Rhodopsin in an Explicit Membrane Bilayer: Coupling between Local Retinal and Larger Scale Conformational Change. *J. Mol. Biol.* **2003**, *333*, 493.

54. Spijker, P.; Vaidehi, N.; Freddolino, P. L.; Hilbers, P. A.; Goddard, W. A. Dynamic behavior of fully solvated β_2-adrenergic receptor, embedded in the membrane with bound agonist or antagonist. *Proc. Natl. Acad. Sci. U.S.A.* **2006**, *103*, 4882.

55. Henin, J.; Maigret, B.; Tarek, M.; Escrieut, C.; Fourmy, D.; Chipot, C. Probing a Model of a GPCR/Ligand Complex in an Explicit Membrane Environment: The Human Cholecystokinin-1 Receptor. *Biophys. J.* **2006**, *90*, 1232.

56. Trent, J. O.; Wang, Z.; Murray, J. L.; Shao, W.; Tamamura, H.; Fuji, N.; Peiper, S. C. Lipid Bilayer Simulations of CXCR4 with Inverse Agonists and Weak Partial Agonists. *J. Biol. Chem.* **2003**, *278*, 47136.

57. Spassov, V.; Yan, L.; Szalma, S. Introducing an Implicit Membrane in Generalized Born/Solvent Accessibility Continuum Solvent Models. *J. Phys. Chem. B* **2002**, *106*, 8726.

58. Im, W.; Feig, M.; Brooks, C. L. An Implicit Membrane Generalized Born Theory for the Study of Structure, Stability, and Interactions of Membrane Proteins. *Biophys. J.* **2003**, *85*, 2900.

59. Still, W. C.; Tempczyk, A.; Hawley, R. C.; Hendrickson, T. Semi-analytical treatment of solvation for molecular mechanics and dynamics. *J. Am. Chem. Soc.* **1990**, *112*, 6127.

60. Gouldson, P. R.; Kidley, N. J.; Bywater, R. P.; Psaroudakis, G.; Brooks, H.D.; Diaz, C.; Shire, D.; Reynolds, C.A. Toward the Active Conformations of Rhodopsin and the β_2-Adrenergic Receptor. *Proteins* **2004**, *56*, 67.

61. Niv, M. Y.; Skrabanek, L.; Filizola, M.; Weinstein, H. Modeling activated states of GPCRs: the rhodopsin template. *J. Comput. Aided Mol. Des.* **2006**, *20*, 437.

62. Salom, D.; Lodowski, D. T.; Stenkamp, R. E.; Le Trong, I.; Golczak, M.; Jastrzebska, B.; Harris, T.; Ballesteros, J. A.; Palczewski, K. Crystal structure of a photoactivated deprotonated intermediate of rhodopsin. *Proc. Natl. Acad. Sci. U.S.A.* **2006**, *103*, 16123.

63. Erlanson, D. A.; Wells, J. A.; Braisted, A. C. TETHERING: Fragment-Based Drug Discovery. *Annu. Rev. Biophys. Struct.* **2004**, *33*, 199.

64. Zartler, E. R.; Shapiro, M. J. Fragonomics: fragment-based drug discovery. *Curr. Opin. Chem. Biol.* **2005**, *9*, 366.

17

Structure-based design of potent glycogen phosphorylase inhibitors

Qiaolin Deng

INTRODUCTION

Diabetes is a disorder of metabolism and is widely recognized as one of the leading causes of death and disability. It is estimated that more than 180 million people worldwide have diabetes.[1] In the United States, more than 20 million people – about 7.0% of the population – have diabetes.[2] Diabetes is a lifelong condition that, if left untreated, can lead to serious complications such as nerve damage, kidney failure, blindness, and cardiovascular diseases.[3] Type 2 diabetes is a chronic metabolic disorder characterized by fed and fasting hyperglycemia. Glycogen phosphorylase (GP) is a key enzyme in the regulation of glycogen metabolism by catalyzing the breakdown of glycogen to glucose-1-phosphate. In muscle, glucose 1-phosphate is used to generate metabolic energy, whereas in liver it is also converted to glucose for export to peripheral tissues. There are three human isozymes of GP: liver, muscle, and brain, named to denote the tissues in which they are preferentially expressed. The muscle and brain isozymes serve the tissues in which they are found, whereas the liver isozyme meets the glycemic demands of the body as a whole. Previous reports have indicated that GP inhibition can lower blood glucose in diabetic models, thus validating it as a potential therapeutic target for treatment of type 2 diabetes.[4–6] The liver isozyme of human glycogen phosphorylase (HLGP) is considered to be the preferred target for therapeutic intervention with GP inhibitors because inhibition of muscle or brain GP could lead to undesirable side effects.

HLGP and human muscle glycogen phosphorylase (HMGP) are dimers composed of two identical monomers, with more than 800 amino acid residues in each. Glycogen phosphorylase exists in two interconvertible forms: a Ser14 phosphorylated high-activity form (GPa) and a dephosphorylated low-activity resting form (GPb). Both forms exist in equilibrium between two different conformational states: a more active R state and a less active T state.[7] The more active R state is induced by the substrate and by allosteric effectors such as adenosine monophosphate (AMP), whereas the less active T state is stabilized by inhibitor binding. X-ray crystallographic studies of inactive and active conformations of HLGPa demonstrated large conformational changes between the two states, including order/disorder transitions and changes in secondary structures.[8] The inactive conformation of GP was used as the target for inhibitor design and optimization.

Glycogen phosphorylase contains at least six potential regulatory sites (Figure 17.1): (1) the Ser14 phosphate recognition site (Ser14 phosphorylation induces conformational changes that alter GP activity); (2) the catalytic site that binds the substrates glycogen and glucose-1-P, as well as glucose and glucose analogs; and (3) the AMP allosteric site that binds AMP, IMP, ATP, and glucose-6-P. This site is about 35Å away from the catalytic site (Figure 17.1). The Bayer diacid compound W1807 [Figure 17.2(a)], a potent inhibitor of rabbit muscle glycogen phosphorylase (RMGP), binds at this site as determined by crystallographic analysis.[9,10] (4) The inhibitor site (also referred to as the purine nucleoside site) binds heterocyclic compounds such as caffeine [Figure 17.2(b)] and flavopiridol. This site is more than 10Å away from the catalytic site.[11] (5) The glycogen storage site. (6) The dimer interface site that binds indole derivative CP320626 [Figure 17.2(c)] and its analogs.[12] This site was identified as a new allosteric site by x-ray crystallographic analysis.[13–15] Four of these six regulatory sites are known to be inhibitor binding sites: the catalytic site, the AMP allosteric site, the inhibition site and the dimer interface site [Figure 17.1].

In this chapter, we describe the use of molecular modeling in the development of a series of potent GP inhibitors. We started from a lead series consisting of phenyl diacids with various substitutions on the pyridine ring (Table 17.1). Of these, the most potent compound is 4-(2-{[(4-nitropyridine-2-yl)carbonyl]amino}phenoxy)phthalic acid [compound **1a**, Figure 17.3(a)]. Due to the lack of competitive binding studies, modeling studies were undertaken to predict the most probable binding site for compound **1a**. These involved superposition[16] of compound **1a** onto inhibitors that are known to bind at different sites based on the x-ray crystal structures, as well as examination of the protein environment to determine the possibility of interaction with nearby residues. Ultimately, these analyses suggested that compound **1a** binds at the AMP allosteric site. The docking of compound **1a** inside the AMP allosteric site was further explored by Internal Coordinates Mechanics (ICM) calculations[17] with subsequent energy optimization.

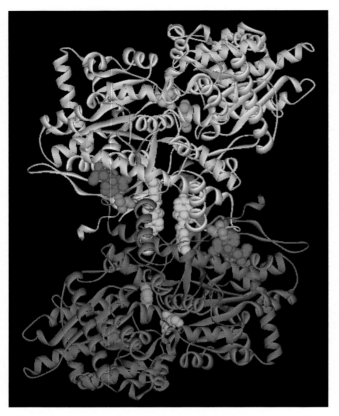

Figure 17.1. Regulatory sites of glycogen phosphorylase. The glycogen phosphorylase (PDB entry 3AMV) is shown in ribbon diagram with the two subunits colored in white and gray, respectively. To show all the regulatory sites in one picture, compounds that bind at different sites are copied from different PDB entries. In CPK models: Ser14 in blue at the phosphate recognition site; glucose in pink at the catalytic site; Bayer W1807 in magenta at the AMP allosteric site (PDB entry 3AMV); caffeine in cyan at the inhibitor site (PDB entry 1GFZ) and Pfizer CP320626 in yellow at the dimer interface site (PDB entry 1C50).

Additional characterization of the binding pocket by grid-based surface calculations[18] revealed a large unfilled hydrophobic region near the central phenyl ring, which provided an opportunity to potentially enhance binding of early leads by increasing the hydrophobic bulk in this

Table 17.1. The activity of phenyl diacid compounds

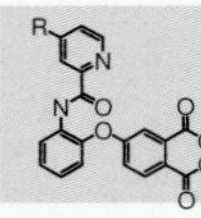	R	HLGPa (IC$_{50}$ nM)	HMGPa (IC$_{50}$ nM)
1a	-NO$_2$	3	25
1b	-Cl	17	181
1c	-OMe	20	200
1d	-CF$_3$	48	591
1e	-Et	56	433
1f	-Me	121	1090
1g	-H	1280	11790

region. A series of naphthyl compounds was designed and synthesized, and they displayed a significant improvement in potency.

STRUCTURE-BASED DESIGN OF GLYCOGEN PHOSPHORYLASE INHIBITORS

Prediction of putative binding pocket

The lead compounds are a series of phenyl diacids with activity on HLGPa ranging from 3 to 1280 nM with various substituents on the pyridine (Table 17.1). The most potent compound in the series incorporates a nitro group on the pyridine, compound **1a** [Figure 17.3(a)], with an IC$_{50}$ of 3 nM for HLGPa and 25 nM for HMGPa (Table 17.1). Two hundred conformers of compound **1a** were generated using our implementation of the distance geometry approach, which incorporates the theory and algorithm as previously described.[19] The conformer set was energy minimized using a distance-dependent dielectric of $2r$ with the Merck Molecular Force Field (MMFF).[20–26] Of the 200 conformers generated and energy minimized, the energetically favored conformation of compound **1a** was found to be in a "V" shape [Figure 17.3(b)]. In this conformation, the NH group of the amide interacts with the nitrogen atom in

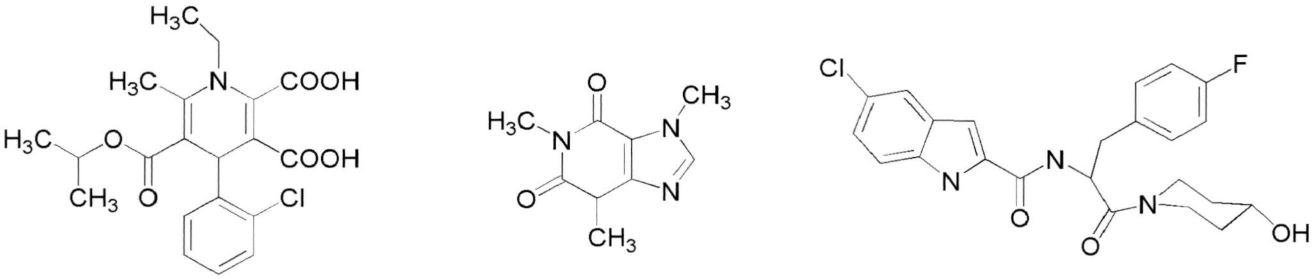

Figure 17.2. Examples of known GP inhibitors. **(a)** Bayer diacid compound W1807 ((-)(S)-3-isopropyl 4-(2-chlorophenyl)-1,4-dihydro-1-ethyl-2-methyl-pyridine-3,5,6-tricarboxylate) that binds at the AMP allosteric site (PDB entry 3AMV). **(b)** Caffeine that binds at the inhibitor site (PDB entry 1GFZ). **(c)** CP320626 (5-chloro-1H-indole-2-carboxylic acid [1-(4-fluorobenzyl)-2-(4-hydroxypiperidin-1-yl)-2-oxoethyl]amide) that binds at the dimer interface site (PDB entry 1C50).

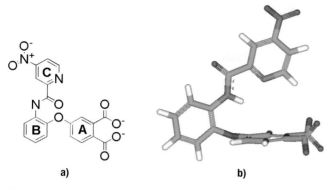

Figure 17.3. Lead compound **1a**. (a) Chemical structure of lead compound **1a**. (b) The lowest energy conformation of compound **1a** from gas phase calculations. The molecule is shown in stick model with carbons in green and noncarbon atoms in standard colors.

the pyridine, presumably in a hydrogen-bonding fashion, to stabilize the molecule. The two aromatic rings at the distal ends of the molecule are nearly perpendicular to each other with an edge-to-face distance of about 4Å, indicating a potentially favorable π-π stacking interaction within the molecule.

Competitive binding studies were not available to identify the binding site of the inhibitors. Before detailed docking studies could proceed, it was therefore necessary to first identify the most likely binding site of compound **1a**. To this end, 3D similarities between conformers of compound **1a** and three probes derived from known crystal structures were assessed. The glucose analog that acts as an inhibitor at the catalytic site was dismissed from consideration because of the obvious lack of similarity between it and compound **1a**. The 3D similarity/superposition tool SQ[16] was employed to superpose conformers of compound **1a** onto three probes derived from publicly available x-ray crystal structures of known inhibitors in complex with GP: Bayer W1807 at the AMP allosteric site [Protein Data Bank (PDB) entry 3AMV[9]], caffeine at the inhibitor site (PDB entry 1GFZ[11]), and Pfizer CP320626 at the dimer interface site (PDB entry 1C50[13]). Each probe represents a class of

inhibitors at a different binding site and their chemical structures are shown in Figure 17.2. The best overlay of compound **1a** onto each of the three probes is depicted in Figure 17.4.

Compound **1a** overlays onto W1807 [Figure 17.4(a)] with the aromatic regions and diacid groups fairly well aligned. W1807 is most similar to compound **1a** among the three probes, so this is not an unexpected result. Like W1807, the diacid moiety of compound **1a** presumably interacts with positively charged arginines at the AMP allosteric site. In contrast, the energetically preferred V shape of compound **1a** precludes it from being able to align well onto the planar structure of caffeine [Figure 4(b)]. Although the superposition of compound **1a** onto CP320626 [Figure 4(c)] is visually appealing, it requires compound **1a** to adopt a conformation energetically disfavored by more than 10 kcal/mol. In this alignment, the diacid groups and the A ring are overlapped onto the 4-hydroxy-piperidyl moiety of CP320626, known to bind in a space filled with water molecules at the dimer interface site.[13] As a result, the diacid group in compound **1a** would not make significant favorable interactions with the enzyme. Based on this analysis of each binding site, it appeared that compound **1a** is likely to bind at the AMP allosteric site.

Docking of compound 1a into AMP allosteric site

Having identified the AMP allosteric site as the most likely binding site for compound **1a** through the SQ overlay, a more extensive docking study was carried out using ICM software.[17] The amino acid sequences of HLGP, HMGP, and RMGP were aligned using Clustal W.[27] HLGP has 80% sequence identity and 90% sequence similarity to HMGP and RMGP. The homology between the two muscle enzymes (HMGP and RMGP) is even higher, with a sequence identity of 97% and sequence similarity of 99%. The residues located within 5Å of W1807 in the AMP allosteric site are conserved among the three enzymes, so it is likely that the binding pocket would be very similar

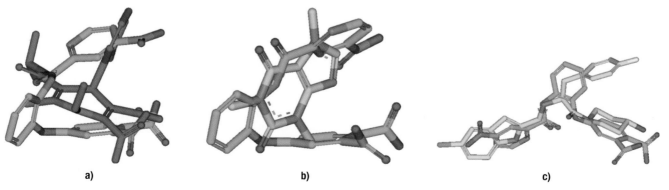

Figure 17.4. Superposition of compound **1a** onto known inhibitors by SQ calculations. Compound **1a** (carbons in green) overlaid onto (a) W1807 (carbons in magenta) at the AMP allosteric site, (b) caffeine (carbons in cyan) at the inhibitor site, and (c) CP320626 (carbons in yellow) at the dimer interface site. Only heavy atoms are shown and noncarbon atoms are in standard colors.

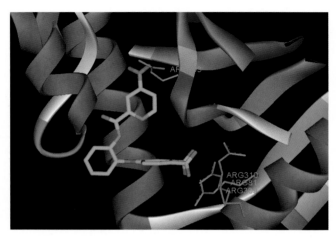

Figure 17.5. Docking model of compound **1a** inside the AMP allosteric site. Compound **1a** is shown in stick model with heavy atoms only, with carbons in green and noncarbon atoms in standard colors. The GP structure is displayed as solid ribbon with helices in red and beta sheets in cyan. Several important arginines in the binding pocket are shown in stick model with standard colors. Hydrogen atoms have been omitted for clarity.

among them. Because of the lack of an x-ray crystal structure of HLGP complexed with an inhibitor bound in the AMP allosteric site at the time of this study, the crystal structures of RMGP complexed with W1807 were used as the templates for docking. Two crystal structures were available for W1807 complexed with RMGP, one in the phosphorylated form GPa (PDB entry 3AMV) and one in the dephosphorylated form GPb (PDB entry 2AMV).[9,10] Both crystal structures are in the less active T state and are structurally similar, with an rmsd for the main-chain atoms of ~0.3Å.[9] Interactions between W1807 and the residues of the AMP allosteric site are essentially identical in the two structures. The most recent crystal structure of T-state GPa complexed with W1807 at high resolution (2.1Å) (PDB entry 3AMV[9]) was selected for use in the docking calculations.

The dimer structure was constructed for docking studies because the AMP allosteric site is formed by residues from both monomers. Starting from the x-ray crystal structure (PDB entry 3AMV), ligand and water molecules were removed. The dimer was built based on crystallographic symmetry operations. In the following context, regular residue numbers will be used to describe residues from the first monomer, and a residue number with a prime (′) will be used to denote residues from the symmetry-related unit. Because the complete dimer structure consists of more than 1,600 amino acids, a smaller enzyme site was created for docking calculations. Residues with any atom falling within a 15Å shell around W1807 were retrieved to construct the enzyme site.

The first docking pose of compound **1a** at the AMP allosteric site was taken from the superposition onto W1807. Ultimately, this pose proved unsuitable as a starting point for further energy minimization and analysis. This was due, in part, to the lack of any consideration of the

nearby protein environment in the superposition calculations. Instead, ICM[17] calculations that perform flexible docking in internal coordinates were carried out to generate initial docking poses to sample various conformations and locations for compound **1a** inside the AMP allosteric binding pocket. One hundred initial docking poses within the AMP allosteric site were generated. Each of the resultant complexes was then energy optimized using the MMFF.[20–26] In the energy optimization, the ligand was fully optimized inside the binding pocket that was allowed limited flexibility. The side chains of residues with any atom located within 5Å of the ligand were fully minimized in conjunction with the ligand. Residues falling within 5–10Å of the ligands were included in the calculations as rigid elements, and the residues beyond a 10Å cutoff from the ligand were ignored in the calculations. The total energy of the complex, the individual energies of the ligand and the enzyme, and the interaction energy between the ligand and the enzyme were calculated. The best docking mode was determined by selecting those poses with the most stabilizing interaction energy and minimal amount of strain on the ligand and by visual inspection of the interactions.

A preferred docking mode of compound **1a** inside the AMP allosteric site is shown in Figure 17.5. The putative binding pocket for compound **1a** is formed by helix 2 (residues 47–78), helix 8 (residues 289–314), beta-sheet 4 (residues 153–160), beta-sheet 11 (residues 237–247), a short beta-sheet 7 (residues 191–193), and a cap′ region (residues 36′–47′) from the symmetry-related unit. The ligand maintained the energetically preferred V shape, with the A and C rings buried inside the AMP allosteric site and the B ring located at the entrance to the binding site. The diacid group of the A ring interacts with a cluster of arginines, Arg81, Arg309, and Arg310, and is near two polar residues, Gln71 and Tyr155, which may provide additional stabilizing interactions. The central phenyl ring B binds in a hydrophobic pocket formed by the aliphatic portion of the Gln72 side chain, the phenyl ring of Tyr75, and the side chain of Val45′. The pyridine (C ring) is bordered by residues Trp67, Ile68, and Val40′. The nitro group on the meta position of the pyridine is close to Arg193, to which it may form a hydrogen bond. This may explain why compound **1a** is the most potent compound in the phenyl diacid series (Table 17.1).

The overlay of docked compound **1a** onto the crystal structure of W1807 (PDB entry 3AMV) and AMP (PDB entry 8GPB) is depicted in Figure 17.6. Compound **1a** and W1807 are both inhibitors, whereas AMP is an allosteric effector. The acid group binding region is the only common region for the three compounds. Compound **1a** is predicted to bind quite differently from AMP by occupying different locations inside the binding pocket. The two inhibitors, compound **1a** and W1807, occupy a similar location inside the AMP allosteric site with their diacid groups interacting with arginines. However, the diacid functionality of

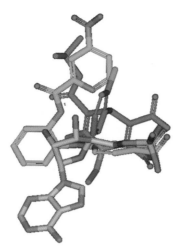

Figure 17.6. Comparison of docked compound **1a** with crystal structure of W1807 and AMP. Compound **1a** (carbons in green), W1807 (carbons in magenta, PDB entry 3AMV), and AMP (carbons in orange, PDB entry 8GPB) are shown in stick model with noncarbon atoms in standard colors. Hydrogen atoms have been omitted for clarity.

compound **1a** is almost perpendicular to that observed with W1807.

Characterization of the binding pocket

Grid-based surfaces were calculated by FLOG[18] using the docking model to further characterize the binding pocket. Each grid was visualized as a series of isoenergetic surfaces that describe the binding pocket by its polar (hydrogen bond donor and acceptor) and hydrophobic nature. The hydrophobic contour and hydrogen bond contour maps are shown in Figure 17.7. For clarity, the docked compound **1a** is shown, whereas the nearby residues in the binding pocket are omitted in the picture.

In the hydrogen bond contour map, the red area shows that the residues in the binding pocket would favor interaction with a hydrogen bond acceptor on the ligand. For example, the large red grid around the diacid on the A ring indicates that the surrounding residues, a cluster of arginines, would prefer to interact with a hydrogen bond donor that is a diacid functional group on the ligand. Similarly, the small red grid around the nitro group on the C ring shows that the residues in this region favor interaction with a hydrogen bond acceptor. In this region, the residue is Arg193 while the hydrogen bond group on the ligand is a nitro group.

In the hydrophobic contour map, the green area around compound **1a** denotes the regions in the binding pocket that would favor interaction with a hydrophobic group on the ligand. For example, the green region near the pyridine (C ring) suggests that activity can be enhanced with appropriate hydrophobic substitutions on the pyridine. This is in good agreement with the SAR in which compounds unsubstituted on the C ring (i.e., compound **1g**) have the least activity while potency increases more than tenfold with

hydrophobic substitutions at the meta position, for example compounds **1e** and **1f** (Table 17.1).

Similarly, there is a large area near the central phenyl ring B that is unfilled by compound **1a** and for which SAR was unavailable. As was the case with the pyridine, this visually suggests that additional hydrophobic groups attached to the central phenyl B ring could fill this space and make favorable interactions with the residues that line this region of the binding pocket, thereby improving the binding and thus the potency.

Design and synthesis

One possible modification was to fuse a hydrophobic ring onto the central phenyl ring B to provide access to the putative hydrophobic region. Both saturated and unsaturated five- and six-member rings were considered. The designed compounds were obtained by modifying compound **1a**. Energy evaluation was carried out by fully optimizing each virtual ligand within the flexible binding pocket, as described before.

The interaction energy between each of the designed compounds and the enzyme was about 5–6 kcal/mol more favorable than that for the parent phenyl compound (Table 17.2). The fused ring moieties are nicely located among the aliphatic portion of the Gln72 side chain, the phenyl ring of Tyr75, and the side chain of Val45′ and make favorable interactions with the hydrophobic pocket. Based on synthetic considerations, compounds fused with an unsaturated six-member ring (naphthyl compounds) were synthesized.

The synthesis of naphthyl compounds was described by Z. Lu et al. in 2003.[28] The potencies of naphthyl analogs

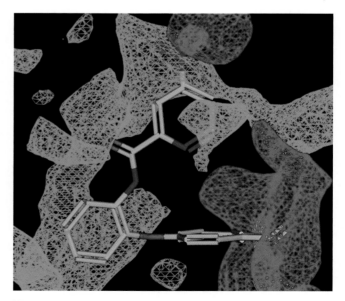

Figure 17.7. Hydrophobic and hydrogen bond acceptor contours from grid-based calculations on the docking model. The hydrophobic surface is shown as a green grid and the hydrogen bond acceptor surface is shown as a red grid. Compound **1a** is shown in stick model with carbons in green and noncarbon atoms in standard colors. Hydrogen atoms have been omitted for clarity.

Table 17.2. Energy calculation on the designed compounds

	Fused ring	Bond	Interaction energy (kcal/mol)
Compound **1a**	no	No	−112.6
Design 1	5	Saturated	−117.6
Design 2	5	Unsaturated	−118.6
Design 3	6	Saturated	−117.5
Design 4	6	Unsaturated	−118.6

are listed in Table 17.3 for a head-to-head comparison with the parent phenyl compounds. Overall, the potency is improved by three- to fourteenfold for HLGP and seven- to nineteenfold for HMGP over the corresponding phenyl compounds. The enhancement in potency is consistent within the entire series and for both HLGP and HMGP. The naphthyl and phenyl series share a similar trend in potency change with different substitutions on the C ring: the unsubstituted compounds (i.e., compounds **1g** and **2g**) are least active while the potency increases over tenfold with hydrophobic substitutions on the meta position (e.g., compounds **1e** and **1f**, **2e** and **2f**); the compounds with a nitro group are most potent (i.e., compounds **1a** and **2a**). This indicates that the naphthyl and phenyl derivatives bind at the AMP allosteric site in a similar manner. The naphthyl series fills more space with the fused ring than the parent phenyl series, making more favorable interactions with the surrounding residues and thereby increasing their potency.[29]

COMPARISON OF THE DOCKING MODEL WITH X-RAY CRYSTAL STRUCTURES

At the time when we finished the design and synthesis of the naphthyl series, an x-ray crystal structure of RMGPb complexed with compound **1a** was solved in-house.[28] The

predicted docking pose of compound **1a** was confirmed by the x-ray crystal structure. Compound **1a** is verified to be bound at the AMP allosteric site. Compared to the x-ray crystal structure, the docked compound **1a** occupies the same location and maintains all major interactions. The ring A and ring B are overlaid well with the diacid groups interacting with the positively charged arginines, Arg81, Arg309, and Arg310. The amide group next to ring B displays a different orientation, which causes the pyridines (ring C) to be poorly overlapped. However, the nitro group on ring C points to the same residue, Arg193, to form favorable interactions. The conformational difference in the amide and ring C region is accompanied by the substantial shift of the side-chain orientation of Arg193 in the binding pockets.

Later on, crystal structures of RMGPb complexed with similar diacid compounds were published by Kristiansen et al.[30] Our proposed binding mode for compound **1a** at the AMP allosteric site is similar to that of the compounds described therein.

SUMMARY

In this chapter we describe modeling aided development of a new series of potent glycogen phosphorylase inhibitors. Due to the lack of suitable competition-based binding assays, superposition was used to predict the potential binding site for the lead compound **1a**. The overlay of compound **1a** onto the crystal structures of inhibitors that are known to bind at different sites in GP, together with analysis of nearby residues at each respective site, correctly determined the AMP allosteric site as the binding site for compound **1a**. By using the x-ray crystal structure of RMGP (PDB entry 3AMV), possible docking modes of compound **1a** were extensively explored by ICM calculations. A reasonable docking model was computationally determined and subsequently confirmed by in-house x-ray crystallography. Further analysis of the binding pocket of the docking model by grid-based surface calculation revealed a large unfilled region near the central phenyl ring of compound **1a**. Fused ring analogs were designed with the goal of increasing hydrophobic bulk in this unfilled region to improve binding. After evaluation of energetics and ease of synthesis for the fused ring analogs, a series of naphthyl compounds was synthesized. As predicted, this exercise resulted in a new series of GP inhibitors with significantly improved potency.

ACKNOWLEDGMENTS

The author thanks Dr. Zhijian Lu and Joann Bohn for the synthesis of compounds; Kenneth P. Ellsworth, Dr. Robert W. Myers, and Wayne M. Geissler for the assay data; Dr. Brian Mckeever for the x-ray crystal structure; and Ralph Mosley for help and support during this work. The author also thanks Dr. Vladimir Maiorov for help with preparation of Figure 17.1 and Dr. Wendy Cornell, Dr. Kate Holloway,

Table 17.3. Comparison of activity of naphthyl and phenyl diacid compounds

R		Phenyl HLGPa (IC$_{50}$ nM)	Phenyl HMGPa (IC$_{50}$ nM)		Naphthyl HLGPa (IC$_{50}$ nM)	Naphthyl HMGPa (IC$_{50}$ nM)
-NO$_2$	**1a**	3	25	**2a**	1	3
-Cl	**1b**	17	181	**2b**	2	12
-OMe	**1c**	20	200	**2c**	2	12
-CF$_3$	**1d**	48	591	**2d**	12	80
-Et	**1e**	56	433	**2e**	4	29
-Me	**1f**	121	1090	**2f**	10	57
-H	**1g**	1280	11790	**2g**	167	844

Dr. Stephen Soisson, and Dr. Andreas Verras for comments on the manuscript.

REFERENCES

1. Diabetes, World Health Organization. Fact Sheet No. 312, 2006.
2. Diabetes overview, National Diabetes Statistics. Fact Sheet, 2005.
3. Talor, S. I. Deconstructing type 2 diabetes. *Cell* **1999**, *97*, 9–12.
4. Treadway, J. L.; Mendys, P.; Hoover, D. J. Glycogen phosphorylase inhibitors for treatment of type 2 diabetes melltus. *Exp. Opin. Invest. Drugs* **2001**, *10*, 439–454.
5. Jakobsen, P.; Lundbeck, J. M.; Kristiansen, M.; Breinholt, J.; Demuth, H.; Pawlas, J.; Torres Candela, M. P.; Anderson, B.; Westergaard, N.; Lundgren, K.; Asano N. Iminosugars: potential inhibitors of liver glycogen phosphorylase. *Bioorg. Med. Chem.* **2001**, *9*, 733–744.
6. Martin, W. H.; Hoover, D. J.; Armento, S. J.; Stock, I. A.; McPherson, R. K.; Danley, D. E.; Stevenson, R. W.; Barrett, E. J.; Treadway, J. L. Discovery of a human liver glycogen phosphorylase inhibitor that lowers blood glucose in vivo. *Proc. Natl. Acad. Sci. U.S.A.* **1998**, *95*, 1776–1781.
7. Johnson, L. N. Glycogen phosphorylase: control by phosphorylation and allosteric effectors. *FASEB J.* **1992**, *6*, 2274–2282.
8. Rath, V. L.; Ammirati, M.; LeMotte, P. K.; Fennell, K. F.; Mansour M. N.; Damley, D. E.; Hynes, T. R.; Schulte, G. K.; Wasilko, D. J. Pandit, Activation of human liver glycogen phosphorylase by alteration of the secondary structure and packing of the catalytic core. *Mol. Cell* **2000**, *6*, 139–148.
9. Oikonomakos, N. G.; Tsitsanou, K. E.; Zographos, S. E.; Skamnaki, V. T.; Goldmann, S.; Bischoff, H. Allosteric inhibition of glycogen phosphorylase a by the potential antidiabetic drug 3-isopropyl 4-(2-chlorophenyl)-1,4-dihydro-1-ethyl-2-methyl-pyridine-3,5,6-tricarboxylate. *Protein Sci.* **1999**, *8*, 1930–1945.
10. Zographos, S. E.; Oikonomakos, N. G.; Tsitsanou, K. E.; Leonidas, D. D.; Chrysina, E. D.; Skamnaki, V. T.; Bischoff, H.; Goldmann, S.; Watson, K. A.; Johnson L. N. The structure of glycogen phosphorylase b with an alkyl-dihydropyridine-dicarboxylic acid compound, a novel and potent inhibitor. *Structure* **1997**, *5*, 1413–1425.
11. Oikonomakos, N. G.; Schnier, J. B.; Zographos, S. E.; Skamnaki, V. T.; Tsitsanou, K. E.; Johnson, L. N. Flavopiridol inhibits glycogen phosphorylase by binding at the inhibitor site. *J. Biol. Chem.* **2000**, *275*, 34566–34573.
12. Hoover, D. J.; Lefkowitz-Snow, S.; Burgess-Henry, J. L.; Martin, W. H.; Armento, S. J.; Stock, I. A.; McPherson, R. K.; Genereux, P. E.; Gibbs, E. M.; Treadway, J. L. Indole-2-carboxamide inhibitors of human liver glycogen phosphorylase. *J. Med. Chem.* **1998**, *41*, 2934–2938.
13. Oikonomakos, N. G.; Skamnaki, V. T.; Tsitsanou, K. E.; Gavalas, N. G.; Johnson, L. N. A New allosteric site in glycogen phosphorylase b as a target for drug interactions. *Structure* **2000**, *8*, 575–584.
14. Rath, V. L.; Ammirati, M.; Danley, D. E.; Ekstrom, J. L.; Gibbs, E. M.; Hynes, T. R.; Mathiowetz, A. M.; McPherson, R. K.; Olson, T. V.; Treadway, J. L.; Hoover, D. J. Human liver glycogen phosphorylase inhibitors bind at a new allosteric site. *Chem. Biol.* **2000**, *7*, 677–682.
15. Oikonomakos, N. G.; Zographos, S. E.; Skamnaki, V. T.; Archontis, G. The 1.76Å resolution crystal structure of glycogen phosphorylase B complexed with glucose, and CP320626, a potential antidiabetic drug. *Bioorg. Med. Chem.* **2002**, *10*, 1313–1319.
16. Miller, M. D.; Sheridan, R. P.; Kearsley, S. K. SQ: a program for rapidly producing pharmacophorically relevent molecular superpositions. *J. Med. Chem.* **1999**, *42*, 1505–1514.
17. ICM-Pro 2.8 docking module. San-Diego: Molsoft LLC.
18. Miller, M. D.; Kearley, S. K.; Underwood, D. J.; Sheridan, R. P. J. FLOG: a system to select 'quasi-flexible' ligands complementary to a receptor of known three-dimensional structure. *Comput. Aided Mol. Des.* **1994**, *8*, 153–174.
19. Crippen, C. M.; Havel, T. F. *Distance Geometry and Molecular Conformation*. New York, NY: Wiley; **1988**.
20. Halgren, T. A. Merck molecular force field. I. Basis, form, scope, parameterization, and performance of MMFF94. *J. Comp. Chem.* **1996**, *17*, 490–519.
21. Halgren, T. A. Merck molecular force field. II. MMFF94 van der Waals and electrostatic parameters for intermolecular interactions. *J. Comp. Chem.* **1996**, *17*, 520–552.
22. Halgren, T. A. Merck molecular force field. III. Molecular geometries and vibrational frequencies for MMFF94. *J. Comp. Chem.* **1996**, *17*, 553–586.
23. Halgren, T. A.; Nachbar, R. B. Merck molecular force field. IV. Conformational energies and geometries for MMFF94. *J. Comp. Chem.* **1996**, *17*, 587–615.
24. Halgren, T. A. Merck molecular force field. V. Extension of MMFF94 using experimental data, additional computational data, and empirical rules. *J. Comp. Chem.* **1996**, *17*, 616–641.
25. Halgren, T. A. MMFF VI. MMFF94s option for energy minimization studies *J. Comp. Chem.* **1999**, *20*, 720–729.
26. Halgren, T. A. MMFF VII. Characterization of MMFF94, MMFF94s, and other widely available force fields for conformational energies and for intermolecular-interaction energies and geometries. *J. Comp. Chem.* **1999**, *20*, 730–748.
27. Thompson, J. D.; Higgins, D. G.; Gibson, T. J. CLUSTAL W: improving the sensitivity of progressive multiple sequence alignment through sequence weighting, position-specific gap penalties and weight matrix choice. *Nucleic Acids Res.* **1994**, *22*, 4673–4680.
28. Lu, Z.; Bohn, J.; Bergeron, R.; Deng, Q.; Ellsworth, K. P.; Geissler, W. M.; Harris G.; McCann, P. E.; McKeever, B.; Myers, R. W.; Saperstein, R.; Willoughby, C. A.; Yao, J.; Chapman, K. A. A New class of glycogen phosphorylase inhibitors. *Bioorg. Med. Chem. Lett.* **2003**, *13*, 4125–4128.
29. Deng, Q.; Lu, Z.; Bohn, J.; Ellsworth, K. P.; Myers, R. W.; Geissler, W. M.; Harris, G.; Willoughby, C. A.; Chapman, K.; Mckeever, B.; Mosley, R. Modeling aided design of potent glycogen phosphorylase inhibitors. *J. Mol. Graph. Model.* **2005**, *23*, 457–464.
30. Kristiansen, M.; Anderson, B.; Iversen, L. F.; Westergaard, N. Identification, synthesis, and characterization of new glycogen phosphorylase inhibitors binding to the allosteric AMP site. *J. Med. Chem.* **2004**, *47*, 3537–3545.

Index